RESEARCH-BASED PRACTICES IN DEVELOPMENTAL DISABILITIES

Second Edition

Howard P. Parette

George R. Peterson-Karlan

Foreword by Ravic Ringlaben and Omowale Akintunde

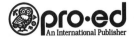

8700 Shoal Creek Boulevard
Austin, Texas 78757-6897
800/897-3202   Fax 800/397-7633
www.proedinc.com

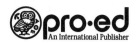

© 1998, 2008 by PRO-ED, Inc.
8700 Shoal Creek Boulevard
Austin, Texas 78757-6897
800/897-3202   Fax 800/397-7633
www.proedinc.com

Library of Congress Cataloging-in-Publication Data

Research-based practices in developmental disabilities/[edited by] Howard P. Parette, George R. Peterson-Karlan, Ravic Ringlaben. —2nd ed.
     p. cm.
Rev. ed. of: Best and promising practices in developmental disabilities/edited by Alan Hilton and Ravic Ringlaben. c1998.
Includes bibliographical references.
ISBN-13: 978-1-4164-0247-3
  1. Developmentally disabled—Education—United States. 2. Developmentally dissabled—Services for—United States. 3. Developmentally disabled—United States—Psychology. 4. Social skills—Study and teaching—United States. 5. Special education teachers—Training of —United States. I. Parette, Howard P. II. Peterson-Karlan, George R. III. Ringlaben, Ravic. IV. Best and promising practices in developmental disabilities.

HV1570.5.U65B47 2007
362.196'8—dc22

2006024726

Art Director: Jason Crosier
Designer: Sandy Salinas
This book is designed in Janson Text and Officina Sans ITC.

Printed in the United States of America

1 2 3 4 5 6 7 8 9 10   17 16 15 14 13 12 11 10 09 08

Research-Based Practices
in Developmental Disabilities

Table of Contents

Contents

vi

Contents

viii

Contributors

Akintunde, Omowale, PhD
Department of Teacher Education
University of Southern Indiana
Evansville, IN

Bakken, Jeffrey P., PhD
Department of Special Education
Illinois State University
Normal, IL

Beck, Ann R., PhD
College of Arts and Science
Illinois State University
Normal, IL

Brown, James, PhD
Department of Vocational and Technical
Education
University of Minnesota
St. Paul, MN

Demchak, MaryAnn, PhD
Department of Educational Specialties
University of Nevada, Reno
Reno, NV

Edelen-Smith, Patricia J., EdD
Department of Special Education
University of Hawaii at Manoa
Honolulu, HI

Edyburn, Dave L., PhD
Department of Exceptional Education
University of Wisconsin–Milwaukee
Milwaukee, WI

Ezell, Dan, EdD
Department of Child, Family, and
Community Sciences
University of Central Florida
Cocoa, FL

Gartin, Barbara C., EdD
Department of Curriculum and
Instruction
University of Arkansas
Fayetteville, AR

Griffith, Kimberly, PhD
Department of Professional Pedagogy
Lamar University
Beaumont, TX

Hider, Alison S., MS
May Institute, Inc.
Newton, MA

Hourcade, Jack J., PhD
Department of Elementary Education and
Specialized Studies
Boise State University
Boise, ID

Hubbard, Anastasia, MS
Autism Asperger Publishing Company
Shawnee Mission, KS

Huer, Mary Blake, PhD.
Department of Speech Communication
California State University, Fullerton
Fullerton, CA

Hutchins, Margaret P., PhD
Department of Special Education
Illinois State University
Normal, IL
(deceased)

Klein-Ezell, Colleen E., PhD
Department of Child, Family, and
Community Sciences
University of Central Florida
Cocoa, FL

x

Knowlton, Earle, PhD
Department of Special Education
University of Kansas
Lawrence, KS

LaRusso, Randy, ME
School Board of Brevard County
Viera, FL

Macfarlane, Christine A., PhD
College of Education
Pacific University
Forest Grove, OR

Maloney, Arthur, EdD
School of Education
Pace University
New York, NY

Martin, James E., PhD
Zarrow Center for Learning Enrichment
University of Oklahoma
Norman, OK

Muellner, Kristin, MS
Niles Township District
Moreton Grove, IL

Munk, Dennis D., EdD
Department of Education
Carthage College
Kenosha, WI

Murdick, Nikki L., PhD
Department of Educational Studies
Saint Louis University
St. Louis, MO

Myles, Brenda Smith, PhD
Department of Special Education
University of Kansas
Lawrence, KS

Parette, Howard P., EdD
Department of Special Education
Illinois State University
Normal, IL

Perner, Darlene E., EdD
Department of Exceptionality Programs
Bloomsburg University
Bloomsburg, PA

Peterson-Karlan, George R., PhD
Department of Special Education
Illinois State University
Normal, IL

Pickett, Anna Lou, BA
National Resource Center for
Paraprofessionals (NRCP)
Utah State, UT and University of Minnesota,
Minneapolis, MN

Porter, Gordon L., LLD
The Education Training Group
Woodstock, NB
Canada

Poston, Denise, PhD
Kansas University Center on Developmental
Disabilities
University of Kansas
Lawrence, KS

Richey, David Dean, PhD
College of Education
Tennessee Tech University
Cookeville, TN

Ringlaben, Ravic P., EdD
Department of Education
Palm Beach Atlantic University
West Palm Beach, FL

Sands, Deanna J., EdD
Division of Technology and
Support Services
University of Colorado at Denver
Denver, CO

Shelden, Debra L., PhD
Department of Special Education
Illinois State University
Normal, IL

Smith, Garnett J., EdD
Department of Special Education
University of Hawaii at Manoa
Honolulu, HI

Smith, J. David, PhD
The University of Virginia's
College at Wise
Wise, VA

Smith, Tom E. C., EdD
Department of Curriculum and Instruction
University of Arkansas
Fayetteville, AR

Sparks, Scott, PhD
Department of Teacher Education
Ohio University
Athens, OH

Stenhjem, Pamela H., MS
Institute on Community Integration
University of Minnesota
Minneapolis, MN

Stodden, Robert A., PhD
Center on Disability Studies
University of Hawaii at Manoa
Honolulu, HI

Stoner, Julia B., EdD
Department of Special Education
Illinois State University
Normal, IL

Summers, Jean A., PhD
Beach Center on Disability
University of Kansas
Lawrence, KS

Thompson, James R., PhD
Department of Special Education
Illinois State University
Normal, IL

Turnbull, Ann P., PhD
Department of Special Education
University of Kansas
Lawrence, KS

Turnbull, H. R., LLB, LLM
Department of Special Education
University of Kansas
Lawrence, KS

Van Laarhoven, Toni, EdD
Department of Teaching and Learning
Northern Illinois University
DeKalb, IL

Wehmeyer, Michael L., PhD
Department of Special Education
University of Kansas
Lawrence, Kansas

Wheeler, John J., PhD
College of Education
Tennessee Tech University
Cookeville, TN

Zager, Dianne, PhD
School of Education
Pace University
New York, NY

Foreword

Research-Based Practices in Developmental Disabilities: Modern and Postmodern Perspectives

Ravic P. Ringlaben and Omowale Akintunde

Many current "research-based practices" related to individuals with developmental disabilities are designed to assist current and future practitioners in the field (Hilton & Ringlaben, 1998). However, any discussion of these practices raises a series of questions, among them (a) How are research-based practices defined? (b) Are certain practices encouraged "politically"? (c) Are practices demonstrated by practitioners solely on basis of the pathologies described within special education (e.g., low intelligence, social incompetence, maladaptive functioning, etc.)? (d) Are current interventions based solely on a deficit/capacity continuum? As noted by Kavale and Mostert (2003), "special education continues to be in a state of flux because, although much is known, there is still room to learn more . . . . The present practice of special education indicates that outcomes for students with disabilities remain unpredictable" (p. 203).

In special education research, the "funding source in power" has a major impact in determining what is researched, along with the influence of particular results. The stage is set to accept only those results that will align with the agenda of the group in power. Political reforms precede research because they "tend to shape policies and practices which in turn shape research" (Sailor & Paul, 2004, p. 40).

In the popular and best-selling novel *State of Fear*, by Michael Crichton (2004), the interaction between politics and science is noted in appendix I, "Why Politicized Science Is Dangerous":

> Imagine there is a new scientific theory that warns of an impending crisis, and points to a way out. This theory quickly draws support from leading scientists, politicians, and celebrities around the world. Research is funded by distinguished philanthropies, and carried out in prestigious universities. The crisis is reported frequently in the media. The science is taught in college and high school classrooms. . . .
>
> Today we know that this famous theory that gained so much support was actually pseudoscience. The crisis it claimed was nonexistent. And the actions taken in the name of this theory were morally and criminally wrong. Ultimately, they led to the deaths of millions of people. (pp. 631–632)

We still speak of this theory in our classes today as a reminder of what science can do—the theory and practice of eugenics. But eugenics is not history. The practice continues throughout the world (Roberts, Stough, & Parrish, 2002; Smith, 1999). Currently, genetic science is practiced and supported governmentally. When does genetic science become eugenics? Will certain developmental disabilities be defined as a defect, disease, disorder, or a normal aspect of human difference (Smith, 2000)? Are there professional practices that we employ today that will seem archaic or even dangerous 100 years or even 50 years after this book is published?

A heated professional debate is evolving in the field of special education between at least two distinct groups of professionals concerning special education philosophy, research, and practice. Each group includes well-respected and "highly published" special education professionals. These two paradigms have been referred to as "modern" and "postmodern." A discussion of these paradigms is imperative because each provides a different and separate rationale for research and services for individuals with disabilities. Each may have different answers to the questions posed earlier. For the sake of space, these distinctions have been oversimplified. Nonetheless, both deserve mentioning. Please refer to the articles referenced in this chapter for additional and more in-depth discussions.

The modernist (behavioral, quantitative, empirical-based) perspective purports that science can answer the questions about what interventions should be used by professional providers. It wants "to confirm or reject general principles and theories about an objective world" (Clear, 1999, p. 440). "Empirical truth is determined by isolating elements, by specifying relationships, and by formulating a sense-making construction unified by testable hypotheses (Kavale & Mostert, 2003, p. 194). This approach evolved with the implementation of scientific inquiry during much of the 20th century. Though initially used in the "hard sciences," the approach was embraced by the social sciences. Modernists believe that we can study specific characteristics of individuals with disabilities and that science will lead us down the road of progress. They are concerned that postmodernists pose a severe threat to science (Sailor & Paul, 2004). Sasso (2001) is concerned that postmodernists "conclude that because logical inquiry and science are not perfect, notions of evidence, truth, fact, reality and knowledge are then ideologically indefensible" (p. 181), and that the postmodernist belief "that science is just a matter of social practice . . . reflects a misunderstanding of the process of logical inquiry" (p. 182). Forness and Kavale (2001) believe that "schools currently misidentify more children with mental or behavioral disorders than they actually identify" (p. 79) and that a major solution would be a return to the medical model. Sasso indicates that the scientific inquiry model has built-in accountability with replication and that results are determined by evidence. "What p value you accept depends how important the result is and what decisions might follow from it" (Sasso, 2001, p. 187).

The postmodernist (constructivist, emancipatory, liberatory, qualitative) perspective emerged as a force in special education in response to the postmodern redefinition of childhood as including children with special needs in federal legislation, especially Public Law 94-142, the Education for All Handicapped Children Act of 1975 (Elkind, 1998; Rhodes, 1995). This group questions the scientific approach and the results of empirical inquiry because they believe the individual is much too complicated and that there is sufficient heterogeneity within disability groups to preclude generalization. This perspective appears to be one reason for changing the name of the organization that publishes this book—from Mental Retardation and Developmental Disabilities to Developmental Disabilities (Smith, 2003). Postmodernism has a radical skepticism for explanations that claim to be valid for all groups, cultures, traditions, or races, choosing instead to investigate the relative truths of each person. In this view, science alone cannot solve all problems; in fact, it often causes the problems or makes them worse. It was empirical research that originally excluded individuals with disabilities from society by determining that they were impure. It is remembered that sterilization, shock therapy, and psychosurgery were promoted as research-based strategies (Hughes, 2002). Postmodernists question the predictive and prescriptive ability of the knowledge base in special education (Gallagher, 1998), and believe that the dominant group has used the scientific method as a means to exclude and oppress others. Research by postmodernists tries to give meaning to the multiple constructions of reality in their environment. Empirical findings are "open to discussion, interpretation, and critical interrogation" (Fawcett & Hearn, 2004, p. 216). Our world is too dynamically interactive for simplistic and formulaic approaches. Those who determine "normal" have the power. We can study an individual only through an investigation of his or her "life-story." The postmodernists focus on "multiple possible forms of anti-oppressive politically engaged agendas around research rather than a more generalizable research methodology" (Fawcett & Hearn, p. 212) and on problem solving by a broader group of stakeholders using a team approach. Facts and values are inseparable. By separating researchers from those studied, a system is developed in which the individuals studied become "others," "invisibles," and "strangers." Akintunde (1999) reports that the modernist multiculturalism position, "through its efforts to increase an 'understanding' of 'others,' actually reinforces and cements 'otherization' " (p. 5). The "people in power" establish an oppressive atmosphere by determining the services that should be delivered to "others."

Skrtic (1991) wonders who benefits most from special education. Is it the consumers or the practitioners and in what proportion? Fawcett and Hearn (2004) suggest that we need to ask the following questions in doing research or serving individuals with disabilities:

Is it possible to research others? If so, how is this to be done? And how does this aspiration and this activity relate to more general questions in social science methodology? Is it possible, and how is it possible for an able-bodied researcher to carry out non-exploitative, participative, qualitative research with people with disabilities. (p. 201)

They also state: "It cannot be assumed that disabled people identify with other disabled people, that a single perspective of disability (or anything else) is shared, or that disability constitutes the most important aspect of a person's identity or social position" (Fawcett & Hearn, 2004, p. 210).

In reality, disability is not just educational. It is also a social, cultural, political, historical, discursive, and relational construct (Goodley, 2001). Bogdan and Taylor recognized this issue in 1982: "Mental retardation is, in fact, a socio-political not a psychological construction. The myth, perpetuated by a society which refuses to recognize the true nature of its needed social reforms, has successfully camouflaged the politics of diagnosis and incarceration" (p. 15).

It is not the purpose of this text to secure supporters of modernist or post-modernist philosophies. However, each paradigm certainly has beliefs that include guidelines for our review of researched-based practices. Elkind (1998) believes that "we have reinvented childhood to encompass difference, particularity, and irregularity, as well as progress, universality and regularity" and that our best practice "incorporates these new themes as well as the older ones" (p. 14). Perhaps Smith (1999) states it best:

The recognition that we are ethical and moral agents—and that the decisions about what we *should* do as opposed to what we *can* do rest with us—is intimidating. . . . As the power of science for human benefit grows, so grows the importance of ethical questions about the use and yield of that power. The great challenge of our age may be to ensure that people who make scientific and medical discoveries interact with those who seek to understand the ethical impact of those discoveries [emphasis added]. (p. 132)

It is up to readers of this text to make informed decisions with regard to individually appropriate practice and accountability.

References

Akintunde, O. (1999). White racism, white supremacy, white privilege, and the social construction of race. *Multicultural Education, 7*(2), 2–8.

Bogdan, R., & Taylor, S. (1982). *Inside out: The social meaning of mental retardation.* Toronto: University of Toronto Press.

Clear, M. (1999). The "normal" and the monstrous in disability research. *Disability & Society, 14,* 435–448.

Crichton, M. (2004). Why politicized science is dangerous. In M. Crichton (Ed.), *State of fear* (pp. 631–638). New York: Avon Books.

Education for All Handicapped Children Act of 1975, 20 U.S.C. § 1400 *et seq.* (1975).

Elkind, D. (1998). Children with special needs: A postmodern perspective. *Journal of Education, 180,* 1–16.

Fawcett, B., & Hearn, J. (2004). Researching others: Epistemology, experience, standpoints, and participation. *International Journal of Social Research Methodology, 3,* 201–218.

Forness, S. R., & Kavale, K. A. (2001). Reflections on the future of prevention. *Preventing School Failure, 45,* 75–81.

Gallagher, D. J. (1998). The scientific knowledge base of special education: Do we know what we think we know? *Exceptional Children, 64,* 493–502.

Goodley, D. (2001). "Learning difficulties," the social model of disability and impairment: Challenging epistemologies. *Disability and Society, 16,* 207–231.

Hilton, A., & Ringlaben, R. (Eds.). (1998). *Best and promising practices in developmental disabilities.* Austin, TX: PRO-ED.

Hughes, B. (2002). Bauman's strangers: Impairment and the invalidation of disabled people in modern and post-modern cultures. *Disability and Society, 17,* 571–584.

Kavale, K. A., & Mostert, M. P. (2003). River of ideology, islands of excellence. *Exceptionality, 11,* 191–208.

Rhodes, W. C. (1995). Liberatory pedagogy and special education. *Journal of Learning Disabilities, 28,* 458–462.

Roberts, C. D., Stough, L. M., & Parrish, C. D. (2002). The role of genetic counseling in the elective termination of pregnancies involving fetuses with disabilities. *Journal of Special Education, 36,* 48–55.

Sailor, W., & Paul, J. P. (2004). Framing positive behavior support in the ongoing discourse concerning the politics of knowledge. *Journal of Positive Behavior Interventions, 6,* 37–49.

Sasso, G. M. (2001). The retreat from inquiry and knowledge in special education. *Journal of Special Education, 34,* 178–193.

Skrtic, T. M. (1991). The special education paradox: Equity as the way to excellence. *Harvard Educational Review, 61,* 148–206.

Smith, J. D. (2003). Abandoning the myth of mental retardation. *Education and Training in Developmental Disabilities, 38,* 358–361.

Smith, J. D. (2000). Looking backward, looking forward: Mental retardation and the question of equality in the new millennium. *Mental Retardation, 38,* 457–459.

Smith, J. D. (1999). Thoughts on the changing meaning of disability: New eugenics or new wholeness? *Remedial and Special Education, 20,* 131–133.

1

Research-Based Practices in Developmental Disabilities

Introduction and Scope of Textbook

Howard P. Parette and George R. Peterson-Karlan

Summary

This chapter presents a brief rationale for the topical approach used in the textbook, coupled with clarifying definitions of research-based and emerging best practices. The scope of the textbook is then presented, with descriptive overviews of each chapter. A standards chart provides readers with a broad overview of specific standards approved by the Division on Developmental Disabilities in April 2005, which are addressed in the chapters.

Learning Outcomes

After reading this chapter, you should be able to:

- Define best practices.
- Define research-based practices.
- Understand the organizational framework for the textbook.

Outline of Context

In the first edition of this textbook (Hilton & Ringlaben, 1998), the term *best practices* was defined as "those overriding practices that direct service provision to individuals with developmental disabilities" (p. 1). The Division on Developmental Disabilities (DDD) of the Council for Exceptional Children has expended considerable effort on developing and disseminating these practices to current and future practitioners in the field (see, e.g., Special Conference, Best Practices for Practitioners, in the September 2005, issue of *Education and Training in Developmental Disabilities*).

In recent years, however, greater emphasis has been placed on the role of research in documenting what should be deemed to be best practice in the field. In fact, the Individuals with Disabilities Education Improvement Act of 2004 authorized greater emphasis on competitive grants for research related to services provided to children with disabilities and to the outcomes/effectiveness of those services (20 U.S.C. § 175). This legislation also created the National Center for Educational Research, which has multiple responsibilities to identify, develop, and support use of *research-based practices* in service delivery to children with disabilities (U.S. Department of Education, 2005). With such legislated emphases on the role of research in special education service delivery (see the foreword in this textbook for a perspective), practitioners are expected to use best practices that have a research basis and to begin to document the effectiveness of their own practices in service delivery settings (i.e., *evidence-based practice*) (Odom, Brantlinger, Gersten, Horner, Thompson, & Harris, 2005).

The sections of this volume address research-based and current best practices, as discussed previously, and are organized around broad themes within the field of developmental disabilities. Each chapter addresses specific standards approved by the Division on Developmental Disabilities in April 2005 (see Table 1.1). The content of each chapter is supplemented by a variety of instructor support materials in the *Research-Based Practices in Developmental Disabilities Instructor's Manual*.

Section 1, Foundations of Developmental Disabilities, begins with an authoritative and comprehensive review of historical and legal issues that affect the field of developmental disabilities by James R. Thompson and Michael L. Wehmeyer (chapter 2). This review is complemented by the reflections of J. David Smith (chapter 3), pertaining to personal and cultural meanings of developmental disabilities. Readers should find both chapters to be of particular relevance, given the current understanding of developmental disabilities as it has evolved.

In section 2, Development and Characteristics of Learners, Tom E. C. Smith presents a broad overview of issues related to definitions of developmental disabilities, as well as a discussion of trends that are supportive of more-generic, functional classification groupings for these individuals (chapter 4). To address the substantive increase in interest in the field of autism spectrum disorders (ASD) in recent years, Brenda Smith Myles, Anastasia Hubbard, Kristin Muellner, and Alison Simonelli provide a cogent overview of ASD, models for assessment, interventions, and educational trends in the United States (chapter 5). Following this chapter, Michael L. Wehmeyer, James E. Martin, and Deanna J. Sands provide an opportunity to examine current thinking regarding the practice of self-determination by persons with developmental disabilities, supported by recommendations emerging in the field for promoting self-determination (chapter 6).

The next section, Individual and Learning Differences, presents two perspectives that emphasize the relationship of culture to the education of students with developmental disabilities. Scott Sparks (chapter 7) shares a broad cultural perspective, with emphasis on the broader facets of diversity (i.e., training needs for professionals, working with families, and cross-cultural adoptions) within special education versus a focus on ethnic issues among students and families from culturally and linguistically diverse backgrounds. Sparks then presents an insightful examination of more-specific cultural considerations that are needed for effective educational decision making and subsequent interventions with children with developmental disabilities and their families from culturally and linguistically diverse backgrounds. Howard P. Parette, Mary Blake Huer, and George R. Peterson-Karlan (chapter 8) examine cultural influences that come into play when working with persons with developmental disabilities and their families, particularly emphasizing three components related to culture and their impact on service delivery: (a) patterns of acculturation (individual change), (b) particular parameters within school systems, and (c) recently recognized generational differences.

Section 4, Instructional Planning and Implementation, offers six contributions. Barbara G. Gartin and Nikki L. Murdick (chapter 9) describe the role of differentiated instruction (i.e., content, process, and product) and its relationship to evidence-based instructional planning. The importance of assistive technology (AT) "consideration" is then explored by George R. Peterson-Karlan and Howard P. Parette (chapter 10) in relation to the practice of technology integration into the curriculum. Earle Knowlton (chapter 11) discusses the underlying intent of legal requirements related to planning for the instruction of students with developmental disabilities and examines longitudinal planning, or "big picture" considerations, as a foundation for all planning. Debra L. Shelden and Margaret P. Hutchins (chapter 12) provide a concise overview of the process of implementing long-term planning by developing a "personalized curriculum" for learners with developmental disabilities,

TABLE 1.1
CEC Knowledge and Skills for Entry-Level Special Education Teachers of Students With Developmental Disabilities

DDD Standard / Chapters	2	3	4	5	6	7	8	9	10	11	12	13	14	15	16	17	18	19	20	21	22	23	24	25	26	27	28	29
Principle 1: Foundations																												
DD1K1 Definitions and issues related to the identification of individuals with developmental disabilities.	X	X	X	X	X													X				X						
DD1K2 Continuum of placement and services available for individuals with developmental disabilities.																								X	X	X		X
DD1K3 Historical foundations and classic studies of developmental disabilities.	X	X			X																							
DD1K4 Trends and practices in the field of developmental disabilities.	X	X	X		X		X	X	X				X		X		X		X			X	X	X	X	X	X	X
DD1K5 Theories of behavior problems of individuals with developmental disabilities.					X							X																
Principle 2: Development and characteristics of learners																												
DD2K1 Medical aspects of developmental disabilities and their implications for learning.																		X										
DD2K2 Psychological, social/emotional, and motor characteristics of individuals with developmental disabilities.			X	X	X																							
DD2K3 Identification of significant core deficit areas for individuals with pervasive developmental disabilities, autism, and autism spectrum disorder.					X	X											X	X										
DD2K4 Factors that influence overrepresentation of culturally/linguistically diverse individuals.							X								X			X										
DD2K5 Complications and implications of medical support services.																						X						

Principle 3: Individual learning differences

DD3K1 Impact of multiple disabilities on behavior.

Principle 4: Instructional strategies

DD4K1 Specialized materials for individuals with developmental disabilities.

DD4K2 Evidence-based practices for teaching individuals with pervasive developmental disabilities, autism, and autism spectrum disorders.

DD4K3 Specialized curriculum specifically designed to meet the needs of individuals with pervasive developmental disabilities, autism, and autism spectrum disorders.

DD4S1 Use specialized teaching strategies matched to the need of the learner.

DD4S2 Relate levels of support to the needs of the individual.

Principle 5: Learning environments/social interaction

DD5S1 Provide instruction in community-based settings.

DD5S2 Demonstrate transfer, lifting and positioning techniques.

DD5S3 Use and maintain assistive technologies.

DD5S4 Structure the physical environment to provide optimal learning for individuals with developmental disabilities.

DD5S5 Plan instruction for individuals with developmental disabilities in a variety of placement settings.

(continues)

TABLE 1.1 (Continued)

DDD Standard	2	3	4	5	6	7	8	9	10	11	12	13	14	15	16	17	18	19	20	21	22	23	24	25	26	27	28	29
DD6S1 Plan instruction on the use of alternative and augmentative communication systems.			X													X												
DD6S2 Use pragmatic language instruction to facilitate ongoing social skills instruction.																	X											
Principle 7: Instructional planning																												
DD7K1 Model career/vocational transition programs for individuals with developmental disabilities including career/vocational transition.															X									X			X	
DD7S1 Plan instruction for independent functional life skills relevant to the community, personal living, sexuality, and employment.					X	X				X	X		X		X						X							
DD7S2 Plan and implement instruction for individuals with developmental disabilities that is both age-appropriate and ability-appropriate.					X			X		X	X										X		X	X				
DD7S3 Select and plan for integration of related services into the instructional program for individuals with developmental disabilities.					X																							
DD7S4 Design, implement, and evaluate specialized instructional programs for persons with developmental disabilities that enhance social participation across environments.					X			X		X	X			X							X			X				
Principle 8: Assessment																												
DD8K1 Specialized terminology used in the assessment of individuals with developmental disabilities.	X				X		X											X										

Code	Description												
DD8K2	Environmental assessment conditions that promote maximum performance of individuals with developmental disabilities.		X		X			X			X	X	
DD8K3	Adaptive behavior assessment.										X		
DD8K4	Laws and policies regarding referral and placement procedures for individuals with developmental disabilities.	X			X			X			X		
DD8S1	Select, adapt and use instructional assessment tools and methods to accommodate the abilities and needs of individuals with mental retardation and developmental disabilities.		X	X		X			X	X			

Principle 9: Professional and ethical practice

| DD9K1 | Organizations and publications in the field of developmental disabilities. | | | | | | | | | | X | | |
| DD9S1 | Participate in the activities of professional organizations in the field of developmental disabilities. | | | | | | | | | | | | |

Principle 10: Collaboration

| DD10K1 | Services, networks, and organizations for individuals with developmental disabilities. | | X | | | | | | | | X | X | |
| DD10S1 | Collaborate with team members to plan transition to adulthood that encourages full community participation. | | X | | | | | | | | | | X |

Source: Division on Developmental Disabilities. (n.d.). *CEC knowledge and skills for entry-level special education teachers of students with developmental disabilities*. Retrieved April 27, 2007, from http://www.dddcec.org/secondarypages/standards/dddstandards.doc

one that includes person-centered planning processes, a long-term vision, a variety of assessments to identify educational priorities, and decision making about short-term and long-term priorities. John J. Wheeler and David Dean Richey (chapter 13) emphasize positive behavior support strategies in the curriculum, with an emphasis on the theoretical framework of positive behavior supports and their application to learners with developmental disabilities. Dennis D. Munk and Toni Van Laarhoven (chapter 14) discuss other aspects of instructional planning by providing a concise review of research on grouping arrangements and delivery of instruction to students with developmental disabilities.

Section 5, Learning Environments and Social Interactions, discusses two important facets of research-based and emerging best practices. Mary Ann Demchak (chapter 15) explores the importance of social relationships and friendships, with particular emphasis on minimizing the negative influence of adults, facilitating positive attitudes, use of peer buddy programs, extracurricular and non-instructional activity involvement, participation in conversations, and friendship circles. Dianne Zager, James Brown, Pamela H. Stenhjem, and Arthur Maloney (chapter 16) advocate for the importance of considering the nature of individual students and their vocational preferences in transition planning, devoting attention to self-determination, the role of assistive technology, independent living, and service learning.

In section 6, Communication, Ann R. Beck (chapter 17) reviews the research on children's attitudes toward and their subsequent impact on the communication needs of peers with developmental disabilities. Additional sections address intervention strategies for altering attitudes and review the characteristics of beginning communicators and strategies for intervention. Julia B. Stoner (chapter 18) focuses on communication skills and strategies for working with children who have ASD and provides classroom recommendations for development of prelinguistic skills, language comprehension, language production, language use, transitions, and communication with families.

In section 7, Assessment, Christine A. Macfarlane (chapter 19) discusses the legal obligations of local education agencies regarding children who enter school or who transition from an early-intervention program. Special emphasis is placed on team-driven and collaborative processes that include parents, with references to legal authority. Dave L. Edyburn (chapter 20) provides an introduction to theoretical and practical issues associated with measuring assistive technology outcomes in education, particularly the application of principles and practices for professionals working with students with developmental disabilities. Colleen E. Klein-Ezell, Randy LaRusso, and Dan Ezell (chapter 21) discuss the role of alternate assessment in the context of legislative mandates to ensure that all students participate and are counted in district- and statewide assessment results. The authors stress the role of Making Action Plans (MAPS) as tools to facilitate the process of collecting information about students to determine effective ways to plan for their futures. Jeffrey P. Bakken (chapter 22) provides an insightful discussion of how teachers of students with developmental disabilities can incorporate a cadre of data-based techniques and decision-making principles into their daily routines to measure how students are performing on content, skills, and behaviors.

In section 8, Professional and Ethical Practice, Ravic P. Ringlaben and Kimberly Griffith (chapter 23) examine the effect of multiple environmental assumptions, biases, stereotypes, and service delivery philosophy on the development of positive and negative attitudes toward persons with developmental disabilities. Strategies that promote positive attitudes are presented.

In section 9, Schools and Community Involvement, Ann P. Turnbull, H. R. Turnbull, Jean A. Summers, and Denise Poston (chapter 24) provide a review of family-related disability policy in the United States, emphasizing that such policies support caregiving efforts and enhance the quality of life for all families. The authors discuss strategies in five areas: disability-related support, physical/material well-being, parenting, emotional well-being, and family interaction. Anna Lou Pickett (chapter 25) addresses a range of issues related to the role of paraeducators in the education of children with developmental disabilities. Specific issues include historical factors contributing to the employment of teacher aides, teacher and principal supervisory roles of these professionals, paraeducator instructional and direct service roles, and administrator responsibilities in developing policies, standards, and systems that affect paraprofessionals. Darlene E. Perner and Gordon L. Porter (chapter 26) describe the importance of establishing a vision and a set of values for inclusive education, and present two models (i.e., support teacher and multilevel instructional approach) that provide support to classroom teachers. In chapter 27, Darlene E. Perner examines the crucial role played by administrators and teachers charged with the responsibility of implementing inclusive education. Emphasis is placed on approaches that develop and maintain inclusive school practices.

Garnett J. Smith, Patricia J. Edelen-Smith, and Robert A. Stodden (chapter 28) describe a field-based and well-researched operational strategic-planning process that initiates, installs, and supports the creation of transdisciplinary (TD) learning organization teams. The authors identify six factors that are crucial to core transformational change in special education and community support systems. Finally, Jack J. Hourcade (chapter 29) discusses professional collaboration—both direct and indirect—along with potential barriers to the effectiveness of this approach (i.e., focus on the present versus the future, resistance to change, lack of administrative support, lack of knowledge and skills, and lack of perseverance).

The Division on Developmental Disabilities of the Council for Exceptional Children hopes that readers find this text to be a valuable tool in increasing their awareness and knowledge of current issues in the field. It is also anticipated that the textbook will help current and future practitioners to better understand educational practices that are deemed effective in working with children with developmental disabilities and their families.

Acknowledgments

This project was undertaken as a service to the Division on Developmental Disabilities (DDD) and to current and future practitioners. It was designed to update the first edition of the textbook *Best and Promising Practices in Developmental Disabilities*, published in 1998, as substantive changes have occurred in the field since that first edition was released. We express our appreciation to all the authors who have contributed to this volume—all experts in the field—for their commitment of time and for their professionalism in bringing this project to completion. Although DDD has underwritten the cost of publishing this textbook, all proceeds from its sale are returned to DDD. Authors have not been compensated for their contributions other than receiving the satisfaction of having made a substantive contribution to the knowledge base of the discipline and thus positively affecting the quality of services provided to children with developmental disabilities and their families nationally.

We wish to thank Dr. Tina Dyches and Dr. Ravic Ringlaben for their early involvement in the project and the assistance that they provided in soliciting proposals for the textbook. We also extend our appreciation to Amanda Giltner for editorial assistance in organizing the vast number of files submitted and for coordinating correspondence with contributors during the final stage of the textbook preparation process. We also acknowledge the support of the DDD board of directors for the intensive effort that went into the completion of this textbook within the targeted time frame.

Glossary

Best practices—Those overriding practices that direct service provision to individuals with developmental disabilities.

Evidence-based practice—Best practices that have a research basis and that have been documented to be effective in service delivery settings.

Research-based practice—Best practices that have a research basis.

References

Hilton, A., & Ringlaben, R. (Eds.). (1998). *Best and promising practices in developmental disabilities.* Austin, TX: PRO-ED.

Individuals with Disabilities Education Improvement Act of 2004, 118 Stat. 2647. (2004).

Odom, S. L., Brantlinger, E., Gersten, R., Horner, R. H., Thompson, B., & Harris, K. R. (2005). Research in special education: Scientific methods and evidenced-based practices. *Exceptional children, 71,* 137–148.

U.S. Department of Education. (2005). *National Center for Educational Research.* Retrieved January 11, 2006, from http://www.ed.gov/about/offices/list/ies/ncer/index.html

SECTION 1

FOUNDATIONS OF DEVELOPMENTAL DISABILITIES

2

Historical and Legal Issues in Developmental Disabilities

James R. Thompson and Michael L. Wehmeyer

If you would understand anything, observe its beginning and its development.

—Aristotle

Summary

This book is titled *Research-Based Practices in Developmental Disabilities*. One might reasonably ask, though, what is meant by the term *developmental disabilities*. To whom does it apply? Where did it come from? Is it a politically correct term? Is it a stigmatizing term? What are the educational, sociological, psychological, and legal implications for how this term is understood and used? Who are people with developmental disabilities and what are their life experiences? The purpose of this chapter is to clarify what *developmental disabilities* has meant historically, how the term is used today, and what it may mean in the future, as well as to review the history of the field of developmental disabilities.

Learning Outcomes

After reading this chapter, you should be able to:

- Understand the evolution of the term *developmental disabilities* with regard to how it has been used over time by different groups.

- Explain current trends and issues with regard to (a) the use of the term *mental retardation*, (b) the alignment of functional definitions with multidimensional models of person competence, and (c) the assessment and measurement of individual support needs.

- Identify milestones and key individuals who contributed to early progress in the field of developmental disabilities.

- Identify differences in contemporary services and supports for persons with developmental disabilities and those provided in earlier eras.

Developmental Disabilities: The Chameleon of Disability Terminology

Federal Legislation Gives Birth to New Terminology

The term *developmental disabilities* was essentially created by the 91st United States Congress in 1970 with passage of the Developmental Disabilities Services and Facilities Construction Amendments (P.L. 91-517), a law that has become commonly referred to as the DD Act (Lakin & Bruininks, 1983; Summers, 1986). Although some people may have used the term informally before 1970, the terms *developmental disabilities* and *developmental disability* were not used in the professional literature (journal articles and textbooks) in the fields of special education and psychology until after this law was passed. A search of the ERIC and PsycINFO databases revealed that before 1971 only 3 documents had included either of these terms in a title or abstract. The earliest entry, published in 1963, focused on issues related to the State of Minnesota's provision of respite care (Minnesota State Planning Agency, 1963). In contrast, since 1971 the ERIC and PsychINFO databases contain 3,006 and 6,659 documents, respectively, that use the term *developmental disabilities* in an abstract or a title.

Congress's creation of a new term in the 1970 legislation was intentional. Congress wanted to amend the Mental Retardation Facilities and Community Mental Health Centers Construction Act of 1963 (P.L. 88-164) to ensure that mental retardation was not the only disability population that the act should benefit (Breen & Richman, 1979). The 1970 DD Act was part of the deinstitutionalization movement, described in great detail subsequently, and was intended to support the growth of community-based service systems, especially community residential opportunities. What was envisioned was the creation of a comprehensive service system in which local organizations provided assistance to a variety of people with both intellectual and physical disabilities that (a) had originated in childhood (the developmental period from birth to age 18), (b) constituted a significant handicap, and (c) were expected to continue indefinitely (Lakin & Bruininks, 1983). The original definition of a developmental disability presented in the 1970 legislation was "a disability attributable to mental retardation, cerebral palsy, epilepsy, or another neurological condition of an individual found by the Secretary to be clearly related to mental retardation or to require treatment similar to that for mentally retarded individuals" (Breen & Richman, 1979, p. 3).

The Federal Definition of DD Changes

The legal definition of developmental disabilities broadened in 1975 when the DD Act was amended. The 1975 version (P.L. 94-103) added autism and dyslexia to the categorical mix and continued to include the catchall phrase "any other condition found to be closely related to mental retardation or that required treatment and services similar to those required by persons with mental retardation." Perhaps the most significant change in the 1975 DD Act was the inclusion of a "Bill of Rights" that indicated the government's commitment to ensuring that individuals with developmental disabilities lived free of neglect and abuse, had access to services that promoted personal independence and growth, lived in the least restrictive environment, and had regular contact with family members or guardians (Lakin & Bruininks, 1983; Summers, 1986). The DD Bill of Rights has continued to be affirmed and updated with each subsequent revision of the DD Act.

Despite the broadening scope of disability conditions subsumed under the umbrella of developmental disabilities in 1975, the term's usefulness was questioned because of the emphasis on disability categories. Specific disabilities were perceived to be problematic for at least two, seemingly paradoxical, reasons. First, populations comprising these disability categories were so heterogeneous that the term did not appear to apply to all the members of these broad groups (Lakin & Bruininks, 1983;

Summers, 1986). For example, *cerebral palsy* refers to a group of conditions that affect control of movement and posture. Depending on the case, it can influence a person's mobility and motor functioning to a small extent or to a great extent. Certainly, individuals with mild cerebral palsy and typical intellectual development are not in need of "treatment and services similar to those required by persons with mental retardation." However, cerebral palsy was one of the disability conditions specifically mentioned in the 1975 DD Act.

The second concern with the DD Act was that many individuals were falling through the cracks. That is, despite being in need of "treatment and services similar to those required by persons with mental retardation," some individuals were unable to get assistance because they did not have the right disability label—one that would provide them with a passport to the service system. To rectify these problems, a task force was formed to recommend revisions to the definition of developmental disabilities (Lakin & Bruininks, 1983; Summers, 1986).

The National Task Force on the Definition of Developmental Disabilities (1977) determined that a functional definition that focused not on clinical disability diagnoses but rather on what people could and could not do would be superior to the categorical approach. Summers (1986) captured the aim of the functional definition approach when she wrote: "The issue is not what sort of disability a person has, but what sort of services a person needs. The question is not one of diagnosis, but of remediation—looking forward to progress, not backward to etiology" (p. 13). As a result of the task force's recommendation, Congress significantly changed its definition of developmental disabilities in the amended DD Act of 1978 (P.L. 95-602). Specifically, a person needed to experience limitations in three of seven life domains as delineated in the law.

Although explicit mention of categorical disability terms (e.g., *mental retardation, dyslexia, autism, epilepsy,* and *cerebral palsy*) was discarded in 1978, language was retained related to age of origin (the disability had to originate in the developmental period) and chronicity (the disability was not temporary). Moreover, severity of the disability was further emphasized in the 1978 DD Act. Summers (1986) reported the 1978 DD Act was intended to support those with more-severe disabilities, and it was assumed that people with mild disabilities could be served under different umbrellas. She specifically mentions that "most authorities would not consider a mildly retarded person [*sic*] to be developmentally disabled under the definition in PL 95-602" (p. 11).

The DD Act has been amended several more times since 1978, but the focus on functional limitations as the defining feature of developmental disabilities has not changed. The current definition is as follows:

> Developmental disabilities (DD) are severe, life-long disabilities attributable to mental and/or physical impairments, manifested before age 22. Developmental disabilities result in substantial limitations in three or more areas of major life activities:
>
> - capacity for independent living
> - economic self-sufficiency
> - learning
> - mobility
> - receptive and expressive language
> - self-care
> - self-direction (Developmental Disabilities Assistance and Bill of Rights Act of 2000, 42 U.S.C. § 15002, 2000)

According to the Administration on Developmental Disabilities (2005), the federal agency responsible for implementation and administration of the DD Act,

> without appropriate services and supports, the choices open to people with developmental disabilities, including where they live, work, and play, are minimal. They are isolated rather than fully integrated and included in the mainstream of society. Persons with developmental disabilities require individually planned and coordinated services and supports (e.g., housing, employment, education, civil and human rights protection, health care) from many providers in order to live in the community. (What Is Developmental Disability? ¶ 1)

Back to the Future: CEC-DDD Casts a Wide Categorical Net

The Council for Exceptional Children's Division on Mental Retardation and Developmental Disabilities (CEC-MRDD) changed its name to the Division on Developmental Disabilities (CEC-DDD) in 2002. The term *mental retardation* was removed from the division's name because it was considered to be an offensive term. Moreover, for several years the division had been addressing the needs of a broad disability population, including individuals with autism. Therefore, highlighting only one specific disability group in the name of the division did not seem appropriate. Also factored into the decision were two trends in the field of special education. Namely, noncategorical special education programs and inclusive classrooms had largely overtaken strictly categorically based programs and classrooms. Finally, many professional and advocacy groups had eliminated the term *mental retardation* from their organizational names (Stodden, 2002).

When the CEC-DDD changed its name, it provided the field with another option for understanding and using the term *developmental disability* by adding the following tag line: "Focusing on individuals with cognitive disabilities/mental retardation, autism, and related disabilities." The tag line is featured prominently at the top of the division's newsletters as well as on its Web page. There is no indication that the division intended to adopt the federal government's "functional" definition of developmental disabilities. Rather, the division wanted *developmental disabilities* to be an umbrella term for a variety of disability populations:

> The Division on Developmental Disabilities (DDD) of the Council on [*sic*] Exceptional Children (CEC) is a professional organization inclusive of educators, therapists, direct service providers, paraeducators, family members, and others providing a full range of supports, services, and accommodations to individuals with cognitive disabilities/mental retardation, autism, and related disabilities in educational, community living, and employment environments. The focus of the Division is on addressing the needs of all persons with developmental disabilities, regardless of the term or "label" used to identify those individuals. This includes persons identified as having high incidence disabilities and/or mild support needs (e.g., *educable mental retardation/mild mental retardation/cognitive impairment, developmental delay/Aspergers* [*sic*]/*high functioning autism/Down syndrome*) through those persons identified as having low incidence disabilities and/or more extensive support needs (e.g., *trainable mental retardation/moderate and severe mental retardation/severe disabilities/dual diagnosis/multiple disabilities/severe*

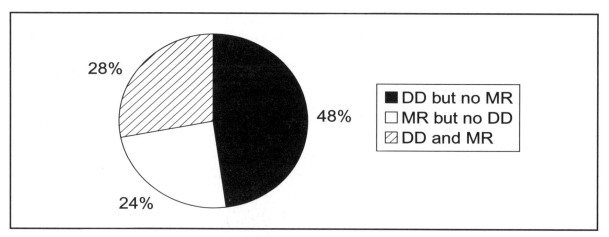

FIGURE 2.1. Overlap between populations of persons with mental retardation and developmental disabilities. Source: Larson et al. (2001). Prevalence of mental retardation and developmental disabilities: Estimates from the 1994/1995 national health interview survey disability supplements. *American Journal of Mental Retardation*, 106, p. 245. Adapted with permission.

developmental delay/organic mental retardation/severe cognitive impairment/low functioning autism) (emphasis in original) (Stodden, 2004, ¶ 3).

It is especially noteworthy that the division indicated that the developmental disabilities umbrella included people with high-incidence disabilities, such as mild mental retardation. As noted earlier, on the basis of the federal government's definition of a developmental disability, a significant number of individuals with "mild mental retardation" would not be included (Garnett, 2003; Summers, 1986). In a study that generated prevalence figures for populations of persons with mental retardation and persons with developmental disabilities, Larson et al. (2001) applied criteria from the DD Act and criteria from leading definitions of mental retardation to data collected from the National Health Interview Survey. They concluded that there is overlap between the populations of people with mental retardation and developmental disabilities, but they are not the same group (see Figure 2.1).

> Across all ages, 28% of people meeting the criteria for either mental retardation or developmental disabilities met both sets of criteria; 24.3% met the criteria for mental retardation but not for developmental disabilities, and 47.7% met the criteria for having developmental disabilities but not for mental retardation. (p. 245)

Put another way, Lawson et al.'s findings indicated that roughly half of the people with mental retardation do *not* qualify under the federal government's developmental disability criteria, and the vast majority of those who do not qualify are people with mild mental retardation. In contrast, according to the CEC-DDD's description of developmental disabilities, 100% of people with "mild mental retardation" would be considered to be people with developmental disabilities.

Keeping Things in Perspective

Determining what exactly does and does not constitute any type of disability is an imprecise process. For example, debates regarding the construct of learning disabilities have raged for years without any final resolution (e.g., see Algozzine, Ysseldyke, &

McGue, 1995; Kavale, Fuchs, & Scruggs, 1994) and special education disability population figures have not been stable over time or across states (Ysseldyke, Algozzine, & Thurlow, 2000). However, developmental disabilities is an especially challenging population to pin down, as there are no standardized assessment instruments or procedures established to make a diagnosis and determine if "substantial limitations" exist in the seven major life activities that are identified in the law. Depending on how one wishes to use the term *developmental disabilities*, this may or may not be a problem.

The intent of the DD Act has been to promote a more coordinated and responsive system of services. Although it is possible for individuals with disabilities to receive support through a demonstration project that is funded through the DD Act, the DD Act has never been a significant source of funding for community services. Rather, the DD Act provides funding to (a) state interagency councils that develop state plans and fund innovative projects, (b) protection and advocacy agencies that support individuals who are attempting to exercise legal rights and/or obtain services, (c) university centers of excellence in developmental disabilities that are involved in either provision of specialized clinical services, technical assistance, and/or research, and (d) special projects of national significance (Administration on Developmental Disabilities, 2005).

Because of the nature of the DD Act, the definition of *developmental disabilities* the act does not serve a significant gate-keeping function regarding who gets assistance and who does not. Thus, the imprecise definition does not have serious ramifications for individuals. In contrast, disability definitions in laws that have extraordinary implications for individuals as well as significant budgetary consequences need to be more precise. For example, the Individuals with Disabilities Educational Improvement Act (P.L. 108-446) determines access to special education services, and the Social Security Protection Act (P.L. 108-203) determines eligibility for Supplemental Security Income (SSI) benefits.

Braddock, Hemp, Parish, and Westrich (1998) pointed out that as a result of the DD Act most states have replaced the term *mental retardation* with *developmental disability* in the name of their state agency. However, few states have adopted the functional criteria included in the DD Act to determine eligibility for state-funded services. Instead, the more concrete disability definitions (e.g., *mental retardation*) have been retained to determine who is and who is not eligible to receive funding. It appears that *developmental disabilities*, as it is currently defined in the DD Act, may be a useful term for advancing broad social policy goals, but it is not perceived to be a very useful term when determining eligibility for services for individuals.

Because the Division on Developmental Disabilities (DDD) of the Council for Exceptional Children (CEC) is a professional organization, it does not have to contend with the messy task of resource allocation (i.e., deciding what a child or a family receives). Therefore, an imprecise umbrella term that applies to a variety of professional interests may work quite well for it, since its membership spans diverse professional backgrounds and roles. Such a term may not, however, be as useful for researchers who are interested in establishing scientifically valid knowledge claims to advance professional practice. Conyers, Martin, Martin, and Yu (2002) reviewed 844 research articles published from 1993 to 2001 in four leading professional journals in the field of special education. They reported that only 4% of the articles described subjects as individuals with developmental disabilities. The remaining articles used a disability diagnosis (e.g., mental retardation, Fragile X syndrome) to describe subjects. Perhaps *developmental disabilities* was simply too imprecise a term to provide the descriptiveness needed to advance knowledge. Regardless, such a low percentage does not bode well for establishing an empirical knowledge base specifically tied to persons with developmental disabilities.

Developmental Disability As It Is Understood Today

In summary, *developmental disability* is an ambiguous term. There are no standardized guidelines to complete an assessment and no explicit criteria to make a diagnosis. When the term was created in the 1970 legislation, it wasn't intended to be a clinical term. However, in time, *developmental disability* "began to assume the properties of a clinical classification, thus creating considerable confusion as to the exact nature of the population being served or studied" (Scheerenberger, 1987, p. 16). The confusion has remained.

Today, *developmental disability* refers to different populations of people, depending on how it is used and who is using it. The CEC-DDD description suggests that the term *developmental disabilities* largely encapsulates mental retardation and autism spectrum disorders but also includes other conditions that results in individuals' needing extraordinary supports to participate in educational, community living, and employment settings. This contrasts with the federal government's definition, which encompasses a smaller, more significantly disabled population that is characterized by experiencing functional limitations in at least three of seven areas. Because the federal description does not operationally define a severe, life-long disability, or indicate what constitutes substantial limitations, there is ample room for different interpretations.

Understanding Developmental Disability Tomorrow: New Directions

One must approach the task of predicting the future with proper humility. The history lesson presented in the next section is replete with stories of individuals who were quite confident they were onto something very useful, but for whom history revealed the opposite. In the words of Socrates, "The only true wisdom is in knowing you know nothing."

Although forecasting the future may be an uncertain undertaking, several trends appear to have the potential to make significant contributions to the way in which developmental disabilities are understood in the coming years. Here we briefly discuss three of these trends: changing terminology, aligning functional definitions with multidimensional models of personal competence, and assessment and planning for support needs.

Changing Terminology

Luckasson et al. (2002) make important distinctions between *naming* (a specific term is attached to something), *defining* (the name or term is explained as precisely as possible), and *classifying* (what is included in the term by definition is divided into subgroups according to stated principles) in the field of mental retardation. Discourse can become very muddled when people fail to make these distinctions. It is important to understand that disagreements over terminology (i.e., what names we should use) have little or nothing to do with issues associated with defining and/or classifying disability conditions.

No terminology associated with developmental disabilities is as controversial as *mental retardation*. Many people consider *mental retardation* to be an outdated, pejorative term and do not want it to be used anymore. The National Service Inclusion Project (2005) indicated that retardation implies that a person cannot learn and therefore mental retardation should be used sparingly. However, there are those who disagree. Richard Garnett (2003) writes that "as the father of a 20 year old son who has severe mental retardation and autism, I do not object to the clear and meaningful term 'Mental Retardation'. As President of The Arc of Texas and a Board member of the Texas Advocates, I have spoken to many self advocates and family members who feel the same" (Last but not least section, ¶ 1).

We believe that *mental retardation* is on its way out. The term has simply acquired too much baggage; too many negative stereotypes are ingrained in the general public's mind. Advocacy groups don't like it and they never will. Unfortunately, at this time in the United States, there is no consensus on an alternative term that (a) facilitates communication as well as *mental retardation*, does but (b) does not have the same degree of stigma. However, alternatives are emerging, among them *cognitive disability* and *intellectual disability*. Once one of these terms begins to be used consistently in the professional literature and everyday conversation, the term *mental retardation* will go the way of *idiocy*, *feeblemindedness*, *mental deficiency*, and other terms that at one time may have been appropriate and/or benign but acquired negative connotations and were therefore discarded.

Aligning Functional Definitions With Multidimensional Models of Personal Competence

Functional definitions of disabilities focus on a person's competency in coping with everyday challenges inherent to successful functioning in school and contemporary society. Functional definitions, also called ecological definitions, present a disability as a mismatch between what the environment (e.g., school, the workplace, home) demands and what the person is able to do. In a functional approach, disability is understood as a *state of being* and not a *personal trait* (Luckasson et al., 1992; World Health Organization, 2001).

Although functional definitions of disabilities are not new, efforts to link functional descriptions with theoretical multidimensional models of intelligence/personal competence are just emerging. The stronger this linkage becomes, the more likely it is that diagnostic and assessment activities will become more directly relevant to intervention and support planning, and the nature of different disabilities will be better understood.

The American Association on Mental Retardation (AAMR, now AAIDD) took a significant step by incorporating personal competence concepts into its latest definition of mental retardation, stating, "Mental retardation is a disability characterized by limitations both in intellectual functioning and in conceptual, social, and practical adaptive skills" (Luckasson et al., 2002, p. 1). Approaching adaptive behavior from a tripartite perspective (i.e., conceptual, social, and practical skills) is supported by over 20 years of research on the factor structure of adaptive behavior (see Thompson, McGrew, & Bruininks, 1999; Widaman & McGrew, 1996). We hope that definitional and diagnostic systems will continue to move forward and that approaches that enable thorough assessment and consideration of all dimensions of personal competence will be developed.

An adapted version of Greenspan's Multidimensional Model of Personal Competence (Greenspan, 1979; Greenspan & Driscoll, 1997; Greenspan & Granfield, 1992) is shown in Figure 2.2. This simplified model attempts to illustrate the nature of a hierarchical personal competence model. It is important to realize that each dimension of personal competence (i.e., physical, conceptual, social, and practical) has subdimensions (represented by the circles). Skill indicators of physical competence

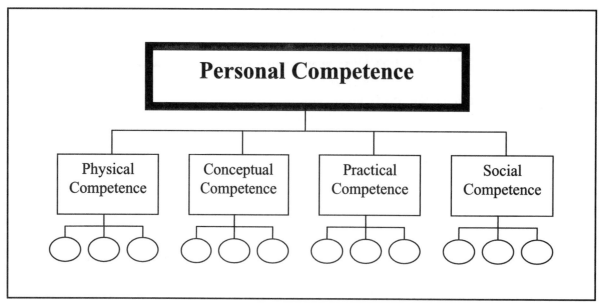

FIGURE 2.2. Greenspan Multidimensional Model of Personal Competence. Adapted.

include ambulation skills, gross motor skills, and fine motor skills. Conceptual competence refers to skills associated with understanding symbolic processes such as language as well as skills needed to master academic tasks. Practical competence is related to the mechanical aspects of life, including self-help skills, daily living skills, and vocational skills. Social competence is concerned with understanding and dealing effectively with social and interpersonal situations and includes skills to protect oneself from exploitation (Greenspan & Driscoll, 1997; Schalock, 2003; Thompson, McGrew, & Bruininks, 2002).

Our understanding of developmental disabilities would be enhanced if individuals were functionally assessed within the context of a valid multidimensional model of personal competence. There is widespread consensus that multiple intelligences exist (e.g., see Carroll, 2005; Sternberg, 2005), as well as multiple dimensions of adaptive behavior (see Thompson et al., 1999; Widaman & McGrew, 1996). Unfortunately, people are rarely assessed in light of multiple dimensions of personal competence; global IQ and adaptive behavior scores simply do not capture the complexity of personal competence.

Being able to identify an individual's relative strengths as well as areas of difficulty across multiple dimensions of personal competence would make disability assessment activities more meaningful than they are today. For example, a person with Asperger's syndrome may lack important skills/competencies in the social and physical dimensions, but may be quite competent in other dimensions. Multidimensional personal competence assessment would allow areas to be identified for special assistance and support. Moreover, it could serve to deemphasize disability labels since the focus would be on personal competence areas with relative strengths and weaknesses instead of disability terminology.

Much work lies ahead before assessment driven by personal competence models can become a reality. Not only do multidimensional models need to be refined and validated, but the significant lack of reliable and valid instrumentation for measuring critical domains of personal competence, in regard to both maximal and typical performance, needs to be addressed. For instance, standardized measures of social competence have not yet been developed (Thompson et al., 2002).

Assessing Support Needs and Developing Support Plans

An advantage to taking a functional approach to understanding disabilities is that it naturally leads to the identification of support needs. For example,

> if a person's competence limits his or her ability to do something that he or she wants to do, such as riding a bus to work, functional descriptions may lead to identifying: (a) the specific skills an individual needs to acquire and the strategies needed to teach the individual these skills, (b) tools (i.e., assistive technologies) that an individual might use to enhance his or her performance in particular settings or activities, (c) strategies for modifying the design or the demands of settings and activities so that individuals of differing abilities can be accommodated, or (d) a combination of any or all of these supports. (Thompson et al., 2004a, p. 3)

A systematic approach to assessment, planning, and monitoring of support needs is shown in Figure 2.3. Component 1, identifying a person's desired life experiences and goals, requires a person-centered planning process (e.g., Butterworth et al., 1993; Mount & Zwernik, 1988). Person-centered planning processes enable the development of a shared vision for a desirable future for an individual, with a focus on what the individual truly wants to do with his or her life. Upon completion of

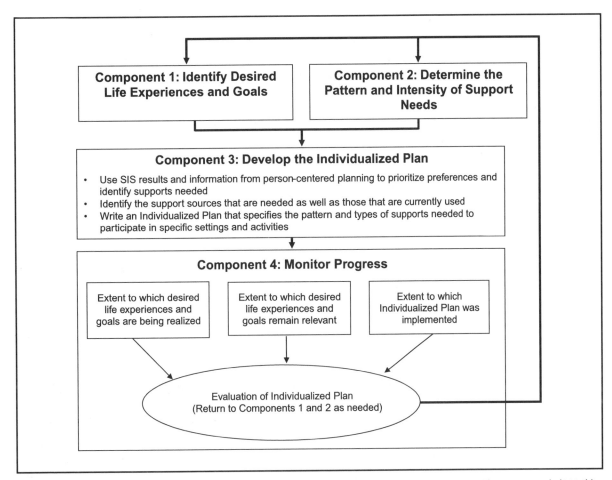

FIGURE 2.3. Four-component support needs assessment, planning, and monitoring process. Source: Thompson et al. (2004b). The Supports Intensity Scale (SIS): Standardization and users manual (p. 79). Washington, DC: American Association on Mental Retardation. Adapted with permission.

Component 1, discrepancies between a person's current life experiences and conditions and his or her preferred life experiences and conditions should be identified. Moreover, a planning team should be able to prioritize desired outcomes and specify which aspects of a person's life are the most important to maintain and/or to change (Thompson et al., 2004a).

The second component involves a formal assessment process that identifies the intensity and patterns of an individual's support needs. This step is completed at the same time as Component 1 (person-centered planning). A standardized scale for measuring support needs, the Supports Intensity Scale, has recently been published by the AAMR (see Thompson et al., 2004b), and can be used to complete Component 2.

Component 3 requires the development of an individualized support plan. It is here that "the rubber meets the road," in the sense that choices need to made at this stage. Both a person's preferences and his or her needs for extraordinary support must be considered, as well as practical issues, such as the resources that are available to support the individual. Completion of Component 3 should result in an unambiguous, individualized plan that specifies the settings and activities in which a person is likely to engage during a typical week, the types and intensities of support that will be provided, and who or what will be providing the support (Thompson et al., 2004a).

Component 4 requires that the planning team monitor the implementation of the support plan and the individual's quality of life. Is the individual plan being implemented as intended? Do the goals remain relevant to the individual? As can be seen in Figure 2.3, the assessment and planning process is cyclical in that if Component 4 reveals that the plan is not working or that the person's support needs or preferences have changed, the team is directed back to the first two components in order to generate a new plan that is responsive to the individual's changing needs.

Perhaps the most significant implication of implementing a supports-based approach is that it will help fuel the shift from a focus on "programs" and "group services" to developing individualized supports. Focusing on support needs as opposed to deficits is more useful for teachers and human service workers who are interested in solving the problem of how to include individuals in activities in settings such as schools and competitive work environments.

Glancing Back to Look Ahead

A consideration of the historical development and use of the term *developmental disabilities*, as well as current trends in terminology, definitions, and conceptual models offers important insights into contemporary approaches to educational and human services. However, attention to the history of people with developmental disabilities and the service system that has been developed to support them can be even more important. That history is, by and large, the history of the fields of mental retardation and autism.

The History of Intellectual and Related Developmental Disabilities

"What is past is prologue." These words, spoken in Act 2 of Shakespeare's *The Tempest* by Antonio, the brother of Prospero, the usurped Duke of Milan, are often quoted to justify the study of history. The quote suggests that unless we know about and understand what has happened in the past, we cannot adequately meet the future. In the area of intellectual and developmental disabilities it is particularly important that we understand the evolution of the field. Specifically, we need to know how people with intellectual and related developmental disabilities have been viewed and treated in the past. Although an exhaustive history of intellectual and related developmental disabilities is not possible or appropriate in the context of this chapter, a brief overview seems warranted, with a particular focus on 19th- and 20th-century developments that contributed to the emergence of special education as a field.

Intellectual and Related Developmental Disabilities in Prehistory and Antiquity

It should not come as a surprise that intellectual and developmental disabilities have existed throughout the history of humankind, although evidence of their presence in prehistory is limited, by necessity, to archaeological and fossil records. Nonetheless, such artifacts show clearly that disability was part of the human condition among *Homo sapiens*, as well as earlier hominids, including Neanderthals (Berkson, 2004); there is no reason to suspect that intellectual and developmental disabilities were not part of the lives of early beings. Records from more recent, though still ancient, eras provide evidence of conditions associated with intellectual and developmental disabilities. The Assyro-Babylonian culture (2800 BCE* recorded instances of birth malformations; the Code of Hammurabi (3700 BCE) mentions epilepsy, and disability is frequently mentioned in Judeo-Christian and Islamic scriptures and texts (Berkson, 2004; Scheerenberger, 1983). More specific to intellectual disability, Berkson described two early reports of people with Down syndrome, one in Saxon, England, and the second in Austria, from as early as 2300 BCE.

Of more relevance than simply the presence of people with disabilities in antiquity are the attitudes toward children and people with disabilities during that time. The truth is, the way in which people with disabilities were perceived and treated varied widely. Evidence from Egyptian writings (4500 BCE) suggests that some people with disabilities were incorporated into their communities and, in fact, were valued members of society (Berkson, 2004). In other cases, people with disabilities were shunned, segregated, or worse. The Old and New Testaments and the Quran all identify populations of people with disabilities who were kept outside of city walls. In general, most religious traditions reveal some negative attitudes about disability, often attributing the disability to sin or viewing it as the punishment meted out by an omnipotent being. However, these traditions also emphasize helping people who are poor, weak, or downtrodden, and thus advocate helping people with disabilities. This religious ethic played an important role in the emergence of disability services in the mid-1800s, as described subsequently. Echoing future eugenic efforts, the Greek city-states Sparta and Rome are frequently identified as practicing infanticide for newborns that were weak or disabled (Scheerenberger, 1983).

---

*BCE refers to "Before the Common Era," and can also be represented as *BP*, or "Before Present." In either case, 1950 is the date associated with the "present" or "common era" because standardizations pertaining to carbon dating techniques were put in place at that time, and thus 1950 became the default "present."

Intellectual and Related Developmental Disabilities From the Middle Ages to the 18th Century

The Middle Ages span roughly 500 to 1500 BCE, and while little is known about broad stretches of time during this era, with the spread of literacy, particularly among religious clerics and the newly emerging European universities (which began to be formed during the 11th and 12th centuries), a written history of disability began to emerge, incorporating religious, medical, and historical documents as well as literature. The medical literature is replete with descriptions of medical conditions associated with intellectual and developmental disabilities (e.g., meningitis, hydrocephalus, and epilepsy). The Swiss physician Paracelsus (1493–1541) linked cretinism with intellectual impairments (Scheerenberger, 1979). Significantly, a distinction began to emerge between people with intellectual disabilities and people with mental illnesses.

The causes of intellectual and developmental disabilities during the Middle Ages were thought to be many and diverse, again focusing on religious or superstitious reasons, from punishment for sin to madness due to lunar cycles. Perhaps the most common representation of people with intellectual disabilities at the time was the so-called village idiot or simpleton. In reviewing the role of people with intellectual disabilities in the late Middle Ages, Scheerenberger (1979) noted:

> In most rural areas, mentally retarded [sic] persons probably toiled long hours alongside their parents, responding to the demands of their lord or nobleman to wage combat at varying intervals. Many undoubtedly died at an early age due to disease or pestilence. The village idiot was common, and mentally retarded [sic] persons of mild temperament were allowed to roam the countryside unmolested, receiving aid and comfort from neighbors. Thus, on an individual basis, they became somewhat of a public responsibility. (p. 33)

However, not all people with intellectual and developmental disabilities were treated with what essentially could be classified as benign neglect. Scheerenberger (1979; 1983) reported that throughout the Middle Ages people with disabilities were paraded about and displayed as objects of ridicule and amusement for others, particularly the elite. In Hamburg, Germany, people with intellectual disabilities were confined to the "Idiot's Cage," located in a tower on the city wall.

As poor laws began to be passed (in Europe in the 1500s), people with intellectual and developmental disabilities were served, although these laws provided only the most basic of services, primarily shelter and food. In 1377 Bethlem Hospital was converted to an asylum for people with mental illness. The English word *bedlam* derives from *Bethlem*, largely because while the hospital housed people with mental illness and intellectual disabilities, it did little else for them. It became fashionable for the elite of society to visit Bethlem Hospital, much as we might visit a zoo, to view the inmates (Scheerenberger, 1983).

Whatever the condition in which people with intellectual and developmental disabilities lived, one universal was applicable. They were viewed as uneducable. Perhaps the person most emblematic of the thinking of this era, particularly during the latter days of the 18th century, was the famous French physician Phillipe Pinel (1745–1826). Pinel, today regarded as the father of psychiatry, was a distinguished physician who was spurred to study mental illness after the suicide of a close friend who had developed a mental disorder. As a physician at the Bicetre, a French asylum for people who were considered insane, he studied mental illness up close. Later he became chief physician for another asylum, the Salpêtrière, in Paris. Many advances in the treatment of people with mental illness and intellectual disabilities are at-tributed to Pinel, including the removal of restraints (chains, straitjackets) and the abandonment of techniques like bleeding and leeches in favor of more humane, ob-servational treatment, the moral treatment method. Pinel's accomplishments were mainly in the area of management of institutional services. He believed that people with intellectual disabilities, who were often still institutionalized with people with mental illnesses, were incurable and uneducable (Blatt, 1987). It was left to historical figures of the 19th century to change this belief, and it was then that the core history of special education began.

Intellectual and Related Developmental Disabilities in the 19th and 20th Centuries

Foundations of Special Education

Several events in the first half of the 19th century shaped the history of special edu-cation and warrant mentioning, but none more than the discovery of a young boy by hunters in the woods near Aveyron, a small village in south-central France, on January 8, 1800 (Lane, 1976). At the time it was thought that the boy, later named Victor, had grown up in the wild for most, if not all, of his 11 or 12 years, thus earn-ing him the epithet "the Wild Boy of Aveyron." Victor was examined by Pinel and declared an "incurable idiot." Eventually, though, Victor came under the care of Jean Marc Gaspard Itard (1775–1838), who was chief physician at the National Institution for Deaf-Mutes in Paris and who had been a student of Pinel's. Itard did not share Pinel's conviction of Victor's uneducability, and so he began a systematic program of intervention to teach Victor to speak, recognize words and letters, and care for himself. Itard's efforts earned him the title "Father of Special Education," and he is recognized as contributing a number of firsts to the field, among them the first individualized education program and the first recognition of the importance of an enriched environment in remediating deficits. Ironically, Itard considered his work with Victor a failure, because his pupil was never able to acquire speech, but in reality Victor did gain a number of social, academic, and independent-living skills. Itard's pioneering work paved the way for future efforts to educate people with intellectual and developmental disabilities (Lane, 1976).

Another one of Pinel's students at the Salpêtrière, Jean Etienne Esquirol, left his own mark on the field by providing the first systematic differentiation between mental illness (dementia) and intellectual disability (amentia). Writing in *Mental Maladies* (Esquirol, 1838/1965), considered to be the first modern text on mental disorders, Esquirol proposed that

> idiocy is not a disease but a condition in which the intellectual facilities are never manifested or have never been developed sufficiently to enable the idiot to acquire such amount of knowledge as persons of his own age reared in similar circumstances are capable of receiving. (p. 26)

At that time the term *idiot* was used to refer to people with intellectual dis-ability and was not yet a pejorative term. Although Esquirol's distinction between mental illness and intellectual disability was an important marker in the history of disabilities, it was perhaps his adherence to Pinel's view of the ineducability of people with intellectual disability that had the most direct effect on the field of special education. "Idiots are what they must remain for the rest of their lives," wrote Esquirol (1838/1965, p. 26).

Pinel, Esquirol, and, indeed, almost all physicians and psychiatrists believed the ineducability of people with an intellectual disability to be a fact, and they viewed Itard as misguided, at best. In 1837, though, the second man to legitimately lay claim to the title "Father of Special Education" was Edouard Seguin (1812–1880), who began the work that would eventually change the view about the educability of people with intellectual disability and prove Itard correct and his teacher, Pinel, and classmate, Esquirol, wrong. That year, an aging Jean Marc Gaspard Itard was approached by the director of a children's hospital about the possibility of taking on another pupil, like Victor, for "his program of demutization and language instruction" (Lane, 1976, p. 261). Itard, whose health was failing and who, by that time, was experiencing considerable pain, declined to accept the opportunity, citing his poor health. He, did, however, suggest that a young doctor who had previously studied under him—Seguin—might be willing to work with the boy.

Seguin was persuaded to take up the cause, though he was not entirely convinced that Itard was correct. He was, however, sympathetic to Itard's devotion to people like Victor, who were so poorly treated. Therefore he began working with the child, adapting, adopting, and refining his mentor's methods, and continuing the work even after Itard's death one year later. Upon the commencement of his work, Seguin consulted Esquirol, who in essence told him that he was wasting his time. Apparently, Seguin was influenced more by Itard's humanistic approach than by the status quo (as represented by the opinion of the influential Esquirol). Instead of dissuading Seguin from embarking on this line of work, Esquirol's comment "goaded Seguin to prove the more experienced and famous doctor wrong" (Blatt, 1987, p. 35). And, unlike Itard's experience with Victor, eighteen months after he began, Seguin's pupil was much improved, having acquired the ability to speak, write, and count (Blatt, 1987).

Burton Blatt (1987), whose name will reappear shortly in this chapter as a key figure in the history of intellectual and developmental disabilities, observed that when Seguin presented his findings to Esquirol, a fairly predictable thing happened. Instead of changing his opinion about the educability of people with intellectual disability, Esquirol concluded that Seguin's pupil must not *really* have had an intellectual impairment.

> To this day, when an individual who has been diagnosed as mentally retarded [*sic*] later performs normally, most clinicians remain wont to conclude ex post facto that the original diagnosis was erroneous, that the person must have been pseudo-mentally retarded, because mental retardation is incurable and irremediable. That resistance to the idea of mental retardation as a *functional designation* [italics added] is reflected in the evolving definitions of this condition, which, until recent years, precluded any possibility for cure, remediation, or amelioration. (p. 35)

It is important to note, in light of the current era's movement toward a functional definition, that the conceptualization of intellectual and developmental disabilities as a function of the relationship between a person's competencies and the environment is *not* a 21st-century notion.

Returning to Seguin, even though Esquirol did not endorse Seguin's findings, he did see potential in Seguin's methods. Seguin had come to believe that "idiocy" was not the result of deficiency or malformation of the brain or nervous system, but simply an arrest of mental development that occurred either before, at, or after birth, for a variety of reasons. Moreover, in Seguin's view, the disability could be overcome by appropriate treatment (i.e., education), and he believed individuals had the potential to become productive members of society. Seguin (1866/1971) advocated for a pedagogy based on careful physiological training of all the senses.

This notion of intellectual disability resulting from arrested mental development that could be overcome by training of the senses did, apparently, resonate with Esquirol, who assisted Seguin in furthering his experimental work at the Hospice des Incurables Bicetre. By 1844, the Paris Academy of Sciences was proclaiming that, with his method, Seguin "had definitely solved the problem of idiot education" (Blatt, 1987, p. 36). Even if Seguin's work did not solve the problem of special education per se, it did launch the field of special education for persons with developmental disabilities.

In America, the news of Seguin's achievements soon spread. In 1842 Horace Mann, the father of the American public school education system, visited Seguin at the Bicetre and wrote about Seguin's work. In 1847 a young physician named Hervey B. Wilbur read about Seguin and Bicetre, and was motivated to emulate Seguin's program in the United States. In July 1848 Wilbur founded the first school for students with intellectual disability in his home in Barre, Massachusetts. Later that same year, Samuel Gridley Howe (1801–1876) opened the first public school (Wilbur's school was private) for students with intellectual disability in a wing of the Perkins School for the Blind in Boston, (Scheerenberger, 1983).

Howe deserves mention for more than just establishing the first public school for students with intellectual disability. In fact, he was one of the most important early advocates for disability services in the United States. A native Bostonian whose paternal grandfather participated in the Boston Tea Party and whose maternal uncle was in charge of fortifying the defenses at the Battle of Bunker Hill, Howe trained as a physician. Upon graduation, however, he became connected with other youth influenced by Lord Byron, and he joined in the battle for Greek independence from Turkey. After achieving hero stature for his actions in Greece, Howe returned to Boston seeking his next conquest.

In 1831 Howe accepted the challenge of establishing a school for the blind in Boston, and following a trip to Paris in 1832 to visit European schools, he established the New England Asylum for the Blind, which later became the Perkins Institute for the Blind. His most famous patient was Laura Bridgman, the "first Helen Keller," who was deaf and blind because she had contracted scarlet fever at an early age. Under Howe's tutelage she became the first person with deaf/blindness to learn language.

Samuel Gridley Howe's social activism took him down many paths before his death in 1876. He married fellow antislavery activist Julia Ward, who later penned the "Battle Hymn of the Republic," and he was part of a small band of progressive Bostonians who funded John Brown's bloody crusade against slavery, which brought the country to the brink of civil war. In addition to founding the first public school for students with intellectual disability, he served on a commission to examine the "problem of idiocy in the Commonwealth," and in 1848 he published an influential report, *On the Causes of Idiocy*, in which he described the causes of intellectual disability (Scheerenberger, 1983).

Howe's (1848/1972) book illustrates how intellectual disability was perceived and understood in his era.

> We regarded idiocy as a disease of society, as an outward sign of an inward malady. It appeared to us certain that the existence of so many idiots in every generation *must* be the consequence of some violation of the *natural laws;* that where there was so much suffering there must have been sin. (p. 4)

It was, however, impious to attribute to the Creator the glaring imperfection of "so many creatures in the human shape, but without the light of human reason"

(p. 4). Instead, idiocy resulted, Howe proposed, from "the chastisements sent by a loving Father to bring back his children to obedience to his beneficent laws" (p. 5).

One cannot, however, acknowledge the contribution of Samuel Gridley Howe as a social reformer without also recognizing his contemporary Dorothea Dix (1802–1887). Dix was one of the most influential pre–Civil War social reformers, tirelessly campaigning for prison reform, reform of the almshouses, the poor system, and orphanages, and services for people with mental disabilities. Dix and Howe, and other social reformers of the era in the United States, reversed the existing neglect and paved the way for the implementation of innovative practices, like those pioneered by Itard and Seguin, to take hold in America. Dix's efforts ultimately led to the establishment of 32 mental hospitals, including 15 schools for the "feebleminded," and a school for the blind. She visited hundreds of almshouses, jails, institutions, and orphanages. She drove herself, literally, to exhaustion and, in the end, was admitted to and died in the State Lunatic Asylum in Trenton, New Jersey, ironically one of the institutions she had founded (Scheerenberger, 1983).

Growth of Institutions and Eugenics

In many ways, the post–Civil War era in the history of intellectual and developmental disabilities in the United States is a history of places (Waverly, Massachusetts; Syracuse, New York; Faribault, Minnesota; Vineland, New Jersey; Elwyn, Pennsylvania) and the institutions that were built in those places (Massachusetts School for the Feeble-Minded; New York State Idiot Asylum at Syracuse; Minnesota Institute for Defectives; Vineland Training School; Pennsylvania Training School for Idiotic and Feeble-Minded Children, respectively). These institutions were established in response to the advocacy of people like Dorothea Dix, and to a large degree they were modeled after Seguin's groundbreaking efforts. In fact, in 1850 Seguin immigrated to the United States (changing the spelling of his first name from Edouard to Edward) and briefly worked with Howe at the Perkins School. He then moved to Syracuse, where Hervey Wilbur had become the superintendent of the New York institution, and, in 1856, was appointed educational director of the Massachusetts School for Idiotic and Feeble-Minded Children in Waverly, where Walter Fernald was superintendent. And just as important, Seguin's text describing his method was translated into English and published in the United States in 1866 as *Idiocy and Its Treatment by the Physiological Method*. The text soon became the bible by which each new institution designed its programming.

Heeding Dix's call, state after state opened residential schools for "idiots" or "the feebleminded." Pinel's early delineations between mental illness and intellectual disabilities had become standard practice, and these institutions were distinct from state asylums for people with mental illness or, even, people with epilepsy. At least, they were as distinct as the classification systems of the era would allow them to be. No measures of intellectual capacity were available, and exactly who would benefit from these educative attempts was still a point of contention. Certainly, by today's standards, the students who were given the opportunity to attend the schools established at Barre and Perkins were students with more capabilities. Part of the problem was a lack of clarity in defining the multitude of terms used to describe intellectual disability. The terms *idiot, imbecile, defective,* and *feebleminded* were all used in varying ways to refer to people with intellectual impairments. The most widely used definition at the turn of the 20th century was one that had been forwarded by Scottish physician William W. Ireland (1832–1909). Ireland was superintendent of the Scottish National Institute for the Training of Imbecile Children at Larbert, Stirlingshire, Scotland, and in 1877 he published what most deem to be the first systematic textbook on intellectual disability, *On Idiocy and*

Imbecility. In this text Ireland defined *idiocy* as "mental deficiency, or extreme stupidity, depending upon malnutrition or disease of the nervous centers, occurring either before birth or before the evolution of mental faculties in childhood. The word imbecility is generally used to denote a less decided degree of mental incapacity" (Ireland, 1877, p. 1).

Hervey Wilbur (1877) also tried his hand at defining intellectual disability, proposing four types of "idiocy": (a) simulative idiocy, which referred to people who might have an intellectual impairment but who could function fairly typically; (b) higher-grade idiocy, referring to those folks who, with some special training, could continue to school and function fairly typically; (c) lower-grade idiocy, referring to people who could be taught some functional skills and eventually live in the community with support; and (d) the so-called incurables, who were not considered appropriate for educative attempts.

The first "schools" for students with intellectual disabilities in the United States, then, were the early manifestations of these institutions. Soon, however, the generosity of the states in their response to social reforms became overwhelmed by the demand. Schools that had begun in the houses of concerned physicians, like Wilbur, or ministers, like the Reverend Olin Garrison, who founded the Vineland Training School, soon outgrew their modest facilities and moved to architecturally grand structures built by the state or, in the case of private institutions like Vineland, through the largesse of civic-minded benefactors. Even these larger buildings, however, were soon insufficient, as were additional institutions. For example, Pennsylvania opened a second institution in 1897 in Polk, situated in the western portion of the state, to relieve the burden on the Pennsylvania Training School for Idiotic and Feeble-Minded Children in Elwyn. Built originally to accommodate 1,000 people (in and of itself indicative of the fact that the small, schoollike institutions were disappearing), by 1906 it housed 1,200 and by 1913 it had grown to 2,300 residents, with a waiting list of 500 people (Wolfensberger, 1975).

With this growth, these institutions began to lose their educative purposes and instead took on the characteristics of medical facilities. Names changed from "school" to "hospital." Living units were called wards. Residents became patients (Wolfensberger, 1975). These facilities were run almost exclusively by physicians (e.g., Dr. Walter Fernald at Waverly, Dr. A. C. Rogers in Faribault, Dr. Isaac Kerlin at Elwyn). In 1876 these superintendents formed an organization, the Association of Medical Officers of American Institutions for Idiotic and Feeble-Minded Persons, which was the precursor to the current American Association on Mental Retardation. Edward Seguin was elected the first president. With the rising numbers of institutions and growing institutional populations came concomitant growth in positions to care for people with intellectual disabilities. Additionally, associations for professionals in the field emerged, and with the associations came annual meetings as well as published journals and books reporting research and practice. A profession that was distinct from other disciplines of medicine or psychology began to emerge.

By the first decade of the 20th century, the transformation of institutions from educational to medical facilities was all but complete. What had also changed were attitudes toward disability, or at least the reasons for acting on behalf of people with disabilities. Reformers like Dix and Howe viewed action on behalf of the less well-off as society's obligation, largely compelled by moral and religious beliefs. Both perceptions about people with disabilities and the reasons for action changed with (a) the emergence of a "system" of services for people with disabilities funded primarily by government, (b) the growth of related professional disciplines, including social welfare and psychology, and (c) the increasing medicalization of the field.

Some of these changes were the inevitable consequences of the structure of institutions. With institutions taking on the aura of hospitals, people who lived there logically became viewed as sick, and the conditions they experienced became categorized as diseases. The routines of workers were governed by hospitallike procedures. Wolfensberger (1975) noted that case records became medical charts and hospital routines, like admission procedures, prevailed. Staff came and went on hospital shifts. Treatments became medically oriented. The sheer growth in numbers of "patients" exacerbated these tendencies and minimized individualized, or even educative, care. Both because of the growing population in institutions and because people were no longer being admitted for habilitation purposes, residents who had more capabilities were put to work to "earn their keep." Older and more capable residents watched over and cared for younger and more disabled residents, scrubbed and mopped the floors, staffed the cafeterias, and even served as nannies for the administrators. Their free labor became too valuable to the superintendents, and instead of preparing them for community living, the existing system transformed the more capable residents into an invisible workforce (Trent, 1994).

Meanwhile, outside the confines of the huge structures that warehoused more and more people, the attitudes of the public toward people with disabilities had begun to change. The Industrial Revolution resulted in the migration of large numbers of rural Americans to urban core areas. Immigration to the United States, particularly from Eastern European countries, increased dramatically, thus exacerbating the conditions in the urban areas. Slums and tenements grew and became social problems. The enthusiasm of professionals in the fields of social work, medicine, and psychology and the belief that their actions could solve the "social problem" of disability began to wane along with the 19th century. Enthusiasm and optimism were replaced by frustration and pessimism. Disenchantment with earlier ideals set in. Soon, it was the people with disabilities themselves, along with the immigrants and the poor, who became the social problem. Efforts that might previously have been educative or habilitative became efforts toward social control.

Perhaps the darkest period for people with intellectual and developmental disabilities since the Middle Ages occurred during the first two decades of the 20th century, which ironically was an era of progressivism and social reform in America. Of most importance was the emergence of the pseudoscience of eugenics and its application to social services. *Eugenics*, a term coined by Charles Darwin's half-cousin, Francis Galton, referred to the supposed study of hereditary improvement of the human race by controlled or selective breeding. By the first decade of the 20th century the most rabid eugenicists were from America. The agendas of men like Charles B. Davenport, Paul Popenoe, and Harry H. Laughlin focused on limiting immigration and curtailing opportunities for people who were seen as "poor genetic stock" to reproduce. Their tools were segregation and sterilization (Gould, 1981; Scheerenberger, 1983).

It was, in some ways, a "perfect storm" that resulted in gross human and civil rights violations of America's most vulnerable citizens. Contributing to the mix were a great array of issues: the massive overcrowding of institutions; the growing sense of futility with regard to solving what seemed to some to be unsolvable social problems; the notion that science, in the form of genetics and eugenics, would provide answers to these social problems; unresolved class and racial issues that had been festering in America since the Civil War; and the growing concern that the "unfit" were flooding the genetic stock of the population with poor genes. People with intellectual and developmental disabilities began to be portrayed as menaces to society, and they were blamed for social problems like prostitution, poverty, crime, alcoholism, and moral decline. Stories about "degenerate" families who propagated generations of "unfit" people reinforced these beliefs, including 1877's *The Jukes* (Dugdale, 1877) and Vineland Training School psychologist Henry Herbert Goddard's 1912 book, *The Kallikak Family* (see Gould, 1981, and Smith, 1985, for critiques of this flawed and infamous study). The general public heard its president and Spanish American war hero Theodore Roosevelt bombastically talk about "race suicide," the idea that the purported watering down of the genetic stock, caused by "unfit" people reproducing at higher rates than the "fit" people, would eventually lead to America's demise.

Thus the already burgeoning institutional population exploded in the first decade of the 1900s as the first line of defense against these dire consequences. Institutionalization was no longer about education or habilitation; rather it was about segregation and control. Still, no systematic means existed by which to determine level of impairment, but that mattered little when the predominant function of institutions was to "protect" society (Kühl, 1994; Scheerenberger, 1983; Trent, 1994).

In 1904 Martin Barr, who was chief physician at the Pennsylvania institution in Elwyn, published what is viewed as the first modern American text on intellectual disability, *Mental Defectives: Their History, Treatment, and Training*. In it he laments the lack of a generally agreed-upon, systematic classification of intellectual disability. That same year, French psychologist Alfred Binet began work on a measure of intelligence intended to assist schools in France in identifying children who needed additional help, which, when published the next year (1905), would become the tool that would eventually be used to classify and diagnose mental impairment. Ironically, instead of providing a means to more accurately diagnose intellectual disabilities and thus narrow the population, the introduction of the Binet-Simon test to a North American audience by Vineland psychologist Goddard actually expanded the range of people labeled as feebleminded (Scheerenberger, 1983).

Goddard learned about the Binet-Simon test on a trip to Europe in 1908, and upon his return, he had it translated and began to use it at the Vineland Training School. It was such a success that he then implemented it with schoolchildren in the New York City public schools. At a meeting in 1910 of the American Association for the Study of the Feebleminded (the new name for the superintendents group), Goddard suggested a classification scheme for intellectual disability that included the levels of "idiot," "imbecile," and "moron." The last, which Goddard defined as people testing with a mental age between 8 and 12 years, was a new category. The term *moron* was derived by Goddard from the Greek word for fool. Soon immigrants, the poor, and, particularly, women of child-bearing age who were viewed as morally loose, were being classified as morons and sentenced to institutions (Scheerenberger, 1983; Trent, 1994).

Eventually, though, eugenicists, including many institution superintendents, saw segregation as insufficient to address the problem (as, of course, they defined the problem). In 1907 Indiana became the first state in the nation to legalize involuntary sterilization, providing for the "prevention of the procreation of 'confirmed criminals, idiots, imbeciles, and rapists'" (Landman, 1932, p. 55). By the late 1920s, more than half the states had laws similar to Indiana's. Propelled by the 1927 U.S. Supreme Court ruling (*Buck v. Bell*) that involuntary sterilization was constitutional, an estimated 50,000 people who were labeled as feebleminded were involuntarily sterilized. Meanwhile, under pressure from eugenicists and the general public, the U.S. Immigration Office added "imbeciles and feeble-minded persons" to its exclusion list (Gould, 1981; Kühl, 1994; Scheerenberger, 1983; Trent, 1994).

In Germany, people with disabilities were among those targeted for eugenic purposes by the Nazi regime. Working from model legislation for sterilization that was developed in the United States, in 1934 the German government subjected more than 32,000 Germans labeled as feebleminded to involuntary sterilization. In the winter of 1939 Hitler began a program of extermination that, by its end 20 months later, had resulted in the murder of 80,000 Germans with disabilities (Kühl, 1994; Trent, 1994).

The horrors of the Holocaust during World War II ended the enthusiasm for eugenics and forced sterilization, but the institutions did not go away. Writing in 2000, Gunnar Dybwad, a pioneer in advocacy for people with intellectual disabilities and a former executive director of what was then called the National Association for Retarded Children, observed:

> Thus I have a vivid memory of conditions that to most readers will only be historical facts which they have read. I saw first hand the dismal conditions in the overcrowded institutions which originated in good intentions, to give asylum and protection and quickly became warehouses to offer society protection from the so-called "mental defectives." I saw in the late 1930s, overcrowding with all its dire consequences was the major problem. In Letchworth Village, considered to be one of the "better" New York State institutions at that time, I found a dormitory with one hundred beds and 125 children in those beds. (p. 431)

The catalyst for change came in several forms. In the economic (and population) boom of the post-WWII 1950s, a parent movement emerged that rejected the notion that their children would be better off in an institution. Again, Dybwad (2000) observed:

> I also vividly remember something else that rose out of the post-war period. Parents of children with intellectual limitations spontaneously came together and organized locally throughout the country, what in 1950, became the National Association for Retarded Children (NARC). The strong voice of this new group was soon heard in Congress and state houses across the nation, effectively challenging the prevailing perceptions of "mental deficiency," and demanding radical changes to meet the needs of the children especially in education. (p. 257)

Advances in science and medicine changed the way disability was perceived and greatly increased the life span of people with disabilities. Influenced by the large number of veterans disabled in the Second World War, which spurred an emphasis on rehabilitation and training, and successes in developing vaccines for diseases like polio, which gave hope for greater cures of disabling conditions, the earlier stereotypes of disability were replaced with more humane, though still in many ways debilitating, stereotypes. People with disabilities were viewed as objects to be fixed, cured, rehabilitated, and at the same time pitied. They were now seen as "victims" worthy of charity, thus precipitating the emergence of the poster child as a fund-raising tool (Shapiro, 1993; Trent, 1994).

This stereotype viewed people with intellectual disabilities as "holy innocents" (e.g., special messengers, children of God) and thus incapable of sin and not responsible for their own actions. Although no longer feared and blamed for all social ills, people with intellectual disability were perceived as children, to be protected, pitied, and cared for (Wolfensberger, 1972). A community-based service system began to emerge, funded by programs initiated by President John F. Kennedy, whose sister, Rosemary, had an intellectual impairment. Legislation was passed providing equal protection under the law for people with intellectual and developmental disabilities (Scheerenberger, 1987; Trent, 1994).

In 1966 Burton Blatt and Fred Kaplan published the photo-essay *Christmas in Purgatory*, which brought to light the horrific conditions in institutions. Blatt and photographer Kaplan gained access to the back wards, through the locked doors, of institutions and surreptitiously photographed the conditions that they saw there.

The stark black-and-white images of people with intellectual and developmental disabilities—huddled in masses, standing naked in sterile rooms furnished only with benches, or rows and rows of beds and children on them—were accompanied by quotes from literature and philosophy depicting human suffering and injustice. *Christmas in Purgatory* began: "There is a hell on earth, and in America there is a special inferno. We were visitors there during Christmas, 1965" (p. i).

Blatt's efforts had been preceded, and to some degree instigated by, visits in the fall of 1965 by Senator Robert Kennedy, whose disgust with the conditions he'd witnessed brought the attention of policy makers to the plight of people who were institutionalized. In 1972 investigative reporter Geraldo Rivera brought his television cameras to the Willowbrook State School in Massachusetts, and, again, the images broadcast brought to light the dismal conditions in which many people lived. The deinstitutionalization movement gained its momentum, and over the last quarter of the 20th century, institutions closed and people moved into the community (Lakin & Bruininks, 1983; Scheerenberger, 1987).

The introduction of the normalization principle to a North American audience in a 1972 text edited by Wolf Wolfensberger and featuring chapters by Bengt Nirje and Robert Perske provided further impetus. In 1969 Bengt Nirje explained that the normalization principle had its basis in "Scandinavian experiences from the field" and emerged, in essence, from a Swedish law on mental retardation that was passed in 1968. In its original conceptualization, the normalization principle provided guidance for creating services that "let the mentally retarded [*sic*] obtain an existence as close to the normal as possible." Nirje stated: "As I see it, the normalization principle means making available to the mentally retarded [*sic*] patterns and conditions of everyday life which are as close as possible to the norms and patterns of the mainstream of society" (1969, p. 36). He identified the following eight "facets and implications" of the normalization principle: the opportunity to (a) experience a normal rhythm of a day; (b) experience a normal routine of life; (c) follow a normal rhythm of the year; (d) experience normal developmental sequences of the life cycle; (e) express preferences and make choices; (f) live in a sexual world; (g) have access to normal economic standards; and (h) live in the same type of housing as ordinary citizens.

Further, the independent-living movement, with activists like Ed Roberts and Judith Heumann, began to show that people with disabilities could live independently in their communities if they had access to adequate supports (Shapiro, 1993). In 1967 the institutional census (the number of people living in institutions for people with intellectual and developmental disabilities) was 194,650 (Wagner, 2002). In 2000, 47,374 people lived in state-funded institutions while 263,359 people with intellectual and developmental disabilities lived in state-supported community-based settings with 1 to 6 people (Braddock, Hemp, Rizzolo, Parish, & Pomeranz, 2002). On the basis of data trends, Braddock and colleagues have projected that by 2025, all state-funded institutions for people with intellectual and developmental disabilities will be closed.

At the forefront of the post-WWII reforms, however, were parents. Two "celebrities" of the era, both of whom had children with disabilities, broke down some of the barriers to parenting children with intellectual disabilities. In 1950, Pearl Buck, the Nobel laureate in literature, published a small book, *The Child Who Never Grew*, which described her life with her daughter, Carol, who was born with phenylketonuria (PKU). Similarly, in 1953, Dale Evans published a book titled *Angel Unaware*, which chronicled the first two years of the life of her daughter, Robin, who was born to Evans and her husband, Roy Rogers, and who had Down syndrome. To a large degree, these two publications made it much more acceptable (i.e., took away the sense of shame) to be the parent of a child with a disability (Scheerenberger, 1987; Trent, 1994).

In 1950 a number of self-organized parent groups from across the country held a meeting in Minneapolis and formed an organization called the National Association of Parents and Friends of Mentally Retarded Children. The impact of that movement on the field during the last half of the 20th century cannot be underestimated. The association, known more readily as the National Association for Retarded Children, or NARC, and now referred to as simply The Arc, waged ongoing battles to change public opinion about and awareness of mental retardation. The Arc benefited from the visionary leadership of executive director Gunnar Dybwad, his wife, Rosemary, and parents like Elizabeth Boggs. The organization facilitated the establishment of a range of services in local communities. Moreover, it was instrumental in securing the passage of the Education for All Handicapped Children Act (P.L. 94-142) in 1975 (arguably the most important outcome of the parent movement) (Dybwad, 2000; Turnbull & Turnbull, 1995).

The Modern Era of Special Education

Although the momentum for the modern era of special education for students with intellectual and developmental disabilities really originated in the 1950s and 1960s with the rise of the parent movement, developments before that time laid some of the groundwork. In 1900 the New York City public school system hired Elizabeth Farrell to teach an ungraded class for students who had what we might now call learning disabilities and physical disabilities, opening what in essence was the first special education class in the United States. Farrell went on to cofound the Council for Exceptional Children (CEC) (Scheerenberger, 1983).

In 1904 administrators at the Vineland Training School started bringing public school teachers from all around the country to the Vineland campus for the summer to learn strategies for working with "the feebleminded." In the 1920s and 1930s, early pioneers in special education like Grace Fernald, Samuel Orton, and Samuel Kirk developed strategies for teaching reading and math to learners with disabilities. According to Scheerenberger (1983), by 1930 sixteen states had legislation that mandated, to one degree or another, public special education. For the most part these were separate, often ungraded classes, where students with diverse disabilities were grouped together. After its introduction by Goddard, the Binet scale became widely used for diagnosis, particularly following the release of a version by Lewis Terman (renamed, then, the Stanford-Binet because Terman was a professor at Stanford University).

Unfortunately, in the 1920s and 1930s, as the special education field began to emerge and develop strategies and methods, it became increasingly common to exclude students who had intellectual and developmental disabilities, particularly students who had IQ scores below 50 (Scheerenberger, 1983). The attitude that students who were less capable needed simply to be institutionalized carried into the public school sector. So although the field was growing, students with intellectual and developmental disabilities were, by and large, shut out.

A Maturing Field

A multidisciplinary field of developmental disabilities emerged during the 20th century, with contributions from many disciplines, including psychology, law, and education. Definitional advancements, the introduction of the concept of autism, and civil rights lawsuits were noteworthy.

In his widely used 1937 text, *Mental Deficiency (Amentia)*, A. F. Tredgold defined *mental deficiency*, a term that used to mean mental retardation, as a "state of incomplete mental development of such kind and degree that the individual is incapable of adapting himself to the normal environment of his fellows in such a way to maintain existence independently of supervision, control, or external support" (Tredgold, 1937, p. 1). Tredgold's definition was to some degree simply a refinement of previous frameworks. The attitudes and beliefs that once again excluded students with intellectual and developmental disabilities from public schools can be seen in statements like "incapable of adapting . . . to normal environments." Indeed, Tredgold's subtitle to the text, which replicates Esquirol's classification of idiocy with "amentia," reflects how little definitions had changed since the 18th century. *Amentia* is derived from Latin and means "without (*a*) mind (*ment*)."

In 1941, however, Edgar Doll, one of Henry Goddard's assistants at Vineland, who by then was director of research, proposed a definitional system that for the first time introduced the element of adaptive behavior in the definition of intellectual disability. Doll's (1941) definition had several criteria for mental deficiency: (a) social incompetence, (b) due to mental subnormality, (c) which has been developmentally arrested and (d) which obtains at maturity. In this definition we see the first version of modern definitions in the emphasis on mental capacity (as measured by IQ scores), social incompetence or adaptive behavior, and the emergence of the disability during the developmental period. Doll also developed the first widely used adaptive behavior measure, the Vineland Social Maturity Scale (Doll, 1935).

In 1961 the American Association on Mental Deficiency, as the association founded by institution superintendents was by then named, released a definition that became the standard for years to come. Heber (1961) defined mental retardation as referring "to subaverage general intellectual functioning which originates during the developmental period and is associated with impairment in adaptive behavior" (p. 1). Revisions by Grossman and colleagues in 1973, 1977, and 1983 essentially tweaked Heber's definition, defining mental retardation as referring "to significantly subaverage general intellectual functioning existing concurrently with deficits in adaptive behavior, and manifested during the developmental period" (Grossman, 1983, p. 1).

In the 1940s two pioneers in autism, Leo Kanner and Hans Asperger, each independently described children with "autistic" symptoms (Sigman & Capps, 1997). For much of the 1950s and 1960s any emphasis on autism viewed it as a psychological disorder and, inaccurately, attributed the condition to parenting styles or strategies, particularly those of mothers. This focus was championed most notably by Bruno Bettelheim, but in the 1960s Bettelheim's work was challenged by researchers like Rimland and Schopler (see Laidler, 2004). Still, focus on the educational needs and strategies was limited, even once P.L. 94-142 was passed. Autism was not added as a categorical area covered under the Individuals with Disabilities Education Act (IDEA) until the 1990 reauthorization.

Advances in definition, however, were not propelling advances in the education of students with intellectual and developmental disabilities, who remained largely unserved by the public school system. It was the advocacy of the parent movement, as it came of age in the 1960s and 1970s, and court action that finally advanced special education opportunities for students with intellectual and developmental disabilities. Parent advocacy had established the right to education for students with intellectual and developmental disabilities in several states by the end of the 1960s; indeed, by 1966 there was a federal Bureau for the Education of the Handicapped. In the early 1970s, though, two major legal rulings paved the way for the passage of P.L. 94-142. *Pennsylvania Association for Retarded Children v. Commonwealth of Pennsylvania* in 1971 and *Mills v. Board of Education of the District of Columbia* in 1972 firmly established the right to an education for all students with disabilities as a matter of case law.

The History of Developmental Disabilities, Post 1975

The chapters that follow, in large part, are a record of the history of disabilities since 1975. From separate settings to inclusive practices, from watered-down curricula to access to general education curricula, and from dependency to self-determination, the last 30 years have seen dramatic progress in the field. What will the next 30 years bring? The answer will depend on the degree of passion, creativity, and commitment that advocates, professionals, researchers, and others in the field bring to their work. In the words of Peter Drucker, "The best way to predict the future is to create it" (BrainyQuote, 2005, ¶ 1).

Glossary

Autism Spectrum Disorder (ASD)—Term that refers to a broad definition of autism, including the classical form of the disorder as well as closely related disabilities that share many of the core characteristics. ASD includes the following diagnoses and classifications: (1) pervasive developmental disorder—not otherwise specified (PDD-NOS), which refers to a collection of features that resemble autism but may not be as severe or extensive; (2) Rett's syndrome, which affects girls and is a genetic disorder with hard neurological signs, including seizures, that become more apparent with age; (3) Asperger's syndrome, which refers to individuals with autistic characteristics but relatively intact language abilities; and (4) childhood disintegrative disorder, which refers to children whose development appears normal for the first few years but then regresses, with loss of speech and other skills, until the characteristics of autism become conspicuous. Although the classical form of autism can be readily distinguished from other forms of ASD, the terms *autism* and *ASD* are often used interchangeably (from ERIC Clearinghouse on Disabilities and Gifted Education, 1999, Autism and Autism Spectrum Disorder, ¶ 2, http://ericec.org/digests/e583.html).

Deinstitutionalization—Public policies focusing on returning individuals with disabilities who are living in institutions to home communities; includes preventing admissions to institutions through developing community service options.

Developmental disabilities—Severe, lifelong disabilities attributable to mental and/or physical impairments manifested before age 22. Developmental disabilities result in substantial limitations in three or more areas of major life activities: capacity for independent living, economic self-sufficiency, learning, mobility, receptive and expressive language, self-care, self-direction (Administration on Developmental Disabilities, 2005, What is Developmental Disability?, ¶ 1; http://www.acf.hhs.gov/programs/add/Factsheet.html).

Eugenics—A social philosophy that advocates the improvement of human hereditary traits through social intervention. The goals have variously been to create more-intelligent people, save society's resources, lessen human suffering, and reduce health problems. Proposed means of achieving these goals most commonly include birth control, selective breeding, and genetic engineering (from Wikipedia, n.d., Eugenics, ¶ 1, http://en.wikipedia.org/wiki/Eugenics).

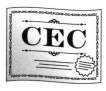

Knowledge and Skills for Entry-Level Special Education Teachers of Students With Developmental Disabilities Standards Addressed in This Chapter

Principle 1: Foundations

DD1K1   Definitions and issues related to the identification of individuals with developmental disabilities.

DD1K3   Historical foundations and classic studies of developmental disabilities.

DD1K4   Trends and practices in the field of developmental disabilities.

Principle 4: Instructional Strategies

DD4S2   Relate levels of support to the needs of the individual.

Principle 8: Assessment

DD8K1   Specialized terminology used in the assessment of individuals with developmental disabilities.

DD8K4   Laws and policies regarding referral and placement procedures for individuals with developmental disabilities.

Web Site Resources

Administration on Developmental Disabilities
http://www.acf.hhs.gov/programs/add/

American Association on Intellectual and Developmental Disabilities
http://www.aamr.org/

Autism Society of America
http://www.autism-society.org/

Disability History Museum
http://www.disabilitymuseum.org/

Image Archive on the American Eugenics Movement
http://www.eugenicsarchive.org/eugenics/

TASH
http://www.tash.org/

The Arc
http://www.thearc.org/

References

Administration on Developmental Disabilities. (2005). *ADD fact sheet.* Retrieved July 5, 2005, from http://www.acf.hhs.gov/programs/add/Factsheet.html

Algozzine, B., Ysseldyke, J. E., & McGue, M. (1995). Differentiating low-achieving students: Thoughts on setting the record straight. *Learning Disabilities Research and Practice, 10,* 140–144.

Barr, M. (1904). *Mental defectives: Their history, treatment, and training.* Philadelphia: Blakiston's & Son.

Berkson, G. (2004). Intellectual and physical disabilities in prehistory and early civilization. *Mental Retardation, 42,* 195–208.

Blatt, B. (1987). *The conquest of mental retardation.* Austin, TX: PRO-ED.

Blatt, B., & Kaplan, F. (1966). *Christmas in purgatory.* New York: Allyn & Bacon.

Braddock, D., Hemp, R., Parish, S., & Westrich, J. (1998). *The state of the states in developmental disabilities.* Washington, DC: American Association on Mental Retardation.

Braddock, D., Hemp, R., Rizzolo, M. C., Parish, S., & Pomeranz, A. (2002). *The state of the states in developmental disabilities.* Washington, DC: American Association on Mental Retardation.

BrainyQuote (2005). *Peter Drucker quotes.* Retrieved July 5, 2005, from http://www.brainyquote.com/quotes/quotes/p/peterfdru131600.html

Breen, P., & Richman, G. (1979). Evolution of the developmental disabilities concept. In R. Wiegerink & J. W. Pelosi (Eds.), *Developmental disabilities: The DD movement* (pp. 3–6). Baltimore: Brookes.

Buck, P. (1950). *The child who never grew.* New York: John Day.

Butterworth, J., Hagner, D., Heikkinen, B., Faris, S., DeMello, S., & McDonough, K. (1993). *Whole life planning: A guide for organizers and facilitators.* Boston: Children's Hospital, Institute for Community Inclusion.

Carroll, J. B. (2005). The three-stratum theory of cognitive abilities. In D. P. Flanagan & P. L. Harrison (Eds.), *Contemporary intellectual assessment: Theories, tests, and issues* (2nd ed., pp. 69–76). New York: Guilford.

Conyers, C., Martin, T. L., Martin, G. L., & Yu, D. (2002). The 1983 AAMR Manual, the 1992 AAMR Manual, or the Developmental Disabilities Act: Which do researchers use? *Education and Training in Mental Retardation and Developmental Disabilities, 37,* 310–316.

Developmental Disabilities Assistance and Bill of Rights Act of 2000, 42 U.S.C. §§ 15001–15002.

Doll, E. A. (1935). A genetic scale of social maturity. *American Journal of Orthopsychiatry, 5,* 180–188.

Doll, E. A. (1941). The essentials of an inclusive concept of mental deficiency. *American Journal of Mental Deficiency, 46,* 214–219.

Dugdale, R. L. (1877). *The Jukes: A study of crime, pauperism, disease, and heredity.* New York: G. P. Putman and Sons.

Dybwad, G. (2000). Mental retardation in the 21st century. In M. L. Wehmeyer & J. Patton (Eds.), *Mental retardation in the 21st century* (pp. 431–433). Austin, TX: PRO-ED.

Esquirol, J. E. (1965). *Mental maladies: A treatise on insanity* (E. Hunt, Trans.). New York: Hafner (Original trans. 1845; original work published 1838).

Garnett, R. (2003). *In opposition to a name change.* Retrieved July 5, 2005, from http://www.aamr. org/Reading_Room/con_memo.shtml

Goddard, H. H. (1912). *The Kallikak family: A study in the heredity of feeble-mindedness.* New York: Macmillan.

Gould, S. J. (1981). *The mismeasure of man.* New York: Norton.

Greenspan, S. (1979). Social intelligence in the retarded. In N. R. Ellis (Ed.), *Handbook of mental deficiency: Psychological theory and research* (2nd ed., pp. 483–532). Hillsdale, NJ: Erlbaum.

Greenspan, S., & Driscoll, J. (1997). The role of intelligence in a broad model of personal competence. In D. P. Flanagan, J. L. Genshaft, & P. L. Harrison (Eds.), *Contemporary intellectual assessment: Theories, tests, and issues* (pp. 131–150). New York: Guilford.

Greenspan, S., & Granfield, J. M. (1992). Reconsidering the construct of mental retardation: Implications of a model of social competence. *American Journal on Mental Retardation, 96,* 442–453.

Grossman, H. J. (Ed.). (1973). *Manual on terminology in mental retardation* (1973 rev.). Washington, DC: American Association on Mental Deficiency.

Grossman, H. J. (Ed.). (1977). *Manual on terminology in mental retardation* (1977 rev.). Washington, DC: American Association on Mental Deficiency.

Grossman, H. J. (Ed.). (1983). *Classification in mental retardation* (1983 rev.). Washington, DC: American Association on Mental Deficiency.

Heber, R. A. (1961). A manual on terminology and classification in mental retardation (2nd ed.). *Monograph Supplement to the American Journal of Mental Deficiency.* Washington, DC: American Association on Mental Deficiency.

Howe, S. G. (1972). *The causes of idiocy* (Reprint ed.). New York: Arno Press. (Original work published 1848).

Ireland, W. W. (1877). *On idiocy and imbecility.* London: J & A Churchill.

Kavale, K. A., Fuchs, D., & Scruggs, T. E. (1994). Setting the record straight on learning disability and low achievement: Implications for policymaking. *Learning Disabilities Research and Practice, 9,* 70–77.

Kühl, S. (1994). *The Nazi connection: Eugenics, American racism, and German national socialism.* New York: Oxford University Press.

Laidler, J. R. (2004). *The "Refrigerator Mother" hypothesis of autism.* Retrieved September 15, 2005, from http://www.autism-watch.org/causes/rm.shtml

Lakin, K. C., & Bruininks, R. H. (1983). Contemporary services to handicapped children and youth. In R. H. Bruininks & K. C. Lakin (Eds.), *Living and learning in the least restrictive environment* (pp. 3–22). Baltimore: Brookes.

Landman, J. H. (1932). *Human sterilization: The history of the sexual sterilization movement.* New York: Macmillan.

Lane, H. (1976). *The wild boy of Aveyron.* Cambridge, MA: Harvard University Press.

Larson, S. A., Lakin, K. C., Anderson, L., Kwak, N., Lee, J. H., & Anderson, D. (2001). Prevalence of mental retardation and developmental disabilities: Estimates from the 1994/1995 national health interview survey disability supplements. *American Journal of Mental Retardation, 106,* 231–252.

Luckasson, R., Borthwick-Duffy, S., Buntinx, W. H. E., Coulter, D. L., Craig, E. M., Reeve, A., et al. (2002). *Mental retardation: Definition, classification, and systems of supports* (10th ed.). Washington, DC: American Association on Mental Retardation.

Luckasson, R., Coulter, D. L., Polloway, E. A., Reiss, S., Schalock, R. L., Snell, M. E., et al. (1992). *Mental retardation: Definition, classification, and systems of supports* (9th ed.). Washington, DC: American Association on Mental Retardation.

Minnesota State Planning Agency. (1963). *Respite care: A supportive and preventive service for families. Issues related to* Welsch v. Levine. Policy analysis series No. 20. St. Paul, MN: Author.

Mount, B., & Zwernik, K. (1988). *It's never too early, it's never too late: A booklet about personal futures planning.* Mears Park Centre, MN: Metropolitan Council.

National Service Inclusion Project. (2005). *Watch your language!* Retrieved September 15, 2005, from http://www.serviceandinclusion.org/web.php?page=language

National Task Force on the Definition of Developmental Disabilities. (1977). *Final report* (Contract No. HEW– 05-77-5005). Cambridge, MA: Abt Associates.

Nirje, B. (1969). The normalization principle and its human management implications. In R. Kugel & W. Wolfensberger (Eds.), *Changing patterns in residential services for the mentally retarded* (pp. 181–194). Washington, DC: President's Committee on Mental Retardation.

Rogers, D. E. (1953). *Angel unaware.* Westwood, NJ: Revell.

Schalock, R. L. (2003). Mental retardation: A condition characterized by significant limitations in practical, conceptual, and social skills. In H. N. Switzky & S. Greenspan (Eds.), *What is mental retardation: Ideas for an evolving disability* (pp. 246–261). Washington, DC: American Association on Mental Retardation.

Scheerenberger, R. C. (1979). *Public residential services for the mentally retarded.* Minneapolis: University of Minnesota, Department of Educational Psychology.

Scheerenberger, R. C. (1983). *A history of mental retardation.* Baltimore: Brookes.

Scheerenberger, R. C. (1987). *A history of mental retardation: A quarter century of progress.* Baltimore: Brookes.

Seguin, E. (1971). *Idiocy: And its treatment by the physiological method.* New York: Augustus M. Kelley. (Original work published 1866).

Shapiro, J. P. (1993). *No pity: People with disabilities forging a new civil rights movement.* New York: Random House.

Sigman, M., & Capps, L. (1997). *Children with autism: A developmental perspective.* Cambridge, MA: Harvard University Press.

Smith, J. D. (1985). *Minds made feeble: The myth and legacy of the Kallikaks.* Rockville, MD: Aspen.

Sternberg, R. J. (2005). The triarchic theory of successful intelligence. In D. P. Flanagan & P. L. Harrison (Eds.), *Contemporary intellectual assessment: Theories, tests, and issues* (2nd ed., pp. 103–119). New York: Guilford.

Stodden, R. A. (2002). Division completes name change process. *MRDD Express, 12*(3), 8.

Stodden, R. A. (2004). *Who we are.* Retrieved July 5, 2005, from http://www.dddcec.org/secondarypages/self_identity.htm

Summers, J. A. (1986). *The right to grow up: An introduction to adults with developmental disabilities.* Baltimore: Brookes.

Thompson, J. R., Bryant, B., Campbell, E. M., Craig, E. M., Hughes, C., Rothholz, D. A., et al. (2004a). *Supports Intensity Scale (SIS).* Washington, DC: American Association on Mental Retardation.

Thompson, J. R., Bryant, B., Campbell, E. M., Craig, E. M., Hughes, C., Rothholz, D. A., et al. (2004b). *The Supports Intensity Scale (SIS): Standardization and users manual.* Washington, DC: American Association on Mental Retardation.

Thompson, J. R., McGrew, K. S., & Bruininks, R. H. (1999). Adaptive and maladaptive behavior: Functional and structural characteristics. In R. Schalock (Ed.), *Adaptive behavior and its measurement: Implications for the field of mental retardation* (pp. 15–42). Washington, DC: American Association on Mental Retardation.

Thompson, J. R., McGrew, K. S., & Bruininks, R. H. (2002). Pieces of the puzzle: Measuring the personal competence and support needs of persons with intellectual disabilities. *Peabody Journal of Education, 77*(2), 23–39.

Tredgold, A. F. (1937). *Mental deficiency (Amentia).* New York: William Wood and Company.

Trent, J. W. (1994). *Inventing the feeble mind: A history of mental retardation in the United States.* Berkeley: University of California Press.

Turnbull, A. P., & Turnbull, H. R. (1995). *Families, professionals, and exceptionality: A special partnership* (3rd ed.). Upper Saddle River, NJ: Merrill.

Wagner, B. (2002). The narrowing role of institutions. In R. L. Schalock, P. C. Baker, & M. D. Croser (Eds.), *Embarking on a new century: Mental retardation at the end of the 20th century* (pp. 101–110). Washington, DC: American Association on Mental Retardation.

Widaman, K. F., & McGrew, K. S. (1996). The structure of adaptive behavior. In J. W. Jacobson & J. A. Mulick (Eds.), *Manual of diagnosis and professional practice in mental retardation* (pp. 97–110). Washington, DC: American Psychological Association.

Wilbur, H. (1877). The classification of idiocy. In *Proceedings of the association of medical officers of American institutions for idiotic and feebleminded persons*, pp. 29–35.

Wolfensberger, W. (1972). *The principle of normalization in human services.* Toronto: National Institute on Mental Retardation.

Wolfensberger, W. (1975). *The origin and nature of our institutional models.* Syracuse, NY: Human Policy Press.

World Health Organization. (2001). *International classification of functioning, disability, and health (ICF).* Geneva: Author.

Ysseldyke, J. E., Algozzine, B., & Thurlow, M. L. (2000). *Critical issues in special education* (3rd ed.). Boston: Houghton Mifflin.

3

Power and Epiphany

Reflections on the Personal and Cultural Meanings of Developmental Disabilities in the 21st Century

J. David Smith

Summary

This chapter presents a philosophical and personal perspective on developmental disabilities. It focuses on stories of disability, how they have been told, and who the tellers have been. It examines the impact of these stories on the lives of the people who have been made the characters of the stories and also asks if it is not time that the characters of the stories be allowed to choose their own narratives and tell their own tales as people with freedom and equality. Indeed, as Bellamy hoped for a truly new time in human history, let us hope that we are living at the beginning of a century that is more than ever the age of the people, including people with developmental disabilities.

Learning Outcomes

After reading this chapter, you should be able to:

- Discuss the impact of both negative and positive stories on the lives of people with disabilities.

- Discuss the hopes and disappointments that have characterized visions of the past for the future of people with disabilities in society.

- Discuss some of the implications of advances in genetic science for people with developmental disabilities.

- Use examples of the positive impact of people with disabilities on the lives of other people.

- Use the story of Montgomery's wishes as a means of illustrating the stigma associated with the term *mental retardation.*

- Define typological thinking and its implications for the field of developmental disabilities.

- Discuss the issue of equality for people with developmental disabilities.

Introduction

Burton Blatt (1987), one of the greatest special educators and advocates of the last century, wrote about the importance of stories to the lives of people with disabilities, to those who care deeply about them, and to those who seek to serve them most effectively. As Blatt noted, "Every story can enhance a life or destroy it. Every story can lift us or depress us. Stories sustain if not make a person's world. And thus, the story teller holds a certain power and responsibility" (p. 141).

Blatt's (1987) observations are certainly true regarding stories of people with disabilities. Heroic stories like that of Helen Keller and Annie Sullivan have encouraged generations of families and professionals. Often, however, the nature and intent of disability stories have been negative and hurtful. This chapter will illustrate how stories about people with developmental disabilities have been constructed and used in powerfully abusive ways. It is also intended, however, to portray the important place that people with disabilities occupy in our individual and social lives. It is an effort to convey the need for caution, clarity, and compassion in the ways that we understand and appreciate each other so that we can transcend differences and reach an ever-renewing epiphany of our shared humanity.

Looking Backward

The Pledge of Allegiance was written in 1892 by Francis Bellamy for the quadricentennial celebration of the arrival of Columbus in America. Bellamy wrote it at the request of a committee of state school superintendents under the auspices of the National Education Association (NEA). The pledge was intended to become part of a flag ceremony that would bring greater attention to the importance of the American flag to schoolchildren who were hardly a generation removed from the Civil War. Bellamy's original draft of the pledge was written as follows: "I pledge allegiance to my Flag and to the Republic for which it stands, one nation, indivisible, with liberty, justice and equality for all" (Baer, 1992, p. 11). After further consideration, however, Bellamy deleted the word *equality*. Through his conversations with members of the NEA committee, he arrived at the conclusion that the word would be unacceptable to the state superintendents. He understood that an American society that in 1892 still denied the vote and most other civil rights to women and to African Americans would not pledge itself to social equality.

In the decades that followed, the wording of the Pledge of Allegiance was twice amended. In 1924 the words *my Flag* were changed to *the Flag of the United States of America*. In 1954, *under God* was added. With this latter change, the pledge became, in a sense, both a patriotic oath and a public prayer. It is important to note, however, that more than a century after its adoption, the pledge is still devoid of a commitment to equality (Baer, 1992).

Francis Bellamy's cousin, Edward Bellamy, was a journalist and novelist. He was also a strident voice for social reform during the late 1800s. His most influential work was *Looking Backward*. Originally published in 1888, this book was a best seller in the years following its release. It was also very influential among America's intellectuals at the time. In 1935, the philosopher and educator John Dewey ranked *Looking Backward* as one of the most important books published during the preceding 50 years.

Bellamy's novel is the story of Julian West, who falls into a trancelike sleep in 1887 and is awakened in the year 2000. West awakens to a United States that has no wars, no political parties, and no poverty. Each citizen is an equal shareholder in the social enterprise of the country, and all citizens have equitable and sufficient incomes. Throughout the book, Bellamy emphasizes that West finds in the year 2000 a society that is deeply committed to the equality of all of its citizens.

Julian West's guide in the new millennium world to which he has awakened is a physician, Dr. Leete. One of the doctor's most profound revelations is that people with disabilities are considered equal members of society. When West expresses surprise that charity has become so prevalent in the United States, an intriguing exchange takes place between the two men:

> "Charity!" repeated Dr. Leete. "Did you suppose that we consider the incapable class we are talking of objects of charity?"
>
> "Why naturally," I said, "inasmuch as they are incapable of self-support." But here the doctor took me up quickly.
>
> "Who are capable of self-support?" he demanded. "There is no such thing in a civilized society as self-support. . . . From the moment that men begin to live together, and constitute even the rudest sort of society, self-support becomes impossible. As men grow more civilized . . . a complex mutual dependence becomes the universal rule." (Bellamy, 1888, p. 178)

Dr. Leete continues his description of the fundamental equality of all people in his society, regardless of their individual needs or limitations in independence and productivity. At this Julian asks, "How can they who produce nothing claim a share of the product as a right?" Dr. Leete answers that each generation in a society inherits most of what it knows and possesses. He asks West:

> How did you come to be possessors of this knowledge and this machinery which represents nine parts to the one contributed by yourself in value to your product? You inherited it, did you not? And were not these others, these unfortunate and crippled brothers whom you cast out, joint inheritors, co-heirs with you? What I do not understand is, setting aside all considerations of justice or brotherly feeling toward the crippled and defective, how the workers of your day could have had any heart for their work, knowing that their children, or grandchildren, if unfortunate, would be deprived of the comforts and even necessities of life? (p. 181)

Edward Bellamy's vision of the year 2000 did not, of course, prove to be prophetic. In many ways the importance of individual achievement and personal competence has become more emphatic than Bellamy could have envisioned during his time. The possibility of scientific and medical enhancement of what are considered the most desirable human traits is also challenging the definition of human difference and complicating our understanding of the meaning of individuality. Looking forward from our own perspective, we see even more complex meanings being assigned to concepts such as normality and health.

Looking Forward

Remarkable developments in molecular biology and genetic engineering are reported in the popular press almost daily. These advances in scientific knowledge and medical technology will almost certainly change the course of human history. The eradication of what are considered diseases, disorders, and defects may become a reality before the end of the present century. A critical question in this pursuit, however, is how diseases, disorders, and defects are defined. Are disabilities, in this context, defects, or are they human differences? Is disability a condition to be prevented in all circumstances, or is it part of the spectrum of human variation? Depending upon the answer, what does this say about the status of people with disabilities in a democracy? What does it say about their fundamental equality as people?

The danger that people with disabilities will be further devalued as genetic intervention techniques increase is illustrated by James Watson (Bhattacharya, 2003), winner of the Nobel Prize and co-discoverer of DNA. Watson was also the first director of the Human Genome Project, and in his capacity as leader of the effort to map and sequence the genetic makeup of human beings, he advocated careful consideration of the ethical, legal, and social implications of the project. Yet, in a 1993 article titled "Looking Forward," Watson dismissed the value of people with severe disabilities when he spoke of the decisions faced by "parents when they learn that their prospective child carries a gene that would block its opportunity for a meaningful life" (p. 314). In the same article, he speaks disapprovingly of parents who do not undergo genetic testing: "So we must also face up to the ethical and practical dilemma, facing these individuals who could have undergone genetic diagnosis, but who for one reason or another declined the opportunity and later gave birth to children who must face up to lives of hopeless inequality" (p. 315). More recently, Watson spoke to the German Congress of Molecular Medicine (Lee, 1998) and condemned the eugenic philosophy that resulted in the atrocities of the Nazi era. Then, in an amazing contradiction, he advocated what might be termed *parental eugenics*. He asserted that the truly relevant question for most families is whether an obvious good will come from having a child with a major handicap. From this perspective, Watson said, "seeing the bright side of being handicapped is like praising the virtues of extreme poverty" (p. 16).

Watson's assertions stand in stark contrast to the questions he raised a few years earlier when he served as the director of the Human Genome Project:

> The question now faces us, as we work out the details of the human genetic message, as to how we are going to deal with these differences between individuals. In the past, at the time of the Eugenics movement in the United States and in England, and during the reign of racist thoughts in Nazi Germany, there was very little genetic knowledge. Most decisions then were made without solid genetic evidence. There were many prejudices, but almost no real human genetics. Now we have to face the fact that we soon will have real facts, and how are we going to respond to them? Who is going to take care of those people who are disabled by the genes they have inherited? How can we compensate them for the fact that many individuals are not as equal genetically as other people? I don't think we know the answers, and that is why we are here for this meeting. (Watson, 1992, p. 27)

An even greater contrast to this statement is evident in Watson's more recent comments concerning people with developmental disabilities and the possibility of a new eugenics movement:

> We must not fall into the trap of being against everything Hitler was for. It was in no way evil for Hitler to regard mental disease as a scourge on society. . . . Because of Hitler's use of the term Master Race, we should not feel the need to say that we never want to use genetics to make humans more capable than they are today. . . . Common sense tells us that if scientists find ways to greatly improve human capabilities, there will be no stopping the public from happily seizing them. (Watson, 1996, p. 15)

Watson has advocated eugenic measures to prevent even mild disabilities, and he argues that most learning problems are genetic in origin:

And what would be the consequences of isolating genes that give rise to the various forms of dyslexia, opening up the possibility that women will take antenatal tests to see if their prospective child is likely to have a bad reading disorder? Is it not conceivable that such tests would lead to our devoting less resources to the currently reading-handicapped children whom now we accept as an inevitable feature of human life?" (Watson, 1996, p. 14)

If you are really stupid, I would call that a disease. The lower 10 percent who really have difficulty, even in elementary school, what's the cause of it? A lot of people would like to say, "Well, poverty, things like that." It probably isn't. So I'd get rid of that, to help the lower 10 percent. (Bhattacharya, 2003, p. 1)

In *Backdoor to Eugenics* (1990), Troy Duster argued that eugenics is alive and well in our society, but in a more subtle manifestation. While it is still presented as an economic and social issue, eugenics is also presented as a matter of parental responsibility or irresponsibility. Although less overt, eugenics in its new form may have an even more powerful impact on the lives of people with disabilities.

The eugenicists of the 19th and 20th centuries looked to evolutionary theory and Mendelian genetics for moral guidelines. They believed that evolutionary theory and science could provide models for social ethics. The failure of this approach was evidenced in the needless institutionalization of people with disabilities, who were deemed to be unfit for social struggle, and in the needless sterilization of people inaccurately assessed to be the carriers of defective genes. Ultimately the moral horrors of the Holocaust evolved from this philosophy. What moral truths will prevail in the current eugenic climate?

The Power of the Powerless

The uses and abuses of power are fundamental concerns of the human condition. Most of us are aware that the challenges of encouraging good and preventing destructive uses of power have been prevailing themes of history. These themes are also central to the most compelling issues we face today. Less obvious to many of us, however, is the question of how the actions and values associated with power may be influenced by people who are thought of as lacking in power themselves. Several stories are offered here as a way of providing insight into the transforming influence of children and adults with disabilities on the lives of others. They are profiles of the "power of the powerless."

In 1992 Floyd Cochran was the chief recruiter for the Aryan Nations. As the fifth-ranking leader of this self-proclaimed neo-Nazi, white supremacist organization, he was admired for his skill in dealing effectively with the public and a critical press. Cochran was very successful in using his media savvy and marketing skills to attract young people to the organization. He became the group's national spokesperson and was described by the Aryan Nations' chief, the Reverend Richard Butler, as being destined to be "the next Goebbels" (Hochschild, 1994, p. 29). In July of that year, however, Floyd Cochran was suddenly ordered off the Nations compound. Butler gave him five minutes to leave.

The rift in Cochran's relationship with the Aryan Nations had begun earlier that year. Shortly before he was to speak at the Hitler Youth Festival in Idaho, Cochran mentioned to the Nations security chief that he was running late because he had been talking to his wife on the telephone. He was very concerned about his four-year-old son, who was having surgery to correct a cleft palate. The chief's response to Cochran was, "He's a genetic defect. When we come to power, he'll have to be euthanized" (Hochschild, 1994, p. 34).

Cochran reported later that he was stunned by this remark. He had studied Ku Klux Klan and Nazi literature for almost 25 years. He had not recognized, nor had he faced until that moment, a sobering fact: The intolerance for difference that he had preached for decades applied to those he loved. When he voiced his concern about this issue, he was ordered to leave Aryan Nations property.

Eldridge Cleaver, who died in May 1998, was the author 30 years earlier of a startling book on race and racism, *Soul on Ice*. During the 1960s and 1970s he was known as a fiery and eloquent voice for the Black Power movement. After the publication of his book, most of which he wrote in prison, he became known as one of the infamous organizers of the Black Panther Party, along with Huey Newton and Bobby Seale.

While serving as minister of information for the Black Panthers, Cleaver was involved in a shoot-out with police officers in Oakland, California. He was wounded in the gun battle and arrested. He later jumped bail and fled to Algeria, where he headed the party's so-called international headquarters until there was a major split in the party in the early seventies, with Newton and Seale advocating nonviolence and Cleaver continuing to preach the use of violent methods. Cleaver returned to the United States in 1975. After a long legal battle, he was convicted of assault, placed on probation, and required to do public service.

In *Soul on Ice*, Cleaver spoke with rage about the experiences of African Americans and with angry disbelief about the oblivious attitudes of most white people regarding their own racism. It is rare to find a line in the book that does not scream with bitterness. And yet Cleaver closes one of his chapters with these words: "The price of hating other human beings is loving oneself less" (Cleaver, 1968, p. 29).

In the years following his return to the United States, Eldridge Cleaver was not visible as a public figure. He was no longer regarded as a symbol of race pride and race rage. Cleaver's historical identity, however, continued to be that of a figure associated with a separatist philosophy and a militant strategy toward race relations. Given that persona, it is interesting to consider some of the public remarks he made in the early 1990s about his youngest child, Riley, who was born with Down syndrome. Cleaver made these statements after he became an activist and advocate for children and adults with disabilities.

In a 1993 speech, Cleaver described his feelings when he learned that his expected son had proven positive for Down syndrome through an amniocentesis test. He spoke candidly of his lack of understanding of the implications of the test, and his insensitivity to the humanity and the needs of the child who was to come into his life. He admitted, in fact, that the only thing he did was to follow the lead of his child's mother in accepting and preparing for Riley.

With Riley's birth came the barrage of terms and decisions that often overwhelm parents of children with disabilities. Cleaver found that the birth of his son coincided with a period when he was questioning his own future. He was no longer a leader of the Black Panther Party, but he did see a role for himself in the civil rights movement in the 1990s. With the birth of a child with Down syndrome, however, Cleaver said,

> I no longer had to wonder what I was going to do, I was doing it. I had my hands full. . . . It was a struggle to understand and comprehend the situation itself, and it was a shock and a struggle to begin to realize that I was involved in a very hostile environment. I began to meet other parents. . . . We began to realize that we were up against the school system, and the legal system, and the medical system. (1993, p. 5)

When Cleaver described his feelings of being "up against" the various social systems of his culture as his son's advocate, his words were reminiscent of the anger he expressed concerning American racism in *Soul on Ice*. And yet, through his struggle to ensure that his son was not the victim of the same kind of prejudice and exclusion that he had raged against decades earlier, Cleaver encountered a new struggle within himself.

He described a situation with a child he encountered when he took his son to a regional center each day after school. He saw that Riley, who typically had an embrace for everyone as he arrived at the center, always had a special kiss for one little girl. Cleaver admitted that he was repulsed by the girl because she drooled saliva constantly. Soon the little girl showed that she was happy to see both Riley and his father each day. At first there were just handshakes for Cleaver; then one day she offered him a hug and a kiss.

> She stood up and came at me, and she was salivating, and I felt myself recoil. I looked at her face . . . and I realized that she was reaching out in faith. And I realized that it would be devastating to her if I . . . rejected her. . . . That confrontation with myself was really a godsend, and it changed me again, and I embraced the little girl, and I'm so glad that I did that, because at that moment of resolving that, it gave me an insight into the condition of humanity! (Cleaver, 1993, p. 7)

People with disabilities have the capacity to enrich our personal and social lives. The deficiency and defect models of disability have, however, often clouded our ability to see their value. More than a decade ago, Wolf Wolfensberger (1988) identified a number of strengths that people with mental retardation may bring to their relationships with others. Among these attributes are (a) spontaneity that is both natural and positive, (b) a tendency to respond to other people with generosity and warmth, (c) a tendency to be honest with others, (d) the capacity to elicit gentleness, patience, and tolerance from others, and (e) a tendency to trust other people.

Many of the disability "stories" that I have told in my writing and in lectures, and many of those that have been told to me, include references to the positive characteristics of people with disabilities. When I reflect on the importance of these children and adults and their qualities, I find I must say something that I have often lacked the courage to say directly and publicly: A disability can be a valuable human attribute. I am not alone in this observation, of course. My thinking in this regard has been shaped by the insights of Blatt, Wolfensberger, and others. I simply share with them the belief that people with disabilities can be powerful in the humanizing influence they have on others. I am glad that I have had friends with disabilities for most of my life.

In his 1988 book *The Power of the Powerless*, Christopher de Vinck describes the experience of growing up with his brother, Oliver, who was born with multiple and severe disabilities. In his work as an English teacher, de Vinck often told his students about his brother:

> One day, during my first year of teaching, I was trying to describe Oliver's lack of response, how he had been spoon-fed every morsel he ever ate, how he never spoke. A boy in the last row raised his hand and said, 'Oh, Mr. de Vinck. You mean he was a vegetable.' . . . Well, I guess you could call him a vegetable. I called him Oliver, my brother. You would have loved him. (de Vinck, 1988, p. 9)

Christopher de Vinck describes Oliver as the weakest human being he ever met. The irony, however, is that he also describes his brother as one of the most powerful human beings he ever knew. When de Vinck assesses the effort and hope that go into teaching and writing and parenting, he thinks of the impact Oliver had on his life: "Oliver could do absolutely nothing except breathe, sleep, eat and yet he was responsible for action, love, courage, and insight. . . . [This] explains to a great degree why I am the type of husband, father, writer, and teacher I have become" (de Vinck, 1988, p. 12).

There is most certainly a human ecology of power and compassion. People with disabilities have an important place in that ecological balance. The power of those who have traditionally been considered powerless may be important to our health as human beings and as cultural groups. A person with a disability may temper hateful and prejudicial attitudes. A person with mental retardation may soften a heart that has become hardened. A person with multiple and severe disabilities may have much to teach us about love.

Montgomery's Wishes

What follows is a story that I treasure. I offer it as an example of how my personal and professional perspectives on developmental disabilities have been shaped by people with these disabilities. In this case it was a lesson taught to me by a young person with Down syndrome.

His name was Montgomery. Of the many people I have known with Down syndrome, he was the most verbally talented. I first met him at a sheltered workshop. He worked there and I served on the board. Later I invited him to attend a weekend respite camp for people with disabilities, staffed by my undergraduate college students. He charmed and amazed them for three days with his jokes and stories.

Montgomery was well aware of the stigma associated with mental retardation. He also clearly understood the term *Down syndrome* and its implications for him. He seemed to be laboring constantly to convince everyone that he was not mentally retarded. From the beginning he made it evident that he did not need help or supervision during the camping weekend. Within a few hours of arriving, in fact, he asked that he be given a job as a counselor. He explained that he would help the college students assist and supervise the "handicapped people" at the camp. His request was granted, and he served as a counselor with distinction throughout the weekend.

Later in that college semester I asked Montgomery to visit one of my classes. He agreed to talk about his experiences as a child, an adolescent, and a young adult. He spoke candidly with the students about the impact of the stereotypes of mental retardation and Down syndrome on his life. He also spoke openly about living with a mother who would not, from his perspective, let him live an adult life. He felt she was treating him like a child even though he was 27 years old. His younger brother was living on his own and doing the things Montgomery wanted desperately to do as a young adult.

That evening after class I drove Montgomery home in my car. On the way he asked if we could stop at a 7-Eleven. In the parking lot he insisted that I wait in the car while he went in for a soft drink. After a few minutes he returned with a Coke for each of us. Soon I delivered him to his front door. His mother greeted us with a glance at her watch. She had apparently been listening for the car and made it obvious that she thought we were a bit late.

The next day Montgomery's mother called me at my office. She was disturbed. She had just discovered a pack of cigarettes and a *Playboy* magazine in his room. She demanded an explanation. I told her that I could only assume that Montgomery had bought these items at the 7-Eleven while I waited in the car. She was furious that I had allowed this to happen.

After several months, numerous apologies, and assurances that there would be no further 7-Eleven stops, Montgomery's mother agreed to allow him to speak with another of my classes. During the ride to the college Montgomery complained to me that his mother wasn't treating him as an adult. He again cited his younger brother as an example of the rights and privileges of adulthood that he longed for. His brother rode a motorcycle; Montgomery was not even allowed to ride as a passenger. He wanted more than anything to experience the feeling of freedom that he imagined riding a motorcycle would give him.

Montgomery talked with my students that evening about his recollections of being in special education classes as a child. He also talked about his experiences at the workshop. He answered each of their questions with care. His observations and reflections were, as always, provocative. My most vivid memory of that evening, however, is of the last question he answered. One of my students asked him what his wishes would be if he had three. Montgomery paused briefly and then replied that he wanted four wishes. "My four wishes," he said, "are to ride a motorcycle, smoke cigarettes, look at *Playboy* if I want to, and not be called retarded."

Along with my students, I was stunned by Montgomery's remarks. Regardless of the wisdom or political correctness of his choices, all of us were moved by his message of a yearning for freedom and a wish to escape the stigma of a term and a concept that were dominating forces in his life. Almost immediately I was lost in thoughts of race and racism, gender bias, and the many devastating stereotypes that pollute our social relationships.

Monty's wish to free himself from the label of mental retardation has been found to be shared widely by those to whom it has been assigned. In an important study and excellent review of the literature, Finlay and Lyons (2005) have found that escape from being labeled in this manner is a common quest for those who are asked for their own opinions of the diagnosis that has been assigned to them by others.

From Typology to Individuality

Typological thinking is the belief that complex individual variations can be reduced to underlying human types or essences. Gelb (1997) found that definitions of mental retardation, regardless of their particulars, are grounded in typological thought. The core of mental retardation as a field is the assumption that somehow there is a "mental retardation essence" that eclipses all of the differences that characterize people described by the term.

Even a brief glance at the panoply of etiologies associated with mental retardation illustrates the allure and power of typological thinking. In 1992 the American Association on Mental Retardation listed more than 350 conditions in which mental retardation occurs. This list of causes does not, of course, take into account the varying degrees of retardation or other disabilities associated with each of the etiologies. When those variables are considered, the universe of human conditions subsumed under the term *mental retardation* is staggering. The only glue that holds mental retardation together as a category is the typological notion that there is some underlying and shared essence to the characteristics and needs of the people identified by the term. Clearly, mental retardation encompasses a vast array of human conditions.

There must be alternatives for conceptualizing the needs of the people who are currently referred to as having mental retardation. It may be helpful to ask ourselves questions about what the abandonment of the term and the definitions associated with it could mean in the lives of individuals and families. We must also ask ourselves what abandoning "mental retardation" as a classification might mean for resource allocations and the provisions of services to people who need them. Finally, we must consider the impact of the deconstruction of retardation in terms of need versus stigma. In other words, is the aggregation of people into this diagnostic category truly necessary to meet their needs? Are services in the name of mental retardation justified, given the risk of stigma associated with the label? How can we provide for those who need assistance without diminishing their identity and integrity as individuals? These are questions that seem to be critical in thinking about the dismantling of the concept.

The time is overdue, however, for a fundamental questioning of the terms and practices associated with retardation. The millions of people with developmental disabilities who have been subsumed under that classification deserve a careful analysis of its impact on the manner in which they are regarded and treated. A thoughtful consideration of the feasibility of disassembling the aggregation that mental retardation has become may enhance our vision of what it should be.

Looking Forward to Equality

As the power of genetic science grows, so does the importance of ethical questions about the implications of that power for human diversity. The greatest challenge for people with developmental disabilities in this century may be that of having their lives understood within the contexts of the civic values of liberty, justice, *and* equality. This challenge, and hope, is embodied in the 1892 address that Francis Bellamy delivered during the unveiling of the Pledge of Allegiance (Baer, 1992). Perhaps borrowing a concept from his cousin Edward, Bellamy spoke of looking forward to a new age:

> We look forward. We are conscious we are in a period of transition. Ideas in education, in political economy, in social science are undergoing revisions. . . . The coming century promises to be more than ever the age of the people; an age that shall develop a greater care for the rights of the weak, and make a more solid provision for the development of each individual. (p. 41)

Glossary

Aryan Nations—A right-wing, anti-Semitic, white supremacist and anti-government organization based in the United States. It was founded in the 1970s by Richard Butler. From the 1970s until 2001 the headquarters of the Aryan Nations was a 20-acre compound at Hayden Lake, Idaho. There are a number of state chapters, loosely tied to the home organization.

Black Panther Party—A revolutionary black nationalist organization formed in the United States in the late 1960s. It grew to national prominence before falling apart as a result of internal problems and arrests by the Federal Bureau of Investigation. It was most famous for its Free Breakfast for Children program, and most infamous for its use of the term *pigs* to describe police officers and for once carrying guns onto the floor of the California Assembly.

Eugenics—A social philosophy and movement advocating the purported improvement of human hereditary qualities. The proposed means of improvement included birth control, institutionalization of so-called mental defectives, and sterilization of those who supposedly carried defective genes. Proponents of eugenics argued that this would lessen human suffering, prevent hereditary health problems, save society money, and create a more intelligent human race. Its scientific credibility tumbled in the 1930s when the Nazis incorporated the principles of eugenics into their racial policies. During the period after World War II both the public and the scientific community associated eugenics with Nazism. Critics have portrayed eugenics as a pseudoscience, and some argue that it constructs disability in completely negative terms. With advances in genetics, however, and the increased ability to locate and modify genes, some scientists and ethicists are speaking more aggressively of the importance of a new eugenics. Usually this is discussed in terms of voluntary measures on the part of prospective parents to prevent the conception or birth of children with genetic diseases or disabilities.

Human Genome Project—Completed in 2003, the Human Genome Project was a 13-year effort coordinated by the U.S. Department of Energy and the National Institutes of Health. The goals of the Human Genome Project were to

- identify all the genes in human DNA
- determine the sequences of the chemical base pairs that make up human DNA
- store this information in databases
- improve tools for data analysis
- transfer related technologies to the private sector, and
- address the ethical, legal, and social issues that may arise from the project.

The mapping and sequencing of the human genome is enabling rapid development of genetic diagnosis and intervention. Efforts to address associated ethical, social, and legal issues has lagged far behind the science and technology that the project produced. The issue of what *should* we do as opposed to what *can* we do is far from resolved.

Mendelian genetics—A set of tenets that underlies much of the genetic science developed by Gregor Mendel in the latter part of the 19th century. Mendel, an Austrian monk, was interested in understanding the varying characteristics in plants. He cultivated some 28,000 plants and observed the results of cross-fertilization in terms of the blossom color, leaf pattern, and stem characteristics produced. Before Mendel's work, the prevailing theory of heredity was that of blending, in which sperm and egg of parent organisms contained an "essence" of the parents. These were thought to somehow blend to form the offspring's characteristics. This theory did not explain, however, why a blue-eyed father and a brown-eyed mother did not produce a child with brownish-blue eyes. Mendel's work eventually led to an understanding of dominant and recessive genes and the patterns of inheritance that constitute the foundation of modern genetics.

Typological thinking—Related to the idea of an essence of a species. As described by Stephen Gelb, however, it portrays the view that there is an underlying essence of mental retardation that somehow binds all of the people described by the term into a common category. If this were accurate, then greater generalities could be found in how to teach, train, socialize, and treat people with mental retardation regardless of their levels of need or the cause of their disabilities. This, of course, is not the case. The needs and characteristics of people categorized by the term *mental retardation* are greatly variable, and meeting their needs requires very individualized strategies.

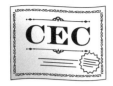

Knowledge and Skills for Entry-Level Special Education Teachers of Students With Developmental Disabilities Standards Addressed in This Chapter

Principle 1: Foundations

DD1K1   Definitions and issues related to the identification of individuals with developmental disabilities.

DD1K3   Historical foundations and classic studies of developmental disabilities.

DD1K4   Trends and practices in the field of developmental disabilities.

Web Site Resources

American Association on Mental Retardation
http://www.aamr.org/

CEC—Division on Developmental Disabilities
http://www.dddcec.org/

Christopher Oliver
http://www.columbia.edu/cu/augustine/arch/devinck.html

Eugenics
http://www.eugenicsarchive.org/

Human Genome Project, Ethics
http://www.ornl.gov/sci/techresources/Human_Genome/home.shtml

References

American Association on Mental Retardation. (1992). *Mental retardation: Definition, classification, and systems of supports* (9th ed.). Annapolis, MD: Author.

Baer, J. (1992). *The pledge of allegiance: A centennial history, 1892–1992.* Annapolis, MD: Free State Press.

Bellamy, E. (1888). *Looking backward.* New York: Ticknor.

Bhattacharya, S. (2003). Stupidity should be cured, says DNA discoverer. Retrieved May 16, 2005, from the NewScientist.com Web site at http://www.newscientist.com/article.ns?id=dn3451

Blatt, B. (1987). *The conquest of mental retardation.* Austin, TX: PRO-ED.

Cleaver, E. (1968). *Soul on ice.* New York: McGraw-Hill.

Cleaver, E. (1993, Fall). Eldridge Cleaver speaks out. *TASH Newsletter, 22,* 4–7.

de Vinck, C. (1988). *The power of the powerless.* New York: Doubleday.

Dewey, J. (1935). *Liberalism and social action.* New York: G. P. Putnam's Sons.

Duster, T. (1990). *Backdoor to eugenics.* New York: Routledge.

Finlay, W., & Lyons, E. (2005). Rejecting the label: A social constructionist analysis. *Mental Retardation, 43,* 120–134.

Gelb, S. (1997). The problem of typological thinking in mental retardation. *Mental Retardation, 35,* 448–457.

Hochschild, A. (1994, May/June). Changing colors. *Mother Jones,* 27–35. Retrieved May 16, 2005, from http://www.motherjones.com/news/update/1994/05/hochschild.html

Lee, T. (1998, March/April). You probably won't like James Watson's ideas about us. *Ragged Edge,* 16. Retrieved July 19, 2005, from http://www.raggededgemagazine.com/mar98/onedge03.htm

Smith, J. (2003). *In search of better angels: Stories of disability in the human family*. Thousand Oaks, CA: Corwin.

Watson, J. (1992). Genetic polymorphisim and the surrounding environment. *In Human Genome Project: Ethics*. Madrid: BBV.

Watson, J. (1993). Looking forward. *Gene, 135*, 309–315.

Watson, J. (1996). *1996 Annual report, president's essay*. Cold Spring Harbor, NY: Cold Spring Harbor Laboratory.

Watson, J. (2003). Stupidity should be cured, says DNA discoverer. *New Scientist, 18*. Retrieved July 19, 2005, from http://www.newscientist.com/article.ns?id=dn345

Wolfensberger, W. (1988). Common assets of mentally retarded people that are not commonly acknowledged. *Mental Retardation, 26*, 64–70.

SECTION 2

DEVELOPMENT AND CHARACTERISTICS OF LEARNERS

4

Developmental Disabilities

Definition, Description, and Directions

Tom E. C. Smith

Summary

This chapter presents information on the broad category called developmental disabilities, along with a rationale for more-generic terms to describe individuals with disabilities. Several trends support the idea of more-generic, functional classification groups. The movement toward generic services is one reason for more-functional disability groups. In addition to this movement, the current AAIDD definition, which focuses more on functional descriptions of individuals with mental retardation than did previous definitions, and the movement toward inclusion have supported the trend toward more-generic services based on functional needs of persons with disabilities. Further, the chapter provides a definition of *developmental disabilities* and some general characteristics of individuals who are classified as having developmental disabilities. Needs and services for individuals with developmental disabilities, as well as legislation that affects individuals with developmental disabilities, are discussed.

Learning Outcomes

After reading this chapter, you should be able to:

- Define developmental disabilities and describe the characteristics and needs of individuals with developmental disabilities.

- Describe the reasons why services for persons with disabilities have been moving to a noncategorical, more-functional service model.

- Discuss legislation that has affected services for persons with developmental disabilities.

Introduction

Whenever society decides that a particular group of individuals wants and/or deserves special recognition, for whatever reason, issues develop with respect to labels, definitions, characteristics, and how the needs of the group will be met. While individuals with disabilities have been designated as such a group and have received a wide variety of services for many years, the nature of how this group is identified and labeled and how services have been provided has been changing almost constantly as new developments, new laws, new court rulings, and new philosophies have become dominant.

One example of this change is how individuals with mental retardation have been identified and labeled. In the past, schools used such terms as *educable mentally retarded (EMR)* and *trainable mentally retarded (TMR)* to label this group, and they used older versions of the definition of mental retardation by the American Association on Intellectual and Developmental Disabilities (AAIDD) to identify students. Now the old *EMR* and *TMR* classifications have given way to *mild* and *moderate*, and the use of IQ as the only criterion for determining mental retardation has changed to using that as only one of several criteria in the process.

Another example of change is in the way individuals with disabilities are served in public schools. Historically, students with disabilities were served by categories in segregated settings, often in self-contained classrooms or special schools. Over the past 25 years, this practice has changed dramatically as inclusive educational programs have become the norm. As services have evolved, the orientation toward providing interventions to students with disabilities has moved away from a categorical approach to a more-generic, or generalized, approach in inclusive settings (Smith, Polloway, Patton, & Dowdy, 2008).

Many programs currently prepare teachers to work with students with various functional abilities, not children with certain clinical labels. Likewise, many states, such as Arkansas, Tennessee, and Alabama, no longer license teachers to work with children who are designated by a particular label. Rather, teacher licensure has also moved to a more-generic, functional model, resulting in teachers' being trained and licensed to teach children with mild disabilities or severe disabilities. Some states have even carried this approach further, to the point of preparing and licensing teachers to work with all children with learning problems in general education settings.

Definining Developmental Disabilities

One of the challenges facing professionals who provide services for individuals with disabilities has been to develop definitions of different groups that provide a focus for research, advocacy, and services. Addressing the needs of individuals with disabilities is much too broad without narrowing the population to different groups with more-specific similarities. The term *developmental disabilities* is used to provide such a focus.

Developmental disabilities is an umbrella category encompassing problems that begin affecting individuals during their development, generally defined as age 5 to the 22nd birthday. The category has a functional orientation, identifying individuals whose disabilities will create needs in specific activities. In 1999 Congress noted that there were between 3.2 and 4.5 million individuals in the United States with developmental disabilities (Developmental Disabilities Assistance and Bill of Rights Act of 2000). Unlike conditions that are short term in duration, developmental disabilities are *chronic* disabilities that will likely continue indefinitely. Therefore, the long-term impact of developmental disabilities is extensive. Individuals with developmental disabilities, because of the lifelong nature of their conditions, will likely require some level of supports and services throughout their lifetime.

The developmental disabilities category, unlike the category of mental retardation and other specific, clinical categories of disabilities, includes a wide variety of conditions that affect people's lives. The 2000 amendments to the Developmental Disabilities Assistance and Bill of Rights Act of 1987 defines developmental disabilities as a severe, chronic disability of an individual that

A. is attributable to a mental or physical impairment or combination of mental and physical impairments;

B. is manifested before the individual attains the age of 22;

C. is likely to continue indefinitely;

D. results in *substantial* functional limitations in three (3) or more of the following areas of major life activity

   i. self care;
   ii. receptive and expressive language;
   iii. learning;
   iv. mobility;
   v. self-direction;
   vi. capacity for independent living; and
   vii. economic self-sufficiency; and

E. reflects the individual's need for a combination and sequence of special, interdisciplinary, or generic services, supports, or other assistance that is of lifelong or extended duration and is individually planned and coordinated, except that such term, when applied to infants and young children means individuals from birth to age 5, inclusive, who have substantial developmental delay or specific congenital or acquired conditions with a high probability of resulting in developmental disabilities if services are not provided. [§ 102(7)]

The definition included in the 2000 Amendments to the Developmental Disabilities Assistance and Bill of Rights Act of 1987 focuses much more on functional than on categorical issues and encompasses a wide variety of possible disabling conditions. While the focus of defining developmental disabilities is in functional issues, some specific conditions would typically be included as developmental disabilities. Among them are the following:

- cerebral palsy (Best, Reed, & Bigge, 2005)
- spina bifida
- epilepsy
- emotional problems (Clark, Reavis, & Jenson, 1992)
- autism (Eaves, 1992)
- deaf-blindness (Marchant, 1992)
- Prader-Willi syndrome (Scott, Smith, Hendricks, & Polloway, 1999)
- fragile x syndrome
- sickle-cell anemia

These are only a few of the many conditions that can be classified as developmental disabilities. Bender (1992) even points out that learning disabilities could be considered a developmental disability, which could enlarge the population significantly, since large numbers of individuals are classified as having learning disabilities.

Although children with many of these conditions have generally been provided appropriate educational programs, the categorical special education system under IDEA has required schools to categorize children into a specific disability group in order to make them eligible for services. In most cases, the requirement of categorical labels has not had a negative impact on the appropriateness of services; however, the mandated categorical system fails to meet the needs of some children (Smith, et al., 2008). For example, children with Prader-Willi syndrome usually have to be classified as having mental retardation in order to be served. Although mental retardation is a frequent characteristic of children with Prader-Willi syndrome, the fact remains that serving a child on the basis of mental retardation may overlook other overall needs related to Prader-Willi syndrome, concerning weight and dietary management (Scott et al., 1999). It is hoped that the more-functional, generic category of developmental disabilities increases the likelihood that school personnel and others providing services to children will structure their interventions on the basis of individual strengths, weaknesses, and needs, rather than on preconceived notions about any categorical disability group.

Characteristics and Needs of Individuals With Developmental Disabilities

As a result of the heterogeneity of the developmental disabilities category, it is difficult to establish universal characteristics and needs for this group of individuals. However, some characteristics and needs are fairly common among individuals with developmental disabilities. Since the primary criteria for developmental disabilities focus on functional deficits, the primary common characteristics of individuals classified as developmentally disabled are functional characteristics. When reviewing the following list, remember that not all individuals with developmental disabilities will exhibit all of the characteristics.

Chronic Disability

By definition, individuals with developmental disabilities manifest a severe, chronic disability that will likely exist throughout the person's life. The result will likely be the need for lifelong specialized services and assistance, provided in a coordinated and culturally competent manner, by many different agencies, professionals, advocates, community representatives, and others (Developmental Disabilities Assistance and Bill of Rights Act of 2000). Therefore, unlike disabilities that have a more time-restricted impact, developmental disabilities are considered a permanent feature of the person.

The chronic nature of developmental disabilities means that services needed by this group of individuals will not terminate when the individual completes high school or other formalized postsecondary education. Rather, services will need to be provided during each stage of adulthood. These could include employment supports, housing supports, and social supports.

Substantial Limitations

Another characteristic of individuals with developmental disabilities, by definition, is that these disabilities result in *substantial* limitations in a variety of functional life activities. Life activities include self-care, language and communication, learning, mobility, self-direction, and economic self-sufficiency. The category of developmental disabilities is thus characterized by functional limitations and impact on routine life activities. If the disability does not result in limitations in at least three of the noted life activities, then the person, by definition, does not have a developmental disability.

Depending on the specific characteristics of persons with developmental disabilities, direct individualized services or environmental supports might be needed. Direct individualized services may include attendant care, educational intervention, and counseling. Environmental supports encompass the many different interventions that can modify the person's environment (e.g., making a particular apartment physically accessible for a person in a wheelchair). Often, individuals with developmental disabilities need both direct individualized services and environmental modifications. However, some individuals may require actions in only one of these areas.

Self-Care Needs

Self-care is directly related to independent living. Individuals with developmental disabilities, while varying a great deal in their self-care needs, frequently require assistance in supported living activities (McDonnell, Hardman, & McDonnell, 2003). The nature of their chronic, severe disabilities frequently affects their ability to live independently. Many individuals with developmental needs may require, for instance, personal assistance services, which are "a range of services, provided by one or more individuals, designed to assist an individual with a disability to perform daily living activities on or off a job that such individual would typically perform if such individual did not have a disability" (Developmental Disabilities Assistance and Bill of Rights Act of 2000).

Self-care skills encompass the repertoire of skills that enable individuals to take care of themselves, "the basic and routine tasks of maintaining personal hygiene: toileting, eating, dressing, and grooming" (Farlow & Snell, 2006, p. 328). Individuals with developmental disabilities often lack self-care skills and will therefore need instruction in these areas and/or lifelong supports.

Language and Communication Needs

Individuals with developmental disabilities frequently display deficits in both receptive and expressive language (Erbas, 2005). Language problems range from mild expressive speech problems to profound dysfunction in both receptive and expressive language abilities. Regardless of the degree of language and communication problems, interventions are almost always warranted because of the critical role that language plays in society (Polloway, Miller, & Smith, 2004). The primary goal of such intervention is the development of functional communication skills (Kaiser & Grim, 2006).

Numerous interventions are related to communication problems, depending on the specific nature of the problem. For example, interventions might be as simple as the development of a language-enriching environment by the teacher or as complex as the use of cochlear implants to facilitate communication skills (Polloway et al., 2004). Depending on the complexity of the intervention, a variety of individuals could be involved in providing services. Speech–language specialists may need to provide support for persons who have severe language and communication problems, whereas positive role models may be the only support needed by persons with mild language and communication problems.

Learning Needs

Of all needs exhibited by individuals with developmental disabilities, learning is probably the most often addressed. Special education services for students with developmental disabilities have expanded rapidly during the past 30 years (Smith et al., 2008). With the beginning of federal mandates to provide a free appropriate public education to children with disabilities in 1975 (Education for All Handicapped Children Act) came a widespread increase in the number and types of children served in special education programs. Indeed, the *Twenty-fifth Annual Report to Congress on the Implementation of the Individuals with Disabilities Education Act (IDEA)* reveals that the number of children served in special education programs increased from 3.7 million in the 1992–1993 school year to more than 5.8 million in the 2001–2002 school year (U.S. Department of Education, 2003).

Special education is directly related to the learning needs of children with developmental disabilities. Through the individualized education program (IEP) process, school personnel develop intervention programs that target the learning needs of each child (Smith et al., 2008). The learning needs of adults are also addressed through various service models. Vocational rehabilitation agencies, adult day-care programs, and adult education programs all assist adults with learning problems in developing skills necessary for independent living.

Mobility Needs

Orientation and mobility training has long been a service provided for individuals with visual disabilities. Recently, however, it has become clear that some individuals with other disabilities also need such services. Many persons with developmental disabilities require training in these areas, especially mobility (Best, Reed, & Bigge, 2005). For example, individuals with cerebral palsy, because of their impairments in posture and movement, frequently require mobility assistance. Also, persons with mental retardation may need assistance in using public transportation resources, and individuals who rely on wheelchairs may need assistance in maximizing their use.

Among the numerous barriers to mobility for persons with developmental disabilities are the following: physical barriers (e.g., stairs without a ramp), social barriers (e.g., restricting some children's participation in certain physical activities), and transportation barriers (e.g., lack of accessible transportation). Mobility needs for individuals with developmental disabilities can take several different forms, among them (a) ambulation within or between settings (walking, running, sliding, pulling, crawling, transferring to/from wheelchair) and (b) conveyance within or between settings (adapted or non-adapted cars and vans, manual or electric wheelchairs, scooters, bicycles, tricycles, public transportation) (Best et al., 2005).

Self-Direction Needs

A significant need for persons with developmental disabilities is self-direction—taking charge of the events that affect one's life and, furthermore, believing that such control is possible (Thoma & Getzel, 2005). Too often, service providers and family members encourage persons with disabilities to be dependent by not respecting their choices in various decisions. This denial of choice keeps individuals with disabilities "in a position of having all aspects of their lives determined through an outer locus of control, thereby denying the person the opportunity to internalize control, which is essential to learning and growth" (Brawner-Jones, 1994, p. 505). Often, the result of such overcontrol is learned helplessness, in which individuals actually learn to believe that they are not capable of participating in the decision-making activities that affect their own life, and are thus not capable of independent living.

Self-advocacy is the process whereby individuals literally advocate for themselves. With training, individuals with developmental disabilities not only make decisions about issues affecting their lives but understand their role in managing and controlling their own lives. "As we move more toward the reality of an inclusive society, it seems inconceivable that such an ideal could ever be fully reached without people with severe disabilities being able to participate in the choices that affect their lives" (McDonnell et al., 2003, p. 54).

Self-adaptability includes exercising one's own abilities and judgments. If too much is done for individuals with disabilities, they are deprived of developing their own adaptability skills (Clark & Bigge, 2005). There is a fine line between providing a proper level of support and doing too much. Learned helplessness can be the result of providing too many supports and not allowing individuals with disabilities to learn how to do things for themselves.

Economic Self-Sufficiency Needs

Economic self-sufficiency is a problem for many Americans, and the presence of a developmental disability compounds this problem. Data indicate that unemployment and underemployment are common problems among adults with developmental disabilities. However, a great deal of the literature in the field suggests that economic self-sufficiency is attainable for many persons with developmental disabilities (McDonnell, et al., 2003). Unfortunately, economic self-sufficiency for these individuals is not automatic; certain services need to be available to assist them in attaining this life goal. Therefore, a primary service need for many such individuals is work-related supports. Transition services to assist individuals with disabilities in moving from school environments to work environments are now mandated by federal law. Though transition programming does not guarantee success as an adult and self-sufficiency, it does provide a support that can facilitate the individual's attainment of this goal.

One of the primary goals of transition programming is to ensure uninterrupted services and supports for individuals with disabilities and their families (Katsiyannis, Zhang, Woodruff, & Dixon, 2005). Schools must develop transition plans and work with adult service agencies to implement those plans (Smith et al., 2008). Transition programs should not only focus on the development of job skills and interests but also include goals and objectives related to independent adult functioning in general. Once the transition from school to the post-school environments has been completed, various programs need to be in place to assist individuals in getting and keeping jobs.

Supported employment is a program for persons with disabilities that facilitates their inclusion in normalized society through employment opportunities. An important concept of supported employment is that the individual with a disability is placed in a regular, competitive job in a community setting instead of in a sheltered employment situation. Supported employment can be described as paid employment for individuals with disabilities whose employment at normal pay rates is unlikely because of their disabilities and who need ongoing support services (McDonnell et al., 2003). The support services are provided at the job site with a job coach who works alongside the individual with a disability, slowly decreasing the amount of intervention required for the employee to successfully complete the task. Another possible component of supported employment includes training other workers at the work site about a person's disability and ways they can provide various supports.

General Needs

In addition to the needs described above, some general needs of individuals with developmental disabilities must be addressed. Foremost is the need for service coordination, which is defined in the Developmental Disabilities Assistance and Bill of Rights Act of 2000 as activities that assist and enable individuals with developmental disabilities and their families to access services, supports, and other assistance, and includes:

   A. the provision of information to individuals with developmental disabilities and their families about the availability of services, supports, and other assistance;

   B. assistance in obtaining appropriate services, supports, and other assistance, which may include facilitating and organizing such assistance;

   C. coordination and monitoring of services, supports, and other assistance provided singly or in combination to individuals with developmental disabilities and their families to ensure accessibility, continuity, and accountability of such assistance; and

   D. follow-along services that ensure, through a continuing relationship, that the changing needs of individuals with developmental disabilities and their families are recognized and appropriately met. (42 U.S.C. 15002 § 102)

Without service coordination, individuals with developmental disabilities and their families are often at a loss about what services are available, how to access services, and how to ensure coordinated intervention efforts related to the disability. While numerous services are available for individuals with developmental disabilities, acquiring these services is often difficult without a coordinated effort.

Still another general need is in the area of technology. Assistive technology can be defined as a large group of aids, tools, and equipment that can enhance functioning for persons with disabilities in classrooms, work sites, home settings, and community locations. Assistive technology can range from very simple to very complex applications

(Best et al., 2005). Appropriate use of assistive technology can be a major asset for professionals, family members, and individuals with developmental disabilities. For further information on this topic, see chapter 17 in this text.

Services for Individuals With Developmental Disabilities

Services for individuals with developmental disabilities have changed a great deal during the past 25 years. The range of services has expanded immensely, and the trend for the past several years has been to provide services in a more-generic way and in inclusive rather than segregated environments. Many factors prompted special education and other services for individuals with disabilities to adopt a more-inclusive, generic service model. These include the movement to functional services, the inclusion movement, provision of individual supports, supported employment, the current approach to defining mental retardation by the American Association on Intellectual and Developmental Disabilities (AAIDD), and the expansion of services to individuals with autism and other developmental disabilities.

Movement to Functional Services

Although states continue to determine student eligibility for special education services under the Individuals with Disabilities Education Improvement Act of 2004 (IDEA) using a categorical model, such as mental retardation and learning disabilities, many have eliminated categorical special education services in favor of services based on more functional skill levels of students. For example, many states provide services to students on the basis of their level of disability, such as mild or severe, rather than on the basis of their clinical classification, such as mental retardation, learning disabilities, or emotional problems (Smith et al., 2008). This generic classification and service model has partly eroded the distinction once held by programs that provided services only to students classified as having mental retardation, learning disabilities, or some other specific type of disability. The generic model is more aligned with the developmental disabilities category than with traditional clinical categories.

Changes in teacher preparation programs also reflect the changing model of providing special education for students with mental retardation, learning disabilities, or other specific categories of disabilities. Whereas there used to be many categorical preparation programs for teachers of students with mental retardation and teachers of students with learning disabilities, more and more teacher preparation programs are now generic in nature, focusing on functional ability levels, such as mild or severe. One has only to look at the decline in the number of college textbooks concentrating on teaching students with mental retardation and the increase in the number of textbooks that emphasize teaching students with mild disabilities to realize the change of focus in special education.

In many public schools no teachers are designated specifically to teach students with mental retardation, learning disabilities, or other categorical disabilities, and no classrooms are specifically for students with these clinical descriptions. Many schools also have eliminated the classrooms that had been designated for students classified as educable mentally retarded or trainable mentally retarded. Resource rooms and resource room teachers have replaced classrooms that were designated by categories of disabilities and staffed by categorically trained and certified teachers (MacMillan, 1989).

The Inclusion Movement

The inclusion movement has also contributed to the generic trend of services and teacher preparation programs. Proponents of the inclusion of students with disabilities emphasize the functionality of each child over categorical labels of any kind. The aim is to provide appropriate services to children in settings with their nondisabled, chronological-age peers, as much as possible, without regard to clinical label. The inclusion movement appears to be a continuing trend (Smith, Gartin, Murdick, & Hilton, 2006). The student receives services and supports, for the most part, in the general education classroom rather than in a separate room. This arrangement represents a major shift from the traditional categorical services provided to students with mental retardation, learning disabilities, and other categorical disabilities during the early period of special education (Smith, Gartin, et al., 2006). This loss of program identity has resulted in more absorption of students with categorical labels into the general special education service system and the broader educational system.

Westling (2004) conducted a study to determine what parents of children with severe disabilities want from schools. After reviewing several studies, he developed recommendations for professionals, among which were to include socialization and friendship development in the curriculum, provide adequate and appropriate supports in inclusive settings, and provide other supports outside the school. Social integration in inclusive settings should definitely be a focus of inclusion (Boutot & Bryant, 2005). These recommendations focus on the inclusion of students not only during the school years but also during adulthood.

Growth of New Disabilities

While not really *new* disabilities, the rapid growth of certain disabilities over the past 20 years has resulted in major changes in the field of developmental disabilities. Two disability areas, attention deficit/hyperactivity disorder and autism, have grown rapidly in recent years, resulting in an influx of students with different types of learning problems. For example, the number of children identified as having autism increased from 15,580 in 1992–1993 to 97,847 in 2001–2002. While the number of children with ADHD is difficult to determine, primarily because they are served under IDEA as other health impaired (OHI), the number of children identified as OHI increased from 66,000 in 1992–1993 to more than 338,000 in 2001–2002 (U.S. Department of Education, 2003). It is likely that a great deal of this increase resulted from the identification of children with ADHD.

One of the reasons the autism category has grown so much is that it was made a separate category under IDEA with the 1990 reauthorization. Before that time, children with autism were definitely provided services but under different disability categories. Making autism a separate category not only created an opportunity to track the number of children with autism who were served in public schools but also increased the category's visibility. The increase in numbers of children identified with Asperger's syndrome, part of the pervasive developmental disorders category, has also increased the number of children served in this category (American Psychiatric Association, 2000).

Provision of Individual Supports

Concomitant with the inclusion trend in schools is the national movement to include individuals with all types of disabilities in normalized community settings (Taylor, Richards, & Brady, 2005). The provision of supports for families and individuals to facilitate community inclusion has helped professionals and adult service agencies move away from the idea of providing services only to persons with a single label, such as mental retardation and toward a model of providing services to individuals who need specific interventions (Walker, 1994). Most individuals with mental retardation and other developmental disabilities will likely need some supports for most of their life (Taylor et al., 2005). For example, rather than working primarily with individuals with physical disabilities, vocational rehabilitation counselors find themselves working with a variety of people with different disabilities in community settings. The result is that programs for adults, similar to programs for children, have lost their identity as serving only individuals with mental retardation or other specific disability categories. Another example is the provision of transition supports for individuals who are moving from public school to post-school environments. Without adequate supports, successful transition is much more difficult (Katsiyannis, et al., 2005).

The new approach that the American Association on Intellectual and Developmental Disabilities (AAIDD) has taken in defining mental retardation focuses on the level of supports needed by the individual. Rather than classifying individuals with mental retardation by the degree of deficit, current classifications focus on the level of supports needed. This refocus of the AAIDD definition underlies the current emphasis on providing supports to individuals rather than emphasizing the degree of deficit presented.

AAIDD Definition of Mental Retardation

The AAIDD has consistently supplied the field of disabilities with the definition of mental retardation that has been the most widely accepted and used. The most recent revision of the definition, published in 2002 (Luckasson et al., 2002), continues a significant shift from early AAMR (now AAIDD) definitions made in 1992 and is compatible with many of the other trends in the field of disabilities. It suggests that it is very difficult to classify an individual on the basis of test scores or other predetermined criteria. Rather, the definition emphasizes the levels of supports (e.g., intermittent or limited) needed by individuals to achieve success rather than degrees of deficits (e.g., mild, moderate, severe, profound) exhibited. The 2002 definition states: "Mental retardation is a disability characterized by significant limitations in both intellectual functioning and adaptive behavior as expressed in conceptual, social, and practical adaptive skills. The disability originates before age 18" (Luckasson et al., 2002, p. 1).

This shift away from early AAIDD definitions, which focused on IQ scores and deficits, emphasizes provision of the appropriate level of supports to enable the individual to live successfully in a normalized community setting rather than the level of disability presented by the person with mental retardation.

Legislation and Individuals With Developmental Disabilities

As noted above, individuals with developmental disabilities exhibit significant needs, many of which are being addressed by schools and other service agencies. The array of services now available for persons with developmental disabilities has developed as the result of parental advocacy, self-advocacy, litigation, and research that has revealed the efficacy of various services. However, the most important reason that services have become available for individuals with developmental disabilities is legislation. Without laws requiring that certain services be made available to persons with disabilities, it is unlikely that the services would be as widespread as they are.

Although state and local governments have made laws and policies that affect individuals with disabilities, the federal government's legislation has had the most impact. Among the landmark federal legislative acts that have had significant impact on services for persons with developmental disabilities are the following:

- Developmental Disabilities Services and Facilities Construction Act of 1970. Introduced the concept of developmental disabilities.

- Title XIX of the Social Security Act (1971). Required intermediate-care facilities for individuals with mental retardation to provide "active treatment" to residents.

- Education for All Handicapped Children Act of 1975. Resulted in mandates for schools to provide appropriate educational services to children with disabilities.

- Rehabilitation, Comprehensive Services, and Developmental Disabilities Amendment (1978). Redefined the term *developmental disability* to focus more on functionality.

- Developmental Disabilities Assistance and Bill of Rights Act of 1984. Included employment-related activities as a focus.

- Developmental Disabilities Assistance and Bill of Rights Act of 1990. Reauthorized the Developmental Disabilities Assistance and Bill of Rights Act of 1984 and put a great deal of emphasis on protection and advocacy.

- Education for All Handicapped Children Act of 1990. Renamed the act Individuals with Disabilities Education Act (IDEA), added autism and traumatic brain injury as disability categories, and required transition planning for students with disabilities.

- Americans with Disabilities Act of 1990. A massive civil rights act for individuals with disabilities, affecting most of U.S. society.

- Individuals with Disabilities Education Improvement Act of 1997. Reauthorized IDEA.

- Developmental Disabilities Assistance and Bill of Rights Act of 2000. Reauthorized the Developmental Disabilities Assistance and Bill of Rights Act of 1984 and put a great deal of emphasis on protection and advocacy.

- Individuals with Disabilities Education Improvement Act of 2004. Most recent reauthorization of IDEA.

Although legislation alone has not resulted in improved services for persons with developmental disabilities, it has created an environment in which professionals, legislators, family members, and individuals with disabilities have begun working together to improve the quality and quantity of services available.

Glossary

American Association on Intellectual and Developmental Disabilities (AAIDD)—The professional organization that provides general guidance on defining and classifying individuals with mental retardation.

Developmental disabilities—umbrella category of disabilities that encompasses individuals who have a severe, chronic mental or physical impairment, manifested before the age of 22, which substantially limits three or more major life activities.

Developmental Disabilities Assistance and Bill of Rights Act—Primary federal legislation that provides services for individuals with developmental disabilities.

Functional services—Services provided that have a practical, functional impact on an individual's life.

Inclusion—Movement to provide services for individuals with disabilities in inclusive, normalized environments.

Major life activity—An activity that is generally considered typical of an individual's daily life.

Mental retardation—A developmental disability characterized by limited cognitive abilities.

Self-direction—Ability to take charge of the events in one's life.

Self-sufficiency—Ability to provide for one's basic needs.

Substantial limitation—A limitation that is considered substantial, resulting in various degrees of dependence.

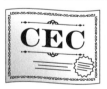

Knowledge and Skills for Entry-Level Special Education Teachers of Students With Developmental Disabilities Standards Addressed in This Chapter

Principle 1: Foundations

DD1K1   Definitions and issues related to the identification of individuals with developmental disabilities.

DD1K4   Trends and practices in the field of developmental disabilities.

Principle 2: Development and Characteristics of Learners

DD2K2   Psychological, social/emotional, and motor characteristics of individuals with developmental disabilities.

Principle 5: Learning Environments/Social Interaction

DD5S1   Provide instruction in community-based settings.

Principle 6: Language

DD6S1   Plan instruction on the use of alternative and augmentative communication systems.

Web Site Resources

Administration for Children and Families

http://www.acf.hhs.gov/programs/add

> Provides services for individuals with developmental disabilities. Includes programs and services, as well as legislation that affects this group of individuals.

American Association on Intellectual and Developmental Disabilities

http://www.aamr.org

> Provides information on mental retardation. Offers publications and other services, as well as information on membership in AAIDD.

Division on Developmental Disabilities of the Council for Exceptional Children

http://www.dddcec.org

> Provides an overview of DDD, publications and position papers, and information on conferences and other activities of the division.

Self-Advocates Becoming Empowered

http://www.sabeusa.org

> Includes the history of the Developmental Disabilities Assistance and Bill of Rights Act and describes its components. Provides a fact sheet on the general provisions of the act.

References

American Psychiatric Association. (2000). *Diagnostic and statistical manual of mental disorders* (4th ed., text rev.). Washington, DC: Author.

Americans with Disabilities Act of 1990, 42 U.S.C. § 12101 *et seq.* (1990).

Bender, W. N. (1992). Learning disabilities. In P. J. McLaughlin & P. Wehman (Eds.), *Developmental disabilities* (pp. 82–95). Boston: Andover Medical.

Best, S. J., Reed, P., & Bigge, J. L. (2005). Assistive technology. In S. J. Best, K. W. Heller, & J. L. Bigge (Eds.), *Teaching individuals with physical or multiple disabilities* (5th ed., pp. 179–224). Columbus, OH: Pearson Merrill.

Boutot, E. A., & Bryant, D. P. (2005). Social integration of students with autism in inclusive settings. *Education and Training in Developmental Disabilities, 40*, 14–23.

Brawner-Jones, N. (1994). Support needs and strategies for adults with profound disabilities. In L. Sternberg (Ed.), *Individuals with profound disabilities* (pp. 485–511). Austin, TX: PRO-ED.

Clark, E., Reavis, H. K., & Jenson, W. R. (1992). Emotional impairments. In P. J. McLaughlin & P. Wehman (Eds.), *Developmental disabilities* (pp. 54–66). Boston: Andover Medical.

Clark, G. M., & Bigge, J. L. (2005). Transition and self-determination. In S. J. Best, K. W. Heller, & J. L. Bigge (Eds.), *Teaching individuals with physical or multiple disabilities* (5th ed., pp. 367–398). Columbus, OH: Pearson Merrill.

Developmental Disabilities Assistance and Bill of Rights Act of 1984, 42 U.S.C. § 6000 *et seq.* Administration on Developmental Disabilities, U.S. Department of Health and Human Services. Washington, DC: U.S. Government Printing Office. (1984).

Developmental Disabilities Assistance and Bill of Rights Act of 1987, 42 U.S.C. § 6000 *et seq.* Administration on Developmental Disabilities, U.S. Department of Health and Human Services. Washington, DC: U.S. Government Printing Office. (1987).

Developmental Disabilities Assistance and Bill of Rights Act of 1990, 42 U.S.C. § 6000 *et seq.* Administration on Developmental Disabilities, U.S. Department of Health and Human Services. Washington, DC: U.S. Government Printing Office. (1990).

Developmental Disabilities Assistance and Bill of Rights Act of 2000, 42 U.S.C. § 15002 *et seq.* Administration on Developmental Disabilities, U.S. Department of Health and Human Services. Washington, DC: U.S. Government Printing Office. (2000).

Developmental Disabilities Services and Facilities Construction Act of 1970, 84 Stat. 1316, 1325.

Eaves, R. E. (1992). Autism. In P. J. McLaughlin & P. Wehman (Eds.), *Developmental disabilities* (pp. 68–80). Boston: Andover Medical.

Education for All Handicapped Children Act of 1975, 20 U.S.C. § 1400 *et seq.* (1975).

Education for All Handicapped Children Act of 1975, 20 U.S.C. § 1400 *et seq.* (1975) (amended 1990).

Erbas, D. (2005). Responses to communication breakdowns by noverbal children with developmental disabilities. *Education and Training in Developmental Disabilities, 40,* 145–157.

Farlow, L. J., & Snell, M. E. (2006). Teaching self-care skills. In M. E. Snell & F. Brown (Eds.), *Instruction of students with severe disabilities* (6th ed., pp. 328–370). Columbus, OH: Merrill.

Individuals with Disabilities Education Act of 1990, 20 U.S.C. § 1400 *et seq.* (1990).

Individuals with Disabilities Education Act of 1990, 20 U.S.C. § 1400 *et seq.* (1990) (amended 1997).

Individuals with Disabilities Education Act of 1990, 20 U.S.C. § 1400 *et seq.* (1990) (amended 2004).

Inge, K. J. (1992). Cerebral palsy. In P. J. McLaughlin & P. Wehman (Eds.), *Developmental disabilities* (pp. 30–52). Boston: Andover Medical.

Kaiser, A. P., & Grim, J. C. (2006). Teaching functional communication skills. In M. E. Snell & F. Brown (Eds.), *Instruction of students with severe disabilities* (6th ed., pp. 447–485). Columbus, OH: Merrill.

Katsiyannis, A., Zhang, D., Woodruff, N., & Dixon, A. (2005). Transition supports to students with mental retardation: An examination of data from the national longitudinal transition study 2. *Education and Training in Developmental Disabilities, 40,* 109–116.

Luckasson, R., Borthwick-Duffy, S., Buntinx, W., Coulter, D., Craig, E., Reeve, A., et al. (2002). *Mental retardation: Definition, classification, and systems of supports* (10th ed.). Washington, DC: American Association on Mental Retardation.

MacMillan, D. L. (1989). Mild mental retardation: Emerging issues. In G. A. Robinson, J. R. Patton, E. A. Polloway, & S. R. Sargent (Eds.), *Best practices in mild mental retardation* (pp. 1–19). Reston, VA: Council for Exceptional Children, Division on Mental Retardation.

Marchant, J. M. (1992). Deaf-blind handicapping conditions. In P. J. McLaughlin & P. Wehman (Eds.), *Developmental disabilities* (pp. 113–122). Boston: Andover Medical.

McDonnell, J. J., Hardman, M. L., & McDonnell, A. P. (2003). *An introduction to persons with severe disabilities* (2nd ed.). Needham Heights, MA: Allyn & Bacon.

Polloway, E. A., Miller, L., & Smith, T. E. C. (2004). *Language instruction for students with disabilities* (3rd ed.). Denver: Love.

President's Committee on Mental Retardation. (1995). *State collaboration for community membership.* Washington, DC: Author.

Rehabilitation, Comprehensive Services, and Developmental Disabilities Amendment of 1978, 92 Stat. 2955.

Scott, E. M., Smith, T. E. C., Hendricks, M. D., & Polloway, E. A. (1999). Prader-Willi syndrome: A review and implications for educational intervention. *Education and Training in Mental Retardation and Developmental Disabilities, 34,* 110–116.

Smith, T. E. C., Gartin, B. C., Murdick, N. L., & Hilton, A. (2006). *Families and children with special needs.* Columbus, OH: Merrill.

Smith, T. E. C., Polloway, E. A., Patton, J. R., & Dowdy, C. A. (2008). *Teaching students with special needs in inclusive settings* (5th ed.). Needham Heights, MA: Allyn & Bacon.

Taylor, R. L., Richards, S. B., & Brady, M. P. (2005). *Mental retardation: Historical perspectives, current practices, and future directions.* Boston: Allyn & Bacon.

Thoma, C. A., & Getzel, E. E. (2005). Self-determination is what it's all about: What postsecondary students with disabilities tell us are important considerations for success. *Education and Training in Developmental Disabilities, 40,* 234–242.

Title IX of the Social Security Act, 42 U.S.C. § 1396 *et seq.* (1935).

U.S. Department of Education. (2003). *Twenty-fifth annual report to Congress on the implementation of the Individuals with Disabilities Education Act.* Washington, DC: Author.

Walker, P. (1994). Housing and support services: Expanding options for people with severe disabilities. *NARIC Quarterly, 4,* 1–4.

Westling, D. (2004). What do parents of children with moderate and severe mental disabilities want? In R. Sandieson & V. Sharpe (Eds.), *Foundations, teachers, and families in developmental disabilities* (pp. 251–279). Austin, TX: PRO-ED.

5

Autism Spectrum Disorders

Brenda Smith Myles, Anastasia Hubbard,
Kristin Muellner, and Alison Simonelli Hider

Summary

After a brief overview of autism spectrum disorders (ASD) and learning characteristics that affect home, school, and community, this chapter provides a model for identifying individuals with ASD and conducting assessments that lead to effective program planning. In addition, it presents a variety of interventions, including environmental supports, instructional interventions, and social and behavioral supports that can be used across environments. Finally, the chapter gives a brief description of educational trends in ASD.

Learning Outcomes

After reading this chapter, you should be able to:

- Define autism spectrum disorders (ASD) and learner characteristics and identify prevalence and causes.

- Explain how ASD are identified.

- Describe environmental supports for students with autism spectrum disorders.

- Identify instructional interventions appropriate for students with ASD across environments.

- List social and behavioral supports that facilitate learning and interaction.

- Identify trends related to ASD.

Introduction

Priya rarely participates in social interactions with others, and she displays behavior that may be perceived as "odd," such as lining up her favorite DVD cases on the floor and becoming upset if someone moves one out of the lineup. When she becomes angry, she mutters, "I can't take it another second." At most other times she appears nonverbal. Priya's mother indicated that she uses this phrase at home and that Priya's grandfather also uses it often. The phrase had become Priya's indication that she was upset. This discovery assisted the teacher in developing a plan for teaching Priya to ask for a break in a more appropriate way, thus decreasing her frustration throughout the school day.

Allen has an intelligence quotient (IQ) score in the very superior range, talks like a little professor, and while he will participate in social interactions, experiences difficulty expanding his conversations beyond his own topic of interest, which is hurricanes. Academically he is at grade level or above. In the hallways between classes peers often ask him, "What's up?" This typically prompts Allen to look toward the ceiling and describe the materials that compose the ceiling tiles. At other times he will "police" the hallway, pointing out rule infractions that students have committed.

Priya and Allen have more in common than it may initially appear. Both have been diagnosed with an autism spectrum disorder (ASD). This chapter will define ASD and describe key issues related to it, including (a) its prevalence, (b) its potential causes, (c) diagnostic assessments and assessments for program planning purposes, (d) evidence-based educational practices, instructional strategies, and social and behavioral supports, and (e) future trends in ASD.

Definition of and Salient Issues Related to Autism Spectrum Disorders

Definitions

Autism spectrum disorders are generally diagnosed by medical professionals using criteria from the *Diagnostic and Statistical Manual of Mental Disorders*, 4th ed., Text Revision [*DSM-IV-TR*; American Psychiatric Association (APA), 2000], which classifies this disability as a Pervasive Developmental Disorder (PDD). According to *DSM-IV-TR*, children and youth with PDD manifest impairments in reciprocal social interaction and communication skills as well as having evidence of stereotypic behavior and restrictive interests and activities. Subcategories of pervasive developmental disorders include Autistic Disorder, Asperger's Disorder, Childhood Disintegrative Disorder, Rett's Disorder, and Pervasive Developmental Disorder—Not Otherwise Specified (PDD-NOS). Because Childhood Disintegrative Disorder and Rett's Disorder are not typically considered a part of the autism spectrum, they are mentioned only briefly.

Autism

Occurring before the age of three, autism, or autistic disorder, is defined by impairments in social interactions and communication as well as by restrictive, repetitive, and stereotyped movements. The majority of children with autism have some degree of cognitive disability, ranging from mild to severe. While 20% of children with autism are reported to have typical development until the age of one or two (APA, 2000), many are thought to have the defining characteristics of this disability from birth. Filipek et al. (1999) labeled the characteristics, shown in Table 5.1, as red flags.

Even with the use of best practice interventions (APA, 2000), only an insignificant percentage of persons with autism live and work independently. According to the APA (2000), approximately one third attain partial independence.

Asperger's Syndrome

In 1944 Hans Asperger published his seminal work on four boys from his clinical practice who exhibited (a) social isolation and awkwardness, (b) self-stimulatory responses, (c) insistence on environmental sameness, (d) normal intellectual development, and

TABLE 5.1
Red-Flag Behaviors That May Denote Autism in Young Children

Communication concerns	Does not respond to his/her name
	Cannot tell me what (s)he wants
	Language is delayed
	Doesn't follow directions
	Appears deaf at times
	Seems to hear sometimes, but not others
	Doesn't point or wave bye-bye
	Used to say a few words, but now (s)he doesn't
Social concerns	Doesn't smile socially
	Seems to prefer to play alone
	Gets things for him-/herself
	Is very independent
	Does things "early"
	Has poor eye contact
	Is in his/her own world
	Tunes us out
	Is not interested in other children
Behavioral concerns	Tantrums
	Is hyperactive/uncooperative or oppositional
	Doesn't know how to play with toys
	Gets stuck on things over and over
	Toe-walks
	Has unusual attachments to toys
	Lines things up
	Is oversensitive to certain sounds or textures
	Has odd movement patterns
Absolute indications for immediate further evaluation	No babbling by 12 months
	No gesturing (pointing, waving bye-bye, etc.) by 12 months
	No single words by 16 months
	No two-word spontaneous (not just echolalic) phrases by 24 months
	ANY loss of ANY language or social skills at ANY age

Source: Filipek et al., 1999.

(e) normal communication development (Asperger, 1944). Currently, the defining characteristic of Asperger's disorder or Asperger's syndrome (AS) is a social interaction impairment. According to Frith (1991), who interpreted the work of Hans Asperger, children with AS have interests in others, yet face severe social challenges. *DSM-IV-TR* stipulates that the predominant features of AS are similar to the characteristics of autism, impaired social interaction accompanied by repetitive and stereotyped behaviors and restricted interests.

Rett's Syndrome

Rett's disorder, or Rett's syndrome (RS), a disability that occurs primarily in girls (Sandberg, Ehlers, Hagberg, & Gillberg, 2000), first appeared in the PDD category of *DSM-IV* in 1994. Five years later, the MeCP2 gene that causes 80% of the cases of RS was identified (Amir, et al., & Zoghbi, 1999). RS most often occurs during the first two years of life and is characterized by head growth deceleration, loss of motor skills (including purposeful hand movements), stereotypic hand wringing or hand washing, and social and communication impairments. Similar to children with autism, children with RS function along a continuum. While the majority are severely challenged, cases of mild RS have been documented (Sandberg et al., 2000).

Childhood Disintegrative Disorder

Childhood disintegrative disorder (CDD), or Heller's syndrome, is a low-incidence disability that is one tenth as common as autism (APA, 2000). Children with this disability manifest behavior patterns similar to children with autism in the areas of social interaction, communication, behavior, and interest impairments. Unlike most children with autism, children with CDD experience at least 2 years (but fewer than 10 years) of typical development, then experience significant regression in language, social skills, adaptive behavior, and motor skills, including loss of bowel or bladder control (APA, 2000). The prognosis for children with CDD is guarded; areas in which regression occurred often are not regained. Empirical evidence on CDD is limited (Malhotra & Gupta, 1999).

Pervasive Developmental Disorder—
Not Otherwise Specified

Another exceptionality category of pervasive developmental disorders in *DSM-IV-TR* (2000) is pervasive developmental disorder—not otherwise specified (PDD-NOS), including atypical autism. As noted by the APA (2000):

> This category should be used when there is a severe and pervasive impairment in the development or reciprocal social interaction association with impairment in either verbal or nonverbal communication skills or with the presence of stereotyped behavior, interests, and activities, but the criteria are not met for a specific Pervasive Developmental Disorder. (p. 84)

For example, a child who manifests the criteria for Asperger's syndrome but experiences late language onset might receive a PDD-NOS classification.

Additional Characteristics Associated With ASD

DSM-IV-TR (APA, 2000) describes the criteria required for a diagnosis of ASD. However, research has identified further characteristics that are common among children and youth with ASD, a selection of which are explained below.

Cognition

The intelligence of students with ASD varies significantly (Manjiviona & Prior, 1999). Students with classic autism typically have IQ scores in the moderate to severe mental retardation range (Simpson & Myles, 1998). Students with AS, however, typically score in the average to above average range, with some scoring in the superior or very superior range (Barnhill, Hagiwara, Myles, & Simpson, 2000; Myles & Adreon, 2001).

Skills such as planning, organizing, prioritizing, multitasking, starting and stopping, and shifting attention may prove extremely challenging for students with ASD (Hughes, Russell, & Robbins, 1994; Ozonoff, Strayer, McMahon, & Filloux, 1995; Pennington & Ozonoff, 1996). Similarly, although students with ASD may be able to memorize large pieces of information, they may not demonstrate understanding of it (Carpentieri & Morgan, 1994; Minshew, Goldstein, Taylor, & Siegel, 1994). For example, a student with ASD may read a book and remember numerous details about what he or she read, perhaps even quoting passages from the book, but may not be able to identify the story's main ideas. This same student might not be able to identify how a character probably felt or what he or she may have been thinking at a particular point in the story. This requires theory of mind, or taking the perspective of another person, a skill that is challenging for most people with ASD (Baron-Cohen, 1992, 1995; Baron-Cohen, Leslie, & Frith, 1985; Baron-Cohen, O'Riordan, Stone, Jones, & Plaisted, 1999; Sicotte & Stemberger, 1999).

Learning Style

Students with ASD tend to be visual, rather than auditory, learners (Harris, Handelman, & Burton, 1990; Quill, 1997; Savner & Myles, 2000). They often experience difficulty with processing information that someone tells them verbally (auditory), but they will have minimal to no difficulty processing this same information if it is presented in a visual format, such as a written note/story, a picture, a list, or a schedule.

Islands of Ability

While many researchers and practitioners focus on the deficits inherent in autism, it should be recognized that children and youth with ASD display numerous relative strengths, such as (a) visual–spatial abilities, (b) physical development, (c) rote memory, (d) attention to detail, and (f) ability to follow rules and routines (Baron-Cohen, 2003; Quill, 2000). These abilities are relative strengths, as they often more well developed than the person's cognitive ability would lead one to indicate, but they may actually be within what is considered an average level (Baron-Cohen, 2003; Quill, 2000).

Self-Stimulatory Behaviors

Self-stimulatory behaviors, such as rocking or flapping of hands, are well-recognized characteristics of children and youth with autism. Defined as repetitive patterns that appear to have little or no discernible function, these behaviors may be pervasive in some children with ASD. According to Quill (2000), these behaviors may help soothe the child, help him or her to focus, or serve as a request for assistance.

Prevalence

The prevalence of ASD is a matter of contention. *DSM-IV-TR* (APA, 2000) reported a 5 per 10,000 prevalence rate of autism and further indicated that similar data on Asperger's syndrome do not exist. Others report different prevalence rates. For example, in a study of all children in one town, Kadesjo, Gillberg, and Hagberg (1999) found a prevalence rate of 60 in 10,000 who manifested classical autism and a rate of 48 per 10,000 for children diagnosed with Asperger's syndrome. According to these researchers, individuals who manifested autism, Asperger's syndrome, and autistic-like behaviors represented 1.21% of the population. In 2002 Scott, Baron-Cohen, Bolton, and Brayne, also studying the children in one town, found that 57 in 10,000 manifested what they termed *autistic spectrum condition*, which included autism, Asperger's syndrome, and PDD-NOS. The Autism and Developmental Disabilities Monitoring (ADDM) Network (2007) recently reported an ASD prevalence rate of 1 in 150. In terms of gender, autism occurs four to five times more often in males than in females, and males are more than five times more likely than females to be diagnosed with Asperger's syndrome (APA, 2000). Kadesjo et al. (1999) reported a male-to-female ratio of 9:1 in ASD, while Scott et al. (2002) reported a 4:1 ratio.

Causes

Researchers have yet to pinpoint a specific cause or constellation of causative factors for ASD. Professionals in fields such as neuropsychology and medicine continue to investigate potential causes, with the reality that ASD is most likely an outcome resulting from many different causes (Gillberg & Coleman, 2000). Three areas are most often discussed in relation to cause: (a) environmental factors, (b) differences in the parts of the brains of individuals with ASD that correlate to their typical strengths and challenges, and (c) genetic factors (Myles, Hubbard, Swanson, Schelvan, & Simonelli, 2007). Immunizations such as the measles-mumps-rubella (MMR) vaccine are potential environmental causes that to date have been researched with mixed results (Dales, Hammer, & Smith, 2001; Stratton, Gable, Shetty, & McCormick, 2001; Wakefield et al., 1988).

Differences in areas of the brain such as the cerebellum, which affects motor and cognitive skills, and the frontal and temporal lobes, which affect communicative and social functioning, have been found in individuals with ASD as compared to neurotypical individuals (Carper & Courchesne, 2000; Courchesne et al., 2001; Pierce & Courchesne, 2001; Piven, Arndt, Bailey, & Anderson, 1996; Piven, Saliba, Bailey, & Arndt, 1997; Ryu et al., 1999), as have differences in brain cell quantity (lower), density (higher), and brain volume (lower) (Aylward et al., 1999; Kemper & Bauman, 1998). Regarding genetics, research has not indicated a single-gene cause, but rather has suggested that multiple genetic factors may combine, with characteristics related to ASD the result, the degree and frequency of which may vary among family members (Gillberg & Coleman, 2000).

Assessment

When one is working with individuals on the autism spectrum, assessment is critical. A broad range of procedures is available to assist in determining a diagnosis, and ongoing assessment is necessary to ensure quality programming that addresses needs in intelligence, language, sensory, and academic skill levels (Myles & Adreon, 2001–2002) throughout the implementation of interventions.

In order for a medical diagnosis of ASD to be established, a person must be evaluated by a licensed physician or a psychologist who will use criteria based on *DSM-IV-TR* to determine if a disability is present (Janzen, 2003). *DSM-IV-TR* provides specific guidelines that aid clinicians and physicians in ensuring reliable and consistent diagnoses (Charak & Stella, 2002). Many formal tools are used in the identification process (see Table 5.2). In addition to formal testing, an individual's developmental history is evaluated through structured interviews and observations (Plotts & Webber, 2001–2002).

Once a child enters the school environment, he or she may be evaluated to determine eligibility for special education services (Janzen, 2003). Again, a battery of formal and informal evaluations may be administered.

Building an appropriate program for a student without ongoing assessment is an impossible task. One needs current knowledge of the student's functioning in the natural environment to develop goals and intervention strategies (Janzen, 2003). The major areas to assess are sensory needs (Myles, Cook, Miller, Rinner, & Robbins, 2000), behavioral concerns (Myles & Southwick, 2005), academic and pre-academic skills, interests and dislikes, tolerance to new experiences, modes of communication, language acquisition, independence, learning style, social awareness, and anxiety levels (Janzen, 2003; Myles & Southwick, 2005).

Observations, interviews, and direct measures of skills are vital throughout intervention because they provide firsthand information regarding the individual's performance levels (Janzen, 2003). Measures such as the *Behavior Assessment System for Children* (BASC) take into account both parent and teacher views of behaviors across settings (Reynolds & Kamphaus, 1992). Self-reports are another option if the student is capable of self-evaluation. For example, Brown and Dunn (2002) created the *Adolescent/Adult Sensory Profile* to provide a measure of responses to typical sensory experiences. Some assessments, such as the *Psychoeducational Profile—III* (PEP-III; Schopler, Lansing, Reichler, & Marcus, 2005) and curriculum-based assessment help to determine learning targets that are appropriate for the student's developmental age (Bock & Hurlbutt, 2002).

The number and breadth of assessments has increased in recent years. Careful assessments can provide a comprehensive picture of an individual's strengths and areas of concern, give parents and educators a place to start, provide methods of monitoring progress, and suggest where to go next.

TABLE 5.2
Sample Diagnostic Assessment Measures

Assessment Measure	Author(s)	Explanation	Features
Asperger Syndrome Diagnostic Scale (ASDS)	Myles, Bock, & Simpson (2001)	Designed to determine diagnosis of AS and rule out other ASD	Comprises 50 items that are rated as "observed" or "not observed"
Autism Diagnostic Observation Schedule—Generic (ADOS)	Lord, Rutter, DiLavore, & Risi, (2001)	Standardized assessment to determine ASD diagnosis	Four modules that provide semi-structured social opportunities
Childhood Autism Rating Scale (CARS)	Schopler, Reichler, & Rochen-Renner (1988)	Behavioral rating scale to assist in determining ASD	Consists of 15 areas that address characteristics associated with classical autism
Gilliam Autism Rating Scale	Gilliam (1995)	Parents or caregivers complete the instrument to determine a diagnosis of autism	Has 50 items that are rated from never to frequently observed

Educational Practices for Students With ASD

Myriad supports are available to ensure that children and youth with ASD are successful in home, school, and community. Among them are (a) environmental supports, such as visual supports and assistive technology, (b) instructional supports, including priming and applied behavior analysis strategies, and (c) social and behavioral supports, including the Power Card strategy and Social Stories™ (Gray Center for Social Learning and Understanding, n.d.). Each of these educational interventions provides structure and support for the learner with ASD.

Environmental Supports

Visual Supports

Students with ASD often think concretely and have difficulty processing verbal instructions. *Visual supports* help students transition from one class to another, complete multi-step tasks, and follow rules and routines (Savner & Myles, 2000). The most commonly used visual support is the visual schedule, which helps students reduce stress and anxiety by providing predictability. The schedule can be handwritten or created by using photographs or line drawings. Posting it in an assigned place or on a student notebook helps make it accessible to the student at anytime during the day. Other visual supports include graphic organizers, lists, and maps. The empirical evidence supports the use of these tools (Bryan & Gast, 2000; Dettmer, Simpson, Myles, & Ganz, 2000; MacDuff, Krantz, & McClannahan, 1993; Schultheis, Boswell, & Decker, 2000; Wilson, Schepis, & Mason-Main, 1987).

Assistive Technology

Assistive technology (AT) enables students with ASD to experience a better quality of life by providing them with additional ways to participate in their daily lives. AT includes any device that aids students with ASD in daily functioning, most often in such areas as communication, social interaction, and executive functioning (Smith, Murphy-Herd, Alvarado, & Glennon, 2005). These devices may be classified as being low-tech, mid-tech, or high-tech.

Low-tech devices are usually easy to implement, look similar to what typically developing peers would use, and are reasonable in cost (Smith et al., 2005; Sweeney, 2003). Mid-tech devices also may be relatively easy to implement, similar in appearance to what a typically developing peer may use, and reasonable in cost, with the difference that they usually involve batteries (Smith et al., 2005). High-tech devices may prove beneficial for students with ASD by providing them with assistance specific to their unique strengths, challenges, and learning characteristics, but this often comes at a cost in both time and financial resources. Using these devices may require a great deal of training on the part of students and the people with whom they interact. They may also be extremely expensive (Smith et al., 2005). Examples of these devices appear in Table 5.3.

TABLE 5.3

Examples of Assistive Technology Devices for Children and Youth With ASD

Low-tech	Mid-tech	High-tech
Picture symbols	Calculators	Voice output
Highlighters	Personal digital assistants	Communication aids
Photo albums	Video recorders	Personal computers
	Audio recorders	

Limited research has been conducted on the use of AT with individuals with ASD. Topics addressed include using AT to (a) increase communication interactions (Bernard-Opitz, Sriram, & Nakhoda-Sapuan, 2001b; Schepis, Reid, Behrmann, & Sutton, 1998), (b) improve social skills (Simpson, Langone, & Ayers, 2004), (c) develop reading skills (Williams, Wright, Callaghan, & Coughlan, 2002), (d) enhance spelling performance (Kinney, Vedora, & Stromer, 2003; Schlosser & Blischak, 2004; Schlosser, Blischak, Belfiore, Bartley, & Barnett, 1998), (e) decrease challenging behavior (Durand, 1999; Plienis & Romanczyk, 1985), (f) teach daily living skills (Shipley, Lutzker, & Taubman, 2002), (g) expand recognition and understanding of emotions (Silver & Oakes, 2001), and (h) teach problem-solving skills (Bernard-Opitz, Sriram, & Nakhoda-Sapuan, 2001a).

Instructional Supports

Priming

Priming was devised by Wilde, Koegel, and Koegel (1992) to (a) familiarize children and youth with academic material prior to its use in school, (b) bring predictability to new tasks by reducing stress and anxiety, and (c) increase the student's success. Priming occurs when a parent, paraprofessional, resource teacher, or trusted peer previews with a student with ASD the actual materials that will be used in a lesson on the day, the evening, or the morning before the activity occurs. In some instances, priming occurs immediately before an activity. Priming is most effective when it is built into the student's routine. It should occur in an environment that is relaxing and be facilitated by a primer who is both patient and encouraging. Finally, priming sessions should be short, providing a brief overview of the day's tasks in 5 to 10 minutes (Myles & Adreon, 2001). Several studies support its use with children with ASD (Bainbridge & Myles, 1999; Schreibman, Whalen, & Stahmer, 2000; Zanolli & Daggett, 1998; Zanolli, Daggett, & Adams, 1996).

Applied Behavior Analysis Strategies

The principles of applied behavior analysis (ABA) provide the foundation for a number of strategies for teaching students with ASD. ABA involves examining behavior specific to the student involved, helping the student replace an undesired behavior with a desired one, and understanding the functional relationship between the student's behavior and the environment (Cooper, Heron, & Heward, 1987).

Discrete Trial Teaching. Discrete trial teaching (DTT) is one of the most common ABA-based strategies for which research has been completed with students with ASD. DTT involves (a) identifying the behavior/skill to be taught, (b) breaking this behavior/skill down into its smaller components, often through a task analysis, and (c) systematically teaching each component. The DTT teaching sequence involves (a) presentation of a cue (the discriminative stimuli [SD]) to the student (which may be presented with or immediately preceding a prompt), (b) the student's response [R]), (c) the instructor's response to the student (the response stimulus, [SR]), and (d) an intertrial interval, or one- to five-second pause before the presentation of the next cue (Leaf & McEachin, 1999; Lovaas, 1987; Smith, 2001). DTT has been used to help students increase skills in the areas of academics, communication, imitation, self-help, and social functioning (Anderson, Taras, & Cannon, 1996; Lovaas, 1987; McEachin, Smith, & Lovaas, 1993).

Pivotal Response Training. Pivotal response training (PRT) builds on the principles of ABA to foster behavior change through naturally occurring situations in the home, school, and community. The PRT teaching sequence is similar to that of DTT: (a) instructor's cue to student, (b) student's response, and (c) instructor's response, but PRT focuses on pivotal areas with the aim that change will then result in untargeted behaviors too. The four pivotal areas are (a) motivation, (b) multiple cues, (c) initiations, and (d) self-management (Koegel et al., 1989). PRT also emphasizes building from activities that the child is interested in at the point of interaction, rather than the adult's preferences or predetermined activities.

PRT has been used to increase skills in the areas of language, joint attention, initiation of play and conversation (Pierce & Schreibman, 1995, 1997), and symbolic play (Stahmer, 1995). Families have also been trained to use PRT with good results, such as high degrees of happiness and interest, low degrees of stress during intervention, and an increase in positive communication (Koegel, Bimbela, & Schreibman, 1996).

Incidental Teaching. Through incidental teaching, instructors can apply the principles of ABA to situations as they occur throughout a student's day, rather than only during structured learning sessions with predetermined goals. For instance, if a preschool teacher notices his or her student with ASD approaching the classroom's play area during choice time, the teacher may seize the opportunity to help the student practice his or her pretend play skills by having the child (and perhaps peers as well) imitate (using ABA-based teaching strategies) kitchen play, such as pretending to cook eggs on the stove and setting the table.

Evidence for the benefits of incidental teaching with individuals with ASD exists in the following areas: (a) expanding speech and communication (Charlop-Christy & Carpenter, 2000; McGee, Krantz, Mason, & McClannahan, 1983; McGee, Krantz, & McClannahan, 1985); (b) increasing social skills, such as reciprocal interactions with peers (McGee, Almeida, Sulzer-Azaroff, & Feldman, 1992), and (c) teaching reading skills (McGee, Krantz, & McClannahan, 1986). Studies on incidental teaching emphasized its positive impact on promoting generalization of target skills (McGee et al., 1985, 1986).

The Picture Exchange Communication System. The Picture Exchange Communication System (PECS) is an ABA-based augmentative and alternative communication (AAC) program that has been used to help individuals with autism increase their communicative abilities (Bondy & Frost, 1994; Charlop-Christy, Carpenter, Lee, LeBlanc, & Kellet, 2002; Ganz & Simpson, 2004; Magiati & Howlin, 2003; Schwartz, Garfinkle, & Bauer, 1998). PECS requires learners to exchange a picture symbol(s) to communicate with others. Training includes six phases: (a) teaching the exchange of a picture symbol, (b) expanding spontaneity of the exchange and increasing the distance between the learner and his communicative partner, (c) discriminating between picture symbols, (d) making/using sentences, (e) responding to questions, and (f) commenting (Bondy & Frost, 1994).

Initial PECS training builds from the learner's interests as determined by a reinforcer assessment. It also involves two instructors. One instructor serves as the learner's communicative partner, while the other provides prompting from behind the learner. Physical prompts are used (no verbal prompts) and are faded as quickly as possible.

Cognitive Learning Strategies

Cognitive learning strategies (CLS) are techniques, rules, or principles that help individuals independently solve problems by applying learned techniques in several environments. (Schumaker, Deshler, & Denton, 1984). CLS typically consist of a series of steps that can be completed to achieve specific and generalized outcomes. For example, only two studies have utilized cognitive learning strategies, both of which were conducted by Bock (1994, 1999). Bock provided strategy instruction that resulted in individuals with autism mastering a tri-phase categorization strategy (Bock, 1994) as well as a vocational task (Bock, 1999). In both studies, generalization and maintenance were consistently achieved.

Structured Teaching

For more than 30 years educators have used structured teaching techniques to create classrooms, homes, businesses, and adult living facilities with individualized environments that foster independence for people with ASD. The base for research and resources for structured teaching was the University of North Carolina, where Schopler founded Division TEACCH—Treatment and Education of Autistic and Related Communication-Handicapped Children (Mesibov, Shea, & Schopler, 2005).

To create an environment that allows meaningful learning to occur, structured teaching concentrates on six pivotal areas: (a) physical structure of the environment, (b) a predictable sequence of activities, (c) visual schedules, (d) routines with flexibility, (e) work/activity systems, and (f) visually structured activities (Mesibov et al., 2005). These supports effectively organize or modify space and time to provide an environment and method that allow individuals with developmental disabilities to be more successful.

Structured teaching has had a positive effect with individuals with ASD. For example, Keel, Mesibov, and Woods (1997) found that with a supported employment program 89% of individuals involved in the study retained job placement in areas such as food service, clerical, and stocking, while without the structure a majority of these individuals were unemployed.

Social and Behavioral Supports

Power Card Strategy

Gagnon's (2001) Power Card strategy is a visual aid that uses a child's special interest to help him or her understand social situations, routines, the meaning of language, and the hidden curriculum. This intervention has two components: a script and the Power Card. A teacher, therapist, or parent develops a brief script written at the child's comprehension level detailing a problem situation or target behavior that includes a description of the behavior and describes how the child's special interest

Angelica Says, "Wash Those Hands"
by Rachele M. Hill

Angelica knows how important it is to keep her hands clean. She does not want to catch any yucky germs from "those babies!" Germs can cause coughing, sneezing, and runny noses. Angelica definitely does not want to catch a cold! She washes her hands often and always after using the bathroom. She knows that washing her hands helps keep her from catching a cold.

Angelica wants you to have clean hands, too. She wants you to remember to wash your hands often and every time after you go to the bathroom.

Angelica wants you to remember these three things:

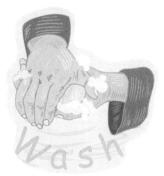

1. Wash your hands after you go to the bathroom.
2. Always use soap.
3. Dry your hands completely.

Angelica can be very bossy, but she does have manners when it comes to having clean hands. Angelica says, "Please wash your hands!"

FIGURE 5.1. Sample Power Card Scenario and Power Card.

has addressed that social challenge. This solution is then generalized back to the child. The Power Card, the size of a business card or trading card, shows a picture of the special interest and a summary of the solution and is portable, to promote generalization. The Power Card can be carried or it can be affixed inside a book, to a notebook, or to a locker. It may also be placed on the corner of a child's desk (Gagnon, 2001). This strategy has been empirically investigated in two studies. In one case, the Power Card strategy resulted in marked behavior change and generalization across settings (Keeling, Myles, Gagnon, & Simpson, 2003); in the second, a child experienced moderate success when the Power Card strategy was used (Myles, Keeling, & Van Horn, 2001). A sample Power Card scenario and a Power Card featuring Angelica from the Rugrats was used to help Marissa, a 7-year-old girl, to remember to wash her hands.

Social Stories™

A Social Story™ (Gray Center for Social Learning and Understanding, n.d.) is an individualized cognitive intervention that describes the salient social cues and appropriate responses associated with a particular social situation. It typically comprises (a) descriptive sentences that provide information about the setting, subjects, and actions, (b) directive statements about the appropriate behavioral response, (c) perspective sentences that describe the feelings and reactions of others in the targeted situation, and (d) control statements that provide analogies with related actions

---

Running

I like to run. It is fun to go real fast. It's okay to run when I am playing outside at recess. I can run when I am on the playground. I can run in the gym during P.E. It is not okay to run when I am inside my school. Running in the classroom or hallway is not safe.

My teacher worries that someone might get hurt if I run into them. When I am inside, I must walk. I will try to walk in my classroom and hallway. I will only run when I am in the gym during P.E. I will only run when I am on the playground at recess.

Correr

Quiero corer. Es divertido ir verdaderamente rapido. Esta bien corer cuando jusgo afuera en el recreo. Puedo corer en el gimnasio durante Educacion Fisica. No es bueno corer cuando estoy dentro de mi escuela. Correr en el aula o en el pasillo no es seguro.

Mi maestro sed preocupa que alguien quizas sea lesionado si choco con ellos. Cuando yo estoy adentro, debo andar. Tratare de andar en mi aula yen el pasillo. Yo solo correre cuando este en el gimnasio durante Educacion Fisica. Yo solo correre cuando este en el campo de juegos en el recreo.

Written by Jan Klein

FIGURE 5.2. Sample Social Story™.

and responses (Gray, 1995; Gray & Garand, 1993). Gray imposed additional structure on Social Stories™ by recommending a ratio of 2:5 descriptive, perspective, and/or control sentences for each directive sentence.

Gray (1995) and Gray and Garand (1993) stressed that Social Stories™ are most appropriate for students with high-functioning autism or Asperger's syndrome when constructed for an individual in a specific situation and that the entire story be presented on one piece of paper without use of visual stimuli. Swaggart et al. (1995) expanded the use of Social Stories™ to individuals with moderate-to-severe autism by using a booklet-style presentation with one sentence per page and icons to enhance students' understanding. Finally, they found that a Social Story™ could be presented to more than one student, thus demonstrating its efficacy in a small-group setting. Figure 5.2 provides a Social Story™ that was created for Mario, who has repeatedly been reprimanded for running. Mario's Social Story™ was written in Spanish, his first language, and English to facilitate understanding.

Social Stories™ have a broad application for children and youth with ASD and have been used successfully to address aggression and precursors to such behavior (Kuttler, Myles, & Carlson, 1998; Lorimer, Simpson, Myles & Ganz, 2002; Swaggart et al., 1995), hand washing (Hagiwara & Myles, 1999), on-task behavior (Hagiwara & Myles, 1999), lunch-time eating behaviors (Bledsoe, Myles, & Simpson, 2003), and social skills training/understanding (Norris & Dattilo, 1999; Rogers & Myles, 2001; Swaggart et al., 1995).

Cartooning

Cartooning helps children with ASD understand social interactions through the presentation of stick figures or similarly presented static drawings, conversation, and thought bubbles. Cartoon figures play an integral role in such intervention techniques as pragmaticism (Arwood & Brown, 1999), Comic Strip Conversations™ (Gray, 1994), and mind reading (Howlin, Baron-Cohen, & Hadwin, 1999). Cartoons, which help children with ASD to understand the messages and meanings that naturally occur in play and conversation (Attwood, 1998), is an emerging practice and has been used successfully by Parsons and Mitchell (1999) and Rogers and Myles (2001).

Stop Observe Deliberate Act (SODA)

Stop Observe Deliberate Act (SODA), a social behavioral learning strategy that uses the *think aloud, think along* model (Andrews & Mason, 1991), was created to help children and youth with AS and related disabilities "attend to relevant social cues, process these cues, ponder their relevance and meaning, and select an appropriate response during novel social interactions" (Bock, 2001, p. 273). Shown to be effective with adolescents with AS (Bock, 2002), SODA relies on using social skills developed through direct instruction or coaching. This flexible visual contains the following steps:

1. *Stop:* During the Stop phase, the user develops an organizational schema related to the event. That is, the child with AS attempts to define the activities and their sequence. In addition, the user identifies an accessible location from which to observe to obtain additional information that will facilitate successful participation in the activity.

2. *Observe:* The individual observes relevant environmental aspects. These may include conversation length, tone, and content; activity routines; nonverbal language; and strategies used to begin and end conversations.

3. *Deliberate:* In this phase, the individual with AS develops an action plan that includes three steps, identifying (a) a conversational topic, (b) strategies that facilitate successful interactions (i.e., eye contact, social distance), and (c) how the individuals thinks he will be perceived by others if he does or does not follow the event's routine.

4. *Act:* At this point, the child carries out the strategies identified in the deliberation phase. The stage serves as a platform for generalizing skills that were learned in another environment, such as in a classroom or community-based social skills group.

SODA is important in that it allows students to approach novel situations without impulsivity or anxiety and to generalize the use of social skills learned in another context.

Future Trends in Autism Spectrum Disorders

The Committee on Education Interventions for Children with Autism (2001) identified the following key areas that affect the field of autism spectrum disorders: (a) diagnosis, assessment, and prevalence, (b) the role of families, (c) effective intervention programs, and (d) ongoing training for educators and other support personnel.

Within the area of diagnosis, assessment, and prevalence, early diagnosis should be stressed, with enhanced discernment of the neurological, behavioral, and developmental characteristics of ASD that facilitate early identification. In order to allocate resources, studies of prevalence are also significant. Within this realm, the Research Council of the Division of Behavioral and Social Sciences and Education (2001) supports dissemination of information about ASD by the National Institutes of Health, the Department of Education's Office of Special Education Programs, and other professional organizations.

As primary, and often lifelong, caretakers, families should have access to the support they need in order to provide instructional and supportive strategies to their children with ASD and to mental health services, if needed. In addition, they should be provided opportunities to understand their rights as specified under the law.

Comparative studies on effective techniques should be conducted to ensure that students with ASD have access to the most appropriate methods to meet their needs. Debate about what ASD practices are most effective is often emotive rather than data-based; thus additional data on effective interventions are required.

Conclusion

Despite a 1000% increase in the prevalence of ASD between 1991–1992 and 1999–2000 (Yell & Katsiyannis, 2003), training and support for educational professionals is deficient. University programs that provide coursework on ASD and regional resource and training centers that support local schools and families are needed. According to the Committee on Educational Interventions for Children with Autism (2001), "Teachers are faced with a huge task. They must be familiar with theory and research concerning best practices . . . including methods of applied behavior analysis, naturalistic learning, assistive technology, socialization, communication, inclusion, adaptation of the environment, language interventions, assessment and the effective use of data collection systems" (p. 225).

Glossary

Applied behavior analysis—The science of human behavior; application of interventions, including discrete trial training, pivotal response training, and incidental teaching, designed to affect individual behavior.

Asperger's syndrome—A spectrum disorder marked by impaired social interactions accompanied by repetitive and stereotyped behaviors and restricted interests.

Assistive technology—Low-tech, mid-tech, or high-tech devices that aid students in daily functioning and provide them with additional means to participate in daily activities.

Autism—A spectrum disorder marked by impairments in social interactions *and* communication, as well as by restrictive, repetitive, and stereotyped movements.

Autism spectrum disorders (ASD)—Complex, lifelong developmental disorders that include autism, Asperger's syndrome, and pervasive developmental disorder—not otherwise specified, in which individuals may display impairments in reciprocal social interaction and communication skills, stereotypic behaviors, and restricted interests and activities.

Cartooning—A strategy that is used to help students with ASD understand social interactions through the presentation of stick figures and conversation/thought bubbles.

Childhood disintegrative disorder (CDD)—Also known as Heller's syndrome. A disorder in which children exhibit behaviors similar to those with autism, yet unlike autism, they experience at least two years of typical development, then experience significant regression in language, social skills, adaptive behavior, and motor skills.

Cognitive learning strategies (CLS)—Techniques, rules, or principles that help individuals independently solve problems by applying learned techniques in several environments.

Fade—Gradually taking away a prompt so that the student does not become dependent on it.

Generalization—The ability to apply information and skills across settings and with different individuals and to integrate learned material and experiences into new situations.

Initiation—A deliberate act, verbal or behavioral, to engage the interest of another person.

Modeling—Providing an example of a task, skill, or behavior for the purpose of giving the student an example of the desired behavior.

Motivation—A child's observable responsiveness to social and environmental stimuli.

Multiple cues—Information gathered from multiple components in the environment.

Pervasive developmental disorder–not otherwise specified (PDD-NOS)—A diagnostic label used to described individuals who meet some, but not all, of the criteria for autism or Asperger's syndrome.

Physical prompt—A physical cue provided to an individual to help him complete a task, such as a tap on the hand.

Power card strategy—A strategy in which a visual aid uses a child's special interest to help her understand social situations, routines, the meaning of language, and the hidden curriculum.

Priming—A strategy in which an adult previews activities to a student prior to their occurrence.

Prompting—Cueing a student either physically or verbally in order to help him complete a task.

Rett's syndrome—A disability that occurs primarily in girls, most often during the first two years of life, and is characterized by head growth deceleration, loss of motor skills (including purposeful hand movements), hand wringing or hand washing, and social and communication impairments.

Self-management—The ability of an individual to monitor and record his own behavior.

Social stories™—An individualized text or story that describes a specific social situation from the point of view of the child.

Stop observe deliberate act (SODA)—A social behavioral strategy that helps students with ASD attend to, process, and respond to social interactions.

Task analysis—Division of a skill or task into small, step-by-step components.

Theory of mind—Ability to take the perspective of another person.

Visual supports—Items that present information to a student in a visual way, such as written schedules and graphic organizers.

Verbal prompt—A verbal cue provided to an individual to help him complete a task, such as repeating the directions.

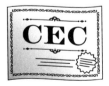

Knowledge and Skills for Entry-Level Special Education Teachers of Students With Developmental Disabilities Standards Addressed in This Chapter

Principle 1: Foundations

DD1K1   Definitions and issues related to the identification of individuals with developmental disabilities.

Principle 2: Development and Characteristics of Learners

DD2K2   Psychological, social/emotional, and motor characteristics of individuals with developmental disabilities.

Principle 4: Instructional Strategies

DD4K1   Specialized materials for individuals with developmental disabilities.

DD4K3   Specialized curriculum specifically designed to meet the needs of individuals with pervasive developmental disabilities, autism, and autism spectrum disorders.

Web Site Resources

Autism Society of America
http://www.autism-society.org

> Lists state and local autism societies, as well as resources for parents and teachers, legislative information, answers to frequently asked questions from parents about autism spectrum disorders, and an overview of the society's annual conference.

MAAP (More Advanced Individuals With Autism, Asperger Syndrome, and Pervasive Developmental Disorder [PDD])
http://www.maapservices.org/

> International support organization that provides resources for individuals with high-functioning autism, Asperger's syndrome, and PDD—not otherwise specified. Quarterly newsletters and an overview of the annual conference are available.

OASIS (Online Asperger's syndrome Information and Support)
http://www.udel.edu/bkirby/asperger/

> A starting point for those who are interested in AS. Includes information related to legal resources, as well as many links to diagnosis information, classroom management, research, parent supports, and projects. Very user-friendly, put together by parents.

Organization for Autism Research (OAR)
http://www.researchautism.org

> Formed and led by parents and grandparents of children and adults with autism. To put applied research to work providing answers to questions that parents, families, individuals with autism, teachers, and caregivers confront each day. Web site includes monthly news-letters, a comprehensive list of resources, and an overview of practical research in autism spectrum disorders.

References

American Psychiatric Association. (1994). *Diagnostic and statistical manual of mental disorders* (4th ed.). Washington, DC: Author.

American Psychiatric Association. (2000). *Diagnostic and statistical manual of mental disorders* (4th ed., text rev.). Washington, DC: Author.

Amir, R. E., Van Den Veyver, I. B., Wan, M., Tran, C. Q., Francke, U., & Zoghbi, H. Y. (1999). Rett Syndrome is caused by mutations in X-linked MECP2, encoding Methyl-CPG-Binding Protein 2. *Nature Genetics, 23*, 185–188.

Anderson, S., Taras, M., & Cannon, B. (1996). Teaching new skills to young children with autism. In C. Maurice, G. Green, & S. Luce (Eds.), *Behavioral interventions for young children with autism* (pp. 181–194). Austin, TX: PRO-ED.

Andrews J. F., & Mason, J. M. (1991). Strategy usage among deaf and hard-of-hearing readers. *Exceptional Children, 57*, 536–545.

Arwood, E., & Brown, M. M. (1999). *A guide to cartooning and flowcharting: See the ideas.* Portland, OR: Apricot.

Asperger, H. (1944). Die "autistischen psychopathen" im kindesalter. *Archiv für Psychiatrie und Nervenkrankheiten, 117*, 76–136.

Attwood, T. (1998). *Asperger's syndrome: A guide to parents and professionals.* London: Jessica Kingsley.

Aylward, E. H., Minshew, N. J., Goldstein, G., Honeycutt, N. A., Augustine, A. M., Yates, K., et al. (1999). MRI volumes of amygdala and hippocampus in non-mentally retarded autistic adolescents and adults. *Neurology, 53*, 2145–2150.

Bainbridge, N., & Myles, B. S. (1999). The use of priming to introduce toilet training to a child with autism. *Focus on Autism and Other Developmental Disabilities, 14*, 106–109.

Barnhill, G., Hagiwara, T., Myles, B. S., & Simpson, R. L. (2000). Asperger syndrome: A study of the cognitive profiles of 37 children and adolescents. *Focus on Autism and Other Developmental Disabilities, 15,* 146–153.

Baron-Cohen, S. (1992). The theory of mind hypothesis of autism: History and prospects of the idea. *Psychologist, 5*(1), 9–12.

Baron-Cohen, S. (1995). *Mindblindness.* Cambridge, MA: MIT Press.

Baron-Cohen, S. (2003). *The essential difference: The truth about the male and female brain.* New York: Basic Books.

Baron-Cohen, S., Leslie, A. M., & Frith, U. (1985). Does the autistic child have a "theory of mind"? *Cognition, 21,* 37–46.

Baron-Cohen, S., O'Riordan, M., Stone, V., Jones, R., & Plaisted, K. (1999). Recognition of faux pas by normally developing children and children with Asperger syndrome or high-functioning autism. *Journal of Autism and Developmental Disorders, 29,* 407–418.

Bernard-Opitz, V., Sriram, N., & Nakhoda-Sapuan, S. (2001a). Enhancing social problem solving in children with autism and normal children through computer-assisted instruction. *Journal of Autism and Developmental Disorders, 31,* 377–398.

Bernard-Opitz, V., Sriram, N., & Nakhoda-Sapuan, S. (2001b). Enhancing vocal imitations in children with autism using the IBM SpeechViewer. *Autism, 3,* 131–147.

Bledsoe, R., Myles, B. S., & Simpson, R. L. (2003). Use of a Social Story™ intervention to improve mealtime skills of an adolescent with Asperger syndrome. *Autism, 7,* 289–295.

Bock, M. A. (1994). Acquisition, maintenance, and generalization of a categorization strategy by children with autism. *Journal of Autism and Developmental Disabilities, 24,* 39–51.

Bock, M. A. (1999). Sorting laundry: Categorization application to an authentic learning activity by children with autism. *Focus on Autism and Other Developmental Disabilities, 14,* 220–230.

Bock, M. A. (2001). SODA strategy: Enhancing the social interaction skills of youngsters with Asperger syndrome. *Intervention in School and Clinic, 36,* 272–278.

Bock, M. A. (2002, April). *The impact of social behavioral learning strategy training on the social interaction skills of eight students with Asperger syndrome.* Paper presented at the YAI National Institute for People with Disabilities 23rd International Conference on MR/DD, New York.

Bock, M. A., & Hurlbutt, K. (2002). Preacademic and vocational assessment: The key to effective educational programming for students with autism. *Assessment for Effective Intervention, 27*(1–2), 81–88.

Bondy, A. S., & Frost, L. A. (1994). The Picture Exchange Communication System. *Focus on Autistic Behavior, 9*(3), 1–19.

Brown, C. E., & Dunn, W. (2002). *Adolescent/Adult Sensory Profile.* San Antonio, TX: Psychological Corporation.

Bryan, L. C., & Gast, D. L. (2000). Teaching on-task and on-schedule behaviors to high-functioning children with autism via picture activity schedules. *Journal of Autism and Developmental Disorders, 30,* 553–567.

Carpentieri, S. C., & Morgan, S. B. (1994). A comparison of patterns of cognitive functioning of autistic and nonautistic retarded children on the Stanford-Binet—4th ed. *Journal of Autism and Developmental Disorders, 24,* 215–223.

Carper, R. A., & Courchesne, E. (2000). Inverse correlation between frontal lobe and cerebellum sizes in children with autism. *Brain, 123,* 836–844.

Centers for Disease Control. (2007). *Prevalence of the autism spectrum disorders in multiple areas of the United States, surveillance years 2000 and 2002.* Retrieved June 27, 2007, from http://www.cdc .gov/ncbddd/dd/addmprevalence.htm

Charak, D. A., & Stella, J. L. (2002). Screening and diagnostic instruments for identification of autism spectrum disorders in children, adolescents, and young adults: A selection review. *Assessment for Effective Intervention, 27*(1–2), 5–17.

Charlop-Christy, M. H., & Carpenter, M. H. (2000). Modified incidental teaching sessions: A procedure for parents to increase spontaneous speech in their children with autism. *Journal of Positive Behavior Interventions, 2,* 98–112.

Charlop-Christy, M. H., Carpenter, M., Lee, L., LeBlanc, L. A., & Kellet, K. (2002). Using the Picture Exchange Communication System (PECS) with children with autism: Assessment of

PECS acquisition, speech, social-communicative behavior, and problem behavior. *Journal of Applied Behavior Analysis, 35,* 213–231.

Committee on Educational Interventions for Children with Autism. (2001). *Educating children with autism.* Washington, DC: Author.

Cooper, J. O., Heron, T. E., & Heward, W. L. (1987). *Applied behavior analysis.* Upper Saddle River, NJ: Prentice-Hall.

Courchesne, E., Karns, C. M., Davis, H. R., Ziccardi, R., Carper, R. A., Tigue, Z. D., et al. (2001). Unusual brain growth patterns in early life in patients with autistic disorder: An MRI study. *Neurology, 57,* 245–254.

Dales, L., Hammer, S. J., & Smith, N. J. (2001). Time trends in autism and in MMR immunization coverage in California. *Journal of the American Medical Association, 285,* 1183–1185.

Dettmer, S., Simpson, R. L., Myles, B. S., & Ganz, J. B. (2000). The use of visual supports to facilitate transitions of students with autism. *Focus on Autism and Other Developmental Disabilities, 15,* 163–169.

Durand, M. (1999). Functional communication training using assistive devices: Recruiting natural communities of reinforcement. *Journal of Applied Behavior Analysis, 32,* 247–267.

Filipek, P. A., Accardo, P. J., Baranek, G. T., Cook, E. H., Dawons, G., Gordon, B., et al. (1999). The screening and diagnosis of autistic spectrum disorders. *Journal of Autism and Developmental Disorders, 29,* 439–484.

Frith, U. (1991). *Autism and Asperger syndrome.* Cambridge, UK: Cambridge University Press.

Gagnon, E. (2001). *The Power Card strategy: Using special interests to motivate children and youth with Asperger syndrome and autism.* Shawnee Mission, KS: Autism Asperger Publishing.

Ganz, J. B., & Simpson, R. L. (2004). Effects on communicative requesting and speech development of the Picture Exchange Communication System in children with characteristics of autism. *Journal of Autism and Developmental Disorders, 34,* 395–409.

Gillberg, C., & Coleman, M. (2000). *The biology of the autistic syndromes* (3rd ed.). London: Mac Keith.

Gilliam, J. E. (1995). *Gilliam Autism Rating Scale.* Austin, TX: PRO-ED.

Gray, C. (1994). *Comic Strip Conversations™: Colorful, illustrated interactions with students with autism and related disorders.* Jenison, MI: Jenison Public Schools.

Gray, C. (1995). *Social Stories™ unlimited: Social Stories™ and Comic Strip Conversations™.* Jenison, MI: Jenison Public Schools.

Gray, C. A., & Garand, J. D. (1993). Social Stories™: Improving responses of students with autism with accurate social information. *Focus on Autistic Behavior, 8,* 1–10.

Gray Center for Social Learning and Understanding. (n.d.). *Social Stories™.* Retrieved November 16, 2005, from http://www.thegraycenter.org/socialstories.cfm.

Hagiwara, T., & Myles, B. S. (1999). A multimedia Social Story™ intervention: Teaching skills to children with autism. *Focus on Autism and Other Developmental Disabilities, 14,* 82–95.

Harris, S., Handelman, J., & Burton, J. (1990). The Stanford-Binet profiles of young children with autism. *Special Services in the School, 6,* 125–143.

Howlin, P., Baron-Cohen, S., & Hadwin, J. (1999). *Teaching children with autism to mind-read: A practical guide.* London: Wiley.

Hughes, C., Russell, J., & Robbins, T. W. (1994). Evidence for executive dysfunction in autism. *Neuropsychologia, 32,* 477–492.

Janzen, J. E. (2003). *Understanding the nature of autism: A guide to the autism spectrum disorders* (2nd ed.). San Antonio, TX: Therapy Skill Builders.

Kadesjo, B., Gillberg, C., & Nagberg, B. (1999). Autism and Asperger syndrome in seven-year-old children: A total population study. *Journal of Autism and Developmental Disorders, 29,* 327–332.

Keel, J. H., Mesibov, G. B., & Woods, A. V. (1997). TEACCH-supported employment program. *Journal of Autism and Developmental Disorders, 27*(1), 3, 7.

Keeling, K., Myles, B. S., Gagnon, E., & Simpson, R. L. (2003). Using the Power Card strategy to teach sportsmanship skills to a child with autism. *Focus on Autism and Other Developmental Disabilities, 18,* 105–111.

Kemper, T. L., & Bauman, M. (1998). Neuropathology of infantile autism. *Journal of Neuropathology and Experimental Neurology, 57,* 645–652.

Kinney, E. M., Vedora, J., & Stromer, R. (2003). Computer-presented video models to teach generative spelling to a child with an autism spectrum disorder. *Journal of Positive Behavior Interventions, 5*, 22–29.

Koegel, R. L., Bimbela, A., & Schreibman, L. (1996). Collateral effects of parent training on family interactions. *Journal of Autism and Developmental Disorders, 26*, 347–359.

Koegel, R. L., Schreibman, L., Good, A., Cerniglia, L., Murphy, C., & Koegel, L. K. (1989). *How to teach pivotal behaviors to children with autism: A training manual*. Santa Barbara: University of California.

Kuttler, S., Myles, B. S., & Carlson, J. K. (1998). The use of Social Stories™ to reduce precursors to tantrum behavior in a student with autism. *Focus on Autistic Behavior, 13*, 176–182.

Leaf, R., & McEachin, J. (1999). *A work in progress: Behavior management strategies and a curriculum for intensive behavioral treatment of autism*. New York: DRL Books.

Lord, C., Rutter, M., DiLavore, P. C., & Risi, S. (2001). *Autism Diagnostic Observation Schedule—Generic*. Los Angeles: Western Psychological Services.

Lorimer, P. A., Simpson, R., Myles, B. S., & Ganz, J. (2002). The use of Social Stories™ as a preventative behavioral intervention in a home setting with a child with autism. *Journal of Positive Behavioral Interventions, 4*(1), 53–60.

Lovaas, O. I. (1987). Behavioral treatment and normal educational and intellectual functioning in young autistic children. *Journal of Consulting and Clinical Psychology, 55*, 3–9.

MacDuff, G., Krantz, P., & McClannahan, L. (1993). Teaching children with autism to use photographic activity schedules: Maintenance and generalization of complex response chains. *Journal of Applied Behavior Analysis, 26*, 89–97.

Magiati, I., & Howlin, P. (2003). A pilot evaluation study of the Picture Exchange Communication System (PECS) for children with autistic spectrum disorders. *Autism, 7*, 297–320.

Malhotra, S., & Gupta, N. (1999). Childhood disintegrative disorder. *Journal of Autism and Developmental Disorders, 29*, 491–498.

Manjiviona, J., & Prior, M. (1999). Neuropsychological profiles of children with Asperger syndrome and autism. *Autism, 3*, 327–356.

McEachin, J. J., Smith, T., & Lovaas, O. I. (1993). Long-term outcome for children with autism who received early intensive behavioral treatment. *American Journal on Mental Retardation, 97*, 359–372.

McGee, G. G., Almeida, C., Sulzer-Azaroff, B., & Feldman, R. S. (1992). Promoting reciprocal interactions via peer incidental teaching. *Journal of Applied Behavior Analysis, 25*, 117–126.

McGee, G. G., Krantz, P. J., Mason, D., & McClannahan, L. E. (1983). A modified incidental-teaching procedure for autistic youth: Acquisition and generalization of receptive object labels. *Journal of Applied Behavior Analysis, 16*, 329–338.

McGee, G. G., Krantz, P. J., & McClannahan, L. E. (1985). The facilitative effects of incidental teaching on preposition use by autistic children. *Journal of Applied Behavior Analysis, 18*, 17–31.

McGee, G. G., Krantz, P. J., & McClannahan, L. E. (1986). An extension of incidental teaching procedures to reading instruction for autistic children. *Journal of Applied Behavior Analysis, 19*, 147–157.

Mesibov, G. B., Shea, V., & Schopler, E. (2005). *The TEACCH approach to autism spectrum disorders*. New York: Kluwer Academic/Plenum.

Minshew, N. J., Goldstein, G., Taylor, H. G., & Siegel, D. J. (1994). Academic achievement in high functioning autistic individuals. *Journal of Clinical and Experimental Neuropsychology, 16*, 261–270.

Myles, B. S., & Adreon, D. (2001). *Asperger syndrome and adolescence: Practical solutions for school success*. Shawnee Mission, KS: Autism Asperger Publishing.

Myles, B. S., & Adreon, D. (Eds.). (2001–2002). Assessment of children and youth with autism spectrum disorders [Special issue]. *Assessment for Effective Intervention, 27* (1–2).

Myles, B. S., Bock, S. J., & Simpson, R. L. (2001). *Asperger Syndrome Diagnostic Scale*. Austin, TX: PRO-ED.

Myles, B. S., Cook, K. T., Miller, N. E., Rinner, L., & Robbins, L. (2000). *Asperger syndrome and sensory issues: Practical solutions for making sense of the world*. Shawnee Mission, KS: Autism Asperger Publishing.

Myles, B. S., Hubbard, A., Swanson, T. C., Schelvan, R. L., & Simonelli, A. (2007). Autism spectrum disorders. In E. Meyen & Y. Bui (Eds.), *Exceptional children in today's school* (4th ed., pp. 245–258). Denver: Love Publishing.

Myles, B. S., Keeling, K., & Van Horn, C. (2001). Studies using the Power Card strategy. In E. Gagnon (Ed.), *The Power Card strategy: Using special interests to motivate children and youth with Asperger syndrome and autism* (pp. 51–57). Shawnee Mission, KS: Autism Asperger Publishing.

Myles, B. S., & Southwick, J. (2005). *Asperger syndrome and difficult moments: Practical solutions for tantrums, rage, and meltdowns* (2nd ed.). Shawnee Mission, KS: Autism Asperger Publishing.

Norris, C., & Dattilo, J. (1999). Evaluating effects of a Social Story™ intervention on a young girl with autism. *Focus on Autism and Other Developmental Disabilities, 14,* 180–186.

Ozonoff, S., Strayer, D., McMahon, W. M., & Filloux, F. (1995). Executive function abilities in autism and Tourette syndrome: An information processing approach. *Journal of Child Psychology and Psychiatry, 35,* 1015–1032.

Parsons, S., & Mitchell, P. (1999). What children with autism understand about thoughts and thought bubbles. *Autism, 3,* 17–38.

Pennington, B. F., & Ozonoff, S. (1996). Executive functions and developmental psychopathology. *Journal of Child Psychology and Psychiatry, 37,* 51–87.

Pierce, K., & Courchesne, E. (2001). Evidence for a cerebellar role in reduced exploration and stereotyped behavior in autism. *Biological Psychiatry, 49,* 655–664.

Pierce, K., & Schreibman, L. (1995). Increasing complex social behaviors in children with autism: Effects of peer-implemented pivotal response training. *Journal of Applied Behavior Analysis, 28,* 285–295.

Pierce, K., & Schreibman, L. (1997). Multiple peer use of pivotal response training to increase social behaviors of classmates with autism: Results from trained and untrained peers. *Journal of Applied Behavior Analysis, 30,* 157–160.

Piven, J., Arndt, S., Bailey, J., & Anderson, N. (1996). Regional brain enlargement in autism: A magnetic resonance imaging study. *Journal of American Academy of Child and Adolescent Psychiatry, 35,* 530–536.

Piven, J., Saliba, K., Bailey, J., & Arndt, S. (1997). An MRI study of autism: The cerebellum revisited. *Neurology, 49,* 546–551.

Plienis, A. J., & Romanczyk, R. G. (1985). Analyses of performance, behavior, and predictors for severely disturbed children: A comparison of adult vs. computer instruction. *Analysis and Intervention in Developmental Disabilities, 5,* 345–356.

Plotts, C., & Webber, J. (2001–2002). The role of developmental histories in the screening and diagnosis of autism spectrum disorders. *Assessment for Effective Intervention, 27*(1–2), 19–26.

Quill, K. A. (1997). Instructional considerations for young children with autism: The rationale for visually cued instruction. *Journal of Autism and Developmental Disorders, 27,* 697–714.

Quill, K. A. (2000). *Do watch listen say: Social communication intervention for children with autism.* Baltimore: Brookes.

Research Council, Division of Behavioral and Social Sciences and Education. (2001). *Educating children with autism.* Washington, DC: National Academy Press.

Reynolds, C. R., & Kamphaus, R. W. (1992). *Behavior Assessment System for Children.* Circle Pines, MN: American Guidance Service.

Rogers, M. F., & Myles, B. S. (2001). Using Social Stories™ and Comic Strip Conversations™ to interpret social situations for an adolescent with Asperger syndrome. *Intervention in School and Clinic, 36,* 310–313.

Ryu, Y. H., Lee, J. D., Yoon, P. H., Kim, D. I., Lee, H. B., & Shin, Y. J. (1999). Perfusion impairments in infantile autism on technetium-99m ethyl cysteinate dimmer brain single-photon emission tomography: Comparison with findings on magnetic resonance imaging. *European Journal of Nuclear Medicine, 26,* 253–259.

Sandberg, A. D., Ehlers, S., Hagberg, B., & Gillberg, C. (2000). The Rett syndrome complex: Communicative functions in relation to developmental level and autistic features. *Autism, 4,* 249–267.

Savner, J. L., & Myles, B. S. (2000). *Making visual supports work in the home and community: Strategies for individuals with autism and Asperger syndrome*. Shawnee Mission, KS: Autism Asperger Publishing.

Schepis, M. M., Reid, D. H., Behrmann, M. M., & Sutton, K. A. (1998). Increasing communicative interactions of young children with autism using a voice output communication aid and naturalistic teaching. *Journal of Applied Behavior Analysis, 31*, 561–578.

Schlosser, R. W., & Blischak, D. M. (2004). Effects of speech and print feedback on spelling by children with autism. *Journal of Speech, Language, and Hearing Research, 47*, 848–862.

Schlosser, R. W., Blischak, D. M., Belfiore, P., Bartley, C., & Barnett, N. (1998). The effectiveness of synthetic speech output and orthographic feedback in a student with autism: A preliminary study. *Journal of Autism and Developmental Disorders, 28*, 309–319.

Schopler, E., Lansing, M. D., Reichler, R. F., & Marcus, L. M. (2005). *Psychoeducational Profile* (3rd ed.). Austin, TX: PRO-ED.

Schopler, E., Reichler, R., & Rochen-Renner, B. (1988). *The Childhood Autism Rating Scale*. Los Angeles: Western Psychological Services.

Schreibman, L., Whalen, C., & Stahmer, A. (2000). The use of video priming to reduce disruptive transition behavior in children with autism. *Journal of Positive Behavior Interventions, 2*, 3–11.

Schultheis, S. F., Boswell, B. B., & Decker, J. (2000). Successful physical activity programming for students with autism. *Focus on Autism and Other Developmental Disabilities, 15*, 159–162.

Schumaker, J. B., Deshler, D. D., & Denton, P. (1984). *The learning strategies curriculum: The paraphrasing strategy*. Lawrence: University of Kansas Center for Research on Learning.

Schwartz, I., Garfinkle, A. N., & Bauer, J. (1998). The Picture Exchange Communication System: Communicative outcomes for young children with disabilities. *Topics in Early Childhood Special Education, 18*, 144–159.

Scott, F. J., Baron-Cohen, S., Bolton, P., & Brayne, C. (2002). Brief report: Prevalence of autism spectrum conditions in children aged 5–11 years in Cambridgeshire, UK. *Autism, 6*, 231–237.

Shipley, B. R., Lutzker, J. R., & Taubman, M. (2002). Teaching daily living skills to children with autism through instructional video modeling. *Journal of Positive Behavior Interventions, 4*, 165–175.

Sicotte, C., & Stemberger, R. M. T. (1999). Do children with PDDNOS have a theory of mind? *Journal of Autism and Developmental Disorders, 29*, 225–233.

Silver, M., & Oakes, P. (2001). Evaluation of a new computer intervention to teach people with autism or Asperger syndrome to recognize and predict emotions in others. *Autism, 5*, 299–316.

Simpson, A., Langone, J., & Ayres, K. M. (2004). Embedded video and computer based instruction to improve social skills for students with autism. *Education and Training in Developmental Disabilities, 39*, 240–252.

Simpson, R. L., & Myles, B. S. (1998). *Educating children and youth with autism: Strategies for effective practice*. Austin, TX: PRO-ED.

Smith, S. J., Murphy-Herd, M., Alvarado, D., & Glennon, N. (2005). Assistive technology supports. In B. S. Myles (Ed.), *Children and youth with Asperger syndrome: Strategies for success in inclusive settings* (pp. 107–126). Thousand Oaks, CA: Corwin.

Smith, T. (2001). Discrete trial training in the treatment of autism. *Focus on Autism and Other Developmental Disabilities, 16*, 86–92.

Stahmer, A. C. (1995). Teaching symbolic play skills to children with autism using pivotal response training. *Journal of Autism and Developmental Disorders, 25*, 123–141.

Stratton, K., Gable, A., Shetty, P., & McCormick, R. (2001). *Immunization safety review: Measles-mumps-rubella vaccine and autism*. Washington, DC: National Academy.

Swaggart, B. L., Gagnon, E., Bock, S. J., Earles, T. L., Quinn, C., Myles, B. S., et al. (1995). Using Social Stories™ to teach social and behavioral skills to children with autism. *Focus on Autistic Behavior, 10*, 1–16.

Sweeney, C. (2003, November). *The CIRCUIT evaluation*. Presentation for the Topeka ARC, Topeka, KS.

Wakefield, A. J., Murch, S. H., Anthony, A., Linnell, J., Casson, D. M., Malik, M., et al. (1988). Ileal-lymphoid-nodular hyperplasia, non-specific colitis, and pervasive developmental disorder in children. *The Lancet, 351*, 637–641.

Wilde, L. D., Koegel, L. K., & Koegel, R. L. (1992). *Increasing success in school through priming: A training manual.* Santa Barbara: University of California.

Williams, C., Wright, B., Callaghan, G., & Coughlan, B. (2002). Do children with autism learn to read more readily by computer assisted instruction or traditional book methods? A pilot study. *Autism, 6*, 71–91.

Wilson, P. G., Schepis, M. M., & Mason-Main, M. (1987). In vivo use of picture prompt training to increase independent work at a restaurant. *Journal of the Association for Persons with Severe Handicaps, 12*, 145–150.

Yell, M. L., & Katsiyannis, A. (2003). Critical issues and trends in the education of students with autism spectrum disorders: Introduction to the special issue. *Focus on Autism and Other Developmental Disabilities, 18*, 138–139.

Zanolli, K., & Daggett, J. (1998). The effects of reinforcement rate on the spontaneous social initiations of socially withdrawn preschoolers. *Journal of Applied Behavior Analysis 31*, 117–125.

Zanolli, K., Daggett, J., & Adams, R. (1996). Teaching preschool age autistic children to make spontaneous initiations to peers using priming. *Journal of Autism and Developmental Disorders, 26*, 407–422.

6

Self-Determination and Students With Developmental Disabilities

Michael L. Wehmeyer, James E. Martin, and Deanna J. Sands

Summary

Promoting and enhancing self-determination has become best practice in the education of children and youth with intellectual and developmental disabilities. This chapter provides a comprehensive overview of the self-determination construct and its application to special education, as well as a synthesis of the findings pertaining to the importance of enhanced self-determination for students with disabilities. The chapter examines four directions for promoting self-determination: (a) infusing instruction on component elements of self-determined behavior into the curriculum, (b) teaching students to self-regulate and self-manage their behavior, (c) implementing available curricular and assessment materials, and (d) involving students in educational planning and decision-making activities.

Learning Outcomes

After reading this chapter, you should be able to:

- Understand the meaning of the construct *self-determination* and its application to the education of students with disabilities.

- Identify why it is important to promote the self-determination of children and youth with disabilities.

- Identify how to infuse instruction to promote self-determination into the general curriculum.

- Implement strategies and an instructional model to teach students to self-regulate learning.

- Locate curricular and assessment resources to assist in teaching students the knowledge and skills they need to be more self-determined.

- Identify the importance of and locate resources pertaining to promoting active student involvement in educational planning and decision making.

Introduction

Since the early 1990s, research and practice in special education has emphasized the importance of promoting the *self-determination* of students with disabilities as a means to achieve the desired outcomes of enhanced self-sufficiency and greater independence. Consequently, a variety of methods, materials, and strategies to promote self-determination have been developed and evaluated for use with students with developmental disabilities. This chapter provides an overview of self-determination, an examination of its importance to students with developmental disabilities, and a summary of educational practices that can be employed to promote self-determination, particularly for students with intellectual disability and autism.

Overview of Self-Determination

What Is Self-Determination?

Webster's Third New International Dictionary of the English Language (Gove, 1967) defined *self-determination* as the "determination of one's acts or states by oneself without external compulsion" (p. 2059). The noun *determination* has a number of meanings that influence one's understanding of this definition. To make a determination means to come to a decision or to render a judgment. To act with determination means to be firm in one's resolve and resolute. One might reasonably conclude that self-determination means to make one's own decisions or to act resolutely. The source of the word *determination* in *self-determination* is, however, the philosophical doctrine of determinism.

The doctrine of determinism posits that actions are caused by events or natural laws that precede the occurrence of the action. Behavior, then, is governed by these other events or natural laws. Consider the role of genetics in human behavior as an example of determinism. We know that people act in certain ways because of their genetic makeup. Thus genes are determinants of human behavior. They cause human behavior. In our modern era, we understand that human behavior has many potential causes or determinants: genes, neurochemicals, past experience, parenting behaviors or cultural norms, religious beliefs, psychological states, emotions, and so forth.

Self-determination refers to actions that are self-caused or volitional. Moreover, self-determined behavior is more than just volitional behavior; it implies that action is in some way caused (e.g., determined) by the "self." This *self*-caused action is, by definition, set in opposition to *other*-caused action. The self-versus-other dichotomy is not just equivalent to saying that self-determination refers to actions that are caused by forces literally inside the person versus forces outside the person—genes, neurotransmitters, and other determinants are, clearly, internal to the person. Instead, the notion of self-determinism is linked to the capacity of humans to, in a sense, override other forces or determinants to act on the basis of their own will. That is why the term *volition* is important in understanding self-determination. *Volition* refers to making conscious *choices* or the actual power to make conscious choices, or will. (For an extensive treatment of definitional and theoretical models of self-determination, see Wehmeyer, Abery, Mithaug, & Stancliffe, 2003.)

Why is this important? Because too often self-determination is misunderstood to mean simply making complex decisions, setting goals, solving problems, and acting independently. The literature reports that self-determined people engage in these often complex, metacognitively based activities as a means to exert control in their lives. Many people with developmental disabilities, however, cannot solve complex problems or make complex decisions independently. If self-determination is understood solely to mean taking such actions and thus controlling one's life, it is unlikely that many people with significant cognitive impairments will be able to become self-determined.

Self-determination, however, refers to self-(versus other-) caused actions. It refers to people acting volitionally, according to their own will. Is this idea applicable to people with developmental disabilities? The clear answer is yes. Even people with severe disabilities can be supported to act more volitionally. Decisions made about their lives can take into account their preferences and interests and, thus, enable them to act according to their own will and of their own volition.

Wehmeyer and colleagues (Wehmeyer et al., 2003) defined self-determined behavior as "acting as the primary causal agent in one's life and making choices and decisions regarding one's quality of life free from undue external influence or

TABLE 6.1

Component Elements of Self-Determined Behavior

Choice-making skills

Decision-making skills

Problem-solving skills

Goal-setting and attainment skills

Independence, risk-taking, and safety skills

Self-observation, evaluation, and reinforcement skills

Self-instruction skills

Self-advocacy and leadership skills

Internal locus of control

Positive attributions of efficacy and outcome expectancy

Self-awareness

Self-knowledge

interference" (p. 177). *Causal agency* implies that it is the person who makes or causes things to happen in his or her life. Thus, people who have severe physical disabilities can employ a personal assistant to perform routine activities and, if such functions are performed under the control of that person (e.g., the person with disabilities), it is really a moot point whether the person physically performed the activity. Likewise, a person with a severe cognitive impairment may not be able to independently (e.g., alone and with no support) make a complex decision or solve a difficult problem. However, to the extent that supports are provided to enable that person to retain control over the decision-making process and to participate to the greatest extent possible, he or she can become more self-determined.

Self-determination emerges across the life span as children and adolescents learn skills and develop attitudes that enable them to be causal agents in their lives. These attitudes and abilities, the component elements of self-determined behavior, are listed in Table 6.1. Although not intended as an exhaustive list, these elements are particularly important to the emergence of self-determined behavior.

Self-Determination, Special Education Practice, and Disability

Promoting the self-determination of students with disabilities became a focal point in special education in the early 1990s along with the establishment of requirements in the Individuals with Disabilities Education Act of 1990 (IDEA) that students 16 and over receive transition services. Those requirements mandated that goals and objectives related to transition be based on student needs, taking into account student interests and preferences (§. 300.344[c]). To assist the development of procedures to involve students with disabilities in educational programming and planning, the U.S. Department of Education's Office of Special Education Programs funded projects to develop methods, materials, and strategies to promote self-determination.

The role of educators in promoting self-determination is to teach students the knowledge and skills they need to become causal agents in their lives. It is important, however, that educators remember that within the context of the disability rights and advocacy movement, the self-determination construct has been imbued with an empowerment and rights orientation. *Empowerment* is a term usually associated with social movements, typically used, as Rappaport (1981) stated, in reference to actions that "enhance the possibilities for people to control their lives" (p. 15). Individuals with disabilities (Kennedy, 1996; Ward, 1996) have been unequivocal in their understanding of self-determination as a form of empowerment.

Importance of Self-Determination to Special Education Practices

The proposition that self-determination is an important outcome if youth with disabilities are to achieve more-positive adult outcomes assumes that students with disabilities are not self-determined, and that self-determination and positive adult outcomes are causally linked. With regard to the former, a growing literature base has now documented that, in particular, people with developmental disabilities are not very self-determined (Wehmeyer, 2001; Wehmeyer et al., 2003).

A few research studies have provided evidence of the relationship between self-determination and more-positive outcomes for youths' transitions to adulthood. Wehmeyer and Schwartz (1997) measured the self-determination (SD) of 80 students with learning disabilities or mental retardation and then examined adult outcomes one year after they left high school. Students in the high SD group were more than twice as likely (80% of sample) as youth in the low SD group to be employed (40% of sample), and they earned, on average, $2.00 per hour more than students in the low SD group who were employed. Wehmeyer and Palmer (2003) conducted a second follow-up study, examining the adult status of 94 students with cognitive disabilities one and three years post-graduation. One year after high school, students in the high SD group were disproportionately likely to have moved from where they were living during high school, and by the third year they were still disproportionately likely to live somewhere other than their high school home and were significantly more likely to live independently. For employed students, those scoring higher in self-determination made statistically significant advances in obtaining job benefits, including vacation, sick leave, and health insurance, an outcome not shared by their peers in the low SD group.

Methods, Materials, and Strategies to Promote Self-Determination

This section provides directions for instruction to promote self-determination. First, we identify instructional approaches that can be infused into instruction across multiple content areas to promote the component elements of self-determined behavior. Second, we review the importance of student-directed learning strategies to achieve this outcome. Third, we examine extant curricular materials and assessments to support teachers. Finally, we discuss means to promote active student involvement in educational planning and decision making.

Infusing Instruction on Component Elements Into the Curriculum

The 2004 Amendments to the Individuals with Disabilities Education Act (IDEA) require the individualized education programs (IEPs) of all students with disabilities to contain statements regarding how the student will access the general curriculum. Wehmeyer, Field, Doren, Jones, & Mason (2004) identified two ways in which promoting self-determination will promote such access. First, school standards frequently include goals pertaining to component elements of self-determined behavior. Second, teaching students skills, such as goal setting or problem solving, that enable them to be more self-determined will also enable them to more effectively interact with the general curriculum.

So, it is more important than ever to address issues pertaining to self-determination across multiple content domains. Fortunately, recent research (Algozzine, Browder, Karvonen, Test, & Wood, 2001) has shown a number of empirically validated methods and strategies that enable students with disabilities to acquire skills and knowledge pertaining to the component elements of self-determined behavior, as listed in Table 6.1, and to learn to self-regulate learning and improve overall self-determination (Wehmeyer, Palmer, Agran, Mithaug, & Martin, 2000).

Goal Setting

Having the skills to set and attain goals is central to one's ability to act in a self-determined manner. The process of promoting goal-setting skills involves working with students to help them learn to: (a) identify and define a goal clearly and concretely, (b) develop a series of objectives or tasks to achieve the goal, and (c) specify the actions necessary to achieve the desired outcome. At each step, students must make choices and decisions about what goals they wish to pursue and what actions they wish to take to achieve their goals. Goal-setting activities can easily be incorporated into a variety of educational activities and instructional domains, as well as in educational planning.

Research has suggested some strategies to make goals both meaningful and attainable for students with disabilities. First, goals should be challenging. If they are too easy to achieve, there is no motivation to do the work necessary, nor is there a feeling of accomplishment after achieving them. Second, while it is preferable for students to set their own goals, if this is not possible and teachers must set the goals, then the student's preferences and interests should be incorporated into the goal to increase the student's motivation to pursue the goal. Goals that have personal meaning for the student are more likely to be attained (Sands & Doll, 2005).

Choice Making

Choice making (e.g., the expression of a preference between two or more options) has received considerable attention in the literature, particularly with respect to students with intellectual disabilities (Wehmeyer & Bolding, 1999, 2001). Opportunities to make choices should be available throughout a student's day, since experiences with making choices "teach" students that they can exert control over their environment. Students should be able to choose instructional activities, those with whom they engage in a task, where they engage in an activity, and whether they complete an activity at all (Brown, Appel, Corsi, & Wenig, 1993). Some students may need to learn how to make choices, particularly if previous opportunities to do so have been restricted (Wehmeyer, 1998). Further, choices can be made more meaningful for students by involving them in decisions about what, how, and why they learn (Mithaug, Mithaug, Martin, Agran, & Wehmeyer, 2003, in press). Research has also found that when students with autism have opportunities to make choices, problem behavior is reduced and adaptive behaviors are increased (Shogren, Faggella-Luby, Bae, & Wehmeyer, 2004).

Problem Solving

A problem is an activity or task for which a solution is not known or readily apparent. The process of solving a problem involves: (a) identifying and defining the problem, (b) listing possible solutions, (c) identifying the impact of each solution, (d) making a judgment about a preferred solution, and (e) evaluating the efficacy of the judgment (Wehmeyer, Agran, & Hughes, 1998). People with intellectual disabilities have been shown to generate fewer potential solutions to problems and to have greater difficulty solving complex problems (Gumpel, Tappe, & Araki, 2000), but they exhibit a greater capacity to apply metacognitive strategies to solve problems than has typically been acknowledged (Erez & Peled, 2001) and they also benefit from instructional efforts to promote this outcome (Agran, Blanchard, Hughes, & Wehmeyer, 2002; Agran & Wehmeyer, 2005; Crites & Dunn, 2004). Developing the skills associated with social problem solving may be particularly important for students with autism, given their characteristic difficulties with social–emotional understanding. Research suggests that students with autism may have difficulty understanding social and emotional cues, which limits their ability to interact with others (Wehmeyer & Shogren, in press), but interventions have been shown to be effective in improving problem-solving skills for this population (Bauminger, 2002; Bernard-Opitz, Sriram, & Nakhoda-Sapuan, 2001).

Decision Making

Decision making involves coming to a judgment about which of a number of potential options is best at a given time. Making effective decisions involves (a) identifying alternative courses of action, (b) identifying the possible consequences of each action, (c) assessing the probability of each consequence's occurrence, (d) choosing the best alternative, and (e) implementing the decision (Furby & Beyth Marom, 1992). Promoting systematic decision-making skills is best addressed at the secondary level, while at the elementary level a focus on choice making and problem solving can support the development of effective decision-making skills later in life (Wehmeyer & Shogren, in press).

Opportunities for making decisions should be embedded in the curriculum. The teacher, by supporting students in making decisions in "real-world" situations, can help them to better develop their ability to conceptualize and generalize the decision-making process. The process of evaluating alternatives is an area in which direct instruction should occur; teachers can provide support for students to develop lists of decision options, to evaluate the risk and benefit associated with a given alternative, and to evaluate biases in their decision making (Furby & Beyth Marom, 1992). Students often evaluate risk somewhat differently than adults do, perhaps because they see the excitement of risk as positive, rather than negative. However, teaching students how to evaluate and conceptualize risk, in terms of both short-term and long-term consequences, can reduce these biases (Sands & Doll, 2005).

Self-Regulation and Student-Directed Learning Skills

Each of the aforementioned areas—goal setting, choice making, problem solving, and decision making—is part of the process of enabling students to self-regulate their behavior and their lives. *Self-regulation* is the process of setting goals, developing action plans to achieve those goals, implementing and following the action plans, evaluating the outcomes of the action plan, and changing action plans if the goal was not achieved (Mithaug, 1993). Because of the importance of teaching students to self-regulate behavior and learning, student-directed learning strategies (which achieve this outcome) are discussed separately in the next section.

Self-Advocacy

Students with disabilities need to learn to advocate on their own behalf. To be an effective self-advocate, students have to learn both how to advocate and what to advocate for. In the context of the educational planning process, ample opportunities exist for students to learn and practice self-advocacy skills. Too often, the perspectives of the students have been lost because the students have not had the opportunities or the skills to express their perspective in the IEP, transition, or general educational planning meetings. A first step to enabling students to express their wants and needs during these meetings is to educate them about their rights and responsibilities in these areas. They can be taught about their educational rights and responsibilities under IDEA, about their civil rights under the Americans with Disabilities Act of 1990 (ADA), and about other rights available to citizens. Instructional strategies have been developed for teaching such knowledge to students with disabilities (Wehmeyer et al., 1998).

When helping students to learn how to advocate for themselves, the teacher should focus on teaching students how to be assertive, how to effectively communicate their perspective (either verbally or in written or pictorial form), how to negotiate, how to compromise, and how to deal with systems and bureaucracies. Students need access to real-world opportunities so that they can practice these skills. This can be done by embedding opportunities for self-advocacy within the school day—allowing students to set up a class schedule, to work out their supports with a resource room teacher or other support provider, or to participate in IEP and transition meetings.

Perceptions of Efficacy and Control

The final component elements of self-determined behavior focus on the attitudes, beliefs, and perceptions that enable people to act in a self-determined manner. Students need to develop perceptions of efficacy and control, along with self-awareness and self-knowledge, so that they will have the motivation and confidence to practice the skills discussed above. Research has shown that students with developmental disabilities tend to have less-adaptive perceptions of efficacy and outcome expectations than do students without disabilities (Wehmeyer et al., 2003). The same has been found with respect to the perceptions of students with disabilities about their ability to exert control over their environment. People who believe they have the ability to exert control over their lives and outcomes tend to be described as having an internal locus of control, whereas people who perceive that others largely control their lives and outcomes are described as having an external locus of control.

Students should be provided opportunities to develop adaptive perceptions of their efficacy in performing given behaviors and their ability to exert control over their lives. One of the simplest ways to do this is to provide students with developmental disabilities opportunities to engage in the skills discussed throughout this section. If students are able to engage in problem solving and goal setting, and to make choices and decisions that are meaningful for them, they can and will learn that they have control over their outcomes, and they will develop confidence in their ability to perform these behaviors and achieve their desired outcomes.

Self-Awareness and Self-Knowledge

For students to become more self-determined, they must possess a reasonably accurate understanding of their strengths, abilities, unique learning and support needs, and limitations. Further, they must know how to utilize this understanding to maximize success and progress. For example, Faherty (2000) developed an approach to guide children and youth with autism spectrum disorders through the process of developing an understanding of their strengths and abilities, and the impact of autism on their lives. The process has activities that encourage students to think about their strengths and abilities and activities that support students in developing and reflecting on how they learn, their sensory experiences, their artistic and technological abilities, their social and communication skills, their thoughts, and the reasons that they sometimes feel upset. It also helps students reflect on the people in their lives, including those at their school. Finally, the approach provides students with facts about autism spectrum disorders. The focus is on promoting adaptive self-awareness and supporting the student in developing both an understanding of autism and its limitations and their unique abilities and strengths as a person.

Student-Directed Learning Strategies to Promote Self-Determination

Students are more likely to become self-determined if they are supported in their efforts to learn strategies that enable them to act in a self-regulated manner, as discussed previously. Individuals can be supported to self-regulate, self-direct, or self-manage their behaviors through external operants, such as visual or audio/verbal prompts or self-recording devices, or through internal operants, such as self-instruction, self-monitoring, self-evaluation, or self-reinforcement (Agran, King-Sears, Wehmeyer, & Copeland, 2003). According to Firman, Beare, and Loyd (2002), "the ultimate goal of self-management is to move from more intrusive/external-oriented and time-consuming work contexts to more intrinsic oriented work context using self-evaluation and self-reinforcement" (p. 165). When students are taught and provided opportunities to use self-directed strategies, they gain more control over initiating tasks, moving through task sequences, evaluating their success on the task, and then reinforcing themselves for task completion. By positioning students to assume these responsibilities, we decrease their need for external support and supervision, thus promoting independence and maintenance of behaviors in classrooms and community settings (Firman et al., 2002).

These strategies can be applied to academic, vocational, community participation, and functional curriculum goals and objectives. A multitude of studies over the years confirm that positive results can be achieved even with students with significant cognitive disabilities (see Hughes et al., 2002). While many strategies can be included under the broad umbrella of "student-directed strategies," we describe here teacher planning and use of self-instruction and then explain three strategies that reflect self-directed instruction: self-monitoring, self-evaluation, and self-reinforcement.

Antecedent Cue Regulation and Self-Instruction

One of the first steps in teaching a student a new skill or behavior is to have a clear plan of the steps and sequence of the task, as well as the cues and stimuli that occur naturally within the task or learning situation. Built within the context of a task analysis, this plan clearly maps out the "instructional cues or directions, setting, teaching and task materials, opportunities for choice making and prompts and procedures for fading prompts, and consequences" (Snell & Brown, 2000, p. 151). Within this analysis, teachers must decide where and when self-directed strategies can be used in order to maximize student independence.

Teacher support can employ a system of graduated prompting using natural cues, modeled cues, physical cues, direct verbal cues, indirect verbal cues, gestural cues, or pictorial cues. The goal is to move toward self-instruction when the student has gained the skills needed to "verbalize cues that direct or maintain his or her own behavior" (Agran, Fodor-Davis, & Moore, 1986, p. 273). Several contemporary models of self-instruction include Did-Next-Now, What/Where, and the Interactive Self-Instructional Model (see Agran et al., 2003 for extensive discussion of these strategies).

Self-Monitoring and Self-Evaluation

Self-monitoring allows a student to track his or her progress through a sequence or task, whereas self-evaluation allows the student to determine that he or she has finished the task and to determine how well it went. When self-monitoring, a student can ask him- or herself a series of questions such as "What's next?" "How am I doing?" "Is it working?" or "Is this getting me to where I need to go?" Typically a student uses a checklist of steps or a set of criteria that have been provided in advance to observe and monitor progress. For example, Sands and Doll (2005) recommended the use of self-monitoring as a support to goal setting and attainment and described several methods that students can use to track their progress, through rubrics, graphs or charts, a series of audio prompts, or checklists. These same tools can be used to teach students to self-record progress. When a desired behavior or skill involves a series of steps, each step may serve as a natural cue, which then serves as a catalyst for the student to take the subsequent step. When a student has difficulty with natural cues, more-permanent prompts may be needed. Permanent prompts are "extra" stimuli or cues, such as pictures, written words, direct verbal prompts, or tape recordings, that students can use to monitor their progress within or between tasks (Browder & Bambara, 2002).

Self-monitoring is a powerful strategy that does not have to be performed with 100% accuracy or accompanied by any other intervention in order to lead to increased performance (reactive effect). For example, in a review of studies that combined the teaching of goal setting and self-monitoring, Copeland and Hughes (2002) cited five studies that found self-monitoring accuracies ranging from 40% to 100%. As had been reported in earlier research (Rosenbaum & Drabman, 1979), the studies reviewed by Copeland and Hughes indicated that not only did students' self-monitoring not have to achieve 100% accuracy in order to achieve gains in performance outcomes, but self-monitoring alone, without any other intervention, provoked changes in performance levels. Even students whose self-monitoring accuracy fell below 80% demonstrated gains in task performance. Hughes and colleagues (2002) found similar results when teaching students with extensive support needs in general education high school classes.

Self-evaluation is a summative process whereby students judge task completion and the quality of their work (Stiggins, Arter, Chappuis, & Chappuis, 2004). Again, students can ask themselves a series of questions when they are self-evaluating— "Am I done?" "How well did I do?" "What helped me the most?" Tracking systems used for self-monitoring can help a student determine that he or she has completed a task. Students can also use a set of criteria to determine task completion and quality. For example, visual models of exemplars and non-exemplars of proficient work can serve as cues to students for work that meets or does not meet expectations.

Self-Reinforcement

With self-reinforcement, students are involved in identifying and administrating their own consequences for having successfully completed a target skill or behavior. In other words, a student is taught how to reward him- or herself for a "job well done" and how to recognize errors that need to be addressed and corrected. The use of self-reinforcement should be consistent with behavioral plans in place for an individual student, with rewards both accessible and immediate.

Instructional Models to Promote Self-Determination

In addition to the strategies described above, two models of teaching have been developed expressly to promote self-determination. These differ from specific curricular approaches, described in the next section, as they are intended to guide instruction but not to curricularize the process. The Self-Determined Learning Model of Instruction (SDLMI) (Wehmeyer et al., 2000) is a model of teaching based on the component elements of self-determination, the process of self-regulated problem solving, and research on student-directed learning. Implementation of the model consists of a three-phase instructional process, depicted in Figures 6.1, 6.2, and 6.3. Each instructional phase presents a problem to be solved by the student.

The student solves each problem by posing and answering a series of four student questions per phase that students learn, modify to make their own, and apply to reach self-selected goals. Each question is linked to a set of teacher objectives. Each instructional phase includes a list of educational supports that teachers can use to enable students to self-direct learning. In each instructional phase, the student is the primary agent for choices, decisions, and actions, even when eventual actions are teacher-directed.

The student questions in the model are constructed to direct the student through a problem-solving sequence in each instructional phase. To answer the questions in this sequence, students must regulate their own problem solving by setting goals to meet needs, constructing plans to meet goals, and adjusting actions to complete plans. Thus, each instructional phase poses a problem the student must solve (What is my goal? What is my plan? What have I learned?). A series of problems is posed by the questions in each phase. The four questions differ in each phase, but they represent identical steps in the problem-solving sequence: (a) identify the problem, (b) identify potential solutions to the problem, (c) identify barriers to solving the problem, and (d) identify the consequences of each solution. These steps are fundamental steps in any problem-solving process, and they form a means–end problem-solving sequence represented by the student questions, enabling the student to solve the problem posed in each instructional phase. The solutions to the problems in each phase lead to the problem-solving sequence in the next phase. The student questions are written in first-person voice in a relatively simple format with the intention that they are the starting point for discussion between the teacher and the student. Some students will learn and use all 12 questions as they are written. Other students will need to have the questions rephrased to be more understandable. Still other students, because of the intensity of their instructional needs, may have the teacher paraphrase the questions for them.

The teacher objectives within the model are just that—the objectives a teacher will be trying to accomplish by implementing the model. In each instructional phase, the objectives are linked directly to the student questions. These objectives can be met by utilizing strategies provided in the educational supports section of the model. The emphasis in the model on the use of educational supports that are student-directed

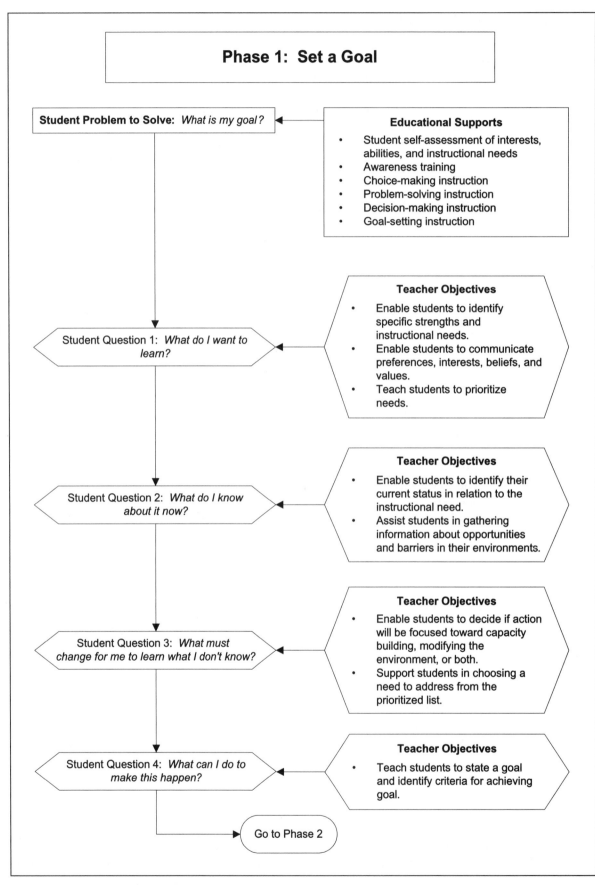

FIGURE 6.1. Phase 1 of the Self-Determined Learning Model of Instruction. Source: Wehmeyer, M. L., Sands, D. J., Knowlton, H. E., & Kozleski, E. B. (2002). *Teaching students with mental retardation: Providing access to the general education curriculum.* Baltimore: Brookes. Used with permission.

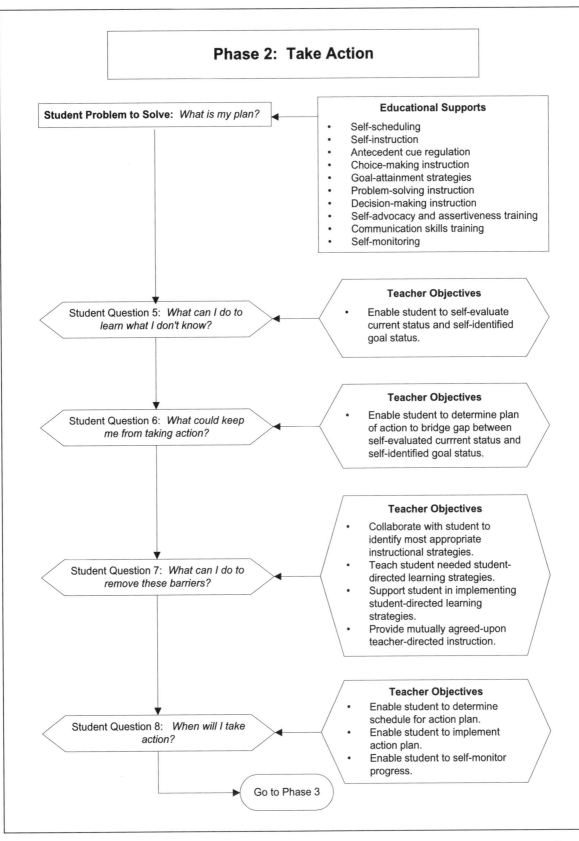

FIGURE 6.2. Phase 2 of the Self-Determined Learning Model of Instruction. Source: Wehmeyer, M. L., Sands, D. J., Knowlton, H. E., & Kozleski, E. B. (2002). *Teaching students with mental retardation: Providing access to the general education curriculum.* Baltimore: Brookes. Used with permission.

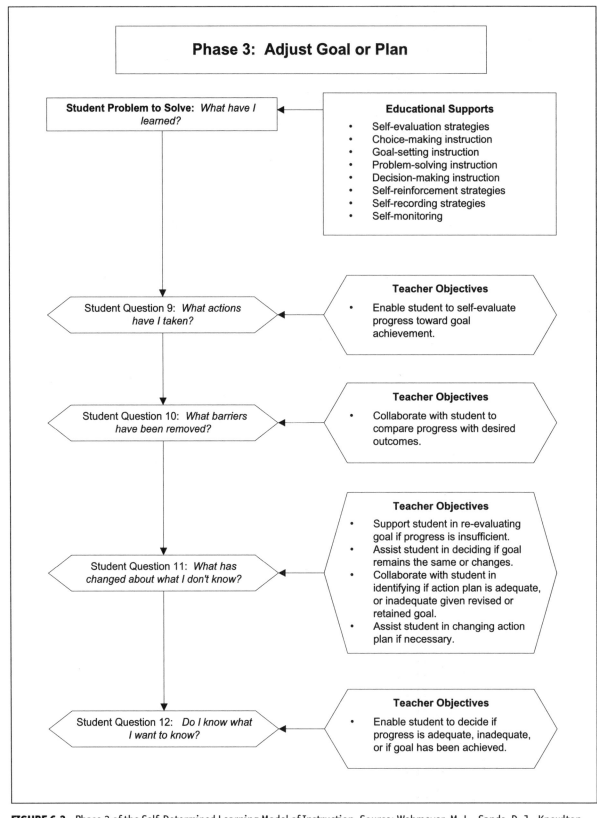

FIGURE 6.3. Phase 3 of the Self-Determined Learning Model of Instruction. Source: Wehmeyer, M. L., Sands, D. J., Knowlton, H. E., & Kozleski, E. B. (2002). *Teaching students with mental retardation: Providing access to the general education curriculum.* Baltimore: Brookes. Used with permission.

provides another means of teaching students to teach themselves. As important as this is, however, not every instructional strategy implemented will be student-directed. In some circumstances the most effective instructional method or strategy to achieve a particular educational outcome will be a teacher-directed strategy. Students who are considering what plan of action to implement to achieve a self-selected goal can recognize that teachers have expertise in instructional strategies and can take full advantage of that expertise.

Wehmeyer et al. (2000) conducted a field test of the SDLMI with 21 teachers who were responsible for the instruction of adolescents receiving special education services in two states. The teachers identified a total of 40 students with mental retardation, learning disabilities, or emotional or behavioral disorders. The field test indicated that the model was effective in enabling students to attain educationally valued goals. Additionally, significant differences were reported in pre- and post-intervention scores on self-determination, with post-intervention scores more positive than pre-intervention scores. Agran, Blanchard, and Wehmeyer (2000) conducted a study using a single-subject design to examine the efficacy of the SDLMI for adolescents with severe disabilities. Students collaborated with their teachers to implement the first phase of the model and, as a result, identified one goal as a target behavior. Before implementing phase 2 of the model, teachers and researchers collected baseline data on student performance of these goals. After baseline data collection, teachers implemented the model with students at staggered intervals, and data collection continued through the end of instructional activities and into a maintenance phase. As before, the model enabled teachers to teach students educationally valued goals. In total, 17 of the participants achieved their personal goals at or above the teacher-rated expected outcome levels. Only 2 students were rated as indicating no progress on the goal.

Students with more-severe disabilities will likely receive educational services through the age of 21. It is important that high-quality 18–21 programs ensure a strong focus on self-determination. To that end we (Wehmeyer, Garner, Lawrence, Yeager, & Davis, in press), have been engaged in the development and evaluation of a multistage model, called Beyond High School, depicted in Figure 6.4, to infuse self-determination into services and supports for 18-to-21-year-olds and to promote active student involvement.

This first stage of the Beyond High School model enables students to establish short- and long-term goals according to their own preferences, abilities, and interests. First, students are taught to self-direct the transition goal-setting, action-planning, and program-implementation process using the SDLMI. Once students learn this self-regulated learning process, they apply the first part of the SDLMI (What is my goal?) to identify goals in key transition areas, including employment, independent living, recreation and leisure, and postsecondary education. The second stage of the model involves a student-directed, person-centered planning meeting that brings together other stakeholders in the instructional process to work with students to refine goals, as needed, to support the student as he or she implements the second phase of the SDLMI (What is my plan?), and to enable the student to provide informed consent with regard to implementation of the instructional program.

During the final stage of the model, the student, with supports identified from the second stage, implements the plan, monitors his or her progress in achieving the goal, and evaluates the success of the plan, revising the goal or the plan as warranted. This is accomplished using the strategies and questions that constitute the third phase of the SDLMI. Students involved in the field test of the model were successful at achieving self-set transition goals across multiple domains (Wehmeyer et al., in press) and increased perceptions of their autonomy after involvement in the process.

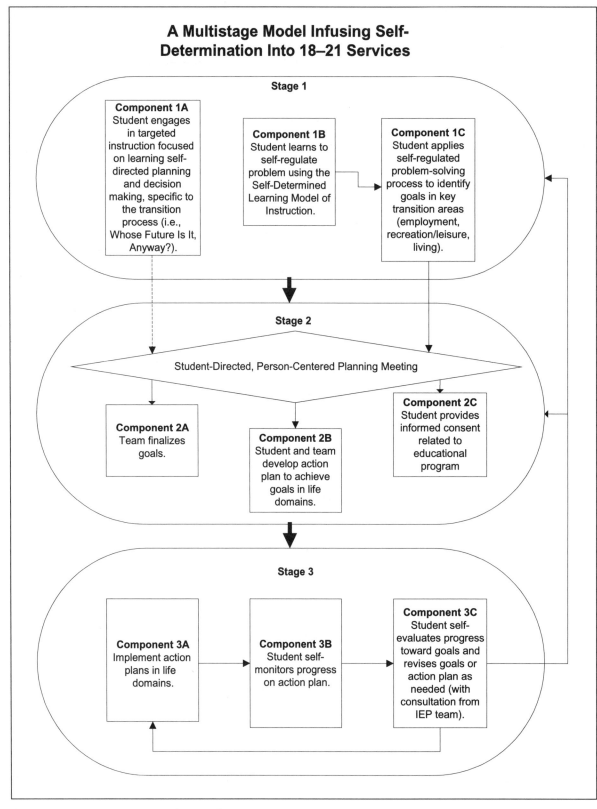

A Multistage Model Infusing Self-Determination Into 18–21 Services

Stage 1

Component 1A
Student engages in targeted instruction focused on learning self-directed planning and decision making, specific to the transition process (i.e., Whose Future Is It, Anyway?).

Component 1B
Student learns to self-regulate problem using the Self-Determined Learning Model of Instruction.

Component 1C
Student applies self-regulated problem-solving process to identify goals in key transition areas (employment, recreation/leisure, living).

Stage 2

Student-Directed, Person-Centered Planning Meeting

Component 2A
Team finalizes goals.

Component 2B
Student and team develop action plan to achieve goals in life domains.

Component 2C
Student provides informed consent related to educational program

Stage 3

Component 3A
Implement action plans in life domains.

Component 3B
Student self-monitors progress on action plan.

Component 3C
Student self-evaluates progress toward goals and revises goals or action plan as needed (with consultation from IEP team).

FIGURE 6.4. A Multistage Model Infusing Self-Determination into 18–21 Services. Source: Wehmeyer, M. L., Bolding, Yeager, & Davis (2001).

Self-Determination-Focused Curricular Materials and Assessments

The strategies discussed previously are intended to be incorporated into instruction across the curriculum. There are, however, several curricular materials and assessments available that provide direction for teachers seeking to promote student self-determination. Test, Karvonen, Wood, Browder, and Algozzine (2000) conducted an extensive review of curricular materials to promote self-determination and located 60 such products. Reviews and information about most of these procedures are available online at http://www.uncc.edu/sdsp, and, readers are referred to that resource for greater detail on the array of materials available.

A few such products have been developed explicitly for students with developmental disabilities and merit highlighting here. The first, the Self-Directed Employment (Martin, Mithaug, Husch, Frazier, & Huber Marshall, 2003; Martin, Mithaug, Oliphant, Husch, & Frazier, 2002) package, uses illustrations to enable individuals with developmental disabilities who cannot read to make basic vocational choices. Using a choose, experience, and choose again format, the person makes choices that produce a cumulative preference profile. First, each person looks at illustrations of job characteristics, job settings, and job tasks and chooses what he or she likes best. Then each person visits a job site to experience his or her choices. Then participants compare their experience to what they chose, and choose again. Teachers or employment specialists repeat this process with their students numerous times until a clear profile emerges of a person's preferred settings, tasks, and job characteristics. The choice-making tools in the Self-Directed Employment program use discrepancy logic to help produce a valid and reliable choice (Martin et al., 2003).

Imagine two illustrations, one that shows a person putting clothes into an industrial-size washing machine and another that depicts a person potting a plant. The student would be asked to mark, circle, or point to the illustration representing what he would like to do. Of course, the student would be told the meaning of the illustration before being asked to choose. Experiences at actual job sites facilitate understanding of the illustrations. After experiencing the activity at a hotel and a nursery, the person would be asked again to circle illustrations representing what he would like to do. When the person consistently circles the same illustration, a strong preference emerges. A discrepancy occurs when a chosen job characteristic, job setting, or job task preference does not match the experience the person had at the job site. This result forces the person to change job characteristics, job settings, or job tasks until he or she becomes consistent in the on-the-job experiences. Individuals with severe disabilities who completed this process were more likely to remain employed for a longer period of time compared to those who simply went to work at the first available job and did not complete the choice-making process (Martin et al., 2002).

A second curricular package, *Choose and Take Action* (Martin et al., (2004), uses the same discrepancy process as the Self-Directed Employment program (Martin et al., 2002). Instead of seeing illustrations, students watch video clips, select a job that matches their interests, try the selected job at a community site, evaluate the experience, and then make new choices on the basis of what they learned. Individuals with developmental disabilities use the *Choose and Take Action* interactive software and matching on-the-job experiences to make practical career choices. The *Choose and Take Action* instructional activities are designed to teach numerous self-determination skills, including choosing from work options, planning what to do, completing the plan, evaluating preferences and work sites, and making career choices. The *Choose and Take Action* software also introduces students to a variety of job and career possibilities and teaches them to identify what is most important to them about a job: the setting, the activity, or the characteristics. Woods, Martin, and Sylvester (2005) found that choices made by individuals with developmental disabilities match those of their parents and teachers less than a third of the time.

Student Involvement in Educational Planning and Decision Making

Research findings are beginning to emerge regarding the extent to which students are becoming involved in educational planning. Unfortunately, much of that research highlights the need to address this issue with greater focus. Zhang, Katsiyannis, and Zhang (2002) reported that most special education teachers do not provide students with opportunities to develop their course schedules and post-school plans. Powers, Turner, Matuszewski, Wilson, and Loesch (1999) reported that most students wanted to participate and become involved in their IEPs, but instead they responded passively because they felt unwelcome and not respected at their respective IEP meetings.

There is evidence, however, of some encouraging trends. In a nationwide survey, parents and school staff reported that 90% of students with mental retardation attended their IEP secondary transition meeting and that about half of the students became moderately active in educational planning discussions (Cameto, Levine, & Wagner, 2004). A three-year study of almost 400 IEP meetings and the perceptions of 1,638 IEP team members found that the students, who attended 70% of their meetings, reported knowing the reason for their meeting, knowing what to do at their meeting, and understanding what was said at these meetings significantly less than all other IEP team members (Martin, Marshall, & Sale, 2004). Martin and colleagues directly observed 109 secondary IEP meetings. They found that students talked 3% of the time and that special education teachers talked 51% of the time. Parents and special educators in this study also talked more about students' interests than students did.

In a statewide survey of special education administrators, Martin et al. (2004) found differing views of student participation, depending on administrative role. Special education directors believed significantly more than principals that students' opinions are solicited at the IEP meetings and that team members involve students in decision making. Special education teachers serving as part-time administrators indicated that the IEP team knows how to facilitate student involvement in the IEP meeting significantly less than the degree indicated by principals and special education directors. The administrators reported that students were somewhat to moderately involved in their IEP meetings.

Teaching Students to Become Involved in Their Educational Planning Meetings

Lehmann, Bassett, and Sands (1999) found that students simply do not engage in planning for their future without a structured process that expects them to become involved. Two research-based instructional tools exist to help teach students with intellectual disabilities how to become active participants in IEP meetings: *The Self-Directed IEP* (Martin, Marshall, Maxson, & Jerman, 1996) and *Whose Future Is It Anyway?* (Wehmeyer, Lawrence, et al., 2004). The Self-Directed IEP program teaches students specific process steps they can use to become active in leading their own IEP meeting. Students learn to begin the meeting by stating its purpose, introducing everyone, reviewing performance on past goals, and completing other process steps. The Whose Future Is It Anyway? program teaches students to understand their disability, make transition-related decisions, identify and secure community supports, become a self-advocate, and other important transition concepts.

Sweeney (1997) found that students with mental retardation who received instruction with the Self-Directed IEP felt more in charge of their meeting, felt more confident that their IEP goals would be attained, shared more of their dreams for life after high school, and attended more of their meetings than students who did not. Allen, Smith, Test, Flowers, and Wood (2001) and Snyder (2002) also taught Self-Directed IEP to students with mental retardation and found that they could use the process steps in their actual IEP meetings. Martin et al. (2005) found that the Self-Directed IEP had a strong impact on increasing the students' starting the meeting, talking during the meeting, and leading their own IEP meetings, compared to students who did not receive Self-Directed IEP instruction. Wehmeyer and Lawrence (1995) used an earlier version of Whose Future Is It Anyway? to improve their participation in the transition-planning process of students with intellectual and developmental disabilities.

Conclusion

Since the early 1990s, when an instructional emphasis on self-determination in special education practices first emerged, quite a bit has been accomplished. First, research has shown that students with intellectual and developmental disabilities who leave school more self-determined achieve more-positive adult outcomes. Second, empirical support validates numerous practices to teach students the component elements of self-determined behavior and shows that doing so is important to ensure student access to the general curriculum. Third, a comprehensive literature base exists to support the implementation of student-directed learning strategies for students with intellectual and developmental disabilities. Finally, a growing evidence base shows that students with intellectual and developmental disabilities can actively participate in their educational planning and decision making, and benefit when they do so. All that remains now is for teachers, like yourself, to put these practices into action. If you do so, it is evident that your students will benefit.

Glossary

Antecedent cue regulation—The use of visual or audio cues that students use to guide their behavior.

Causal agency—Acting in a way that will cause something to happen in one's life.

Choice—The expression of a preference between two or more options.

Component elements of self-determined behavior—Basic skills, knowledge, and beliefs that lead one to be more self-determined. Includes problem solving, decision making, goal setting, self-advocacy, and other skills.

Determinism—The philosophical doctrine that all actions are caused by events or natural laws that precede the occurrence of the action.

Empowerment—Usually associated with social movements; refers to actions that enhance the potential that people who have limited control over their lives will gain greater control.

Problem—An activity or a task for which a solution is not known or readily apparent.

Self-determination—Ability to act as the causal agent in one's life and to make choices and decisions that affect one's quality of life, free from undue influence or interference.

Self-evaluation—Comparison by a student of his or her performance (as tracked through self-monitoring), with a desired goal or outcome.

Self-instruction—Ability to provide verbal cues before the execution of target behaviors.

Self-monitoring—Ability to observe whether a targeted behavior has been performed and whether the response met existing, mastery criteria.

Self-regulation—Ability to set goals, developing action plans to achieve those goals, implement and follow the action plans, evaluate the outcomes of the action plan, and change action plans if the goal was not achieved.

Self-reinforcement—Ability to administer consequences to oneself.

Volition—Ability to make conscious choices about one's behavior or actions.

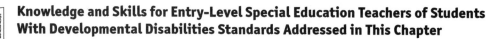

Knowledge and Skills for Entry-Level Special Education Teachers of Students With Developmental Disabilities Standards Addressed in This Chapter

Principle 1: Foundations

DD1K1   Definitions and issues related to the identification of individuals with developmental disabilities.

DD1K3   Historical foundations and classic studies of developmental disabilities.

DD1K4   Trends and practices in the field of developmental disabilities.

DD1K5   Theories of behavior problems of individuals with developmental disabilities.

Principle 2: Development and Characteristics of Learners

DD2K2   Psychological, social/emotional, and motor characteristics of individuals with developmental disabilities.

DD2K3   Identification of significant core deficit areas for individuals with pervasive developmental disabilities, autism, and autism spectrum disorder.

Principle 3: Individual Learning Differences

DD3K1   Impact of multiple disabilities on behavior.

Principle 4: Instructional Strategies

DD4K2   Evidence-based practices for teaching individuals with pervasive developmental disabilities, autism and autism spectrum disorders.

DD4K3   Specialized curriculum specifically designed to meet the needs of individuals with pervasive developmental disabilities, autism, and autism spectrum disorders.

DD4S1   Use specialized teaching strategies matched to the need of the learner.

DD4S2   Relate levels of support to the needs of the individual.

Principle 5: Learning Environments/Social Interaction

DD5S1   Provide instruction in community-based settings.

DD5S3   Use and maintain assistive technologies.

DD5S4   Structure the physical environment to provide optimal learning for individuals with developmental disabilities.

DD5S5   Plan instruction for individuals with developmental disabilities in a variety of placement settings.

Principle 7: Instructional Planning

DD7S1   Plan instruction for independent functional life skills relevant to the community, personal living, sexuality, and employment.

DD7S2   Plan and implement instruction for individuals with developmental disabilities that is both age-appropriate and ability-appropriate.

DD7S3   Select and plan for integration of related services into the instructional program for individuals with developmental disabilities.

DD7S4   Design, implement, and evaluate specialized instructional programs for persons with developmental disabilities that enhance social participation across environments.

Principle 8: Assessment

DD8K1   Specialized terminology used in the assessment of individuals with developmental disabilities.

DD8K2   Environmental assessment conditions that promote maximum performance of individuals with developmental disabilities.

DD8S1   Select, adapt, and use instructional assessment tools and methods to accommodate the abilities and needs of individuals with mental retardation and developmental disabilities.

Web Site Resources

Beach Center on Disability

http://www.beachcenter.org

Access to articles, books, and assessment materials, including the Arc's Self-Determination Scale, all available for download.

Self-Determination Synthesis Project at the University of North Carolina at Charlotte

http://www.uncc.edu/sdsp/home.asp

Product of a project funded by the U.S. Department of Education Provides numerous resources, including a searchable database of publications on self-determination.

References

Agran, M., Blanchard, C., Hughes, C., & Wehmeyer, M. L. (2002). Increasing the problem-solving skills of students with severe disabilities participating in general education. *Remedial and Special Education, 23,* 279–288.

Agran, M., Blanchard, C., & Wehmeyer, M. L. (2000). Promoting transition goals and self-determination through student-directed learning: The Self-Determined Learning Model of Instruction. *Education and Training in Mental Retardation and Developmental Disabilities, 35,* 351–364.

Agran, M., Fodor-Davis, J., & Moore, S. (1986). The effects of self-instructional training on job-task sequencing: Suggesting a problem-solving strategy. *Education and Training in Mental Retardation, 21,* 273–281.

Agran, M., King-Sears, M., Wehmeyer, M., & Copeland, S. (2003). *Teachers' guides to inclusive practices: Student-directed learning.* Baltimore: Brookes.

Agran, M., & Wehmeyer, M. (2005). Teaching problem solving to students with mental retardation. In M. Wehmeyer & M. Agran (Eds.), *Mental retardation and intellectual disabilities: Teaching students with innovative and research-based strategies* (pp. 255–271). Columbus, OH: Merrill/Prentice Hall.

Algozzine, B., Browder, D., Karvonen, M., Test, D. W., & Wood, W. M. (2001). Effects of intervention to promote self-determination for individuals with disabilities. *Review of Educational Research, 71,* 219–277.

Allen, S. K., Smith, A. C., Test, D. W., Flowers, C., & Wood, W. M. (2001). The effects of "self-directed IEP" on student participation in IEP meetings. *Career Development for Exceptional Individuals, 24,* 107–120.

Americans with Disabilities Act of 1990, 42 U.S.C. § 12101 *et seq.* (1990).

Bauminger, N. (2002). The facilitation of social-emotional understanding and social interaction in high-functioning children with autism: Intervention outcomes. *Journal of Autism and Developmental Disorders, 32,* 283–298.

Bernard-Opitz, V., Sriram, N., & Nakhoda-Sapuan, S. (2001). Enhancing social problem solving in children with autism and normal children through computer-assisted instruction. *Journal of Autism and Developmental Disorders, 31,* 377–398.

Browder, D. M., & Bambara, L. M. (2002). Home and community. In M. Snell & F. Brown (Eds.), *Instruction of students with severe disabilities* (5th ed., pp. 543–589). Upper Saddle River, NJ: Prentice Hall.

Brown, F., Appel, C., Corsi, L., & Wenig, B. (1993). Choice diversity for people with severe disabilities. *Education and Training in Mental Retardation, 28,* 318–326.

Cameto, R., Levine, P., & Wagner, M. (2004). *Transition planning for students with disabilities.* Menlo Park, CA: SRI International.

Copeland, S. R., & Hughes, C. (2002). Effects of goal setting on task performance of persons with mental retardation. *Education and Training in Mental Retardation and Developmental Disabilities, 37,* 40–54.

Crites, S. A., & Dunn, C. (2004). Teaching social problem solving to individuals with mental retardation. *Education and Training in Developmental Disabilities, 39,* 301–309.

Erez, G., & Peled, I. (2001). Cognition and metacognition: Evidence of higher thinking in problem solving of adolescents with mental retardation. *Education and Training in Mental Retardation and Developmental Disabilities, 36,* 83–93.

Faherty, C. (2000). *What does it mean to me? A workbook explaining self awareness and life lessons to the child or youth with high functioning autism or Aspergers.* Arlington, TX: Future Horizons.

Firman, K. B., Beare, P., & Loyd, R. (2002). Enhancing self-management in students with mental retardation: Extrinsic versus intrinsic procedures. *Education and Training in Mental Retardation and Developmental Disabilities, 37,* 163–171.

Furby, L., & Beyth Marom, R. (1992). Risk taking in adolescence: A decision-making perspective. *Developmental Review, 12*(1), 1–44.

Gove, P. B. (Ed.). (1967). *Webster's third new international dictionary of the English language unabridged.* Springfield, MA: Merriam-Webster.

Gumpel, T. P., Tappe, P., & Araki, C. (2000). Comparison of social problem-solving abilities among adults with and without developmental disabilities. *Education and Training in Mental Retardation and Developmental Disabilities, 35,* 259–268.

Hughes, C., Copeland, S. R., Agran, M., Wehmeyer, M. L., Rodi, M. S., & Presley, J. A. (2002). Using self-monitoring to improve performance in general education high school classes. *Education and Training in Mental Retardation and Developmental Disabilities, 37,* 262–272.

Individuals with Disabilities Education Act of 1990, 20 U.S.C. § 1400 *et seq.* (1990) (amended 1991).

Individuals with Disabilities Education Improvement Act of 2004, 118 Stat. 2647. (2004).

Kennedy, M. (1996). Self-determination and trust: My experiences and thoughts. In D. J. Sands & M. L. Wehmeyer (Eds.), *Self-determination across the life span: Independence and choice for people with disabilities* (pp. 35–47). Baltimore: Brookes.

Lehmann, J. P., Bassett, D. S., & Sands, D. J. (1999). Students' participation in transition related actions: A qualitative study. *Remedial and Special Education, 20,* 160–169.

Martin, J. E., Marshall, L. H., Maxson, L. M., & Jerman, P. L. (1996). *The self-directed IEP.* Longmont, CO: Sopris West.

Martin, J. E., Marshall, L. H., & Sale, P. (2004). A 3-year study of middle, junior high, and high school IEP meetings. *Exceptional Children, 70,* 285–297.

Martin, J. E., Marshall, L. H., Wray, D., Wells, L., O' Brien, J., Olvey, G. H., et al. (2004). *Choose and take action: Finding the right job for you.* Longmont, CO: Sopris West.

Martin, J. E., Mithaug, D. E., Husch, J. V., Frazier, E. S., & Huber Marshall, L. (2003). Optimal opportunities and adjustments during job searches by adults with severe disabilities. In D. E. Mithaug, D. Mithaug, M. Agran, J. E. Martin, & M. Wehmeyer (Eds.), *Self-determined learning theory: Predictions, prescriptions, and practice* (pp. 188–205). Mahwah, NJ: Erlbaum Associates.

Martin, J. R., Mithaug, D. E., Oliphant, J. H., Husch, J. V., & Frazier, E. S. (2002). *Self-directed employment: A handbook for transition teachers and employment specialists.* Baltimore: Brookes.

Martin, J. E., Van Dycke, J. L., Christensen, W. R., Greene, B. A., Gardner, J. E., & Lovett, D. L. (2005). *Increasing student participation in their transition IEP meetings: Establishing the self-directed IEP as an evidenced-based practice.* Manuscript submitted for publication.

Mithaug, D. E. (1993). *Self-regulation theory: How optimal adjustment maximizes gain.* Westport, CT: Praeger Publishers/Greenwood Publishing Group.

Mithaug, D. E., Mithaug, D., Agran, M., Martin, J., & Wehmeyer, M. L. (Eds.). (2003). *Self-determined learning theory: Construction, verification, and evaluation.* Mahwah, NJ: Erlbaum.

Mithaug, D. E., Mithaug, D., Agran, M., Martin, J., & Wehmeyer, M. L. (in press). *Self-instruction pedagogy: How to teach self-determined learning.* Springfield, IL: Thomas.

Powers, L. E., Turner, A., Matuszewski, J., Wilson, R., & Loesch, C. (1999). A qualitative analysis of student involvement in transition planning. *Journal for Vocational Special Needs Education, 21,* 18–26.

Rappaport, J. (1981). In praise of a paradox: A social policy of empowerment over prevention. *American Journal of Community Psychology, 9,* 1–25.

Rosenbaum, M. S., & Drabman, R. S. (1979). Self-control training in the classroom: A review and critique. *Journal of Applied Behavioral Analysis, 12,* 467–485.

Sands, D. J., & Doll, B. (2005). Teaching goal setting and decision making to students with developmental disabilities. In M. Wehmeyer & M. Agran (Eds.), *Mental retardation and intellectual disabilities: Teaching students with innovative and research-based strategies* (pp. 273–296). Columbus, OH: Merrill/Prentice Hall.

Shogren, K., Faggella-Luby, M., Bae, S. J., & Wehmeyer, M. L. (2004). The effect of choice-making as an intervention for problem behavior: A meta-analysis. *Journal of Positive Behavior Interventions, 6,* 228–237.

Snell, M., & Brown, F. (2000). Development and implementation of educational programs. In M. Snell and F. Brown (Eds.), *Instruction of students with severe disabilities* (5th ed., pp. 115–172). Upper Saddle River, NJ: Prentice Hall.

Snyder, E. P. (2002). Teaching students with combined behavioral disorders and mental retardation to lead their own IEP meetings. *Behavioral Disorders, 27,* 340–357.

Stiggins, R. J., Arter, J. A., Chappuis, J., & Chappuis, S. (2004). *Classroom assessment for student learning: Doing it right, using it well.* Portland, OR: Assessment Training Institute.

Sweeney, M. A. (1997). The effects of self-determination training on student involvement in the IEP process. *Dissertation Abstracts International, 58* (03), 821. (UMI No. 9725019).

Test, D. W., Karvonen, M., Wood, W. M., Browder, D., & Algozzine, B. (2000). Choosing a self-determination curriculum: Plan for the future. *Teaching Exceptional Children, 33*(2), 48–54.

Ward, M. J. (1996). Coming of age in the age of self-determination: A historical and personal perspective. In D. J. Sands & M. L. Wehmeyer (Eds.), *Self-determination across the life span: Independence and choice for people with disabilities* (pp. 1–16). Baltimore: Brookes.

Wehmeyer, M. L. (1998). Self-determination and individuals with significant disabilities: Examining meanings and misinterpretations. *Journal of the Association for Persons with Severe Handicaps, 23,* 5–16.

Wehmeyer, M. L. (2001). Self-determination and mental retardation. In L. M. Glidden (Ed.), *International review of research in mental retardation* (Vol. 24; pp. 1–48). San Diego, CA: Academic Press.

Wehmeyer, M. L., Abery, B., Mithaug, D. E., & Stancliffe, R. J. (2003). *Theory in self-determination: Foundations for educational practice.* Springfield, IL: Thomas.

Wehmeyer, M. L., Agran, M., & Hughes, C. (1998). *Teaching self-determination to students with disabilities: Basic skills for successful transition.* Baltimore: Brookes.

Wehmeyer, M. L., & Bolding, N. (1999). Self-determination across living and working environments: A matched-samples study of adults with mental retardation. *Mental Retardation, 37,* 353–363.

Wehmeyer, M. L., & Bolding, N. (2001). Enhanced self-determination of adults with intellectual disability as an outcome of moving to community-based work or living environments. *Journal of Intellectual Disability Research, 45*(5), 371–383.

Wehmeyer, M. L., Field, S., Doren, B., Jones, B., & Mason, C. (2004). Self-determination and student involvement in standards-based reform. *Exceptional Children, 70*, 413–425.

Wehmeyer, M. L., Garner, N., Lawrence, M., Yeager, D., & Davis, A. K. (2006). Infusing self-determination into 18–21 services: A multistage model. *Education and Training in Developmental Disabilities, 41*, 3–13.

Wehmeyer, M. L., & Lawrence, M. (1995). Whose future is it anyway? Promoting student involvement in transition planning with a student-directed process. *Career Development for Exceptional Individuals, 18*, 69–83.

Wehmeyer, M., Lawrence, M., Kelchner, K., Palmer, S., Garner, N., & Soukup, J. (2004). *Whose future is it anyway?: A student-directed transition planning process* (2nd ed.). Lawrence, KS: Beach Center on Disability.

Wehmeyer, M. L., & Palmer, S. B. (2003). Adult outcomes for students with cognitive disabilities three years after high school: The impact of self-determination. *Education and Training in Developmental Disabilities, 38*, 131–144.

Wehmeyer, M. L., Palmer, S. B., Agran, M., Mithaug, D. E., & Martin, J. (2000). Teaching students to become causal agents in their lives: The self-determined learning model of instruction. *Exceptional Children, 66*, 439–453.

Wehmeyer, M. L., Sands, D. J., Knowlton, H. E., & Kozleski, E. B. (2002). *Teaching students with mental retardation: Providing access to the general education curriculum.* Baltimore: Brookes.

Wehmeyer, M. L., & Schwartz, M. (1997). Self-determination and positive adult outcomes: A follow-up study of youth with mental retardation or learning disabilities. *Exceptional Children, 63*, 245–255.

Wehmeyer, M. L., & Shogren, K. (in press). Self-determination and learners with autism spectrum disorders. In R. Simpson & B. Myles (Eds.), *Educating children and youth with autism: Strategies for effective practice* (2nd ed.). Austin, TX: PRO-ED.

Woods, L. P., Martin, J. E., & Sylvester, L. (2005). *Choose and take action: Match between caregiver and choices made by individuals with developmental disabilities.* Unpublished manuscript, University of Oklahoma, Zarrow Center.

Zhang, D., Katsiyannis, A., & Zhang, J. (2002). Teacher and parent practice on fostering self-determination of high school students with mild disabilities. *Career Development for Exceptional Individuals, 25*, 157–169.

SECTION 3

INDIVIDUAL LEARNING DIFFERENCES

7

Culturally and Linguistically Diverse Learners With Developmental Disabilities

Scott Sparks

Summary

This chapter discusses issues faced by students with developmental disabilities from backgrounds that are culturally and linguistically diverse. Rather than presenting issues from the perspective of various ethnic groups, the chapter focuses on the broader facets of diversity within special education. Such issues include training needs for professionals, working with families, and cross-cultural adoptions. A continuing theme throughout the chapter is the critical need to respect diversity. Respect for diversity will benefit the child who has a developmental disability, since society often deals with such people as being separate from their own *culture*. Communication patterns are also discussed at some length, along with a number of curricular adaptations for use with children from culturally and linguistically diverse populations who are developmentally disabled. These adaptations focus on multicultural education as an ongoing part of the curriculum and not as a special-theme phenomenon (e.g., the birthday of a famous person from a particular ethnic group). The chapter gives suggestions for the education professional in the field of developmental disabilities with respect to teaching and working with students and families from culturally and linguistically different backgrounds. It also presents specific ideas to assist professionals in providing a truly appropriate education and a professional development package, Culture: Differences? Diversity!

Learning Outcomes

After reading this chapter, you should be able to:

- Be aware of the importance of giving respect to and displaying cultural sensitivity toward students with developmental disabilities who are culturally and linguistically diverse.

- Identify a variety of issues that present challenges to students with developmental disabilities who come from various cultural backgrounds.

- Understand factors contributing to overrepresentation of students from culturally and linguistically different backgrounds in special education.

- Appreciate the importance of "localizing" multicultural education.

- Appreciate the value of understanding a family's cultural background and values in order to provide more appropriate services.

Introduction

Today's society might be characterized as being extremely diverse. One can travel across the United States, for example, and confront a plenitude of cultural differences. More and more, this cultural diversity is evident around the world, and educators are beginning to recognize the challenges and benefits of the global range of beliefs and values (Goor,

1999; Kimberly, 1999). Education professionals who serve children and adults who have developmental disabilities need responsive, multicultural educational environments in order to facilitate appropriate growth of both learners and educators. Such learning is the focus of this chapter, from the perspectives of both the learner and the education professional.

Learning in today's classrooms brings with it the same demands that previous generations dealt with. For the child with developmental disabilities who comes from a culturally and linguistically diverse background, many individuals (e.g., school staff, fellow students, and classroom personnel) must demonstrate understanding before meaningful multicultural education can occur (Obiakor, Rotatori, & Utley, 2004).

Grossman (1995) notes that to increase respect and reduce prejudice, education professionals must "teach students that all people have similar needs, desires, and problems, but have different ways of satisfying and solving them" (p. 106). Kimberly (1999) states that respect is critical to achieving cultural sensitivity. By including aspects of a student's culture in the curriculum, educators can build respect and reduce prejudice.

Defining Culturally and Linguistically Diverse Learners with DD

In this chapter, the term *developmental disabilities* will be consistent with the constituents identified by the Division on Developmental Disabilities of the Council for Exceptional Children (CEC-DDD). Using the Vocational Rehabilitation Act of 1973 as amended in P.L. 95-602 as the source definition, the term *developmental disabilities* means:

> a severe chronic disability of an individual that (a) is attributable to a mental or physical impairment or combination of mental and physical impairments; (b) is manifested before the individual attains age 22; (c) is likely to continue indefinitely; (d) results in substantial limitations in 3 or more of the following areas of major life activity (self-care, receptive and expressive language, learning, mobility, self-direction, capacity for independent living, economic self-sufficiency); and (e) reflects the individual's needs for a combination and sequence of special, interdisciplinary, or generic services, individualized supports, or other forms of assistance that are of lifelong or extended duration and are individually planned and coordinated. (Center on State Systems and Employment, 2001)

This definition may include children and adults with cognitive disabilities, severe disabilities, autism, and other pervasive developmental disabilities. A *multicultural learner* with developmental disabilities is a learner who is culturally and linguistically diverse, with such specific cultural identifiers as race, ethnicity, gender, sexual orientation, and linguistic differences. While many ideas presented are worthwhile and relevant for any person with any disability, the chapter will not focus on other types of disabilities, such as children with sensory, behavioral, and physical disabilities.

Teacher Perspectives on Multiculturalism

Teachers' perceptions of multicultural education constitute a critical variable in the success or failure of multiculturalism. It is important for education professionals to understand students' needs in a specific classroom or learning environment and how culture affects students' learning. For instance, does cultural identification have an impact on learning style? Certainly, children with cognitive disabilities exhibit their own individual learning styles, but how much can be attributed to their cultural affiliation? Diaz (2001) notes that cultural experiences can have an effect on a child's learning style and should be considered within a multicultural curriculum. However, he notes that while certain characteristics can be attributed to culture, the education professional must be careful not to stereotype all persons within a culture just because they belong to that particular cultural group. Diaz offers excellent insights regarding the learning styles and preferences of the African American, Native Indian, Asian American, and Hispanic American cultures. Gilliland and Reyhner (1999) observe that though the auditory approach of the standard school curriculum may work well for non-Native urban students, Native Americans are highly visual learners because of their cultural upbringing, and they need modifications in the curriculum that support visual learners. This type of learning and instructional style difference is just one of countless culturally related differences in a wide variety of cultural groups (Grossman, Obiakor, & Utley, 2003).

It is critical that educators know and use the terminology of multicultural education in a curriculum that serves students from cultural and linguistically diverse backgrounds. Education professionals must develop awareness of this language in order to interpret research and to better serve children in an appropriate and sensitive manner. Issues related to the use of appropriate language will be discussed later in the chapter.

As noted earlier, showing respect for the cultural values of others is an integral aspect of becoming culturally sensitive. The education professional who works with people with developmental disabilities who are from culturally and linguistically diverse groups must be culturally sensitive especially in view of the disproportionate number of minorities who receive special education services (Taylor & Whittaker, 2003). Giving respect allows the professional to break through barriers (e.g., understanding that the word *disability* and other such nomenclature may be laden with a range of positive and negative implications from the family's perspective) and facilitate more-positive interactions with the student.

In many cultures, having a family member with a disability may bring shame and have other negative consequences in the family's community. Before an education professional can work effectively with a child from such a background, it is of paramount importance that he or she understands the family's value system and other cultural characteristics. Key behaviors that the education professional should demonstrate include (a) assuring confidentiality, (b) keeping language focused on positive future goals rather than dwelling on past negative experiences, and (c) making sure that actions and words are consistent.

When interacting with others from culturally different backgrounds, one must be careful not to stereotype them on the basis of ethnicity or other cultural factors. For example, Klein (1995) points out several stereotypical misconceptions about people from the Appalachian culture. While those who live in Appalachia are not viewed as a distinct ethnic cultural group, the region does represent a wide range of behaviors that are identified with Appalachian culture. People from Appalachia are often referred to as "hillbillies" or "poor whites," and it has been a common misconception that they inbreed and produce a large number of children with serious disabilities. Such myths about Appalachia have one thing in common: They have mostly negative connotations. Every culturally and linguistically diverse group is a target for such misconceptions, and unfortunately the overwhelming result of such stereotypes is a negative viewpoint. An open mind and a positive attitude are prerequisites for education professionals who may be working with students from a culturally and linguistically different background. These attributes can increase the probability that professionals and family members can agree on shared meaning and appropriate outcomes for children with developmental disabilities.

To understand any culturally or linguistically diverse group requires some degree of personal effort. No one individual can know everything about all the individual cultures represented worldwide, even those in the United States. Thus, it seems more reasonable that the education professional should focus his or her efforts on raising personal awareness by examining specific groups of individuals that he or she will encounter in professional and private venues. This localization of multiculturalism serves to make it (a) less daunting (i.e., less overwhelming), (b) more meaningful, and (c) immediately relevant to what is being presented.

Baruth and Manning (2004) offer the following ideas to assist the professional in developing an understanding of culturally and linguistically diverse learners:

1. Read textbooks, journal articles, and other written material on cultural diversity and teaching/learning in multicultural settings.

2. Request information from organizations that disseminate objective information and promote the various cultures.

3. Meet on a first-hand basis culturally diverse learners and their families (perhaps in their homes) to gain a better understanding of what it means to be a culturally different learner.

4. Attend conferences that focus on cultural diversity and working with children and adolescents from the various cultures.

5. Read about cultural diversity in books and magazines that are written primarily for children and adolescents. (p. 163)

Dong (2005) reinforces the notion of using reading and literature in a cultural response approach. This approach utilizes small-group reading and discussion about different cultures in a classroom or other learning setting. The small-group experiences facilitate student empathy and understanding.

The manner in which education professionals communicate with persons from culturally and linguistically different backgrounds makes a significant difference in being accepted or rejected by them. The language one uses to refer to an ethnic group, for instance, can clearly indicate a particular cultural bias (e.g., using insulting terms when referring to another person's ethnicity). Lynch and Hanson (1998) suggest that communication effectiveness may be improved when the professional:

1. Respects individuals from other cultures

2. Makes continued and sincere attempts to understand the world from others' points of view

3. Is open to new learning

4. Is flexible

5. Has a sense of humor

6. Tolerates ambiguity well

7. Approaches others with a desire to learn. (p. 77)

Likewise, the body language that a professional uses in working with culturally and linguistically different people may exhibit cultural bias (e.g., unwillingness to shake hands, hesitancy to use the same water fountains). Such nonverbally communicated biases are typically presented in very subtle ways, and often the education professional who exhibits such behaviors is unaware that he or she is projecting cultural bias to others. To the person who is culturally and linguistically different, however, these signals can be very apparent, whether or not a disability is present.

The above suggests the importance of developing a level of self-awareness regarding one's own culture (Goor, 1999). By thinking of oneself in cultural terms, a person develops sensitivity to a variety of cultural issues such as family heritage, beliefs, and values. Chapter 8 presents a more detailed description of many of these variables.

Family Perspectives on Multiculturalism

A family's cultural values and beliefs have powerful influences on the growth and development of its family member who has developmental disabilities. Education professionals who work with students with developmental disabilities are mandated to work with parents to develop individualized education programs (IEPs) for children receiving special education services (Individuals with Disabilities Education Improvement Act of 2004). Working with families who are culturally and linguistically different requires a clear understanding of family cultural values and beliefs, coupled with best practices that reflect sensitivity to student and family differences. An important consideration when working with culturally and linguistically different families is to avoid making unfounded generalizations on the basis of perceived involvement in their child's education. For example, Grossman (1995) observed that migrant Hispanic children often miss a great deal of school, and as a result, education professionals may erroneously assume that Hispanic Americans generally devalue education. While the economic realities of being a migrant worker seem obvious, such overgeneralizations are frequently made with regard to low-income families who are culturally and linguistically diverse. Many families cannot take the time to attend meetings at schools or to attend scheduled parent/teacher nights because of "survival" considerations (e.g., transportation, child-care scheduling, the costs of feeding a family). In rural areas, distance alone represents a major barrier when the school is a considerable distance away and fuel costs are high in the region.

Harry (1992) noted that another common misconception among education professionals serving children with developmental disabilities is that they have an obligation to "train" or "educate" parents in terms of education issues and best practice parenting strategies. Many Web sites currently accessible on the Internet reflect such a mind-set, offering parenting education and training programs (see, e.g., Kid-Source Online, 2000, and Educator's Reference Desk, n.d.). However, such practices reveal a lack of respect for diverse parenting styles and are not appropriate in relationships that strive to be sensitive to cultural and linguistic diversity. To assume that a parent needs parenting education is both egocentric and an invasion of privacy. A preferred best practice approach is for the education professional to learn from individual families by (a) listening to what family members say about their respective cultural values and (b) gaining insights and trust before giving advice about private lives (Roach, 1994). Home visits can be an excellent way to develop trust and gain the needed cultural insight into a family.

Learning From and Empowering the Family

The process of gathering information about a particular family's cultural habits and values involves a high level of continuous learning on the part of the education professional. By making observations in the home and talking with family members, an education professional can gain valuable information about (a) the learning habits of individual children and (b) the expectations of parents for their children. When families come to realize that the education professional's goal is to provide the best possible education that will maintain cultural integrity for their children, they may become more cooperative. Barbour and Barbour (2005) suggest that education professionals involve parents by asking them to contribute materials about their culture for use in the classroom. They also encourage education professionals to invite minority parents to speak about their cultures and beliefs, or perhaps to demonstrate skills they have learned in their culture (e.g., basket making, cooking, silver work). Inviting family members into a classroom for a participation visit in which they share or read a story or some other cultural activity with the class is a positive way of involving the family. Learning from and involving families helps to increase family interest in their children's education and assists education professionals in delivering more meaningful curricula to students.

Hildebrand, Phenice, Gray, and Hines (2000) discuss several principles for empowering families. This philosophy is designed to assist individuals and families in taking charge of their future by encouraging decision making and weighing alternatives.

> The four principles put forth are: (1) The professional's task is one of identifying a family's strengths and building upon those strengths for the good of the individual family member as well as the family as a whole, (2) The methods and strategies selected by professionals to achieve goals will enable and empower families to make informed decisions themselves, (3) The approach will be one of a cooperative partnership with families, as families recognize their own needs and decide what steps they want to take to fulfill their needs, and (4) The goal is to strengthen the available human and material resources in the total community—within the individual, family, school, service clubs, religious organizations and neighborhood. (pp. 40–41)

The concept of empowering parents implies that they will become actively involved in their child's education and gain the tools to overcome the negative images and stereotypes often portrayed by the media regarding minority communities. However, many families will still need information about teaching in order to work effectively at home with their children (Berger, 2003).

Cross-Cultural Foster Care and Adoption

A disturbing trend both abroad and in the United States is the increase of cross-cultural foster-care placements and adoptions (Timpson, 1993; Van Krieken, 1999). In many of these situations, families who have different backgrounds from those of the children being considered for adoption may take children into their family while (a) ignoring the child's unique cultural and linguistic background, and (b) expecting the child to adopt the value systems of the parents of the new family. Because of such practices, considerable social breakdown has occurred among many culturally and linguistically different groups, and children have subsequently experienced serious identity crises. Timpson notes that the child welfare system itself has been a cause of social breakdown by taking children away from their culture and placing them in culturally different settings. Today, most minority groups oppose this type of foster placement or adoption, because the foster or adoptive family cannot pass the child's culture on to the child unless they have experienced it and identify with it themselves. This includes using native language, following cultural traditions, and actively living the culture of the child. The current trend in this area has a strong international aspect, as it has been estimated that international adoptions in the United States have increased by 300% since 1992 (Coughlin & Abramovitz, 2005).

In the case of Native Americans, placement in non-Native families was seen as necessary, given the reluctance of Native American adults to become foster or adoptive parents. Once in non-Native living situations, however, many Native American youth suffered an identity crisis and had difficulty defining their own cultural being.

Mannes (1993a) reports that by 1974 approximately 25% to 35% of Native American young people had been separated from their families. Families play crucial roles in (a) socializing children in their Native culture, (b) helping them define their eventual place in the social order, and (c) helping to shape and mediate family members' definitions of themselves as individuals. Separating large numbers of children only serves to perpetuate self-concept difficulties for children and frequently leads to placement in a special education setting and a developmental disabilities label.

In 1978 passage of the Indian Child Welfare Act (P.L. 95-608) established a number of procedural directives and standards aimed at strengthening tribal sovereignty and stopping transracial placement practices (Mannes, 1993a). However, tribally based child welfare programs seem to be responding to their increasing caseloads by acting just as other jurisdictional units have historically behaved—they are breaking up Native American families, separating children from their parents, and making extensive use of out-of-home care. This perpetuation of bad practices in foster placement for Native Americans only serves to alienate these children further from their indigenous culture. One can assume that many children from other culturally and linguistically diverse backgrounds who are placed outside their respective cultures feel the same kinds of effects.

Creating motivation to achieve among children requires a great deal of encouragement from family members and school personnel. Children need role models in their families who will encourage their achievement and recognize it appropriately in culturally sensitive ways. Children with developmental disabilities often have difficulties with both the academic and the social aspects of school and need motivation provided by others to help them develop their own internal motivation. However, achievement motivation is significantly compromised when a child's family (a) is very poor, (b) is living at a subsistence level, (c) has alcohol and/or drug problems, or (d) frequently mistreats children in the family.

Mannes (1993b) notes that "adults who spent much of their childhood in some form of out-of-home care . . . are now establishing a new wave of troubled families, producing a new cohort of children experiencing difficulties, and forcing child welfare programs to deal with the placement of children in out-of-home care" (p. 143). This vicious cycle of troubled families must be addressed before any significant achievement motivation can be developed in the child's own native culture.

The family preservation approach calls for creating a service continuum that will deliver services concerned with basic life skills and environmental problems to children and parents in normalized settings such as the home, render services that support and strengthen families, and employ the person-in-environment perspective (Mannes, 1993b). Likewise, efforts at developing self-determination within the context of a child's culture, such as that used in the Dine (Navajo) culture, should be encouraged (Frankland, Turnbull, & Wehmeyer, 2004).

The teacher's role in serving these children is no different than the role in serving any other child from a culturally and/or linguistically different background. Teachers should make every effort to ascertain the child's "whole reality" and work within its confines while still giving positive cultural images.

Language

Within the context of the curriculum, language can be a useful tool for infusing multiculturalism into the classroom routine of children with developmental disabilities. Children with developmental disabilities may feel alienated because of poor English skills and may not be able to keep up with their classmates either academically or socially. The task of the education professional in this case is to help the student develop specific competencies that his or her peers can see and appreciate. One of the most obvious methods to use in this situation is to have the student highlight his or her strengths by utilizing native language skills. For example, reading a book in another language may impress peers, and speaking fluently in his or her native tongue may be perceived favorably. The student might also take part in helping other students learn words and phrases in his or her language. The education professional can develop activities about the student's home country to foster understanding and ultimately acceptance. Through such activities, peers will more likely model behavior and accept the language-different student.

Rodriguez and Higgins (2005) cite research that supports the notion that children must practice English with English-speaking peers in order to develop these language skills most efficiently. This "sharing" of language enables children to practice linguistic and social skills that are important in mainstream society. As an example, Marcus and Ames (1998) describe how cross over training and a whole-school approach can help preschool children with disabilities to develop language skills. When working with students from culturally and linguistically diverse backgrounds, the education professional should create a language-rich environment in the classroom, in which both English and other languages are spoken frequently and encouraged.

It is also best practice for the education professional to be aware of language differences *between* students in specific cultural and linguistic groups. For example, some Asian cultures give great deference to adult authority and place value on individuals' remaining "quiet" in the presence of others, while other Asian groups may place great emphasis on active inquiry by the individual (Parette & Huer, 2002). The education professional must be aware of such communication differences when planning the curriculum for an individual class and when making decisions about communication styles to be used with particular students.

One must be realistic about expectations for students with developmental disabilities who come from non-English-speaking backgrounds, particularly with regard to learning to speak English like a natural speaker. Banks and Banks (2004) note that it takes a typically developing student five to seven years to reach the native-like facility with the English language that is needed to perform well on academic tasks. An important implication of this timeline is the need for language education that embraces the cultural needs of non-English speakers while at the same time emphasizing English as the dominant language in the United States and the need for its mastery. Banks and Banks suggest that at least 50% of academic instruction should be in the student's native tongue so that the student will be able to meet the cognitive demands of the curriculum until English usage is appropriate for total academic instruction. However, other ideas have been presented that emphasize immersion in English with little use of the child's native language.

By building language into the curriculum, the education professional is sending a message that the language of every student is important and should be preserved. The culturally sensitive education professional will identify and build on the learner's strengths and interests (Lenters, 2004). Grossman (1995) points out that "rejecting students' native languages can alienate students and lead them to develop poor self-concepts" (p. 187).

Traditions and Conflict

Certain cultural beliefs of persons with developmental disabilities may come into conflict with U.S. law (using peyote for Native American religious rituals, for example). When such conflict occurs, the minority culture must either change or accept the legal and social consequences of its continued cultural practices. Of course, such a situation raises a legitimate concern about who makes such cultural decisions and how they are made. The education professional who works with students with developmental disabilities should be aware of such legal conflicts and seek positive solutions rather than treating traditional cultural practices with disrespect. Sometimes the health-care practices of families or minority communities may deviate markedly from what is practiced in the dominant, mainstream society. When this occurs, those practices may sometimes be scrutinized, viewed negatively, and deemed inappropriate by people who represent the dominant culture. Children with developmental disabilities within the minority communities that demonstrate and value "unacceptable" practices may be made to feel that their culture and practices are unacceptable. For example, in such instances where the individual chooses to disrespect traditional cultural experiences because of the "perceived inappropriateness" of those in the mainstream, the individual can potentially be made to view his or her own experiences as something that is "not good." The purpose of multicultural education is not to judge another's culture but to gain understanding from another's perspective. While conflicting values should be confronted and discussed in the classroom so that students will be able to make a cultural choice with full understanding of the consequences, the educator's personal judgments should be muted.

Developmental Disability as a Culture

For the person with a developmental disability, the disability is often seen as a predominant feature of the individual's culture. In American society, it is common to group people with disabilities in what has been referred to as a "handicapped culture." Indeed, because of this cultural identification, this issue should be dealt with in the context of multicultural education (Baruth & Manning, 2004). In a multicultural perspective, a disability would be accepted as a part of the normalcy of the individual. If the concept of "normal" is embraced from an individual perspective rather than a group perspective, being normal becomes the everyday experience of every person. It is difficult to define "normal" from a group perspective. The reader is encouraged to ask a group of people who among them is normal and what beliefs are acceptable within the context of normalcy. The perceptions of normalcy that would be offered might include such diverse responses as "having sex before marriage," "recreational drugs are okay," "aliens exist," or "women in wheelchairs cannot bear children." Defining a developmental disability as a part of a person's normal culture would seem to gain a greater likelihood of acceptance by others.

The Role of the Community

Minority communities have the potential to address many of the problems that families of children with developmental disabilities face in dealing with school systems. By supporting curricula that are culturally sensitive and celebrate the many facets of culture, a community can send a positive message about the importance of maintaining one's cultural identity. As Baruth and Manning (2004) put it, "the home and community can serve as powerful and positive forces to help reinforce the efforts of the school" (p. 190). Lynch and Hanson (1998) point out that by engaging in such activities as cultural celebrations and holidays, worship, and community projects a person may increase his or her understanding and appreciation of different cultures. Important community landmarks exist in all locales, and members of the community have an obligation to make children aware of these sites and to encourage their visits to them. Communities have material resources that education professionals and parents can use in teaching children about culturally and linguistically diverse groups (Barbour & Barbour, 2005). Through positive community involvement, families, teachers, and community members learn about the role that schools and a good education play in building strong communities. This type of collaboration is a significant statement of support for students and their individual cultures.

Culture: Differences? Diversity!

The Division on Developmental Disabilities (DDD) of the Council for Exceptional Children (CEC) has been updating and using a professional development package—Culture: Differences? Diversity! (CDD)—developed by the Ohio Federation Council for Exceptional Children (OFCEC) Standing Committee on Multicultural and Ethnic Concerns (Lockwood, Ford, Sparks, & Allen, 1991). Based on several years of study by the committee members who developed CDD, the framework for this professional development package was presented by DDD in 2003 at the CEC International Convention in Seattle, Washington (Lockwood, 2003). The professional development materials employ a "trainer of trainers" model to allow for rapid dissemination to practitioners in the field. The materials are also designed so that the content may be adapted, or "localized," for specific cultural groups in communities where it is to be used. Because many recipients of the professional development will serve in positions across the United States and abroad, the teacher preparation programs and in-service providers using CDD may have to "globalize" CDD content to address the needs of unique groups of people in varying communities. As noted earlier, however, it is practically impossible to become culturally knowledgeable about the thousands of cultures represented within the United States and internationally. By localizing multicultural professional development experiences, the education professional does not feel so overwhelmed and sees an immediate relevance to what is being presented. Naturally, CDD focuses on serving learners who have developmental disabilities by helping education professionals become culturally sensitive and better able to meet the diverse needs of the students with whom they are working.

CDD trainings have two parts: Part A is designed to develop an awareness mind-set. Part B is designed to provide in-depth exploration related to the designated topics to be infused with multicultural concepts. This is important because values and attitudes of educators have a direct impact on the design and implementation of learning environments/services for culturally and linguistically diverse learners as well as interactions with their families. Before conducting the professional development activity, the leader should (a) have actively participated in at least one structured multicultural training program, (b) be familiar and comfortable with a multicultural frame of reference and concepts as discussed in CDD, (c) have completed independent research and readings in the area of cultural diversity, (d) have knowledge of multicultural resources/references (written and human), and (e) familiarize himself or herself with the local cultural groups included in the schools of professional development participants.

The professional development activity consists of exploration activities in five component areas that serve as the foundation for CDD:

1. Acquiring cultural awareness of culturally and linguistically diverse groups as well as gaining knowledge about one's own culture. Awareness is always the first step in becoming culturally accepting.

2. Understanding cultural differences that learners bring to the educational environment (different values and belief systems) that will allow them to respond differently from each other and also the teachers they may have. Educators must be aware of and understand the differences, identify the many similarities between cultures, and begin to respect the right to be different.

3. Appreciating the diversity of culturally and linguistically diverse learners and their families and being culturally sensitive. Educators have a responsibility to identify what is important to individual groups and to demonstrate respect as they, the educators, work with the students and their families in the learning environment.

4. Valuing diversity, which begins with self-valuing and discovering what and how individuals feel about themselves. Examining one's own value systems and attitudes is a prerequisite for understanding the role that self-knowledge plays in self-valuing. Educators who demonstrate a clear cultural self-identity can assist culturally and linguistically diverse learners with this important need, with the end result being improved self-esteem.

5. Making a commitment to appropriately educate culturally and linguistically diverse learners, to address the unique educational needs of these learners and to be motivated to provide quality education and services to and for them.

Each area is progressive, building on previously addressed areas so that the educational professional begins with awareness and ends with commitment. This progression of cultural exploration cannot be changed. It is a crucial part of CDD. Ideally, the professional development activity is conducted over a two-day period and focuses primarily on the awareness component, with the understanding that participants will complete the other four areas on their own, since the timeline for moving from awareness to commitment varies for each individual. CDD can be used without the formal professional development approach, but it is most effectively utilized in conjunction with the training.

A videotape used as a visual support for CDD addresses definitions to facilitate initial discussions and identifies nine characteristics of all cultural groups. It also shows several vignettes of education professionals in different school settings as they share their experiences with culturally and linguistically diverse learners and their parents. The nine characteristics that were identified as existing across all cultural groups are (a) family systems, (b) roles and responsibilities, (c) child-rearing, (d) communication, (e) religious beliefs, (f) lifestyles, (g) health practices, (h) learning styles, and (i) parental attitudes about education.

Individual groups exhibit responses to developmental disabilities ranging from complete acceptance to non-acceptance. Some typical responses or feelings expressed about a disability may be "the disability is fate," "it's my/our fault," or "it's our responsibility." Culturally and linguistically diverse parents and family members can also share feelings of shame and/or embarrassment. Individual families may not seek assistance for their children and may be reluctant to accept assistance when it is offered. CDD attempts to bring these issues to the forefront for discussion purposes during training.

A typical CDD professional development activity begins with an "icebreaker" to facilitate group involvement. For example, a person's first name is written vertically and a descriptive word about the person connected to each letter of his or her name. This generates discussion and provides insight for individual participants. Following the short icebreaker activity, small-group activities are initiated. In the awareness stage, activities can include preparing family trees, developing self-profiles, and using self-identification circles. Each small-group activity is followed by a large-group discussion of each small group's activities. The video shows characteristics of culture and other sensitivity issues.

CDD represents a resource that addresses a frequently mentioned weakness in multicultural education: lack of professional development experiences for pre-service and in-service educators. It provides a guide for users, but does not incorporate stereotypical or easy answers for becoming culturally sensitive. The professional development is designed to provoke thought and understanding that will lead to the ultimate goal of commitment to quality multicultural education.

Conclusion

Multicultural education for people who have developmental disabilities is important, but it is especially critical for those education professionals who serve such students in school settings. Development of this cultural sensitivity holds the potential to create a world with fewer culturally insensitive people and more people who have greater appreciation of cultural diversity.

People with developmental disabilities are frequently regarded as having their own handicapped culture. Educators must dispel misconceptions about these students in order to serve them appropriately. For instance, a person's disability has an impact on learning style, but that person's primary culture may have an even greater impact. To focus on the disability alone serves to devalue the cultural aspects of a person's life. It is hoped that educators of people with developmental disabilities will adopt a holistic perspective when developing curricula and will learn to serve and understand the "whole person"—not just the person's disability. Every special educator should embrace the concept of individual normalcy.

Modifying instruction to accommodate culturally and linguistically diverse students is crucial for their academic success. By incorporating cultural and language differences into the curriculum, the educator can foster understanding between students. Further, by being aware of one's own language usage with respect to cultural and linguistic differences, the education professional can recognize and better appreciate those students with linguistic differences. The same approach should be used on the cultural side of this equation. Language usage can demonstrate acceptance, rejection, and a multitude of emotional feelings between these two extreme reactions. Use of interpreters and translators can avoid common misunderstandings. Bilingual education gives linguistically diverse students a chance to succeed academically and socially. When bilingual instruction is unavailable, English as a Second Language (ESL) instruction is preferable to having little or no language accommodation whatsoever.

Respecting cultural values different from one's own is a hallmark in multicultural education in both typical and special education settings. Respecting values that differ from one's own can be difficult, but it pays tremendous dividends with regard to understanding and appreciating diversity. Respect and sincere listening skills can lead to trust and effective multicultural educational practice.

There is a lack of appropriate multicultural preservice preparation and in-service professional development programs. Culture: Differences? Diversity! was discussed as one program that targets the higher-education community and serves as a resource for in-service leaders as well. CDD emphasizes five stepwise components that lead to a commitment to quality multicultural education for children with developmental disabilities. Skilled professionals are in demand in multicultural education, and higher education must answer the call to deliver such training.

Multicultural sensitivity is the result of a *process*; it does not happen without personal effort. One must study cultural issues, become familiar with culturally different individuals and groups in one's own geographical region, and develop a positive awareness of one's own culture. In order to effectively and appropriately serve students with developmental disabilities, the education professional must become a learner and embrace the positive concepts of multiculturalism.

While much of this chapter has presented information in terms of language *or* culture, the context is really one of language *and* culture. One aspect should not be emphasized over the other. While we embrace the term *culturally and linguistically diverse learners*, the challenge to today's education professional is to be true to our calling—to treat culture and language equally.

Glossary

Body language—Nonverbal messages communicated through body movement.

Cultural bias—Unfounded beliefs and values, as well as insulting terms that refer to someone's ethnicity.

Cultural differences—Differences that are based solely upon one's cultural identity.

Cultural identification—The primary culture with which one identifies.

Culturally and linguistically diverse populations—Groups of people that are from different cultures and speak different languages.

Culturally different—A person who does not share your cultural identity or values.

Culturally sensitive—Feeling empathy with someone from a culturally different group.

Cultural response approach—A method that utilizes small-group reading and discussion about different cultures in a classroom or other learning setting.

Culture: Differences? Diversity!—A trainer-of-trainers model for teaching about multiculturalism in special education.

Disability culture—Persons who share a similar disability and form cultural bonds on the basis of that disability.

Diversity—Differences that exist between groups of people.

Dominant language—The language used by the dominant cultural group in a society.

Ethnicity—Identification with a recognized ethnic group.

Family heritage—The background, history, and values of a family group.

Family preservation approach—Services concerned with basic life skills and environmental problems, delivered to children and parents in normalized settings such as the home, to support and strengthen families by employing the person-in-environment perspective.

Localization—Defining multicultural education from a regional perspective rather than a global one.

Minority communities—Groups of people who share a common ancestry or ethnicity.

Multicultural education—A school curriculum that includes cultural information.

Multicultural learner with DD—Learners who are culturally and linguistically diverse, with such specific cultural identifiers as race, ethnicity, gender, sexual orientation, and linguistic differences.

Native language skills—The ability to speak the language of one's identified cultural group.

Parenting education—Education designed to improve parenting skills.

Prejudice—Negative attitudes toward someone from a different cultural or ethnic identity.

Stereotypes—Behaviors that are attributed to a cultural group and believed to apply to all within that group.

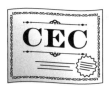

Knowledge and Skills for Entry-Level Special Education Teachers of Students With Developmental Disabilities Standards Addressed in This Chapter

Principle 2: Development and Characteristics of Learners

DD2K4   Factors that influence overrepresentation of culturally/linguistically diverse individuals.

Principle 5: Learning Environments/Social Interaction

DD5S1   Provide instruction in community-based settings.

Principle 7: Instructional Planning

DD7S1   Plan instruction for independent functional life skills relevant to the community, personal living, sexuality, and employment.

Principle 8: Assessment

DD8K2   Environmental assessment conditions that promote maximum performance of individuals with developmental disabilities.

Principle 10: Collaboration

DD10S1   Collaborate with team members to plan transition to adulthood that encourages full community participation.

Web Site Resources

Center on State Systems and Employment
http://www.communityinclusion.org/rrtc/Research/StateProfiles/Glossary.htm

> Rehabilitation research and training center (RRTC), located at the Institute for Community Inclusion/UAP and funded by National Institute on Disability Rehabilitation Research (NIDRR), studies how state agencies provide employment supports to people with disabilities.

Educator's Reference Desk
http://www.eduref.org/cgibin/print.cgi/Resources/Specific_Populations/Disabilities/Parenting.html

> Lesson ideas, resources, and information on disability-specific topics.

Indian Child Welfare Act of 1978—P.L. 95-608
http://www.ssa.gov/OP_Home/comp2/F095-608.html

> Regulations of P.L. 95-608, approved November 8, 1978, which recognize the special relationship between the United States and the *Indian* tribes and their members and the federal responsibility to *Indian* people.

References

Banks, J., & Banks, C. (2004). *Multicultural education: Issues and perspectives* (5th ed.). Boston: Allyn & Bacon.

Barbour, C., & Barbour, N. (2005). *Families, schools, and communities: Building partnerships for educating children* (3rd ed.). Columbus, OH: Merrill.

Baruth, L., & Manning, M. (2004). *Multicultural education of children and adolescents* (4th ed). Boston: Allyn & Bacon.

Berger, E. (2003). *Parents as partners in education: Families and schools working together* (6th ed.). Columbus, OH: Merrill.

Center on State Systems and Employment. (2001). *Glossary of key terms.* Retrieved November 2, 2005, from http://www.communityinclusion.org/rrtc/Research/StateProfiles/Glossary.htm

Coughlin, A., & Abramowitz, C. (2005). *Cross-cultural adoption.* Washington, DC: Lifeline Press.

Diaz, C. (2001). *Multicultural education for the 21st century* (2nd ed.). Washington, DC: National Education Association.

Dong, Y. (2005). Taking a cultural-response approach to teaching multicultural literature. *English Journal, 94*(3), 55–60.

Educator's Reference Desk. (n.d.). *Disabilities/special education parenting.* Retrieved November 2, 2005, from http://www.eduref.org/cgi-bin/print.cgi/Resources/Specific_Populations/Disabilities/Parenting.html

Frankland, H., Turnbull, A., & Wehmeyer, M. (2004). An exploration of the self-determination construct and disability as it relates to the Dine (Navajo) culture. *Education and Training in Developmental Disabilities, 39,* 191–205.

Gilliland, H., & Reyhner, J. (1999). *Teaching the American Indian* (4th ed.). Dubuque, IA: Kendall/Hunt.

Goor, M. (1999). Preparation of teachers and administrators for working effectively with multicultural students. *Advances in Special Education, 12,* 183–203.

Grossman, H. (1995). *Special education in a diverse society.* Boston: Allyn & Bacon.

Grossman, H., Obiakor, F. E., & Utley, C. A. (2003). Multicultural learners with exceptionalities in general and special education settings. *Advances in Special Education, 15,* 445–463.

Harry, B. (1992). Restructuring the participation of African-American parents in special education. *Exceptional Children, 59,* 123–131.

Hildebrand, V., Phenice, L., Gray, M., & Hines, R. (2000). *Knowing and serving diverse families* (2nd ed.). Columbus, OH: Merrill.

Indian Child Welfare Act of 1978, 25 U.S.C. § 1901 *et seq.* (1978).

Individuals with Disabilities Education Improvement Act of 2004, 118 Stat. 2647. (2004).

KidSource Online. (2000). *Parenting a child with special needs: A guide to readings and resources*. Retrieved November 2, 2005, from http://www.kidsource.com/NICHCY/parenting.disab.all.4.6.html

Kimberly, M. (1999). Cooperative learning experiences: Meeting the needs of culturally diverse students. *Journal of Family and Consumer Sciences, 91*(2), 50–53.

Klein, H. (1995). Urban Appalachian children in northern schools: A study in diversity. *Young Children, 50*(3), 10–16.

Lenters, K. (2004). No half measures: Reading instruction for young second-language learners. *Reading Teacher, 58*, 328–336.

Lockwood, R. (2003, April). *Developing a multicultural training package*. Poster presented at the Council for Exceptional Children Annual Convention and Expo, Seattle, WA.

Lockwood, R., Ford, B., Sparks, S., & Allen, A. (1991). *Culture: Differences? Disability!* Columbus, OH: Ohio Federation Council for Exceptional Children.

Lynch, E., & Hanson, M. (1998). *Developing cross-cultural competence: A guide for working with young children and their families* (2nd ed.). Baltimore: Brookes.

Mannes, M. (1993a). Factors and events leading to the passage of the Indian Child Welfare Act. *Child Welfare, 74*, 264–282.

Mannes, M. (1993b). Seeking the balance between child protection and family preservation in Indian child welfare. *Child Welfare, 72*, 141–151.

Marcus, S., & Ames, M. (1998). Reaching linguistically and culturally diverse young learners with disabilities. *TESOL Journal, 7*(4), 10–17.

Obiakor, F., Rotatori, A., & Utley, C., (Eds.). (2004). *Advances in special education: Effective education for learners with exceptionalities*. Oxford, England: Elsevier Science/ JAI Press.

Parette, P., & Huer, M. B. (2002). Working with Asian American families whose children have augmentative and alternative communication (AAC) needs. *Journal of Special Education Technology, 17*(4), 5–13.

Roach, D. (1994). My grandma's house: Reaching out to underserved families of children and youth with neurobiological, emotional, or behavioral differences. *Focal Point, 8* (2), 21–23.

Rodriguez, C., & Higgins, K. (2005). Preschool children with developmental delays and limited English proficiency. *Intervention in School and Clinic, 40*, 236–242.

Taylor, L., & Whittaker, C. (2003). *Bridging multiple worlds: Case studies of diverse educational communities*. Boston: Allyn & Bacon.

Timpson, J. (1993). Four decades of literature on native Canadian child welfare: Changing themes. *Child Welfare, 74*, 525–546.

Van Krieken, R. (1999). The stolen generations and cultural genocide: The forced removal of Australian indigenous children from their families and its implications for the sociology of childhood. *Childhood: A Global Journal of Child Research, 6*, 297–311.

8

Meeting the Educational Needs of Persons With Developmental Disabilities Across Cultures

Howard P. Parette, Mary Blake Huer, and George R. Peterson-Karlan

Summary

The chapter explores the complexity of cultural influences on working with persons with developmental disabilities and their families, with particular emphasis on three components related to culture and the impact of each for service delivery: (a) related patterns of acculturation (individual change), (b) particular parameters within school systems, and (c) recently recognized generational differences.

Learning Outcomes

After reading this chapter, you should be able to:

- Understand the complexity of culture and its relationship to the education of students with developmental disabilities.

- Identify various components of culture in American society.

- Identify difficulties in studying culture.

- Understand the effects of acculturation on children with disabilities and their families.

- Identify generational influences on teaching practices.

- Explain the process of cultural reciprocity in working with families.

The Changing Context Within the School Setting

In our diverse society, education professionals have increasingly noted the heterogeneity of children with developmental disabilities and their families who are served in public school and other settings. For example, Civilrights.org (2002), in interpreting 2000 U.S. Census data reported the following trends:

1. There are currently 35.4 million African Americans in the United States. (12.5% of the total population), reflecting an increase from the 30 million (12.1% of the total population) in 1990. A growth rate of 16% in the African American population since 1990 exceeds the growth rate of the American population as a whole (10.7% overall).

2. Hispanics number approximately 35.3 million people (12.5% of the total U.S. population), reflecting a 38% growth rate since 1990. This growth is up from 22.4 million

(9% of the total population in 1990). Hispanics are the fastest-growing segment of the population (Economic Research Service, 2002).

3. Asian/Pacific Islanders number approximately 11.3 million (4% of the U.S. population), an increase from 7.3 million and 2.9% of the total population in 1990. This group exhibited the highest rate of population growth (45%) of all racial/ethnic groups.

4. Native Americans reflected a population of approximately 2.5 million (less than 1% of the total U.S. population), though this group increased by 2 million since 1990, and has also grown by 18% during the past decade (versus 10.7% for the U.S. population as a whole).

School as an Intersection of Culture

Differences among children in schools from these various population groups are often attributable to an array of cultural influences that are still little understood by well-intentioned practitioners. Such influences are frequently powerful determinants of children's learning and their acceptance by peers and others, and affect the nature and quality of interactions that education professionals have with family members and their children. Racial groups are becoming a larger proportion of the U.S. population base, and education professionals cannot afford to continue using the Euro-American dimension of culture as the primary referent against which other cultural groups are compared, as it results in a competitive dichotomy (Hains, Lynch, & Winton, 2000) and has important implications for service delivery to persons with developmental disabilities. Although schools have been described as having their own culture (as discussed later), it is clear that American schools have come to be an intersection of cultures. While this chapter is intended to provide an overview of important cultural facets that all practitioners educating these children and interacting with their families should know, a caveat to this discussion is that the complexity of culture prevents a truly comprehensive treatment of any of these issue areas. Each area could arguably be discussed in a treatise, and those interested in exploring more in-depth readings are directed to other sources (see e.g., Kalyanpur & Harry, 1999; Lynch & Hanson, 1997; National Center for the Dissemination of Disability Research, 1999).

Understanding the Concept of Culture

Culture permeates and substantively influences all aspects of the worldviews of individuals within particular groups of people. Thus, who we are, how we see ourselves in the world, and how we view our relationships to others are functions of culture. This is true of family members who have children with developmental disabilities, their children, and all education professionals with whom they come in contact. Yet there is not a consensus regarding the definition of culture (see e.g., Kroeber & Kluckhohn, 1952).

Defining Culture

On a simplistic level, *culture* has been defined as a "lens" through which people see themselves and their relationships to others in the world (Battle, 2002; Soto, Huer, & Taylor, 1997). Such a rudimentary definition of culture would include a set of beliefs, values, behaviors, and communication patterns that are shared by a particular group of people and learned as a function of social membership (Miraglia, Law, & Collins, 1999; Soto, 1994; Soto et al., 1997; Sue & Sue, 1990). Since cultures are influenced by social factors and are learned phenomena, they are constantly changing in response to forces and events that may affect people (e.g., legislation, migration, immigration, assimilation, marginalization; Venkatesh, 1995) or interactions between cultures (Smedley, 1993).

Identifying Cultures

In the United States, our identification of culture is perhaps most influenced by commonly used geographic terms, e.g., American, European, Middle Eastern, South American, or terms associated with "racial groups," e.g., Hispanic, African American, Asian-Pacific Island, Native American. We also identify cultural groups by country of origin, e.g., Japanese, Korean, Russian, Mexican, Indian.

Ethnicity

Understanding culture to be purely geographic area, country of origin, or major racial group is far too simplistic. Within racial and ethnic categories, groups and individuals vary in terms of nationality, language, religion, and other characteristics. As an example, Leung (1996) identified 47 different cultural groups within the broad category of Asian Pacific Americans. Similarly, Hispanics are often broadly grouped together as a distinctive cultural group, even though individuals within the group may have come from Mexico, Puerto Rico, Central America, South America, or Spain (McNaughton, 2003; World Book, 2004). Many also point out that culture is only "one of several significant variables" that influence human interactions (Duarte & Rice, 1992, p. 42); for example, people within one ethnic group may differ greatly in their beliefs, values, and practices based upon their religious affiliation (Christian, Muslim, etc.).

Macrocultures and Microcultures

A more fluid way to think about cultural groups in the United States is to consider the observation of Banks and McGee Banks (1997) that there is a "national culture as well as ethnic and other subsocieties and institutions" (p. 6). To better understand this statement, one might think in terms of what it means to be an "American." This notion of a national, or *macro* culture means different things to different individuals, but shared or common values—such as freedom, rights, and consumer orientation—are characteristics of U.S. society that most Americans would agree upon. Most Americans are familiar with the term *mainstream* and have a general sense of core values of mainstream macroculture. Within this broad national framework, or macroculture, and its related core value and belief systems, however, are many *micro* cultural groups (e.g., race, ethnicity, nationality, language, social status, rural/urban, disability), each participating to varying degrees in the macroculture while also retaining to differing degrees elements of their respective microcultural traditions (Kalyanpur & Harry, 1999). Education professionals thus face a particular challenge to understand not only the degree of affiliation held by family members of children with disabilities (and the children themselves) with mainstream values and beliefs but also the importance placed on their respective microculture's values and beliefs.

Public Schools as a Microculture

Public schools have been recognized for decades as being distinct cultural entities that have values, behaviors, and characteristics consistent with the profiles of communities within which they reside (Goodlad, 1984; Rossman, Corbett, & Firestone, 1988; Thomas & Loxley, 2001; Welch, 1989). Inherent in the cultural characteristics of schools is an instinctive resistance to change, resulting in the educational establishment's remaining essentially the same since the late 19th and early 20th centuries (Casey, 2000).

Interestingly, people may also belong to several professional or "personal-interest groups" that have their own unique values and rules regarding membership and participation (e.g., public schools, parent organizations). Their participation in these groups may vary depending upon the extent of the meaningful socialization and interactions that occur (Banks, 1997a, 1997b). Sleeter and Grant (2003) have observed that the extent of cultural continuity between home and school often varies markedly and can have a variety of effects on children's learning (Pheelan, Davidson, & Cao, 1991).

Culture and Disability

Disability is a condition of individuals regardless of cultural membership; race and ethnicity do, however, have a very strong association with the occurrence of disability (Smart & Smart, 1997). For example, a higher incidence of persons with disabilities (ages 15–64) is found among African Americans and American Indians (U.S. Census Bureau, 2002; also see Table 8.1). Walker and Brown (1996) reported that African Americans and Hispanic Americans are overrepresented in *all* disability

TABLE 8.1
Numbers of Individuals With Disabilities

Subject	Population (Thousands)	N With Disability (Thousands)	% With Disability	N With Self-Care Difficulty (Thousands)	% With Self-Care Difficulty
Race					
White	205,620	30,853	15.00	5,379	2.60
African American	32,942	5,525	16.80	1,167	3.50
Asian/Pacific Islander	12,619	1,072	8.50	187	1.50
American Indian/Alaska Native	3,590	850	23.70	170	4.70
Ethnicity					
Hispanic	35,127	3,658	10.40	661	1.90
Non-Hispanic	228,188	35,277	15.50	6,361	2.80

Source: U.S. Census Bureau. (2002). *American community survey*. Retrieved April 21, 2005, from http://pascenter.org/state_based_stats/state_statistics_2003.php?state=us

categories, including chronic health conditions; physical, sensory, and language impairments; and nervous and mental disorders. Similarly, most Asians and Pacific Islanders do not fit the disability or socioeconomic profile of other minorities, though recent immigrants (e.g., Hmongs, Laotians, Vietnamese, and Cambodians) are exceptions and tend to be both poorer and less well educated than other Asians in the United States. Hispanics and Asians are the fastest-growing minority groups in the United States (Economic Research Service, 2002). An examination of data on public health reveals similar disparities in risk rates between white and minority populations (National Center for the Dissemination of Disability Research, 1999; Williams & Jackson, 2005).

As noted by LaVeist (1996), race and ethnicity among minority groups cannot be viewed as causative factors in the higher incidence of disabilities and chronic or life-threatening health problems, but they are factors in health risks that are influenced primarily by social and political parameters, such as education level. Higher incidences of disability, for example, have been reported among persons who do not complete high school, and markedly lower rates among college graduates (Smart & Smart, 1997; Traustadottir, 2000). Education, income, and discrimination (which often results in disparities in employment, education, and income) may be more-primary influences on disability than race or ethnicity per se (National Center for the Dissemination of Disability Research, 1999).

However, the human condition of developmental disability cannot be fully understood without also understanding the cultural context in which such disabilities are perceived. Numerous sources have noted that perceptions of disability vary markedly across ethnic groups (Ingstad & Whyte, 1995; Lynch & Hanson, 1997; Parette, 1998; Roseberry-McKibben, 2002), ranging from such diverse perspectives as (a) having multiple causes and being fixable/treatable (e.g., Euro American; Duarte & Rice, 1992; Harry, 1992; Roseberry-McKibben, 2002); (b) being a punishment from God, influence of evil spirits or the devil, and/or bad luck (e.g., African American; Willis, 1997); (c) being a function of fate or resulting from sins committed by parents/ancestors (e.g., Asian Americans; Chan, 1997); (d) being attributable to external, nonmedical causes, such as witchcraft; part of an incomprehensible divine plan; or punishment for wrongdoing (e.g., Hispanic Americans; Alper, Schloss, & Schloss, 1994; Loridas, 1988); and (e) being a divine gift to be shared with others (e.g., Native Americans; Richardson, 1981).

Responsiveness of Schools to Culture

What is problematic with these diverse perspectives of disability within the broad cultural fabric of the United States, is that our service delivery system has historically been influenced by and responsive to white (Euro-American) value systems (i.e., the "mainstream"; Hains et al., 2000; National Center for the Dissemination of Disability Research, 1999), which are often represented in many of our public schools across the country. Such assumptions pose substantive challenges to the field of developmental disabilities given the current shift in population growth.

Growing awareness of cultural influences on school decision making has also called attention to the discrepancies between values of family members, their children, and the school culture (Boykin, 1994; Gordon & Yowell, 1994; Lamorey, 2002; Valdivieso & Nicolau, 1994; Vogt, Jordan, & Tharp, 1992; Parette, 2005). For example, African American children, both with and without developmental disabilities, often prefer and do better in cooperative learning settings, while Euro-American students prefer and do better in competitive learning settings (Boykin & Bailey, 2000; Parette, 1998). Other research suggests a relation between cultural differences in child-rearing environments and intelligence test performance (Moore, 1985). Cultural dissonance, or evident differences in value systems, may also lead to erroneous interpretations of parent behaviors (e.g., head nodding during conferences that might be interpreted as agreement versus affirmation of having heard and giving deference to the professional position), creating misunderstandings between home and school (Misra, 1994; Valdivieso & Nicolau, 1994).

Special Education Services and Culture

As noted above, cultural differences have also been reported to affect the responses that family members have to disability (i.e., they may perceive disability more or less favorably than school professionals do) (Chan, 1986; Hanline & Daley, 1992; Zborowsky, 1969). These differences may also affect their willingness to receive interventions from professionals who use interaction styles that differ from those used by families (e.g., authoritarian or nonauthoritarian) (Harry et al., 1995; McGoldrick, Pearce, & Giordano, 1982). Specific cultural differences have also been reported to have potentially powerful influences on the effectiveness of education team planning, such as in the area of assistive technology (Kemp & Parette, 2000; Parette, 1999; Parette, Huer, & VanBiervliet, 2005; Parette & Petch-Hogan, 2000).

Despite the presence of dissonance among families from varying cultural and ethnic backgrounds, however, professionals in special education have historically expected families to adapt to the expectations of the broader, mainstream school culture, which reflects white, middle-class values (Douthit, 1997; Kalyanpur & Harry, 1999; Soto, 1994) such as individuality, control of one's environment, and value of the future. When a family member or person with a developmental disability from a cultural background has different values (e.g., values group behavior rather than individuality, harmony with the environment rather than control over it, and the past or present rather than the future), substantive problems may be anticipated both in seeking and in receiving educational services (Douthit, 1997). Unfortunately, as Lamorey (2002) has noted, "Optimal outcomes for children with disabilities can only occur when professionals bridge from the culture of schooling to parents' multifaceted perceptions of disability, its cause, its acceptable treatments, and the available sources of formal and informal support" (p. 67). Strategies for making this "bridge" will be discussed later in the chapter.

Influences on Culture

Throughout these discussions it should be clear that culture is not a static, monolithic structure that uniformly affects people, families, and persons with disabilities. As noted initially, the influences of culture on a person are learned and thus are subject to myriad societal forces and events. Religion can have a major impact in influencing individual and family values and practices within a culture (Emmons & Paloutzian, 2003). Schools have come to recognize the impact of a student's religious background and make accommodations such as alterations to dress codes, changes in food options, and observance of holidays. As demonstrated by the role of socioeconomic status (SES) within a specific culture as a determinant of the incidence of disability, wealth can have a significant influence upon culture, especially in the school context.

Economic Influences on Culture

In the American culture, wealth is viewed as something that everyone can have or accumulate. Television commercials for building wealth through real estate investment, home businesses, little-known government grants and programs, and even the lottery are a testament to this fundamental belief. And while there remain stories of self-made millionaires (e.g., Sam Walton of Wal-Mart, or Dave Thomas of Wendy's), it is also clear that our U.S. society (as well as in many other parts of the world), also includes people who experience lifelong poverty. Ruby Payne (1998) has extensively explored the effects of poverty that extends across multiple generations of people in the United States and has found that cross-generational poverty in fact produces similar values, practices, and patterns of behavior.

Culture of Poverty

Payne's (1998) work focuses on the operational assumption that middle-class mores and norms conflict with the "hidden" rules of persons from low SES backgrounds. She refers to "generational poverty," or values passed from one generation to the next that are simply assumed because of circumstances and conditions in which individuals live over time. If persons in low SES environments do not have certain educational services and are accustomed to not having such services available, that can become an expectation or assumption of lifestyle that may not resonate with Anglo-European American professionals who believe strongly that specific types of services and interventions are necessary. It is particularly important to understand the rules (and values) of individuals from diverse backgrounds if professionals are to maintain effective interactions during educational decision making.

Disability—Culture or Influence?

Not only is an understanding of the complexity of culture important to planning an appropriate education for students with developmental disabilities, but also an awareness of the "culture of disability," separate from knowledge regarding racial/ethnic identities, is essential. Smart (2001) provides a comprehensive work explaining the sources and effects of prejudice and discrimination by individuals, their parents, and society whenever an individual with a disability participates in an environment where there are persons without disabilities.

Acknowledging Assumptions and Perceptions of Disabilities

It is important to recognize the assumptions and perceptions that operate among persons without disabilities in order to better interpret the actions, societal influences, and expectations of families who have children with disabilities, as encountered by professionals within school systems. Smart (2001) notes: "In the past, disability was thought of as a private or family concern" (p. xiv), but now, because of changes in public laws giving access to education and advocacy efforts by many, disability is "a universal concern" (p. xiv).

What this means for educators is that they are now serving a culturally and linguistically diverse population of students with a variety of disabling conditions. Persons with disabilities have been identified as a "devalued group" (Smart, 2001, p. xiv) in American society. Thus, in essence, service providers must now not only gain knowledge about the consequences for service delivery of ethnic and linguistic diversity; they must also acquire an understanding of other factors that stem from perceptions of disabilities in American culture, which affect the success or failure of their planned transformation of targeted skills and abilities for the students they serve in daily educational intervention experiences. An understanding of culture and cultural influence is becoming even more complex and necessary for educators.

Parents of Children With Developmental Disabilities

When a child is born with a disability, parents experience a period of adjustment/response (Smart, 2001). They go through stages of responding to the disability, as well as adapting to the sense of loss of the child they expected to have—a child without a disability. Whatever ethnic/racial group parents represent, they typically need time to adjust to the effects of the disability on their own feelings and perceptions, as well as to respond to their family members, neighbors, and friends about the disability. No doubt their cultural beliefs, values, religion, and educational history regarding etiology, causes, and prognosis come into play during the stages of responding. But parents are typically bombarded with a tremendous amount of information that may be contradictory but may nevertheless represent the opinions and traditional actions of members of different communities (medical, educational, religious) that they encounter.

It is important, therefore, to consider "the family's cultural values before automatically assuming that the family responds to the child with a disability in the same way that Euro-American, middle-class families do" (Smart, 2001, p. 267). Research reveals that children with congenital disabilities may experience abuse and neglect, may interact with a variety of different caregivers (medical as well as educational) without forming long-term relationships, and may be at risk for emotional maladaptation, behavior problems, and low self-esteem, as well as prejudice and discrimination by persons without disabilities. "There is a stigma in attending 'special' classes" (Smart, 2001, p. 282). Finally, the consequence of loss of functions also has cultural ramifications with respect to gender. For example, males with developmental disabilities are viewed differently than females are. Knowledge of such different viewpoints is important for education professionals who work with persons with developmental disabilities and their families.

Generational Influences on Macro- and Microcultures

In both the macroculture of American society and the microculture of the school, children, adolescents, and young adults, including those with developmental disabilities, are part of a generation that is markedly different from the generations of teachers with whom they are working. These children, born between 1978 and 1982, are often referred to as Digital Children (Edyburn, 2002), the Net Generation/ N-Gens (Oblinger & Oblinger, 2005; Tapscott, 1998), or Millennials (Howe & Strauss, 2000; Miller & Norton, 2003). They have been described as being confident, hopeful, achievement-oriented, civic-minded, and inclusive (Howe & Strauss, 2000; Mask, 2002; Raines, 2001; Tapscott, 1998), but they vary most markedly from their parents and teachers with regard to the way in which technology is perceived and used (Peterson-Karlan & Parette, 2005). These children particularly have grown up in a world rich with a range of technology (e.g., DVD players, high-definition television, MP3 players, cell phones, high-speed Internet connectivity) (Parette, 2004; Peterson-Karlan & Parette, 2005; Woodard, Emory, & Gridina, 2000).

What is especially important about recent research conducted regarding this group of children (Howe & Strauss, 2000; Oblinger, 2003; Oblinger & Oblinger, 2005), particularly those with developmental disabilities, is the fundamental question of whether current educational approaches reflect an understanding of their learning styles and preferences. The area of technology usage may hold especially far-reaching implications for practitioners. As Peterson-Karlan and Parette observed in an insightful analysis of the literature, children of this generation are so exposed to and comfortable with technology that it is both transparent and an accepted part of their lives.

Most education professionals have observed students in public school settings using a range of technologies, often in "multitasking situations" (e.g., listening to music on a MP3 player while instant-messaging, conducting searches on the Internet, using word processing and various graphics programs, and talking on a cell phone). It can be argued that from a marketing perspective, vendors have acknowledged the generational differences and technology use patterns of these children. For example, CNNMoney .com (2007) observed: "Personal computers, MP3 players, digital cameras have all become a critical component of a student's back-to-school survival gear."

Unfortunately, little is known regarding the extent to which the technology involvement and use patterns demonstrated by Millennial students without disabilities are also characteristic of students with developmental disabilities in today's classrooms. Friedman (2004), for example, reporting on a sample of 53 school-age children with cognitive disabilities, noted a wide array of technologies used by the students. However, when asked what strategies/technologies were used for specific school tasks, children with disabilities indicated that they are being influenced by and expecting technology to a greater extent in public school settings than in the past (Lahm & Sizemore, 2002; Parette, Huer, & Scherer, 2004; Parette & Peterson-Karlan, 2005).

The lack of understanding exhibited by education professionals about the technology use patterns and preferences of students with developmental disabilities is alarming in light of the mandate to consider AT in the development of their IEPs [Individuals with Disabilities Education Act Amendments of 1997, § 1414(d)(3)(B)(iv)]. As noted by Peterson-Karlan and Parette (2005), "Assistive technology is inherently still technology and we know little of their comfort with and assimilation of technology" (p. 32). Some education professionals might question why such understanding is important, though it has the potential to affect (a) the selection of instructional and assistive technology; (b) the ways that students interact and learn with the technology; (c) the amount of instruction the students will need in the use of technology, especially computer-based and other digital AT; and (d) the acceptance or rejection of specific types of AT. This knowledge may clarify the varying "cultural" perspectives that adults and Millennial children bring to the selection and implementation of instructional and assistive technology (Peterson-Karlan & Parette, 2005).

Finally, the process of determining what kinds of technology students want, prefer, and use can affect self-determination, one of the domains that has been found to be important to the attainment of post-school outcomes. Lack of consumer preference and choice has been shown to be the most important factor in technology abandonment (Galvin & Scherer, 1996; Phillips & Zhao, 1993), and the literature is replete with support for the active involvement of consumers in the AT decision-making process (Carroll & Phillips, 1993; Freeman & Field, 1994; Phillips & Broadnax, 1992; Riemer-Reiss & Wacker, 1999; Turner et al., 1995). Personal choice and preference are also fundamental components of self-determination (Field & Hoffman, 1994; Wehmeyer, 1999), in student involvement in planning educational programs (Wood, Karvonen, Test, Browder, & Algozzine, 2004), in transition planning (Field & Hoffman, 1998), and in achieving post-school success (Wehmeyer & Schwartz, 1997). To omit the technology preferences and choices is to ignore students' preferences during longitudinal educational planning related to the development of both their IEPs (primary through the high school grades) and their school to post-school transition plans (middle and high school grades).

Within school cultures, substantive differences often exist between skills that are taught and valued in the schools and skills that are valued in the larger society. For example, in some states standards emphasize knowledge of facts more than application of facts and processes. In the workplace importance may be attached to manipulating digital information using information technologies, whereas in the schools greater emphasis is often placed on processes (e.g., the process of completing math problems rather than using calculators to solve problems or the process of developing dictionary skills rather than using an online dictionary and word-prediction software). Such differences suggest a cultural dissonance, or tension, between the larger community culture and the school culture.

Generational Influences on Family Culture

Differences among individuals across generations have frequently been addressed in the professional literature (see, e.g., Mannheim, 1952; Mitchell, 2002; Zemke, Raines, & Filipczak, 1999). Not only do persons from various ethnic and other microculture groups hold different perspectives on education, but differences within these groups across generations are also evident. For example, Baby Boom generation parents would have grown up with access to very different educational resources and experiences than their children who were Gen Xers (born in the 1960s and 1970s). It is not uncommon for many of these Baby Boomers to have had limited exposure to computer and other information technologies until later in their lives, and thus to be less inclined to use such technologies than are their children, who have grown up in a world rich with technology. Similarly, Gen Xers would have had differing educational experiences from Millennial children (born after 1978–1982), and the nature of their family values and behaviors, while sometimes similar to those of their parents, are often markedly different.

Cultural Change

When people give up "old ways" and adopt "new ways" of thinking or behaving, they have been affected by the process of *acculturation* (Ruiz, 1981). From the perspective of mainstream culture, acculturation might be understood as the extent to which microcultural groups participate in the cultural traditions, values, assumptions, and practices of the dominant white society (Landrine & Klonoff, 1995).

Acculturation—Synthesis or Dissonance?

Inherent in the process of acculturation is the assumption of *individual change* in response to various influences (Parette et al., 2004). All persons change certain behaviors across time depending on the timing and strength of various forces that confront them. Certainly, for family members of children with developmental disabilities, and for the children themselves, acculturation can wield immense influences on behavior when working with school or other service system personnel. For example, members of a particular family unit may differ from one another with regard to the extent of their acculturation (e.g., how they perceive assistive technology, education in general, the school system specifically). Similarly, the family's (or child's) acculturation experience, and thus their perceptions of a range of important education-related processes, may be markedly different from the viewpoints of the education professionals with whom they are involved. What is especially important for education professionals to recognize is that every person changes across time. This change is sometimes linear (i.e., persons lose their own culture and language as they adopt those of the mainstream; Keefe, 1980; Schumann, 1986), but it may also be nonlinear (Masgoret & Gardner, 1999; Parette et al., 2004) and can vary at different points in time. At the core is their response to macrocultural influences, that is, the extent to which family members and/or their children with developmental disabilities approach or avoid interaction with the macroculture and the degree to which these persons maintain or relinquish attributes of the microculture (Parette et al., 2004).

Outcomes of Acculturation

Berry and colleagues (Berry, Kim, Power, Young, & Bujaki, 1989; Berry, Poortinga, Segall, & Dasen, 1992; Berry & Sam, 1997) have described four acculturation outcomes that occur in response to change forces: (a) assimilation, (b) integration, (c) separation, and (d) marginalization (see Figure 8.1).

Assimilation

Assimilation results from the extent to which a person desires contact with the macroculture while not necessarily maintaining an identity with a relevant microculture. For example, an immigrant family may feel so strongly about being a part of the American mainstream, or being accepted into the school community, that they accept all recommendations and go to great lengths to adopt and practice the prevailing values and beliefs. Unfortunately, this often may be what education professionals expect for families of children with developmental disabilities. Such a mind-set fails to recognize that some cultural groups prefer not to be assimilated (Pew Hispanic Center/Kaiser Family Foundation, 2002; Salins, 1997; Swaidan & Marshall, 2001) into some aspects of American society. The extent to which families from diverse cultural backgrounds may reasonably be anticipated to be accepting of mainstream-weighted, educationally recommended services is relatively unknown at this time, though efforts have been made to identify both family and service provider goals and preferences for specific educational services, such as assistive technology (Parette, Brotherson, & Huer, 2000; Parette, Huer, & Brotherson, 2001).

Integration

Integration occurs when family members and/or their children with developmental disabilities desire both to maintain their cultural identity and to engage in a high level of interaction with a macroculture. Many ethnic groups prefer integration versus assimilation into American culture (Laroche, Kim, Hui, & Joy, 1996; Swaidan &

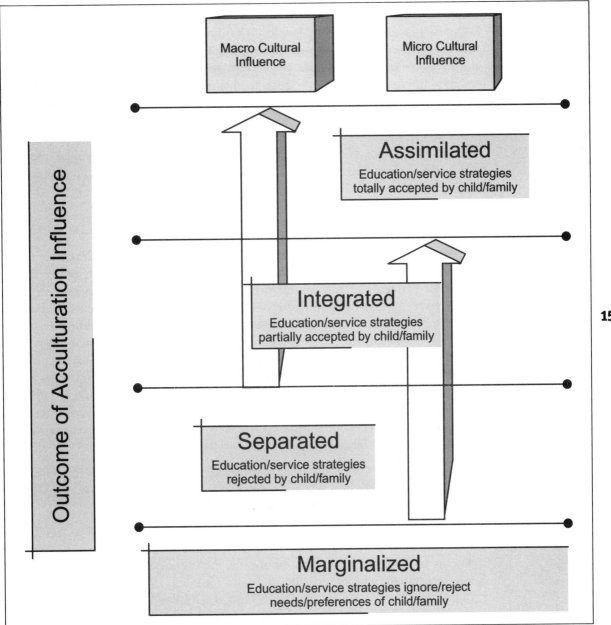

FIGURE 8.1. Outcome of acculturation influence.

Marshall, 2001), though there is lack of consensus regarding the exact meaning of integration and its defining characteristics (Ray, 2002). Historically, many immigrants have tended to be more concerned than second and subsequent generations of family members about fitting into the dominant culture versus maintaining their cultural roots (Zhang & Carrasquillo, 1995), even though immigrants may practice their own native culture at home.

Although first-generation migrants (who have immigrated to the new society) typically change their values to a certain extent, second and subsequent generations (as a result of being raised in the new country) may differ markedly with regard to their acceptance of traditional values (Citrin & Highton, 2004; Georgas, Berry, Shaw, Christakopoulou, & Mylonas, 1996; Phinney, Du Pont, Espinosa, Revill, & Sanders, 1994). Contingent upon influential variables, a relatively high degree of value maintenance may also be expected in the second generation (Georgas et al., 1996; Nauck, 2001).

Separation

Separation is characterized by low levels of interaction with the macroculture (and related microcultural groups) while also maintaining a close connection with and affirmation of the native culture. Separation involves resistance to the macroculture and its value systems, as well as efforts to change the environment where the person lives (Swaidan & Marshall, 2001). In the United States, such a change is difficult to achieve, as it would require creating an environment where the original culture dominates in the midst of powerful macrocultural forces like established standards for living in a democratic, consumer-oriented society, a range of individual freedoms within the culture, the influence of friends within the community, a competitive economy, and influence of the media.

Marginalization

Marginalization occurs when persons do not identify with either their native culture or the dominant culture (e.g., enforced cultural loss combined with enforced segregation). Elements of the culture that somehow survive every attempt at being destroyed are systematically belittled or denigrated by the dominant culture. Persons from the dominant culture may label indigenous practices as pagan religions, primitive art, and folk medicine. Though they concede that such belief systems exist, they regard them as inferior to the prevailing mainstream culture (e.g., what occurred in the United States with indigenous Native American tribes). This country has a long history of marginalizing persons with disabilities (Hahn, 2000). Similarly, rejection of (or failure to acknowledge) important cultural values held by family members may result in the family's unwillingness to participate in educational decision-making processes (Parette & Petch-Hogan, 2000).

Acculturation Reflected Through Preferences

Inherent in the definition of acculturation is the notion of individual change in response to contact with other cultural groups (Kunkel, 1990; Pomales & Williams, 1989; Ponce & Atkinson, 1989; Wells, Hough, Golding, & Burnam, 1987; Woods et al., 2002). These studies suggest that (a) individual acculturation may be an important consideration during education decision making, especially when various family members at different stages of acculturation are asked for input and participation in decision-making processes, and (b) team members must take such influences into account during decision making, as family members may vary markedly in their degree of alignment with white cultural values. The degree to which a particular decision maker in the family has been acculturated to specific education-driven preferences, such as technology, may have a marked effect on the extent to which he or she is familiar with and responsive to particular devices and services recommended or implemented by white professionals. In addition, the student who was born to a culturally different background but has been living in this country since a young age, may differ from either or both of the parents with respect to generational differences such as technology preference and use; the student may be closer to his or her peers in technology preferences, especially in school and outside the home.

With regard to education practices, all persons in our society are familiar with changing, or becoming acculturated to the wide range of strategies and options currently available. For example, many individuals who decades ago were hesitant to use computers to increase productivity now would have great difficulty working in a business environment that did not have such tools. Similarly, the increasing popularity of other modern devices, such as VCRs, cell phones, and fax machines reflects acculturation among people. In a general sense, students with disabilities and their families may be viewed as becoming more acculturated to the presence of specific educational strategies, such as technology, in classroom and other environments/milieus—and expecting it with greater frequency (Lahm & Sizemore, 2002).

It is important to recognize, however, that not all persons respond to acculturation influences in the same way. Some elements of our society continue to resist using new and emerging practices in favor of earlier, learned ways of doing things. One example of such resistance may be families of children with disabilities with whom professionals must collaborate in the process of developing individualized service plans. The family's resistance to accepting and implementing assistive technologies recommended for children may undermine the intent of the AT decision-making team and create tension or dissonance. A range of factors may be at work in such a situation. For example, with regard to AT service delivery, some families may accept some AT strategies and reject others, depending on the environmental context in which the strategies are to be implemented. As has been noted, "Perhaps the greatest obstacle to school change efforts is the attitudes of the individuals who must implement the change" (Fieldler, 2000, p. 119). The next section addresses strategies for bridging the gap between professionals who must implement the change and families with whom professionals collaborate.

Making the Bridge to Practice

Bridging the gap between the macro- and microcultures that intersect in the school context acknowledges that all cultures possess diverse cultural sets, often conflicting symbols, rituals, stories, and guides to action. This is true of all institutions in the United States, including special education (i.e., a subsystem of culture in special education exists within the larger education system) (Kalyanpur & Harry, 1999). Special education as a system reflects a culture of sets of behavior that have become ingrained among professionals who work with families. When conflicts with existing cultural sets occur in the school environment, students with disabilities and their families must employ a cultural tool kit (Swidler, 1998) to mediate the conflicts. Individuals need access to tools for constructing different strategies of action in response to conflicts, or environmental demands. Both individuals and groups actively use different tools from this kit to do different things in different situations.

Strategies for Culturally Responsive Professional Practice

To have an adequate understanding of service delivery needs for any family of a child with disabilities, it is necessary to examine the culture that shapes the family, as well as the culture of the school system in which the child is enrolled. With such understanding, "family and multicultural theoretical constructs may be viewed not as mutually exclusive but rather as complementary approaches to treatment" (Gushue

& Sciarra, 1995, p. 586). Drawing from the counseling literature, Gushue and Sciarra use a multidimensional approach as the basis for a suggested educator's tool kit that includes strategies for becoming knowledgeable about the student and family cultural background, identity, values, and preferences, as well as processes for applying this knowledge to educational decision making with children from culturally diverse families who have disabilities.

Cultural Identity

Various strategies from the field of multicultural counseling have been suggested for understanding the multidimensional components of ethnic identity brought by families who are culturally and linguistically diverse (Sodowsky, Kwan, & Pannu, 1995). Before the education professional begins any plan of intervention with families, it is necessary that he or she identify the culture of the family. Approximately 19 different ethnic portraits of family patterns have been identified in the United States (Gushue & Sciarra, 1995); thus the educator will need to determine the behaviors, values, and beliefs of the family's normative ethnic group before proceeding with a plan for the child with disabilities.

As noted by Gushue and Sciarra (1995), the educator will want to ask two questions: "First, to what extent does this particular family conform to or differ from the 'typical' patterns of family functioning for its culture? Secondly, what cultural differences may exist within the family itself?" (p. 589). These questions remind the professional to consider the extent of acculturation of the family. For example, it may be useful for professionals to establish how closely a family identifies with their ethnic group. It may also be helpful to examine their participation in various cultural activities, e.g., food, religion, language use. Further, it also seems necessary for education professionals to observe families' external ethnic identities (e.g., "these behaviors are manifested in the areas of ethnic language, ethnic group friendship, participation in ethnic group functions and activities, ethnic media, and ethnic traditions"; Sodowsky et al., 1995, p. 138), and internal ethnic identities, i.e., the person's self-image and image of the ethnic group (cognitive dimension), "feelings of group obligations" (moral dimension; Isajiw, 1990, p. 36), and affective dimension, which refers to an associative preference or feeling of attachment or comfort with one's own ethnic group. These two identities (external and internal) together more closely represent the whole identity of each family.

Through the two identities, scholars have begun to examine the various characteristics of ethnic identities. For example, researchers do not believe that each identity is interdependent (Isajiw, 1990); rather, the internal and external aspects may vary independently. Ethnic identity inquiry has yielded a comprehensive literature, beyond the scope of this chapter, but it is important to comment that each ethnic identity orientation evolves over time and not always linearly. What is probably most important for educators to understand is that when a family is asked or expected to act according to or between two different ethnic identity orientations, the process "can make an ethnic individual's life complex and difficult because many options are available for the individual, and these put pressure on him or her to make many decisions" (Sodowsky et al., 1995, p. 145).

Linguistic Differences

Finally, knowledge of the "linguistic differences within the family system" (Gushue & Sciarra, 1995, p. 596) is important to an understanding of the child's cultural context. To further examine this dimension, educators would ask questions about the languages spoken by the family and the child, when the second language was acquired/lost, the dominant language, the age when the language(s), was learned, and linguistic competencies in each language, both spoken and written.

Cultural Reciprocity

Simply being knowledgeable about families' cultural identity, practices, and linguistic differences is not enough to ensure collaboration with families and effective decision making. If the family and the professional are from different ethnic/racial groups, it is important to understand the feelings between members of each group. Is one group the dominant group and the other a non-dominant culture in the United States? If so, how will members of the family feel about movement toward, or practices within, another cultural identity model? Careful consideration of the attitudes, past experiences with, and interactions between cultural issues during assessment and treatment of members of groups will be necessary in order to create "cultural maps" that explain all the various intervention parameters to the family (Huer, 2005). Cultural maps will help to explain the patterns of thinking of the professionals, the patterns of thinking of the family, and the different orientations to the child's intervention plan.

To construct and then use such a map for cultural understanding as a guide to educational decision making, Kalyanpur and Harry (1999) suggest a four-step process for professionals to develop a "posture of *cultural reciprocity*" (p. 118, emphasis added). By combining this four-step process with knowledge of research-based and emerging best practices and a family-centered approach, the education professional may achieve cultural reciprocity with the family.

Step 1. Identify the cultural values reflected in the education professional's interpretation of the family and/or student's needs or in the recommendation for service. This step essentially requires the professional to ask "why" a specific perception is held (Parette, Huer, & VanBiervliet, 2005). For example, a Hispanic student with a developmental disability acts out when competitive activities are conducted in the classroom. Despite discussions about the importance of individual excellence and achievement in the classroom, the student displays a perceived inability or unwillingness to participate in such activities. At this point, the professional should ask him/herself why competitiveness is deemed important. If the professional is from a white cultural background, the perception may simply be that this is a strongly held value in the mainstream culture and necessary for success in the workplace.

Step 2. Determine whether the family recognizes and values these assumptions, and if not, how their perception differs from that of the education professional. In this second step, the professional approaches the family and presents his or her perception of the "issue" to them. This can become problematic in working with some families if an interpreter is needed in order for interactions with school personnel to occur. Some families are uncomfortable discussing family matters in the presence of others, and they may also feel that probing questions from professionals are intrusive (Chan, 1986; VanBiervliet & Parette, 1999; Zuniga, 1997). Issues related to working with interpreters are beyond the scope of this chapter, but resources are available elsewhere (see, e.g., Lynch & Hanson, 1997; VanBiervliet & Parette, 1999). Once appropriate contact is made with the family, the professional should present his or her perception in a culturally sensitive way for the family's consideration and response. In this example, the family may reveal that they see nothing wrong with the child's behaviors and that cooperative activities (versus competitive) in the family and other settings are typical.

Step 3. Acknowledge and provide specific respect to any cultural differences identified and fully explain the cultural basis of the education professional's assumptions. In this step, the professional should explain to the family his or her own assumptions and beliefs and how they are different from those of the family (Kalyanpur & Harry, 1999). For the previous example, the education professional would clarify that competition is important for some learning tasks and activities to provide the practitioner with a means of evaluating the student's progress. Further, the professional would note that failure to demonstrate a willingness to compete with others communicates disrespect for the structure of the classroom and for the wisdom of the teacher. The professional must also acknowledge that the family feels (a) that competitiveness is not emphasized in their family setting and (b) that cooperation with others is an important way of learning and achieving targeted goals.

Step 4. Determine the most effective way to adapt the education professional's interpretations or recommendations to the value system of the family. For example, through discussion and collaboration, all parties work out an alternative solution that is acceptable to the professional *and* to the family. In this student's case, both the professional and the family members agree that acceptable outcomes are for the teacher to be certain that the child has "heard" the teacher when asked to participate in competitive activities and understands that this is a valued classroom activity.

Conclusion

The multidimensional approach outlined here emphasizes the exploration of both between-group cultural differences and within-group differences of families participating within the educational activities available through the school system. Taking into account differences across the four dimensions of ethnic groups, cultural identities, extent of acculturation, and linguistic abilities will provide a solid foundation for professionals working with families with children having disabilities. The multidimensional approach contributes to helping education professionals "gain a more accurate assessment of the families they serve and a better understanding of their own role and responses; it will also enable them to devise more appropriate and effective family interventions" (Gushue & Sciarra, 1995, p. 604).

Glossary

Assimilation—Outcome resulting from the extent to which a person desires contact with the macroculture while not necessarily maintaining an identity with a relevant microculture.

Cultural reciprocity—A four-step process of professional and family values clarification that can culminate in enhanced understanding of all parties in educational decision-making processes.

Culture—A common set of beliefs, values, behaviors, and communication patterns that are shared by a particular group of people and *learned* as a function of social membership.

Dissonance—Evident differences in value systems that are perceived by an individual or groups.

Generational poverty—Values that are passed from one generation to the next and are simply assumed because of circumstances and conditions in which individuals live over time.

Integration—Outcome of family members and/or their children with developmental disabilities who desire both to maintain their cultural identity and to engage in a high level of interaction with a macroculture.

Macroculture—A large cultural group that has broad values (e.g., Americans).

Marginalization—Outcome reflected by persons not identifying with either their native culture or the dominant culture (e.g., enforced cultural loss combined with enforced segregation).

Microculture—A subgroup within a macroculture that has shared values (e.g., race, ethnicity, nationality, language, social status, rural/urban location).

Separation—Outcome reflected in low levels of interaction by individuals with the macroculture (and related microcultural groups) while maintaining a close connection with and affirmation of their native culture.

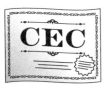

Knowledge and Skills for Entry-Level Special Education Teachers of Students With Developmental Disabilities Standards Addressed in This Chapter

Principle 1: Foundations

DD1K4   Trends and practices in the field of developmental disabilities.

Principle 2: Development and Characteristics of Learners

DD2K4   Factors that influence overrepresentation of culturally/linguistically diverse individuals.

Principle 5: Learning Environments/Social Interaction

DD5S3   Use and maintain assistive technologies.

DD5S5   Plan instruction for individuals with developmental disabilities in a variety of placement settings.

Principle 8: Assessment

DD8K1   Specialized terminology used in the assessment of individuals with developmental disabilities.

Web Site Resources

Culture, Disability, and Family Policy

http://thechp.syr.edu/dfpbcult.htm

     A quick overview of family issues relevant to culture and disability.

Disability, Diversity, and Dissemination

http://www.ncddr.org/du/products/dddreview/toc.html

     A comprehensive examination of cultural issues related to disability: What is culture? A nice compilation of theoretical perspectives of culture, Web site resources, definitions, and other supplemental information.

The Implications of Culture on Developmental Delay

http://www.ericec.org/digests/e589.html

     An ERIC information document that explores background cultural issues related to developmental delay.

Perspectives on Culture

http://www.wsu.edu:8001/vcwsu/commons/topics/culture/culture-definition.html

     A definition of culture and various theoretical positions.

What Is Culture?

http://www.wsu.edu:8001/vcwsu/commons/topics/culture/culture-index.html

     A definition of culture and some examples of different cultures.

References

Alper, S. K., Schloss, P. J., & Schloss, C. N. (1994). *Families of students with disabilities: Consultation and advocacy.* Boston: Allyn & Bacon.

Banks, J. A. (1997a). Multicultural education: Characteristics and goals. In J. A. Banks & C. A. Mc-Gee Banks (Eds.), *Multicultural education: Issues and perspectives* (3rd ed., pp. 3–31). Needham Heights, MA: Allyn & Bacon.

Banks, J. A. (1997b). *Teaching strategies for ethnic studies* (6th ed.). Needham Heights, MA: Allyn & Bacon.

Banks, J. A., & Mc Gee Banks, C. A. (Eds.). (1997). *Multicultural education: Issues and perspectives* (3rd ed.). Needham Heights, MA: Allyn & Bacon.

Battle, D. E. (2002). *Communication disorders in multicultural populations* (3rd ed.). Boston: Andover Medical.

Berry, J. W., Kim, U., Power, S., Young, M., & Bujaki, M. (1989). Acculturation attitudes in plural societies. *Applied Psychology, 38,* 185–206.

Berry, J. W., Poortinga, Y. H., Segall, M. H., & Dasen, P. R. (1992). *Cross-cultural psychology: Research and application.* Cambridge: Cambridge University Press.

Berry, J. W., & Sam, D. L. (1997). Acculturation and adaptation. In J. W. Berry, M. H. Segall, & C. Kagitcibasi (Eds.), *Handbook of cross-cultural psychology: Vol. 3. Social behaviour and applications* (2nd ed., pp. 291–326). Boston: Allyn & Bacon.

Boykin, A. W. (1994). Harvesting talent and culture: African American children and educational reform. In R. Rossi (Ed.), *Schools and students at risk* (pp. 116–138). New York: Teachers College Press.

Boykin, A. W., & Bailey, C. T. (2000). *The role of cultural factors in school relevant cognitive functioning: Description of home environmental factors, cultural orientations, and learning preferences* Report No. 43. Baltimore: Center for Social Organization of Schools, Johns Hopkins University. Retrieved September 21, 2004, from http://www.csos.jhu.edu/crespar/techReports/Report43.pdf

Carroll, M., & Phillips, B. (1993). *Survey on assistive technology abandonment by new users* (Cooperative Agreement No. H133E0016). Washington, DC: National Institute on Disability and Rehabilitation Research.

Casey, J. M. (2000). *Early literacy: The empowerment of technology* (Rev. ed.). Englewood, CO: Libraries Unlimited.

Chan, S. (1986). Parents of exceptional Asian children. In M. K. Kitano & P. C. Chan (Eds.), *Exceptional Asian children and youth* (pp. 36–53). Reston, VA: Council for Exceptional Children.

Chan, S. (1997). Families with Asian roots. In E. W. Lynch & M. J. Hanson (Eds.), *Developing cross-cultural competence. A guide for working with children and their families* (2nd ed., pp. 251–353). Baltimore: Brookes.

Citrin, J., & Highton, B. (2004). Latino political integration follows European pattern. *Public Affairs Report, 43*(4). Retrieved June 9, 2005, from http://www.igs.berkeley.edu/publications/par/winter2002/latino%20integration.htm

Civilrights.org. (2002). *Civil rights 101. Demographics.* Retrieved April 22, 2005, from the Civilrights.org Web site, http://www.civilrights.org/research_center/civilrights101/demographics.html

CNNMoney. com. (2007). Revving up for back to school. Retrieved July 9, 2007, from http://money.cnn.com/2004/07/28/news/fortune500/backtoschool/

Douthit, C. (1997). *Problems of providing services to persons with disabilities from minority groups.* Retrieved June 8, 2005, from http://www.dinf.ne.jp/doc/english/Us_Eu/ada_e/pres_com/pres-dd/douthitt.htm

Duarte, J. A., & Rice, B. D. (1992, October). *Cultural diversity in rehabilitation.* Nineteenth Institute on Rehabilitation Issues. Fayetteville, AR: Arkansas Research and Training Center in Vocational Rehabilitation.

Economic Research Service. (2002). *Race and ethnicity in rural America: The demography and geography of rural minorities.* Retrieved April 22, 2005, from http://www.ers.usda.gov/Briefing/RaceAndEthnic/geography.htm

Edyburn, D. L. (2002). Born digital: Technology in the life of students starting kindergarten, high school, and college. *Special Education Technology Practice, 4*(4), 48.

Emmons, R. A., & Paloutzian, R. F. (2003). The psychology of religion. *Annual Review of Psychology, 54,* 377–402.

Field, S., & Hoffman, A. (1994). Development of a model for self-determination. *Career Development for Exceptional Individuals, 17,* 159–169.

Field, S., & Hoffman, A. (1998). Self-determination: An essential element of successful transitions. *National Educational Service, 2*(4), 37–40.

Fieldler, C. (2000). *Making a difference: Advocacy competencies for special education professionals.* Boston: Allyn & Bacon.

Freeman, S. A., & Field, W. E. (1994). Selection of rural assistive technology using a hypercard-based knowledge system. *Assistive Technology, 6,* 126–133.

Friedman, M. (2004, March). *Assistive technology research and development collaborative on cognitive disabilities.* Paper presented at the 2004 CSUN Technology and Persons with Disabilities Conference, Northridge, CA. Retrieved February 9, 2005, from http://www.biausa.org/word. files.to.pdf/good.pdfs/CSUN2004finalused.pdf

Galvin, J. C., & Scherer, M. J. (Eds.). (1996). *Evaluating, selecting, and using appropriate assistive technology.* Gaithersburg, MD: Aspen.

Georgas, J., Berry, J. W., Shaw, A., Christakopoulou, S., & Mylonas, K. (1996). Acculturation of Greek family values. *Journal of Cross-Cultural Psychology, 27,* 329–338.

Goodlad, J. (1984). *A place called school: Prospects for the future.* New York: McGraw-Hill.

Gordon, E., & Yowell, C. (1994). Cultural dissonance as a risk factor in the development of students. In R. Rossi (Ed.), *Schools and students at-risk: Context and framework for positive change* (pp. 51–59). New York: Teachers College, Columbia University.

Gushue, G. V., & Sciarra, D. T. (1995). Culture and families: A multidimensional approach. In J. G. Ponterotto, J. M. Casas, L. A. Suzuki, & C. M. Alexander (Eds.), *Handbook of multicultural counseling* (pp. 586–606). Thousand Oaks, CA: Sage.

Hahn, H. (2000). Accommodations and the ADA: Unreasonable bias or biased reasoning? *Berkeley Journal of Employment and Labor Law, 21*(1), 166–192.

Hains, A. H., Lynch, E. W., & Winton, P. J. (2000, October). *Moving towards cross-cultural competence in lifelong personnel development: A review of the literature.* CLAS Early Childhood Research Institute (Technical Report No. 3). Retrieved April 22, 2005, from http://clas.uiuc. edu/techreport/tech3.html#culture

Hanline, M. F., & Daley, S. E. (1992). Family coping strategies and strengths in Hispanic, African-American, and Caucasian families of young children. *Topics in Early Childhood Special Education, 12,* 351–366.

Harry, B. (1992). *Cultural diversity, families, and the special education system: Communication and empowerment.* New York: Teachers College Press.

Harry, B., Grenot-Scheyer, M., Smith-Lewis, M., Park, H. S., Xin, F., & Schwartz, I. (1995). Developing culturally inclusive services for persons with severe disabilities. *Journal of the Association for Persons with Severe Handicaps, 20,* 99–109.

Howe, N., & Strauss, W. (2000). *Millennials rising: The next great generation.* New York: Vintage Books, Random House.

Huer, M. B. (2005). Using concept maps for educational-based implementation of assistive technology: A culturally inclusive model for supervision in special education. *Journal of Special Education Technology, 20*(4) 51–61.

Ingstad, B., & Whyte, S. R. (Eds.). (1995). *Disability and culture.* Berkeley: University of California Press.

Isajiw, W. W. (1990). Ethnic-identity retention. In R. Breton, W. W. Isajiw, W. E. Kalbach, & J. G. Reitz (Eds.), *Ethnic identity and equality* (pp. 34–91). Toronto: University of Toronto Press.

Kalyanpur, M., & Harry, B. (1999). *Culture in special education: Building reciprocal family-professional relationships.* Baltimore: Brookes.

Keefe, S. E. (1980). Acculturation and the extended family. In A. M. Padilla (Ed.), *Acculturation: Theories, models, and some new findings* (pp. 85–109). Boulder, CO: Westview.

Kemp, C., & Parette, H. P. (2000). Barriers to minority parent involvement in assistive technology (AT) decision-making processes. *Education and Training in Mental Retardation and Developmental Disabilities, 35*(4), 384–392.

Kroeber, A. L., & Kluckhohn, C. (1952). Culture: A critical review of concepts and definitions. *Papers of the Peabody Museum of American Archaeology and Ethnology 47.* Cambridge, MA: Harvard University.

Kunkel, M. A. (1990). Expectations about counseling in relation to acculturation in Mexican-American and Anglo-American student samples. *Journal of Counseling Psychology, 37,* 286–292.

Lahm, E. A., & Sizemore, L. (2002). Factors that influence assistive technology decision-making. *Journal of Special Education Technology, 17,* 15–25.

Lamorey, S. (2002). The effects of culture on special education services: Evil eyes, prayer meetings, and IEPs. *Teaching Exceptional Children, 34*(5), 67–71.

Landrine, H., & Klonoff, E. A. (1995). The African American Acculturation Scale II: Cross-validation and short form. *Journal of Black Psychology, 21,* 124–152.

Laroche, M., Kim, C., Hui, M. K., & Joy, A. (1996). An empirical study of multidimensional ethnic change. *Journal of Cross-Cultural Psychology, 27,* 114–131.

LaVeist, T. A. (1996). Why we should continue to study race…but do a better job: An essay on race, racism, and health. *Ethnicity and Disease, 6*(1), 21–29.

Leung, P. (1996). Asian Pacific Americans and Section 21 of the Rehabilitation Act Amendments of 1992. *American Rehabilitation, 22*(1), 2–6.

Loridas, L. (1988). *Culture in the classroom: A cultural enlightenment manual for educators.* Detroit: Michigan State Department of Education, Wayne County Intermediate School District. (ERIC Document Reproduction Service No. ED 303 841).

Lynch, E. W., & Hanson, M. J. (Eds.). (1997). *Developing cross-cultural competence. A guide for working with young children and their families* (2nd ed.). Baltimore: Brookes.

Mannheim, K. (1952). The problem of generations. In K. Mannheim (Ed.), *Essays on the sociology of knowledge* (pp. 276–320). New York: Oxford University Press.

Masgoret, A., & Gardner, R. C. (1999). A causal model of Spanish immigrant adaptation in Canada. *Journal on Multilingual and Multicultural Development, 20,* 216–236.

Mask, T. (2002). *Are millennials smarter?* Retrieved February 8, 2005, from http://www.millennials.com/CognitiveMask.html

McGoldrick, M., Pearce, J. K., & Giordano, J. (Eds.). (1982). *Ethnicity and family therapy.* New York: Guilford.

McNaughton, W. A. (2003). *Ten mistakes to avoid in working with Latin Americans.* Retrieved April 22, 2005, from http://interamerican-understanding.freewebspace.com/mistakes.htm

Miller, C. K., & Norton, M. P. (2003). *Making God real for a new generation: Ministry with millennials born from 1982 to 1999.* Nashville, TN: Discipleship Resources.

Miraglia, E., Law, R., & Collins, P. (1999). *A baseline definition of culture.* Retrieved October 10, 2005, from http://www.wsu.edu:8001/vcwsu/commons/topics/culture/culture-definition.html

Misra, A. (1994). Partnership with multicultural families. In S. K. Alper, P. J. Schloss, & C. N. Schloss (Eds.), *Families of students with disabilities* (pp. 143–179). Boston: Allyn & Bacon.

Mitchell, S. (2002). *American generations: Who they are, how they live, what they think.* Ithaca, NY: New Strategists Publications.

Moore, E. G. J. (1985). Ethnicity as a variable in child development. In M. B. Spencer, G. K. Brookins, & W. R. Allen (Eds.), *Beginnings: The social and affective development of black children* (pp. 201–214). Hillsdale, NJ: Erlbaum.

National Center for the Dissemination of Disability Research. (1999). *Disability, diversity, and dissemination: A review of the literature on topics related to increasing the utilization of rehabilitation research outcomes among diverse consumer groups.* Austin, TX: Southwest Educational Development Laboratory. Retrieved June 15, 2005, from http://www.ncddr.org/du/products/dddreview/index.html

Nauck, B. (2001). Intercultural contact and intergenerational transmission in immigrant families. *Journal of Cross-Cultural Psychology, 32,* 159–173.

Oblinger, D. (2003). Boomers, Gen-Xers, and millennials: Understanding the new students. *Educause Review, 38*(4), 36–47.

Oblinger, D. G., & Oblinger, J. (2005). *Educating the Net generation*. Washington, DC: Educause. Retrieved June 21, 2005, from http://www.educause.edu/EducatingtheNetGeneration/5989

Parette, H. P. (1998). Cultural issues and family-centered assistive technology decision-making. In S. L. Judge & H. P. Parette (Eds.), *Assistive technology for young children with disabilities: A guide to providing family-centered services* (pp. 184–210). Cambridge, MA: Brookline.

Parette, H. P. (2004, April). *Millennial children in a digital age: Assistive technology futures in special education. Program Chair Invited Presentation.* Paper presented at the Council for Exceptional Children Annual Convention and Expo, New Orleans.

Parette, H. P., Brotherson, M. J., & Huer, M. B. (2000). Giving families a voice in augmentative and alternative communication decision-making. *Education and Training in Mental Retardation and Developmental Disabilities, 35,* 177–190.

Parette, H. P., Huer, M. B., & Brotherson, M. J. (2001). Related service personnel perceptions of team AAC decision-making across cultures. *Education and Training in Mental Retardation and Developmental Disabilities, 36,* 69–82.

Parette, H. P., Huer, M. B., & Scherer, M. (2004). Effects of acculturation on assistive technology service delivery. *Journal of Special Education Technology, 19*(2), 31–41.

Parette, H. P., Huer, M. B., & VanBiervliet, A. (2005). Cultural issues and assistive technology. In D. L. Edyburn, K. Higgins, & R. Boone (Eds.), *The handbook of special education technology research and practice* (pp. 81–103). Whitefish Bay, WI: Knowledge by Design, Inc.

Parette, H. P., & Petch-Hogan, B. (2000). Approaching families: Facilitating culturally/linguistically diverse family involvement. *Teaching Exceptional Children, 33*(2), 4–10.

Parette, P. (1999). Transition planning with families across cultures. *Career Development for Exceptional Individuals, 22,* 213–231.

Parette, P. (2005). Restrictiveness and race in special education: The issue of cultural reciprocity. *Learning Disabilities: A Contemporary Quarterly, 3*(1), 17–24.

Parette, P., & Peterson-Karlan, G. (2005, January). *Issues in building a national assistive technology coalition.* Paper presented at the Assistive Technology Industry Association 2005 Conference and Exhibition, Orlando, FL.

Payne, R. K. (1998). *A framework for understanding poverty.* Highlands, TX: aha! Process, Inc.

Peterson-Karlan, G. R., & Parette, H. P. (2005). Millennial students with mild disabilities and emerging assistive technology trends. *Journal of Special Education Technology, 20* (4), 27–38.

Pew Hispanic Center/Kaiser Family Foundation. (2002). *2002 national survey of Latinos.* Retrieved October 10, 2005, from http://pewhispanic.org/reports/report.php?ReportID=15

Pheelan, P., Davidson, A. L., & Cao, H. T. (1991). Students' multiple worlds: Negotiating the boundaries of family, peer, and school cultures. *Anthropology and Education Quarterly, 22,* 224–250.

Phillips, B., & Broadnax, D. D. (1992). *National survey on abandonment of technology* (Cooperative Agreement No. H133E80016). Washington, DC: National Institute on Disability and Rehabilitation Research.

Phillips, B., & Zhao, H. (1993). Predictors of assistive technology abandonment. *Assistive Technology, 5,* 36–45.

Phinney, J. S., Du Pont, S., Espinosa, C., Revill, J., & Sanders, K. (1994). Ethnic identity and American identification among ethnic minority youths. In A. M. Bouvy, F. J. R. Van de Vijver, P. Boski, & P. Schmitz (Eds.), *Journey into cross-cultural psychology* (pp. 167–183). Amsterdam: Swets and Zeitlinger.

Pomales, J., & Williams, V. (1989). Effects of level of acculturation and counseling style on Hispanic students' perceptions of counselors. *Journal of Counseling Psychology, 36,* 79–83.

Ponce, F. Q., & Atkinson, D. R. (1989). Mexican-American acculturation, counselor ethnicity, counseling style, and perceived counselor credibility. *Journal of Counseling Psychology, 36,* 79–83.

Raines, C. (2001). *Managing millennials.* Retrieved February 8, 2005, from http://www.generationsatwork.com/articles/millenials.htm

Ray, B. (2002). *Immigrant integration: Building to opportunity.* Retrieved from the Migrant Policy Institute Web site June 8, 2005, http://www.migrationinformation.org/Feature/display.cfm?ID=57

Richardson, E. H. (1981). Cultural and historical perspectives in counseling American Indians. In D. W. Sue (Ed.), *Counseling the culturally different: Theory and practice* (pp. 216–255). New York: John Wiley & Sons.

Riemer-Reiss, M. L., & Wacker, R. R. (1999). Assistive technology use and abandonment among college students with disabilities. *International Electronic Journal for Leadership in Learning, 3*(23). Retrieved November 28, 2004, from http://www.acs.ucalgary.ca/~iejll/volume3/riemer.html

Roseberry-McKibben, C. (2002). *Multicultural students with special language needs: Practical strategies for assessment and intervention* (2nd ed.). Oceanside, CA: Academic Communication Associates.

Rossman, G., Corbett, D., & Firestone, W. (1988). *Change and effectiveness in schools: A cultural perspective.* Philadelphia: Research for Better Schools.

Ruiz, R. A. (1981). Cultural and historical perspectives in counseling Hispanics. In D. W. Sue (Ed.), *Counseling the culturally different: Theory and practice* (pp. 186–215). New York: John Wiley & Sons.

Salins, P. D. (1997). *Assimilation, American style.* New York: Basic Books.

Schumann, J. H. (1986). Research on the acculturation model for second language acquisition. *Journal on Multilingual and Multicultural Development, 7,* 379–392.

Sleeter, C. E., & Grant, C. A. (2003). *Making choices for multicultural education: Five approaches to race, class, and gender* (4th ed.). New York: John Wiley & Sons.

Smart, J. (2001). *Disability, society, and the individual,* Gaithersburg, MD: Aspen Publishers.

Smart, J. F., & Smart, D. W. (1997). The racial/ethnic demography of disability. *Journal of Rehabilitation, 63*(4), 9–15.

Smedley, A. (1993). *Race in North America: Origin and evolution of a world view.* Boulder, CO: Westview.

Sodowsky, G. R., Kwan, K-L. K., & Pannu, R. (1995). Ethnic identity of Asians in the United States. In J. G. Ponterotto, J. M. Casas, L. A. Suzuki, & C. M. Alexander (Eds.), *Handbook of multicultural counseling* (pp. 123–154). Thousand Oaks, CA: Sage.

Soto, G. (1994). A cultural perspective on augmentative and alternative communication. *American Speech-Language-Hearing Association Special Interest Division 12, 3*(2), 6.

Soto, G., Huer, M. B., & Taylor, O. (1997). Multicultural issues. In L. L. Lloyd, D. H. Fuller, & H. H. Arvidson (Eds.), *Augmentative and alternative communication* (pp. 406–413). Boston: Allyn & Bacon.

Sue, D. W., & Sue, D. (1990). *Counseling the culturally different: Theory and practice.* New York: John Wiley & Sons.

Swaidan, Z. P., & Marshall, K. P. (2001, November). *Acculturation strategies: The case of the Muslim minority in the United States.* Paper presented at the Society of Marketing Advances, annual meeting, New Orleans.

Swidler, A. (1998). Culture and social action. In P. Smith (Ed.), *The new American cultural sociology.* Cambridge: Cambridge University Press.

Tapscott, D. (1998). *The rise of the Net generation: Growing up digital.* New York: McGraw-Hill.

Thomas, G., & Loxley, A. (2001). *Deconstructing special education and constructing inclusion.* Buckingham, PA: Open University Press.

Traustadottir, R. (2000). *Women with intellectual disabilities: Finding a place in the world.* Philadelphia: Jessica Kingsley Publishers.

Turner, E., Barrett, C., Cutshall, A., Lacy, B. K., Keiningham, J., & Webster, M. K. (1995). The user's perspective of assistive technology. In K. F. Flippo, K. J. Inge, & J. M. Barcus (Eds.), *Assistive technology: A resource for school, work, and community* (pp. 283–290). Baltimore: Brookes.

Valdivieso, R., & Nicolau, S. (1994). Look me in the eye: A Hispanic cultural perspective on school reform. In R. J. Rossi (Ed.), *Schools and students at risk: Context and framework for positive change* (pp. 90–115). New York: Teachers College Press.

VanBiervliet, A., & Parette, H. P. (1999). *Families, cultures, and AAC* (CD-ROM). Little Rock: Southeast Missouri State University and University of Arkansas for Medical Sciences.

Venkatesh, A. (1995). Ethnoconsumerism: A new paradigm to study cultural and cross-cultural consumer behaviour. In J. A. Costa & G. J. Bamossy (Eds.), *Marketing in a multicultural world* (pp. 26–67). Thousand Oaks, CA: Sage.

Vogt, L. A., Jordan, C., & Tharp, R. G. (1992). Explaining school failure, producing school success: Two cases. In E. Jacob & C. Jordan (Eds.), *Minority education: Anthropological perspectives* (pp. 53–66). Norwood, NJ: Ablex.

Walker, S., & Brown, O. (1996). The Howard University Research and Training Center: A unique resource. *American Rehabilitation, 22*(1), 27–33.

Wehmeyer, M. L. (1999). A functional model of self-determination: Describing development and implementing instruction. *Focus on Autism and Other Developmental Disabilities, 14*(1), 53–61.

Wehmeyer, M. L., & Schwartz, C. A. (1997). Self-determination and positive adult outcomes: A follow-up study of youth with mental retardation or learning disabilities. *Exceptional Children, 63,* 245–255.

Welch, M. (1989). A cultural perspective and the second wave of educational reform. *Journal of Learning Disabilities, 22,* 537–540, 560.

Wells, R. B., Hough, R. L., Golding, J. M., & Burnam, M. A. (1987). Which Mexican Americans underutilize health services? *American Journal of Psychiatry, 144,* 918–922.

Williams, D. R., & Jackson, P. B. (2005). Social sources of racial disparities in health. *Health Affairs, 24,* 325–334.

Willis, W. (1997). Families with African American roots. In E. W. Lynch & M. J. Hanson (Eds.), *Developing cross-cultural competence: A guide for working with children and their families* (2nd ed., pp. 165–207). Baltimore: Brookes.

Wood, W. M., Karvonen, M., Test, D. W., Browder, D., & Algozzine, B. (2004). Promoting student self-determination skills in IEP planning. *Teaching Exceptional Children, 36*(3), 8–16.

Woodard, I. V., Emory, H., & Gridina, N. (2000). *Media in the home 2000: The fifth annual survey of parents and children. Survey Series No. 7.* Philadelphia: The Annenberg Public Policy Center of the University of Pennsylvania. Retrieved February 15, 2005, from http://www.annenbergpublicpolicycenter.org/05_media_developing_child/mediasurvey/survey7.pdf

Woods, V. D., Montgomery, S. B., Belliard, J. C., Belle, S. M., Nortey, J. J., & Ramírez, J. (2002, November). *Cultural health beliefs, attitudes, and fears of African American men and the associated impact on their willingness to participate in prostate cancer screening. Preliminary report.* Paper presented at the 130th annual meeting of the American Public Health Association, Philadelphia.

World Book. (2004). *Cultural backgrounds of Hispanic Americans.* Retrieved April 22, 2005, from http://www2.worldbook.com/wc/popup?path=features/cinco&page=html/cultural.htm&direct=yes

Zborowsky, M. (1969). *People in pain.* San Francisco: Jossey-Bass.

Zemke, R., Raines, C., & Filipczak, B. (1999). *Generations at work: Managing the clash of veterans, boomers, Xers, and Nexters in your workplace.* New York: AMACOM Books.

Zhang, S. Y., & Carrasquillo, A. L. (1995). Chinese parents' influence on academic performance. *New York State Association for Bilingual Education Journal, 10,* 46–53.

Zuniga, M. E. (1997). Families with Latino roots. In E. W. Laynch & M. J. Hanson (Eds.), *Developing cross-cultural competence. A guide for working with children and their families* (2nd ed., pp. 209–249). Baltimore: Brookes.

SECTION 4

INSTRUCTIONAL PLANNING AND IMPLEMENTATION

9

Meeting the Needs of All Students Through Instructional Design

Barbara C. Gartin and Nikki L. Murdick

Summary

This chapter describes the differentiated instruction model and its relationship to the principles of evidence-based instructional planning. A discussion of the three components of differentiated instruction (content, process, and product) is included.

Learning Outcomes

After reading this chapter, you should be able to:

- List four evidenced-based findings that should direct instructional planning.

- Give the three components of differentiated instruction that must be considered in evidenced-based instructional planning.

- Know the questions to apply in each of the three components of differentiated instruction to direct the planning process.

Introduction

Given the increasingly diverse student population schools today are challenged to serve, we should not still be asking whether it is feasible to provide for student diversity in heterogeneous classes. The question at hand is how we can best respond to student diversity so that outcome standards are upheld for every student, including the most difficult to teach and most challenging to motivate. (Issue, 1994, p. 7)

This call to respond to diversity through curriculum design and the instructional process continues to be one that educators must address to meet the needs of *all* students. The challenge to meet the needs of *all* students is the foundation of our democratic values, principles, and values based on equity and excellence (Hitchcock, Meyer, Rose, & Jackson, 2002; Kluth, Straut, & Biklen, 2003; Tomlinson, 1999). The foundation is reinforced by recent legislation (Individuals with Disabilities Education Improvement Act of 2004; No Child Left Behind Act of 2001), with its intricately involved standards-based reform movement and focus on student learning (Nolet & McLaughlin, 2000; Tomlinson, 2000).

Evidence-Based Instruction

In order to respond to this call, the informed educator must understand and use evidence-based research to direct the selection of curriculum and instructional methods. *Curriculum*, according to Mercer and Mercer (2001), "primarily involves what is taught in the school and consists of learning outcomes that society considers essential for success" (p. 170). Meyen (1981) defined curriculum as "the courses offered, the overall experience provided a child by the school, the program included in a particular subject field, or in some cases, the sum total of experiences afforded school-age children regardless of school sponsorship" (pp. 20–21). *Instruction*, on the other hand, is the method by which curriculum is presented to the students. According to Oliva (2001), the distinction between curriculum and instruction is that curriculum is "a program, a plan, content, and learning experiences, whereas we may characterize instruction as methods, the teaching act, implementation, and presentation" (p. 8). Thus it is clear that the informed and effective educator must understand what constitutes the curriculum in his or her school [United Nations Educational, Scientific, and Cultural Organization (UNESCO), 2004], how to design evidence-based instruction (Ormrod, 2006), and how to identify effective instructional strategies that will assist in the acquisition of instructional goals of the curriculum (Mastropieri & Scruggs, 2002).

Research on evidence-based instruction was begun early in the 1970s and continued through the 1980s under the umbrella of teacher planning processes. In 1986, Clark and Peterson presented the first important summary of this research base. Orlich, Harder, Callahan, and Gibson (2001) use this summary and the results of recent research to identify four important components in instructional planning.

The first evidence-based finding is that instructional planning can be used to accomplish multiple purposes, including serving as a guide to instruction, a directional focus, or a content organizational process (see Borko & Niles, 1987; Borko & Shavelson, 1991; Clark & Peterson, 1986; Kagan & Tippins, 1992; Price & Nelson, 1999; Sardo-Brown, 1988; Shavelson & Stern, 1981; and Wiggins & McTighe, 1998). According to Algozzine, Ysseldyke, and Elliott (1997), instructional planning also occurs at two levels: strategic and tactical. Strategic planning involves developing the basic structure and emphasis of the rationale for instruction, i.e., the overall curriculum. Tactical planning, on the other hand, involves the day-to-day planning that most commonly takes the form of daily or weekly lesson plans (Rosenberg, O'Shea, & O'Shea, 2006). The intended use (or level) of the planning process thus dictates how and in what format the instruction will eventually occur.

The second evidence-based finding is that instructional planning does not always occur in a linear format, as described, for example, in seminal work by Ralph Tyler (1949) and Saylor, Alexander, and Lewis (1981). This linear format, also known as a rational-logical process (Sowell, 2000), has been used as the basis for curriculum and instructional planning since that time. A circular format was proposed by Taba (1962) as a way to move from the linearity of Tyler's rational-step format in developing curriculum to one in which ongoing evaluation occurred by educators within the schools (Marshall, Sears, & Schubert, 2000). Research has noted that effective teachers often do not use the linear format espoused by most curriculum developers, but instead use the more circular spiral format for instructional planning (Bruner, 1960; Burden & Byrd, 2003; Glickman, Gordon, & Ross-Gordon, 2001; Wolcott, 1994; Yinger & Clark, 1982).

Effective teachers use reflective planning both to improve their teaching and to select and plan instructional strategies (Cruickshank & Haefele, 2001; Good &

Brophy, 2000; Stronge, 2002). Reflective planning may not occur in a written format, for as Orlich et al. (2001) state, "teachers tend to carry much of their planning in their mind rather than on paper" (p. 127). This "intellectual" planning, or "mental-image approach," more often occurs as educators become more skilled and experienced in planning instruction to meet the perceived needs of the students (Clark & Yinger, 1987; Juarez, 1992; Stronge, 2002). But one caveat has been identified—mental planning without some form of written planning "leaves a high probability that objectives and activities will be vague and loosely structured" (Rosenberg et al., 2006, p. 129).

The third evidence-based finding is the need for flexibility in instructional planning. The research indicates that effective teachers are not only skilled in instructional planning but also willing to change those plans as required to meet the needs of their students (Gettinger & Stoiber, 1999). Some researchers label this ability "withitness," along with the ability to make moment-by-moment adjustments during the application of their instructional plan (Kounin, 1970; Lampert & Clark, 1990).

The fourth evidence-based finding is that research has not supported any specific instructional planning model as being more effective than another. Research continues in this area, but it appears that the effectiveness of instructional planning models is dependent on "the selection of learning activities, instructional objectives, content, students' age, available time, and teaching strategies" (Orlich et al., 2001, p. 127). Thus the individual teacher's skill in completing the above activities will have a significant impact on the effectiveness of the instructional planning model being used.

Evidence-Based Instructional Planning and Differentiated Instruction

Numerous models of instructional planning have been described and researched. Four of the more well known are the unit planning model (Orlich et al., 2001), the diagnostic teaching model (Rosenberg et al., 2006), the universal design for learning model (Council for Exceptional Children, 2005), and the differentiation of instruction model (Tomlinson, 1999). Each of these models is based on the concept of differentiating the instruction provided to students within the classroom setting. According to Tomlinson (2000), "differentiation is simply attending to the learning needs of a particular student or group of students, rather than the more typical pattern of teaching the class as though all individuals in it were basically alike" (p. 149). In fact, when one discusses the concept of differentiation within the instructional arena, it includes all forms of changes within the curriculum, no matter how small. In other words, individualized planning can take numerous forms, and no perfect example presently exists (Pettig, 2000).

For this chapter, the authors have chosen the differentiation of instruction model, known as differentiated instruction, as a model that is effective when planning instruction for students with developmental disabilities who are included in the general education classroom. Differentiated instruction is defined as "the planning of curriculum and instruction using strategies that address student strengths, interests, skills, and readiness in flexible learning environments" (Gartin, Murdick, Imbeau, & Perner, 2002, pp. 1–8). In other words, it is not a teaching plan, nor an instructional strategy, but a philosophy that guides the teacher's thoughts and actions with the children who are in the classroom (Tomlinson, 2000).

Differentiated instruction is considered to be a "global strategy" that occurs in some format in most heterogeneous classrooms (CEC, 2005). When students in a classroom present extreme variance in their learning abilities, some form of individualized instruction and planning is essential. Research during the 1980s and 1990s focused on the issues presented by this heterogeneity and the effectiveness of the methods used by teachers (see Brantlinger, 1993; Cohen & Lotan, 1995; Evans, 1985; Evertson, Sanford, & Emmer, 1981; Mevarich & Kramarski, 1997; Newmann, 1992; Rothenberg, McDermott, & Martin, 1998). From this research certain evidence-based principles for differentiating instruction were identified: (a) matching assignments to student ability levels; (b) using multiple levels of reading materials, including textbooks; (c) preparing assignments on different ability levels; and (d) planning instruction to accommodate the needs of individual students (Good & Brophy, 2000; Janney & Snell, 2000). The research indicates that teachers might be more effective if they incorporate these principles or practices in a planning format known as differentiated instruction (Good & Brophy, 2000).

Components of Differentiated Instruction

The differentiated instruction model is a model that uses a "backward design" technique (Greece Central School District, 2005). As in all models for planning instruction, there is an overarching learning goal, and the teacher begins with the end in mind. In a forward design technique, though, the teacher sees the goal and works toward it by planning activities and lessons that are designed to lead the students to that goal. Opponents of the forward planning model state that when all the activities have been implemented, not all students understand and know the requisite information. The backward planning model, on the other hand, poses a series of questions at the beginning that focus the instructional planning process not only on the end goal but on the steps leading up to that goal. Questions are used as the basis for designing instruction in the differentiated model because "when questions are used strategically, they help frame ideas, lead to new ideas, and promote learning" (Bay Area School Reform Collaborative, 2005).

The differentiated instruction model includes three specific curricular components that provide the basis for developing questions to be answered during the planning process (UNESCO, 2004):

> (1) the content—the curriculum and the materials and approaches used for students to learn the content, (2) the process—the instructional activities or approaches used to help students to learn the curriculum, and (3) the products—the assessment vehicles through which students demonstrate what they have learned. (Burden & Byrd, 2003, p. 151)

In the differentiated instruction model, the *content* of the curriculum is considered first. Content is defined as "what we teach," or the specific information that the student is expected to learn (UNESCO, 2004). The first step in the differentiated instruction model begins with a review of the content to be studied, including the required information or "enduring understandings" (Greece Central School District, 2005) that students should have acquired when the end of the lesson has been reached. In other words, the "what" of the curriculum is the core foundation for any changes that must be made to address the individualized needs of students. Marshall et al. (2000), citing Schubert's 1992 quote, epitomize this concept when they state:

> My important school teaching experience taught me that the question of greatest import was a philosophical curriculum question: What is worthwhile to know and experience? This Spencerian question (Spencer, 1861) must flow in the lifeblood of teachers in their daily activities. Everything they do is contingent upon some image of what is worth knowing and experiencing. (p. 174)

Examples of the type of questions that might be used are: (a) What is essential that *all* students learn of this curricular content? (b) What is essential that *most*, but not all, students learn of this curricular content? And (c) What is essential that *some* students learn of this curricular content? The answers to these questions will assist the teacher in selecting a framework for presenting the curricular content material— for example, Schumm, Vaughn, & Leavell's (1994) Planning Pyramid. Other methods that teachers might use in differentiating the content are concept-based teaching, or curriculum compacting (Tomlinson, 1995). In some instances the teacher may not have the freedom to change the curriculum significantly, as the content may be prescribed by a required curriculum guide developed by the local school district or the state department of education. In that case, the teacher may have to expand the other two components (process and product) of the differentiated instruction model.

Once the content has been addressed, the teacher can develop questions that assist in the *process* of deciding how best to differentiate the process of the instruction. According to the CEC (2005), the process is defined as the method that the teacher selects, or designs, to present the content, as well as the method by which the students are to respond to the content. The differentiated instruction model uses the questioning technique to identify the most appropriate method for introducing the content while at the same time meeting the diverse needs of the students. Examples of questions to ask include: (a) What is the purpose of the lesson? (b) What are the specific individualized needs and strengths of the students? (c) How do the students learn best? (d) What methods would best guide them in understanding the essential ideas or concepts of the content? and (e) What methods would be most effective in assisting the students to relate the new information to previous information they have learned? The answers to these questions will help the teacher to identify the most appropriate process, or teaching method, for students with diverse learning needs. Examples of process methods that might be used in differentiating instruction include tiered lessons (Tomlinson, 1999), entry points (Gardner, 1993), learning centers, cubing strategy, tic-tac-toe menus, and the RAFT strategy (Billmeyer & Barton, 1998).

After the questions concerning the content and the process have been answered, the teacher must identify *product* questions, that is, questions whose answers indicate the student's "understanding performance" (Perkins, 1991). In other words, no instructional design is complete without a means of demonstrating that the instructional goal has been attained. In the differentiated instruction model, this demonstration of the student's knowledge of the content, and therefore, the effectiveness of the process, is known as the "product." In other words, the product that is selected indicates the means by which the student demonstrates that he/she has learned the content, or achieved mastery (CEC, 2005). Questions to ask in order to use the differentiated instruction model to review the products of the lesson being designed include: (a) What should students have learned at the end of the lesson or unit? (b) What should students understand? (c) What application of the knowledge should students be able to do? (d) How will successful completion of the lesson be recognized? To differentiate instructional products teachers might use concrete products such as "essays, videos, dramatizations, and experiments" (Gartin et al., 2002, pp. 6–52) that fit into Renzulli's seven categories—artistic products, performance products, spoken products, visual products, model/construction products, leadership products, and written products (Renzulli, Leppien, & Hays, 2000). Or teachers might use abstract products that are identified as teacher indicators, such as cognitive structures and affective structures that verify that student learning has occurred (Gartin et al., 2002). This component of differentiated instruction includes the various assessment options that can be used and/or modified to meet students' diverse needs. For example, the teacher might use assessment procedures other than the typical paper and pencil tests, such as authentic assessment, portfolio assessment, student work presentations, or scoring guides and rubrics. The teacher selects the assessment procedure according to the answers that result from the questions.

Since teachers often use various methods and modifications in the general classroom, they may expect the differentiated instruction model to be a simple model. But in fact it can be difficult to implement. According to Tomlinson and Allan (2000), the use of the differentiated instruction model requires that teachers "move toward expertise" (p. 13). For opponents of this model, this statement is the crux of the concern. Gartin et al. (2002) agree when they state that "teachers see differentiated instruction as a means of lesson planning, not as a method for developing curriculum for successful learning and instruction. The focus on lessons without an overarching plan can result in a disjointed curriculum" (pp. 1–10).

Because of the perceived simplicity of the differentiated planning model, some researchers believe that teachers are misled into believing that instructional design for students with diverse needs will be both simple to develop and simple to implement. This, of course, is not the case. In this era of an expanded focus on inclusion and on standardized testing, it may become detrimental to the actual students whose needs we are attempting to meet (Kauffman, McGee, & Brigham, 2004).

In the end, these challenges are not new. Adequately meeting the needs of diverse learners, particularly students with disabilities in mainstreamed classrooms, has been a problem under traditional circumstances (Baker & Zigmond, 1990; Schumm et al., 1994). The challenges are simply more acute in an era of high standards and student outcomes. We can begin to achieve greater educational equity through better curricular materials and pedagogical strategies. But we also need to attend to a range of contextual variables—from improved preservice preparation through coordinated general and special education services—if teachers are to be successful in classrooms with diverse learners. (Kame'enui, Carnine, Dixon, Simmons, & Coyne, 2002, p. 230)

Glossary

Circular format, as in planning curriculum—An inductive curriculum developed by creating teaching-learning units rather than by developing a general curricular design.

Content—Facts, concepts, generalizations, principles, attitudes and skills being taught.

Curriculum—What is taught; consists of learning outcomes valued by society and includes the learning environment, content, and learning experiences.

Differentiated instruction—A method of differentiation that chooses content, process, and products based on individual student strengths, interests, skills, and readiness in flexible learning environments.

Differentiation—The process of modifying content, process, and product to meet the individual student's learning preferences.

Evidenced-based, or research-based, instruction—Instruction that utilizes strategies found to have a statistically positive effect on student learning. Instruction that is evidenced-based, or research-based, has been found to have a high probability of enhancing student achievement for all students in all content areas across all grades.

Instruction—How one presents curriculum to students; the act of teaching.

Instructional planning—Setting up instruction while acting as a content organizer and giving directional focus to the actions of the teacher. Instructional planning occurs on two levels: strategic and tactical.

Linear format, as in planning curriculum—A rational-logical process of curriculum development that moves step by step toward the end goal.

Process—How students make sense of, understand, and internalize the content. Examples include activities, exercises, assignments, and tasks based on the learning goal.

Product—How the student demonstrates knowledge, understanding, or doing that has resulted from instruction and the subsequent study of content.

Reflective planning—A mental process that occurs in teachers' heads as they consider the responses of students to instruction and then plan and implement changes in the instructional plan.

Spiral format, as in planning curriculum—Repetition of concepts, skills, and knowledge at successive levels of competency.

Strategic planning—The development of curriculum, including the rationale for instruction and the overall structure for its delivery.

Tactical planning—Daily or weekly lesson plans.

Withitness—A characteristic of teachers that allows them to be simultaneously cognizant of individual student responses and aware of the response of the group and to make moment-by-moment instructional adjustments that allow the needs of the individual as well as the needs of the group to be met.

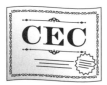

Knowledge and Skills for Entry-Level Special Education Teachers of Students With Developmental Disabilities Standards Addressed in This Chapter

Principle 1: Foundations

DD1K4   Trends and practices in the field of developmental disabilities.

Principle 3: Individual Learning Differences

DD3K1   Impact of multiple disabilities on behavior.

Principle 4: Instructional Strategies

DD4S1   Use specialized teaching strategies matched to the need of the learner.

DD4S2   Relate levels of support to the needs of the individual.

Principle 5: Learning Environments/Social Interaction

DD5S4   Structure the physical environment to provide optimal learning for individuals with developmental disabilities.

Principle 7: Instructional Planning

DD7S2   Plan and implement instruction for individuals with developmental disabilities that is both age-appropriate and ability-appropriate.

DD7S4   Design, implement, and evaluate specialized instructional programs for persons with developmental disabilities that enhance social participation across environments.

Web Site Resources

Association for Supervision and Curriculum Development (ASCD)

http://www.ascd.org/portal/site/ascd/index.jsp/

> Homepage for ASCD (Association on Supervision and Curriculum Development). Links to articles related to curriculum and instruction, including differentiated instruction. Also includes a catalog of materials related to differentiated instruction that can be previewed and are for sale on this site.

Differentiated Instruction

http://tst1160-35.k12.fsu.edu/mainpage.html

> Links to sites for articles on differentiated instruction, samples of differentiated lessons at the elementary, middle, and secondary school level, and links to other academic resources that may be useful when differentiating instruction.

Differentiated Instruction Resources

http://www.middleweb.com/MWLresources/rickdiffbiblio.html

> Resources on differentiated instruction.

Differentiating Instruction

http://www.wall.k12.nj.us/staff_dev/differentiating_instruction.htm

> A description of the ASCD's differentiation model, a description of strategies for differentiating instruction, and ways to differentiate content, process, and product.

Enhance Learning with Technology: Strategies for Differentiating

http://members.shaw.ca/priscillatheroux/differentiatingstrategies.html

> A description of the various learning strategies used when one implements the differentiated instruction planning model.

Greece Central School District

http://www.greece.k12.ny.us

> Description of backward design, including the specific steps in how to use it in a secondary classroom setting.

References

Algozzine, B., Ysseldyke, J. E., & Elliott, J. (1997). *Strategies and tactics for effective instruction.* Longmont, CA: Sopris West.

Baker, J. M., & Zigmond, N. (1990). Are regular classes equipped to accommodate students with learning disabilities? *Exceptional Children, 56,* 515–526.

Bay Area School Reform Collaborative. (2005). *Inquiry in curriculum design.* Retrieved May 24, 2005, from http://www.wested.org/basrc/bank/Institue99/design/curriculumframework.pdf

Billmeyer, R., & Barton, M. L. (1998). *Teaching reading in the content areas: If not me, then who?* (2nd ed.). Aurora, CO: Mid-continent Regional Educational Laboratory (MCREL).

Borko, H., & Niles, J. (1987). Planning. In V. Richardson-Koehler (Ed.), *Educator's handbook: A research perspective* (pp. 167–187). New York: Longman.

Borko, H., & Shavelson, R. J. (1991). Teacher decision making. In B. Jones & L. Idol (Eds.), *Dimensions of thinking and cognitive instruction* (pp. 311–346). Hillsdale, NJ: Lawrence Erlbaum.

Brantlinger, E. (1993). *The politics of social class in secondary school: Views of affluent and impoverished youth.* New York: Teachers College Press.

Bruner, J. S. (1960). *The process of education.* Cambridge, MA: Harvard University Press.

Burden, P. R., & Byrd, D. M. (2003). *Methods for effective teaching* (3rd ed.). Boston: Allyn & Bacon.

Clark, C. M., & Peterson, P. L. (1986). Teachers' thought processes. In M. C. Wittrock (Ed.), *Handbook of research on teaching* (3rd ed., pp. 255–296). New York: Macmillan.

Clark, C. M., & Yinger, R. J. (1987). Teacher planning. In D. C. Berliner & B. Rosenshine (Eds.), *Talks to teachers* (pp. 342–365). New York: Random House.

Cohen, E., & Lotan, R. (1995). Producing equal-status interaction in the heterogeneous classroom. *American Education Research Journal, 32,* 99–120.

Council for Exceptional Children (CEC). (2005). *Universal design for learning: A guide for teachers and education professionals.* Arlington, VA: CEC and Merrill/Prentice Hall.

Cruickshank, D. R., & Haefele, D. (2001). Good teachers, plural. *Educational Leadership, 58*(5), 26–30.

Evans, J. (1985). *Teaching in transition: The challenge of mixed ability grouping.* Philadelphia: Open University Press.

Evertson, C., Sanford, J., & Emmer, E. (1981). Effects of class heterogeneity in junior high school. *American Education Research Journal, 18,* 219–232.

Gardner, H. (1993). *Multiple intelligences: The theory in practice.* New York: Basic Books.

Gartin, B. C., Murdick, N. L., Imbeau, M., & Perner, D. E. (2002). *How to use differentiated instruction with students with developmental disabilities in the general education classroom.* Arlington, VA: Division on Developmental Disabilities, CEC.

Gettinger, M., & Stoiber, K. C. (1999). Excellence in teaching: Review of instructional and environmental variables. In C. R. Reynolds & T. B. Gutkin (Eds.), *The handbook of school psychology* (3rd ed., pp. 933–958). New York: John Wiley & Sons.

Glickman, C. D., Gordon, S. P., & Ross-Gordon, J. M. (2001). *Supervision and instructional leadership: A developmental approach* (5th ed.). Boston: Allyn & Bacon.

Good, T. L., & Brophy, J. E. (2000). *Looking in classrooms* (8th ed.). New York: Longman.

Greece Central School District. (2005). *Backward design: Beginning with the end in mind to design multi-genre thematic units.* Retrieved May 24, 2005, from http://www.Greece.k12.ny.us

Hitchcock, C., Meyer, A., Rose, D., & Jackson, R. (2002). Providing new access to the general curriculum: Universal design for learning. *Teaching Exceptional Children, 35*(2), 8–17.

Individuals with Disabilities Education Improvement Act of 2004, 20 U.S.C. 1400 *et seq.* (2004).

Issue: In heterogeneous classrooms, is it feasible to modify instruction to meet students' individual needs—and if so, how? (1994). *ASCD Update Newsletter, 36*(7), 7.

Janney, R. E., & Snell, M. E. (2000). *Teachers' guide to inclusive practices: Modifying schoolwork.* Baltimore: Brookes.

Juarez, T. (1992). Helping teachers plan: The role of the principal. *NASSP Bulletin, 75*(541), 63–70.

Kagan, D. M., & Tippins, D. J. (1992). The evolution of functional lesson plans among twelve elementary and secondary student teachers. *Elementary School Journal, 92,* 477–489.

Kame'enui, E. J., Carnine, D. W., Dixon, R. C., Simmons, D. C., & Coyne, M. D. (2002). *Effective teaching strategies that accommodate diverse learners* (2nd ed.). Upper Saddle River, NJ: Merrill/Prentice-Hall.

Kauffman, J. M., McGee, K., & Brigham, M. (2004). Enabling or disabling? Observations on changes in special education. *Phi Delta Kappan, 85,* 613–620.

Kluth, P., Straut, D. M., & Biklen, D. P. (2003). Access to academics for all students. In P. Kluth, D. Straut, & D. Biklen (Eds.), *Access to academics for all students: Critical approaches to inclusive curriculum, instruction, and policy* (pp. 1–31). Mahwah, NJ: Erlbaum.

Kounin, J. S. (1970). *Discipline and group management in classrooms.* New York: Holt, Rinehart & Winston.

Lampert, M., & Clark, C. M. (1990). Expert knowledge and expert thinking in teaching: A response to Floden and Klinzing. *Educational Researcher, 19*(5), 21–23.

Marshall, J. D., Sears, J. T., & Schubert, W. H. (2000). *Turning points in curriculum: A contemporary American memoir.* Upper Saddle River, NJ: Merrill/Prentice-Hall.

Mastropieri, M. A., & Scruggs, T. E. (2002). Designing effective instruction. *Effective instruction for special education* (3rd ed., pp. 27–47). Austin, TX: PRO-ED.

Mercer, C. D., & Mercer, A. R. (2001). *Teaching students with learning problems* (6th ed.). Upper Saddle River, NJ: Merrill.

Mevarich, Z., & Kramarski, B. (1997). IMPROVE: A multidimensional method for teaching mathematics in heterogeneous classrooms. *American Education Research Journal, 34,* 365–394.

Meyen, E. (1981). *Developing instructional units for the regular and special education teachers* (3rd ed.). Dubuque, IA: Brown.

Newmann, F. (Ed.). (1992). *Student engagement and achievement in American secondary schools.* New York: Teachers College Press.

No Child Left Behind Act of 2001, 20 U.S.C. 6301 *et seq.* (2002).

Nolet, V., & McLaughlin, M. J. (2000). *Accessing the general curriculum: Including students with disabilities in standards-based reform.* Thousand Oaks, CA: Corwin.

Oliva, P. F. (2001). *Developing the curriculum* (5th ed.). New York: Longman.

Orlich, D. C., Harder, R. J., Callahan, R. C., & Gibson, H. W. (2001). *Teaching strategies: A guide to better instruction* (6th ed.). Boston: Houghton Mifflin.

Ormrod, J. E. (2006). *Educational psychology: Developing learners* (5th ed.). Upper Saddle River, NJ: Pearson/Merrill.

Perkins, D. N. (1991). Educating for insight. *Educational Leadership, 49*(2), 4–8.

Pettig, K. L. (2000). On the road to differentiated practice. *Educational Leadership, 58*(1), 14–18.

Price, K. M., & Nelson, K. L. (1999). *Daily planning for today's classroom.* Belmont, CA: Wadsworth.

Renzulli, J. S., Leppien, J. H., & Hays, T. S. (2000). *The multiple menu model: A practical guide for developing differentiated curriculum.* Mansfield Center, CT: Creative Learning Press.

Rosenberg, M. S., O'Shea, L. J., & O'Shea, D. J. (2006). *Student teacher to master teacher: A practical guide for educating students with special needs* (4th ed.). Upper Saddle River, NJ: Pearson/Prentice-Hall.

Rothenberg, J., McDermott, P., & Martin, G. (1998). Changes in pedagogy: A qualitative result of teaching heterogeneous classes. *Teaching and Teacher Education, 14,* 633–642.

Sardo-Brown, D. S. (1988). Twelve middle-school teachers' planning. *Elementary School Journal, 89*(1), 69–87.

Saylor, J. G., Alexander, W. M., & Lewis, A. J. (1981). *Curriculum planning for better teaching and learning* (4th ed.). New York: Holt, Rinehart & Winston.

Schumm, J. S., Vaughn, S., & Leavell, A. G. (1994). Planning Pyramid: A framework for planning for diverse students' needs during content instruction. *Reading Teacher, 47,* 608–615.

Shavelson, R. J., & Stern, P. (1981). Research on teachers' pedagogical thoughts, judgments, decisions, and behavior. *Review of Educational Research, 51,* 455–498.

Sowell, E. J. (2000). *Curriculum: An integrative introduction.* Upper Saddle River, NJ: Merrill/Prentice-Hall.

Stronge, J. H. (2002). *Qualities of effective teachers.* Alexandria, VA: Association for Supervision and Curriculum Development.

Taba, H. (1962). *Curriculum development: Theory and practice.* New York: Harcourt Brace Jovanovich.

Tomlinson, C. (1995). *How to differentiate instruction in mixed-ability classrooms.* Alexandria, VA: Association for Supervision and Curriculum Development.

Tomlinson, C. (1999). Mapping a route toward differentiated instruction. *Educational Leadership, 57*(1), 12–16.

Tomlinson, C. (2000). Reconcilable differences: Standards-based teaching and differentiation. *Educational Leadership, 58*(1), 6–11.

Tomlinson, C. A., & Allan, S. D. (2000). *Leadership for differentiating schools and classrooms.* Alexandria, VA: Association for Supervision and Curriculum Development.

Tyler, R. W. (1949). *Basic principles of curriculum and instruction.* Chicago: University of Chicago Press.

United Nations Educational, Scientific and Cultural Organization. (UNESCO). (2004). *Changing teaching practices using curriculum differentiation to respond to students' diversity.* Paris, France: Author.

Wiggins, G., & McTighe, J. (1998). *Understanding by design.* Alexandria, VA: Association for Supervision and Curriculum Development.

Wolcott, L. L. (1994). Understanding how teachers plan: Strategies for successful instructional partnerships. *School Library Media Quarterly, 22,* 161–165.

Yinger, R. J., & Clark, C. M. (1982). *Understanding teachers' judgments about instruction: The task, the method, and the meaning* (Research Series No. 121). East Lansing: Institute for Research on Teaching, Michigan State University.

10

Integrating Assistive Technology Into the Curriculum

George R. Peterson-Karlan and Howard P. Parette

Summary

The concept of assistive technology as an element to be considered in developing individualized educational plans (IEPs) was introduced in 1990. Since then, changes have occurred in both education and society with regard to the role that technology plays in our schools, our work, and our lives. Today, there is an expectation that the tools of technology will be taught to and used by all students, both those with and those without disabilities. This chapter provides an overview of the role of assistive technology (AT) in supporting the progress of students with disabilities in the academic and life skills curricula. It examines the knowledge and skills that teachers need in order to integrate AT into the curriculum as well as the impact upon the IEP of such integration.

Learning Outcomes

After reading this chapter, you should be able to:

- Summarize influences on and the changing role of various types of technology in 21st-century school settings.

- Provide a rationale for technology proficiency among education professionals and give an example of a knowledge or performance standard for teachers related to technology use.

- Compare and contrast instructional technology (IT) and assistive technology (AT) and articulate their roles in remedial and compensatory interventions.

- Describe differences between an academic and a life skills curriculum and the manner in which AT is used to support the curriculum.

- Provide a rationale for multiple levels of technology professional development.

Introduction

A convergence of influences has created both new opportunities (Silver-Pacuilla, 2006) and new demands to integrate learning and assistive technologies into curriculum development and implementation to benefit students with disabilities (see Figure 10.1). The digital information age has transformed the world; "accelerating technological change, rapidly accumulating knowledge, increasing global competition, and rising workforce capabilities" (Partnership for 21st Century Schools, n.d.a, p. 2) have created the need for students to leave school prepared with "21st-century skills." This same digital revolution has given rise to a new generation of students and future teachers, referred to as the *Millennial* (Howe & Strauss, 2000) or *Net Generation* (Tapscott, 1998), who have grown up with and are substantively shaped by technology (Peterson-Karlan & Parette, 2005a).

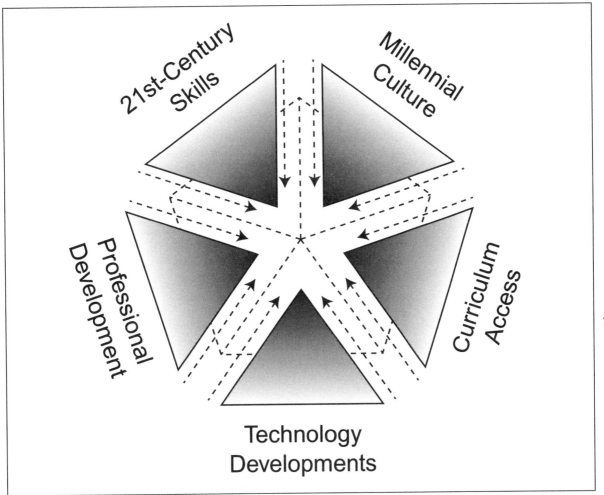

FIGURE 10.1 Integration of technology into the curriculum. © 2006, George R. Peterson-Karlan and Howard P. Parette.

Another factor is the "stunning innovation of technology; it has become easier to use and customize, more powerful and robust, and available at lower costs, making it attractive as part of a schoolwide solution" (Silver-Pacuilla, 2006, p. 11). Increased accountability for the outcome of our educational systems (Anderson & Anderson, 2005; Wehmeyer, Lattin, & Agran, 2001), along with increased accountability for the progress of students with disabilities within our schools (Silver-Pacuilla, 2006; Wehmeyer et al., 2001), have created a demand to improve curriculum access.

Convergence has also occurred in national legislative mandates related to special education. While consideration of the needs of every student with disabilities to have assistive technology was mandated by the Individuals with Disabilities Education Act Amendments of 1997 (IDEA, 1997), a national mandate to use universally designed curriculum materials and to make digitally accessible print materials has emerged from the Individuals with Disabilities Education Improvement Act of 2004 (IDEA, 2004). Finally, while the improvement of educational access and outcomes for students with developmental disabilities is a critical task, it cannot be accomplished without the preparation of personnel who can use technology to meaningfully educate students for 21st-century outcomes.

21st-Century Skills
for 21st-Century Learners

Integration of assistive and learning technologies into the curriculum requires the fundamental recognition that successful, productive citizenship now uses and depends on technological tools (Partnership for 21st Century Skills, n.d.a), that diverse learners require diverse tools to support learning (Rose & Meyer, 2002), and that the learners themselves have changed in substantive ways (Peterson-Karlan & Parette, 2005a).

Learning for the 21st Century

The educational reform movement of the past decade has focused public attention at the local, state, and national levels on improvement of student achievement accompanied by rigorous academic standards, large-scale assessments, and increased accountability. However, while the No Child Left Behind Act of 2001 (NCLB) emphasizes student achievement in foundational core subjects,

> the world in which students live has changed. . . . The explosion of powerful technology has altered traditional practices in workplaces and communities. . . . Today, it is not only business that demands a drastically different set of skills. Rapidly evolving technologies have made new skills a requirement for success in everyday life. Effectively managing personal affairs, from shopping for household products to selecting health care providers to making financial decisions, often requires people to acquire new knowledge from a variety of media, use different types of technologies and process complex information. Participating effectively in communities and democracy requires people to use more advanced knowledge as well. (Partnership for 21st Century Skills, n.d.a, p. 6)

As an initial response to such demands, NCLB has required that in addition to core subject competence, students must be proficient in technological literacy by the eighth grade, but education for the world as it is evolving requires more than basic competence. Together with new models for learning, new skill sets have been defined that students need in order to achieve success in the information age (International ICT Literacy Panel, 2002). At the core of these 21st-century skill sets are lifelong learning skills and technology tools that students need to learn.

The new learning skills that information age students need encompass three broad areas (see Table 10.1): (a) information and communication skills, (b) thinking and problem-solving skills, and (c) interpersonal and self-directional skills. These are not core content knowledge; rather, they are broader application skills that permit successful individuals to think critically, apply knowledge and skills to new situations, analyze new information, communicate, collaborate, solve problems, and make decisions. The ability to use recent and emerging technologies such as computers, networking, audio, video, and other media and multimedia tools, to learn and use 21st-century skills is known as *information and communication technology (ICT) literacy* (International ICT Literacy Panel, 2002). Table 10.2 illustrates the relationship of ICT tools to the core 21st-century learning skill domains. While such tools are certainly not required—students can and do communicate or collaborate in and outside the classroom without using technology—ICT tools increasingly are *enablers* of learning skills (International ICT Literacy Panel, 2002), and students, both those with and those without disabilities, are using them on their own outside the classroom to communicate and collaborate with peers.

Such higher-level thinking skills combined with technology use as described in Table 10.2 should certainly not be seen as beyond the capabilities of students with developmental disabilities. Students with developmental disabilities have used handheld computers that provided audio and digital images to support self-instruction, time management, and personal scheduling, resulting in increased independence and productivity in community-based employment (Davies, Stock,

TABLE 10.1
Key Elements of 21st Century Learning

Learning in core subjects	As defined by No Child Left Behind: • English, reading, or language arts; mathematics; science; foreign language; civics/government; economics; arts; history; geography As defined by 21st-century needs: • Understanding at higher levels of reasoning and use, which exceeds basic competence

Use of 21st-century learning skills	• Information and communication skills
	  • Information and media literacy
	  • Communication skills
	• Thinking and problem-solving skills
	  • Critical thinking and systems thinking
	  • Problem identification, formulation, and solution
	  • Creativity and intellectual curiosity
	• Interpersonal and self-directional skills
	  • Interpersonal and collaborative skills
	  • Self-direction
	  • Accountability and adaptability
	  • Social responsibility

Use of 21st-century tools	Use of digital and communication tools to access, manage, integrate, evaluate information, construct new knowledge, and communicate with others to participate effectively in society
Learning in 21st-century contexts	Learning content in the context of real-world examples both in and out of the classroom using 21st-century tools to communicate and collaborate
Learning 21st-century content	Emerging content areas critical to community and workplace success: • Global awareness • Financial, economic, and business literacy • Civic literacy
Use of 21st-century assessments	Measurement of student performance of 21st-century skill performance using 21st-century tools that include both standardized and classroom-based alternatives

Source: *The Road to 21st Century Learning*. Partnership for 21st Century Skills, n.d. Adapted with permission.

TABLE 10.2
21st-Century Learning Skills and ICT Literacy

Learning Skill Domain	Learning Skills & 21st-Century Tools	Information and Communication Technology Literacy
Information and Communication Skills	**Information and media literacy skills** Analyzing, accessing, managing, integrating, evaluating, and creating information in a variety of forms and media in society **Communication skills** Understanding, managing, and creating effective oral, written, and multimedia communication in a variety of forms and contexts	Using **communication, information processing, and research tools,** such as word processing, e-mail, groupware, presentation, Web development, and Internet search tools *to access, manage, integrate, evaluate, create, and communicate information*
Thinking and Problem-Solving Skills	**Critical thinking and systems thinking** Exercising sound reasoning and making complex choices, understanding the interconnections among systems **Problem-identification, formulation, and solution** Framing, analyzing, and solving problems **Creativity and intellectual curiosity** Developing, implementing, and communicating new ideas to others, staying open and responsive to new and diverse perspectives	Using **problem-solving tools** such as spreadsheets, decision support, design tools, *to manage complexity, solve problems, and think creatively and systematically*
Interpersonal and Self-Directional Skills	**Interpersonal and collaborative skills** Demonstrating teamwork and leadership, adapting to varied roles and responsibilities, working productively with others, exercising empathy, respecting diverse perspectives **Self-direction** Monitoring one's own understanding and learning needs, locating appropriate resources, transferring learning from one domain to another **Accountability and adaptability** Exercising personal responsibility and flexibility in personal, workplace, and community contexts; setting and meeting high standards and goals for one's self and others; tolerating ambiguity **Social responsibility** Acting responsibly with the interests of the larger community in mind; demonstrating ethical behavior in personal, workplace, and community contexts	Using **personal development and productivity tools** such as e-learning, time management/calendar, collaboration tools, *to enhance productivity and personal development*

Source: Partnership for 21st Century Skills, n.d., reprinted by permission

& Wehmeyer, 2002). A specialized Web browser has also supported independent Internet access by students with developmental disabilities to search and retrieve information (Davies, Stock, & Wehmeyer, 2001). Active engagement in the planning of meetings, leading meetings, or communicating preferences, goals, and employment interests during IEP meetings by students with developmental disabilities has been supported by switch-accessed computers (Wehmeyer, 2002); augmentative and alternative communication technologies (Leuchovious, 2006); presentation technologies such as PowerPoint (Laughlin, 2006); and electronic portfolios constructed by students with presentation and digital image technologies (Glor-Scheib & Telthorster, 2006).

Addressing 21st-century skills and tools meets two major needs. First, it has been shown to increase students' educational performance, as evidenced by higher test scores (Partnership for 21st Century Skills, n.d.a). Second, it bridges the gap with contemporary culture, where students already use the latest technologies to communicate, work, and play. "Whether looking up a book on a computerized card catalogue at the public literary, making a withdrawal from an automated teller machine, or accessing telephone messages" (International ICT Literacy Panel, 2002, p. 1), the impact of the new technologies on those who are in today's schools, both those students with disabilities and those without, as well as those who are preparing to be teachers, cannot be underestimated and must be explored in greater detail.

21st-Century Learners

Today's learners and tomorrow's teachers have grown up in a technologically rich world that currently includes a range of popular technologies such as DVD players, high-definition television, MP3 players, cell phones, and high-speed Internet connectivity (Peterson-Karlan & Parette, 2005a). While Parette, Peterson-Karlan, and Huer have explored this topic in greater detail in Chapter 8, we offer here a brief sketch of the impact of this development.

- In 2000, there were more than 11 million cell phone users ages 10–24, with projections of such usage approximating 30,000 in 2004 (Georgia Tech Research Corporation, 2004).

- The Kaiser Family Foundation (1999) reported that 99% of middle school children had a television, 97% had a VCR, 96% had an audio system, 82% had a video game player, 74% had a satellite TV connection, and 69% had a computer.

- By 2001, about 90% of 5- to 17-year-olds used computers and 59% used the Internet (DeBell & Chapman, 2004). By 2003, home computer ownership for children, for example, increased to 76%. In addition, the number of children who use the Internet at home increased from 22% in 1997 to 42% in 2003 (Child Trends Databank, 2003).

- Peterson-Karlan & Parette (2005b) examined technology use among seventh and eighth graders in a Midwestern community; 88% reported having cable or satellite TV, 92% reported having a DVD player, and 50% reported having more than one computer in the home, with 31% reporting having it in their bedroom and 21% reporting an Internet connection on that bedroom computer.

The results of these influences are that this "Net Generation" (Tapscott, 1998) is comfortable using technology, is highly connected to the world, and sees technology as a tool for acquiring information and for learning (Peterson-Karlan & Parette, 2005a).

Persons with disabilities are also influenced in similar ways. Friedman (2004) reported that school-age children with cognitive disabilities used a wide range of technology devices at higher rates than their adult counterparts, including computers, the Internet, cell phones, and e-mail. In Canada, younger persons with disabilities used cell phones more frequently than older individuals did (Canadian Council on Social Development, 2002). Though fewer people with disabilities have computers compared to their typical peers, they are less likely to want to give up a range of technologies at home (Fallows, 2004). Of particular importance is the finding that persons with disabilities feel that the Internet is an important venue for socialization with others. They have been reported to use the Internet at more than twice the rate of their typical peers (Hendershot, 2001). A National Organization on Disability/Harris Survey on Community Participation (2001) reported that the Internet was effective in helping people with less-severe disabilities to make contact and develop social relationships, as reflected in the finding that 52% of participants stated the Internet has significantly increased such ability.

The Digital Divide in the Information Age

While 21st-century learning by "tech ready" students using new technological tools holds great promise, professional attention has focused on the Digital Divide, or existing disparities across groups of people with regard to access to information and communication technology (Blau, 2002; Carvin, 2000; Guice & McCoy, 2001; ICT, 2002; Kalyanpur & Kirmani, 2005; National Telecommunications and Information Administration, 1995; Pearson, 2001; Shapiro & Rohde, 2000). As noted by Kalyanpur and Kirmani, these disparities in the United States are primarily "based on geography, income and race" (p. 9). More generally, Digital Divide discussions have tended to focus on the fact that poor minority children were least likely to have a computer or access to the Internet (Wilhelm, Carmen, & Reynolds, 2002), though persons with disabilities have also been included in more recent discussions. Even given the trends noted above, for persons with developmental disabilities the disparities regarding actual computer ownership and access to the Internet remain (National Telecommunication and Information Administration, 2002; Lenhart et al., 2003). They may be less likely to own a computer or to use the Internet when compared to the general population (Cullen, 2001; Gorski, 2005; Katsinas & Moeck, 2002; Kaye, 2000) and have less interest in using or gaining access than typical peers (Lenhart et al., 2003; National Telecommunication and Information Administration, 2002).

Despite arguments that disparities exist across income, ethnic, and disability groups, some data suggest that the Digital Divide may be closing, with significant gains in computer ownership and Internet access being exhibited across various demographic groups and geographic locations (Cooper & Victory, 2002; Marks, 2000; Shields, 2005). Yet, even with the increasing availability of technology in both schools and homes, some have argued that the Digital Divide has widened for many groups, and that we are misunderstanding the definition of the term *access*. As Kalyanpur and Kirmani (2005) noted, mere availability of the technology cannot be the sole determinant of access. People can have physical access but not true access to technology. For example, providing DSL lines in rural areas may bring the potential of physical access to low-income families, but the costs of the connections may be prohibitive for them (Malecki, 2003).

Similarly, merely placing computers in schools or having them available in homes does not ensure that children use software applications and resources to develop needed skills for employment in 21st-century settings (e.g., communication, research, problem-solving, and decision-making skills; Swain & Pearson, 2003).

The impact of these influences has not been as rapid or as widespread on schools as on students in schools, creating another kind of Digital Divide. It is problematic with regard to this cultural shift in technological comfort and assimilation of use, exhibited even by children with disabilities, that schools are often resistant, or unable to respond appropriately, being composed of technologically uncomfortable adults who must work hard to accommodate to the ever-increasing pressure to use technology themselves (Rosenthal, 1999). Numerous investigators (e.g., Becker & Ravitz, 1999; Gorski, 2005; Swain & Pearson, 2003; Wilhelm et al., 2002) assert that differences in teachers' levels of comfort, familiarity, and expertise with educational technology are important contributing factors to the digital literacy divide. Compounding these problems, fewer fiscal resources are often available to rural and low-income schools, and administrators must make choices regarding how scarce resources are distributed. For example, administrators faced with the reality of limited funding might have to choose between spending money on computer labs and state-of-the-art learning software (Gorski, 2005) or using those funds for basic school operations needs (salaries, building, and bus maintenance, for example). Even when computer labs are available in many minority school settings, the sheer student-to-computer ratio negates regular access for individual students (Pearson, 2001).

For students with developmental disabilities, physical access to technology continues to be limited (Jackson, 2003; Kaye, 2000; Lenhart et al., 2003). As a result of an ongoing lack of adequate funding for many school systems, general education classrooms may often be far better equipped than their special education counterparts (Bergstahler, 2001; Gorski, 2005; Jackson, 2003). In school settings, where there is a hesitancy to commit resources to technology for general education, there may also be a tendency not to expend resources on AT devices and services for students with developmental disabilities (Kalyanpur & Kirmani, 2005). This may be attributed in part, to the perception that technology for students with developmental disabilities must be individualized and/or modified, thereby incurring additional expenses (Jackson, 2003; SEAT Center, 2004). While this seems to be a contradiction to the spirit of IDEA—which mandates that AT be considered in developing individualized education programs (IEPs)—the reality is that cost is often a significant administrative factor in team decision making. When such fiscal concerns are a prominent issue, they may take precedence over costs associated with certain types of AT that help students benefit from special education or gain access to the curriculum.

Accessing the Curriculum

The previous sections have examined the convergence of information and communication technologies, skills for an information age, and technology-immersed learners. Such convergence broadens the view of technology in relation to the curriculum. Technology becomes a means of engagement and participation in everyday living, as well as an enabler of lifelong learning. It also creates the need for the acquisition and application of technology literacy. While technology developments have transformed the curriculum, they have also transformed curriculum implementation and access. *Instructional technology* (IT) has transformed the way in which learning is designed, delivered, and evaluated (Newby, Stepich, Lehman, & Russell, 2000), while AT and *universal design* have transformed access to learning and the curriculum (Rose, Hasselbring, Stahl, & Zabala, 2005). But living and learning in the information age also transforms the context for learning. As noted by the Partnership for 21st Century Skills (n.d.a), this is because "children now live in a world of almost unlimited streams of trivial and profound information, of enormous opportunity and difficult choices; helping students make vital practical, emotional, and social connections to skill and content is more important than ever" (p. 12).

To get learners to see the connections between their classroom learning and their lives outside of the classroom, teachers must make content relevant to their lives by bringing the world into the classroom, by taking students out into the world, and by creating opportunities for students to interact with teachers, with peers, and with other knowledgeable adults in authentic learning experiences (Partnership for 21st Century Skills, n.d.a). For learners with developmental disabilities, the need for such a learning context converges with the increased focus on curriculum access that has arisen from IDEA 1997, standards-based educational reforms, and the accountability reforms of NCLB (Wehmeyer et al., 2001).

IDEA 1997 mandated that the IEP team (a) determine how the student's disability affected his or her opportunity to be involved in and make progress in the general curriculum; (b) develop goals to involve the student in the general curriculum; and (c) identify services, program modifications, and supports necessary for the student to be involved in and progress in the general curriculum (Wehmeyer et al., 2001). While some have argued that the *general curriculum* represents all those activities of school life that constitute a school day, including general education classes and participation in noncurricular (lunch, assemblies) and extracurricular (clubs, sports) activities (Cushing, Clark, Carter, & Kennedy, 2005), others have argued that such a perspective defines the curriculum in terms of both the "what" (the content) and the "where" or "how" (the implementation; Wehmeyer et al., 2001). Standards-based educational reform has clearly established the content standards that define the curriculum and the performance standards that define what students should learn (Wehmeyer et al., 2001). This formal curriculum is clearly different from the "informal or unplanned curriculum" offered by noncurricular and extracurricular activities (Doll, as cited in Wehmeyer et al., 2001).

Thus, for students with developmental disabilities, access to the curriculum is based on the extent of their participation and progress in the content of the standards-based curriculum while also considering their individual needs for challenging and high-quality functional content that links performance outcomes to an array of transitional needs and post-school futures (Wehmeyer et al., 2001). Such an approach requires that curriculum content and implementation consider the need to *adapt implementation of the general curriculum* to provide access to students with developmental disabilities (Cushing et al., 2005; King-Sears, 2001; Wehmeyer et al., 2001). It also necessitates (a) *the augmentation of the general curriculum* with content representing important self-direction and self-determination skills that provide the learners with important strategies for succeeding in school (Wehmeyer et al., 2001) or in life outside of school (Partnership for 21st Century Skills, n.d.a) or (b) *the alteration of the general curriculum* to address content that is important for the student and not addressed in the general curriculum (Wehmeyer et al., 2001).

The result of such curriculum access is a focus both on student attainment of standards in the general education (academic) curriculum (Anderson & Anderson, 2005) and on student outcomes in a community-referenced, life-skills curriculum (Ford et al., 1989; Sitlington, 1996). A comprehensive curriculum (see Figure 10.2) addresses attainment of core academic content, attainment of critical post-school outcomes (Sitlington, Clark, & Kolstoe, 2000; Test, Aspel, & Everson, 2006), and

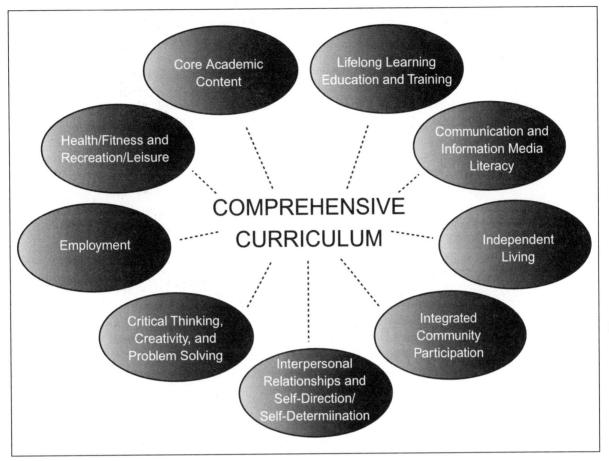

FIGURE 10.2 Comprehensive knowledge and skill domains.

attainment of information age skills (Partnership for 21st Century Skills, n.d.a). It has been argued that only by addressing a comprehensive curriculum that is concerned with critical independent living, employment, residential, community and social and interpersonal skills as well as communication and academic development can positive post-school outcomes for students with disabilities be improved (Test et al., 2006) and their goal of becoming productive 21st-century citizens be achieved.

Development into a successful and productive citizen is not assured simply by increasing the scope of the curriculum, however. Students must be able to access the curriculum and learn from it. Just as ICTs have developed to improve the ability to engage in critical information age activities, so too have IT and AT tools developed to improve ability to engage in critical educational and life activities (Blackhurst, 2005). Such tools improve access to and implementation of the curriculum (Wehmeyer et al., 2001) so that students with developmental disabilities might achieve more positive educational outcomes.

Instructional and Assistive Technology—
Tools for Curriculum Access

IT has been defined as "applying scientific knowledge about human learning to the practical tasks of teaching and learning" (Newby et al., 2000, p. 10). Application and use of IT addresses the three desired learning outcomes of instruction: increased instructional effectiveness, increased instructional efficiency, and increased instructional appeal (Newby et al., 2000). *Instructional effectiveness* results in the student's learning in a better way than would have been accomplished without the experience. *Instructional efficiency* results in the same amount (or more) of learning occurring, but in a shorter amount of time. *Instructional appeal* enhances the possibility that students will devote time and energy to the learning task. To attain these outcomes, instructional technology focuses not only on teaching—that moment of communicating the curriculum content—but also on the planning and evaluation of instruction. Thus the tools of IT are used to *plan* instructional interventions, to *prepare* print, audio, video, or digital instructional materials, to *instruct* the relevant content (knowledge and skills), and to *assess* student learning (Newby et al., 2000). The applications and uses of these technologies can be best understood by examining specific identified categories of IT.

Instructional Technologies

Media technologies (Blackhurst, 2005) are those tools such as computers, CDs, DVDs, projection devices, digital audio and video recording or editing devices or software, used by teachers to prepare or present information in order to connect the learner to the instructional experience (Newby et al., 2000). Instructional *systems technology* (Blackhurst, 2005), or instructional *process technology* (Newby et al., 2000) are those systematic principles of instructional design and delivery that include strategies, methods, and techniques.

In special education, this process of systematic design and precise delivery of instruction has been referred to as the "technology of teaching" and it includes the use of (a) well-defined objectives, (b) precise instructional procedures based upon the tasks that students are required to learn, (c) small units of instruction that are carefully sequenced, (d) high levels of teacher activity and student involvement, and (e) reinforcement and careful monitoring of student performance (Blackhurst, 2005). Among the systems technology applications cited by Blackhurst are applied behavior analysis to teach social, behavioral, and academic skills (Alberto & Troutman, 1999), direct instruction of academic skills (Carnine, Silbert, & Kameenui, 1990), teaching students to apply learning strategies (Deshler & Schumaker, 1986) or to self-regulate during academic tasks (Harris & Graham, 1996), and teaching special educators through competency-based instruction (Blackhurst, 2001).

Distinct from instructional technologies are technology *productivity tools* (Blackhurst, 2005) or *information and communication technologies* (Partnership for 21st Century Skills, n.d.a). Productivity, information, and communication tools are those technologies that help us to communicate and interact with others, work, solve problems, find information, and manage our lives more efficiently and effectively in a variety of home, school, work, and community settings.

Assistive Technologies

Assistive technologies (AT) have been developed for people with disabilities to assist them in learning, to make the environment more accessible, to enable them to compete in the workplace, to enhance their independence, or otherwise to improve their quality of life (Blackhurst, 2005). An AT *device* is "any item, piece of equipment or product system, whether acquired commercially or off the shelf, modified, or customized, that is used to increase, maintain, or improve functional capabilities of individuals with disabilities" [20 U.S.C. § 1401(251)]. There are now more than 25,000 AT items, equipment, and product services (Abledata, as cited in Edyburn, 2000) to consider for use with more than 6 million students ages 6–21 with disabilities.

AT has its roots in the technologies developed for people with physical, sensory, or severe communication impairments. The potential of technology to positively affect the lives of people with disabilities was first highlighted as public policy in *Technology and Handicapped People* (U.S. Congress, Office of Technology Assessment, 1982). The powerful stories of how technology changed the lives of people with disabilities documented in this report advanced the argument that public investment in research and development would reap individual and public benefit (Edyburn, 2000). The first AT products focused on physical, sensory, and communication impairments; examples include communication wallets, electronic communication devices, wheelchairs, prone standers, adapted eating utensils, large-print books or books on tape, Braille watches, CCTV units, hearing aids, sound-filed amplification systems, and alternatives to the mouse or keyboard. For such items, a clear relationship exists between the person's function that is lost or impaired and the function that the technology replaces or enhances (e.g., the ability to communicate; to grasp, point, or hold; to perceive printed text; to hear others speak; to manipulate the keyboard). The functions for which AT enhances, improves, or maintains the individual's performance capabilities include (a) existence (activities of daily living), (b) communication, (c) bodily support, (d) protection and positioning, (e) travel and mobility, (f) environmental interaction, and (g) sports, fitness, and recreation (Blackhurst, 2005).

Existence, or *activities of daily living*, includes those basic responses needed to maintain everyday life, activities such as eating, dressing, bathing, grooming, and sleeping (Blackhurst), while AT that can assist persons with developmental disabilities in these areas includes such tools as adapted eating utensils, dressing aids, specialized clothing or fasteners, personal hygiene and grooming aids.

A distinction should be made here between AT and medical technology. *Medical technologies* are used to sustain life outside of hospitals or medical settings. Such technologies would include ventilators, devices to treat physical conditions (e.g., cardiac pacemakers, blood glucose monitors, dialysis machines), or devices that replace vital functions (e.g., cochlear implants for hearing). Certain medical technologies, specifically those that are surgically implanted or that must be replaced surgically, have been specifically excluded by IDEA 2004.

Communication includes the abilities to receive and express communication in both oral and written or visual form or to engage in social interactions (Blackhurst, 2005). AT that can assist students with communication includes augmentative and alternative communication devices, hearing aids and assisted listening devices, telephone amplifiers, captioned video, and writing and drawing aids.

Bodily support, protection, and positioning refers to the needs for assistance that some students with disabilities have when they attempt to sit, stand, align or stabilize their bodies, or protect themselves when falling (Blackhurst, 2005). Technologies that can help students with disabilities include braces, chair inserts, prone standers, furniture adaptations, and protective headgear.

Travel and mobility includes the ability of the person to navigate the environment by walking, driving, climbing stairs, or transferring position, e.g., from a sitting to a standing position, from lying prone to standing (Blackhurst, 2005). AT that can help students with travel and mobility includes wheelchairs, walkers, crutches, canes for the visually impaired, adapted tricycles, scooters, car or bus lifts, and adaptations to automobile steering, acceleration, and braking controls.

Environmental interaction includes many of the indoor and outdoor settings associated with daily living (e.g., food preparation, use of appliances, alterations to living spaces, operation of lighting controls) or access to community, school, and workplace environments (e.g., accessible doors, door or drawer handles, adjustable desks, grabbers to reach items on high shelves; Blackhurst, 2005).

Sports, fitness, and recreation includes those abilities and functions associated with individual participation in sports, physical fitness, hobbies or crafts, and any other productive use of leisure time (Blackhurst, 2005). AT that can help these students includes balls that beep audibly, skis for individuals with single-leg amputations, adapted aquatics, Braille playing cards, and specialized wheelchairs for basketball or "off-road" travel. Note how closely several of these functions align with the comprehensive curriculum depicted in Figure 10.2; they provide means to access or perform important areas of life-skill functioning.

Instructional vs. Assistive Technologies

The development of technology has more recently evolved from physical or sensory functions described above to encompass educational functions (Blackhurst, 2005) often associated with academic deficiencies and learning disabilities (Behrmann & Jerome, 2002; Edyburn, 2000; Thompson, Bakken, Fulk, & Peterson-Karlan, 2005). There is a range of technology that can support reading, writing, math, information acquisition, organization, and cognitive processing (Thompson et al., 2005). However, the distinctions between IT and AT can be confusing when applied to the development or evaluation of educational abilities and functions. For example, the calculator has been advocated to be an important tool in the mathematics curriculum (National Council of Teachers of Mathematics, 2003, 2005). The goal is use of the calculator as a learning tool to explore and discover certain properties, increasing the emphasis on the mathematical process of problem solving (instructional effectiveness) while decreasing the emphasis on the computational aspect (increased efficiency). Most students in this situation would likely be able to learn the process while performing the calculations needed for problem solving without using the calculator. When used in this way, calculators are instructional tools that *supplement* student learning.

However, with a student whose cognitive or learning disability may impair computational ability by decreasing recall of mathematical facts or causing frequent transposition of numbers when writing or solving a math problem, a calculator may provide a *necessary* means to circumnavigate the effects of his or her disability and allow the student to access the mathematics curriculum content. Without using a calculator, the student would probably be unsuccessful in meeting math objectives, thus the calculator becomes AT when the student requires it to permit educational progress. Some AT, then, is the same technology used for everyone (e.g., the calculator or a book on CD); other AT uses quite different technology (e.g., a voice output screen reader) to enhance the performance of individual students (Blackhurst, 1997).

The key is that the student with disabilities requires the continued use of the tool after its use in typical "learning situations" is completed for the student without disabilities. AT is individually matched to and uniquely required for a student to make educational progress or participate in the curriculum and/or classroom (Lewis, 1993; Rose et al., 2005).

To fully understand the differences between IT and AT as noted above, it is necessary to identify the central goal of each. The outcome of instruction in a standards-based curriculum is for students to be proficient in targeted skills at their grade level; in those instances in which the student struggles to learn at and within grade level, remediation is introduced to help students to "catch up." *Remediation* concentrates upon re-teaching the information, using alternative instructional strategies, breaking down the task into smaller components, or engaging in one-to-one tutoring (Edyburn, 2002). Instructional technologies are used as tools to (a) accomplish the instructional or remedial process, e.g., to increase reading comprehension, phonemic skills, or vocabulary skills (Strangman & Dalton, 2005);

(b) teach or improve organization of thoughts and ideas before writing, transcribing ideas into written text or editing or revision of written compositions (Sitko, Laine, & Sitko, 2005); or (c) increase mathematical skills and their use in problem solving (Maccini & Calvin-Magnon, 2005). The goal in using such technology is clear—to develop underlying reading, writing, and math skills by enhancing "teaching performance" (Newby et al., 2000) or by enhancing "specified student performance" (Edyburn, 2002).

But when instructional technologies, including direct systematic instruction approaches, fail to achieve the specified level of performance, e.g., oral reading fluency, then a *compensatory* approach utilizing assistive technology is needed (Edyburn, 2002; Strangman & Dalton, 2005). In rehabilitation, it is understood that when a person loses the function of the lower extremities, he or she might need gait training and a crutch (remediation) and, further, that after prolonged therapy, a manual wheelchair might be needed permanently (compensation). The loss of leg function to walk is compensated by the remaining ability to use the arms to propel a wheelchair in order to produce mobility (the functional outcome). Consider the example in education of a sixth-grade student who needs to acquire and use information in science or social studies but who has such a severe reading impairment that print is functionally inaccessible. This student might benefit from a voice-output screen reader that can "read" both transformed print and information from the Internet, allowing the student to access and participate in grade-level instruction. In this instance, AT is used as a compensatory means of achieving a *functional level of performance* (or outcome).

Educationally, AT is used to augment the student's strengths or to provide an alternate mode of performing tasks (Lewis, 1993). The goals of the student's educational program would be for the student to (a) learn to read, write, or compute (remediation) and (b) successfully acquire information, record thoughts and ideas, or solve problems (compensation) at grade level if possible. This is not an either/or scenario. For example, writing instruction with a computer while providing voice-recognition software for voice dictation are *not* mutually exclusive. Continued instruction in writing skills, in organizing thoughts, and in creating grammatical sentences will support writing by dictation.

IT and AT converge upon the goal of enhancing the progress of students with developmental disabilities in the academic curriculum. IT increases the effectiveness and efficiency of the instruction in the curriculum (Newby et al., 2000), while AT permits students to access the classroom, materials, media, and instructional activities, to enhance their productivity by increasing the amount, frequency, rate, or duration of communication and work output while decreasing cognitive or physical effort or time, and, ultimately to improve the quality or accuracy of their communication, interaction with others, and work products (King, 1999; Smith, 2000).

Integrating Technology Into the Curriculum

The earlier sections of this chapter have presented the view that technology enters the curriculum both as a content (e.g., information and communication technology skills) and as a means of accessing and implementing the curriculum. How do such curriculum content and implementation look when technology integration is achieved for learners with developmental disabilities?

Curriculum Implementation in a 21st-Century School

Twenty-first-century schools are created when ICT tools are used in every core class of every grade level to learn core subject content and to meet the 8th-grade technology literacy requirement (Partnership for 21st Century Skills, n.d.b). Three examples from those collected by the Partnership for 21st Century Skills illustrate how this occurs. Schools in the Bronx borough of New York were provided with laptops and camcorders so that 5th- through 12th-grade students could research, direct, and produce their own public service announcements or documentary videos examining local issues or historical events while addressing social studies and language arts standards. At Lawrence North High School in Indiana, freshman with low-level algebra skills helped third graders to learn math skills while reinforcing their own math skills. This was accomplished by examining the problem-solving process, reading elementary picture books with math themes, creating math dictionaries for third graders, and working with them on math problem solving. Test scores on the statewide assessments of math for the high school students showed a 22.9% increase after participation in the project. In Avery Middle School in Somers, Connecticut, students use ICT skills to plan a one-week trip to the amusement park by researching local parks and hotels, developing a budget, mapping their findings, and presenting them in words, graphs, images, and charts. Using IT combined with systematic instruction to break skills into smaller, manageable units, students with developmental disabilities could potentially participate in any of these activities, but they may also need to have curricular content modified to meet their needs (Wehmeyer et al., 2001). A further example will illustrate this in greater detail.

A content map for geography instruction at the 4th-grade level (Partnership for 21st Century Skills, n.d.b) incorporates reasoning, critical thinking, and making complex choices with ICT tools. Students

- use information gathered from newspapers, television, and the Internet to describe how weather and climate influence activities in the region on a daily, seasonal, and permanent basis,

- map and analyze the spatial aspects of routes to and from school and choose the most desirable and safe route to school, and

- describe the relationship between population growth and air pollution by interpreting a graph displaying information on both topics.

To meet the needs of students with more-significant developmental disabilities, these outcomes could be modified so that the students

- use information gathered from television or the Internet to select clothing to wear on a daily basis or to pack for a weeklong trip to an amusement park,

- use a visual route map with digital pictures of critical landmarks loaded into a handheld PDA to learn to go to and from school safely using neighborhood sidewalks, and

- use a PowerPoint presentation with images from the Internet to explain how air pollution causes breathing and health risks.

Modified content that relates to the concepts and ideas but is different from standards-based content has been referred to as *standards-related content* (Ryndak & Alper, 2003). Tasks are selected that meet the educational needs of learners with more-significant developmental disabilities but that still represent the use of information, decision making, and digital tools.

Curriculum Implementation
With Universally Designed Learning

Not only do the previous examples represent learning activities that are connected to the thinking, reasoning, and problem-solving skills of the information age, but they also reflect a convergence of recent knowledge of how the brain learns (Rose & Meyer, 2002) and the digital information age tools that are transforming education as well as the world (Rose et al., 2005); *universally designed learning*, the name for this convergence, is an approach that can increase access to the curriculum for the diverse learners found in today's schools (Rose & Meyer, 2005) including learners with developmental disabilities (Wehmeyer et al., 2001).

Universally designed learning (UDL) is based on the principles of universal design found in engineering and architecture but emphasizes the special purpose of learning environments to support and foster changes in knowledge and skill (Rose et al., 2005). Universal design is a process for designing general products or structures so as to reduce barriers for any individual, with or without a disability, and to increase opportunities for the widest possible range of users; it is flexible so as to anticipate the need for alternatives, options, and adaptations when serving groups or whole communities of individuals (Rose et al., 2005). Examples of universal design include curb cuts, automated doors, and ramps designed into the architecture of buildings. When applied to learning, universal design seeks flexible means of representing information, of expressing information, and of engagement in learning (Rose & Meyer, 2002; Rose et al., 2005). Using many of the same "21st-century technologies," UDL employs digital content to provide multiple representations (image and sound), to transform one medium to another (printed text to digital speech), to alter the characteristics of the presentation (size, color, contrast), and to provide the same basic content at different levels of difficulty (Hitchcock, 2001).

An example from a 1st-grade science unit on the life cycle of plants illustrates how these principles are applied in a UDL classroom (Center for Applied Special Technology, n.d.). After introducing science concepts about plants and having students find seeds inside fruits and vegetables and plant some seeds, the teacher introduces the science content into guided reading, a science workshop, and "read alouds." During guided reading, four different books are provided on the same topic but at different levels of difficulty; students preview all four and select one. Two questions printed on a large chart are used to guide reading; students are given sticky notes to attach to the pages where information relevant to the questions appears, and later they are asked to write, draw, or dictate answers to the two questions using the sticky notes or to use the word processor to write an answer. Sticky notes (or printed answers) are posted next to the question being answered. Finally, multiple media and formats are introduced in the form of digital versions of each book for use on the classroom computer with text-to-speech options, audiotape versions of each book to be used with the text, partner reading of the print version, and independent reading of the print version.

Such an approach permits learners to select and use digitally produced materials or digitally based forms of expression that provide scaffolds for their own skills and strengths (Hitchcock, 2001). UDL differs from AT in that it is not a uniquely designed solution for one learner; rather, it attempts to anticipate the needs and learning styles of a diverse range of learners (Rose et al., 2005). However, UDL solutions for the needs of all learners with disabilities, especially those with significant cognitive, sensory, or physical disabilities, may not be available or may be too cumbersome, complex, or cost-effective to provide to all learners as a UDL solution, and so assistive technologies are needed to provide access and to support learning (Rose et al., 2005).

Integrating AT Into Curriculum Implementation

Blackhurst (2005) provides an example that illustrates how the convergence of technologies can benefit learners with disabilities:

> Carrie had a horseback-riding accident that damaged her spinal cord. She has breathing difficulties and is unable to use her hands to operate a computer keyboard. Carrie must use a respirator to help her breathe (*medical technology*). She also uses a voice-operated computer (*assistive technology*) that delivers instruction from a software program that was designed to deliver spelling instruction (*instructional technology*) using a constant time delay prompt fading instructional procedure (*technology of teaching*). Her teacher stores progress reports in an electronic gradebook program and uses a word processing program to prepare progress reports for Carrie's parents (*technology productivity tool*). She also uses the Web to conduct ERIC searches related to assistive technology and to obtain information about resources that she can use to improve Carrie's instruction (*information technology*). (p. 11)

While providing a comprehensive view of the application of technology to the issues of educating students with developmental disabilities, the preceding account is perhaps too common a representation of limited use of AT. Carrie's use of AT is limited to promoting access to instructional activities and experiences, while her teacher gains greater productivity and access to information age resources. AT is typically considered when students with developmental disabilities also exhibit physical, sensory, or communication impairments, since it can increase their access to environments, materials, and activities with peers. But technology developments have created opportunities for students with developmental disabilities to gain more than just access. They have also enhanced opportunities to improve productivity (amount of work) as well as quality or accuracy of work in school, home, professional, and community settings. There are now AT devices having research-based evidence of effectiveness designed to scaffold (Hasselbring, Lott, & Zydney, n.d.) existing skills and abilities and produce functional increases in the ability to read (Silver-Pacuilla, Ruedel, & Mistrett, 2004; Strangman & Dalton, 2005), write (Sitko et al., 2005), and use math (Hasselbring et al., n.d.; Maccini & Clavin-Magnon, 2005) through remedial instructional and compensatory AT.

While it is beyond the scope of this discussion to provide a detailed summary of AT tools and strategies currently available to support and increase the reading, writing, and math skills of students with developmental disabilities, reviews of the literature and tool-finding matrices are available for math, reading, and writing at www.techmatrix.org (a Web site maintained by the National Center on Technology Innovation (NCTI) at www.nationaltechcenter.org). These information tools focus upon the application of rapidly advancing digital and computer-based technologies to improve student functioning. While the role of adaptive strategies and low-tech devices (e.g., pencil grips, slant boards, or raised lien paper for writing, or book holders, highlighting tape, and reading ruler guides for reading) is not to be dismissed or diminished in meeting the needs of students with developmental disabilities, the increased use of computers in general education classrooms and the increased availability of instructional materials in digital formats (Rose et al., 2005; Silver-Pacuilla et al., 2004) combined with continued declining costs suggest that computer-based approaches offer the most flexibility and are able to address more learning needs (Silver-Pacuilla et al., 2004).

A key to implementing technological solutions that increase curricular access, productivity, and quality of students' learning experiences and products is the preparation of the current and future teachers who serve them. Preparation of new teachers and the continuing professional development of teachers must address the selection, application, and use of not only information and communication technologies (Partnership for 21st Century Skills, n.d.a) but also IT and AT for students with developmental and other learning disabilities (Wojcik, Peterson-Karlan, Watts, & Parette, 2004).

Technology and Professional Development

Digital Literacy Issues

Even if schools and households have computers, digital literacy—those skills needed to effectively use information technologies for productivity—continues to be a barrier (Blau, 2002; Hargittai, 2002). Knowing how to use technology effectively is integral to success in many of today's work settings (SEAT Center, National Center for Technology Innovation, and University of Kansas, 2006). Both teachers *and* students have needs for digital literacy skill sets. If teachers are not trained to use information age technologies effectively, do not have adequate support to maintain the technologies, and do not teach needed digital literacy skills to students, diminished access to technologies may be anticipated for students (Carvin, 2000; Hargittai, 2002; Menard-Warwick & Dabach, 2002; Swain & Pearson, 2003). Given that Millennial students have different learning styles and technology experiences than the teachers with whom they work in public schools, teachers' failure to understand these learning styles and technology-use preferences may result in decreased access for students (Parette, 2004; Peterson-Karlan & Parette, 2005a; see Chapter 8). Similarly, failure to acknowledge the needs that students with developmental disabilities have with regard to accessible information (e.g., enlarged text, text-to-speech features, talking word processors, symbol-based word processors, universally designed Web sites), may result in students' being denied access to learning opportunities (Bergstahler, 2001, 2002; Meyer & Rose, 2000).

Professional Development and Digital Literacy Skills

Numerous investigators (e.g., Becker, 2000; Gorski, 2005; Swain & Pearson, 2003; Wilhelm et al., 2002) assert that differences in teachers' levels of comfort, familiarity, and expertise with respect to educational technology are important contributing factors to the digital literacy divide. Teachers need professional development not only on how to use technology and how to teach students to use it (Gorski, 2005;

Hinson & Daniel, 2001; Hughes & Coyne, 1996; Litton, 2002; Parette & Brotherson, 2004; Pearson & Swain, 2001), but also on how to integrate it into classroom settings (Wojcik et al., 2004). The NCLB mandate for student achievement, coupled with the IDEA mandate that AT be considered during IEP decision making places even greater pressure on the educational community to develop a broad base of well-trained education professionals who have expertise with technology and its integration in the school curriculum.

Unfortunately, the current state of AT service delivery in the United States reflects a reliance on an "expert model," in which school systems tend to depend on one or a few well-trained AT specialists. This results in a "funneling effect" in which the broad knowledge base of those who have AT skills sets is diluted, since only small portions of the expert's knowledge base can be passed on to others in the system (SEAT Center, 2004). As a result, expanded AT capacity within the school system is never achieved.

The Emerging Role of Technology Standards

Despite the broader societal recognition of the importance of technology skills in order to be productive members of society in the 21st century (Partnership for 21st Century Skills, n.d.a), fewer than half of teacher preparation programs have stringent technology requirements and few preservice training programs include coursework or experiences on AT applications and issues for students with developmental disabilities (Lahm, 2003; SEAT Center, 2004; SEAT Center et al., 2006; Wojcik et al., 2004). As a result, education professionals are often unprepared to effectively use and integrate AT into the school curricula (Ashton, 2004; Hasselbring & Bausch, 2004; Jackson, 2003; McGregor & Pachuski, 1996) and the ability of school systems to fully implement the IDEA mandate of AT consideration is minimized (Hasselbring & Bottge, 2000). This can often mean that students with developmental disabilities do not acquire the requisite skills to be competitive in an information age workforce.

In response to these needs for increasing capacity at the school level, standards have been established for the preparation of teachers to use educational technology, in general (ISTE, 2006a, 2006b), and for the preparation of special education teachers to use technology and AT, specifically (CEC, in press; Lahm, 2003). These standards incorporate the principles of the standards-based reform movement in K–12 education (cf. McDonnell, McLaughlin, & Morison, 1997; Thurlow, 2000). Two important sets of standards that are relevant for education professionals working with students with developmental disabilities are (a) the International Society for Technology in Education (ISTE) National Educational Technology Standards (NETS); and (b) the Council for Exceptional Children Technology Specialist Standards.

ISTE NETS Standards

In partnership with many stakeholders, ISTE created the NETS Project in response to emerging needs for educational technology standards, guidelines, and tools. A focus of the project was to develop national standards for pre K–12 educational uses of technology that culminate in school improvement. Specifically, standards have been developed to guide educational leaders in recognizing and addressing the essential conditions for effective use of technology to support pre K–12 education. The first standards developed by the NETS Project were *technology foundation standards for students*. These standards—designed to be introduced, reinforced, and mastered by students—are divided into six broad categories and provide a framework for linking performance indicators to the standards. As noted by the NETS Project (2005), teachers may use these standards and indicators as guidelines for planning technology-based activities in which students achieve success in critical 21st-century learning, communication, and life skills. These standards, adopted by 49 states as of May 2004 (NETS Projects, 2004), are presented in Table 10.3. Additional standards have been developed for teachers and administrators.

Generally, the standards address 21st-century skills that should be developed among Millennial students in today's schools and that will be increasingly necessary in the workplace if one is to be successful there (see, e.g., SEAT Center et al., 2006; Partnership for 21st Century Skills, n.d.a).

CEC Technology Standards

The Council for Exceptional Children (CEC, in press) has also developed 10 standards that address both a knowledge and a skills base for beginning special education technology specialists (see Table 10.4). Generally, these standards embrace many of

TABLE 10.3
Technology Foundation Standards for Students

Standard	Indicators
	Students:
Basic operations and concepts	• demonstrate a sound understanding of the nature and operation of technology systems • are proficient in the use of technology
Social, ethical, and human issues	• understand the ethical, cultural, and societal issues related to technology • practice responsible use of technology systems, information, and software • develop positive attitudes toward technology uses that support lifelong learning, collaboration, personal pursuits, and productivity
Technology productivity tools	• use technology tools to enhance learning, increase productivity, and promote creativity • use productivity tools to collaborate in constructing technology-enhanced models, prepare publications, and produce other creative works
Technology communications tools	• use telecommunications to collaborate, publish, and interact with peers, experts, and other audiences • use a variety of media and formats to communicate information and ideas effectively to multiple audiences
Technology research tools	• use technology to locate, evaluate, and collect information from a variety of sources • use technology tools to process data and report results • evaluate and select new information resources and technological innovations based on the appropriateness for specific tasks
Technology problem-solving and decision-making tools	• use technology resources for solving problems and making informed decisions • employ technology in the development of strategies for solving problems in the real world

Source: National Educational Technology Standards Projects. (2000–2005). *ISTE national educational technology standards for students*. Retrieved February 26, 2006, from http://osx.latech.edu/students/s_stands.html (reprinted with permission)

TABLE 10.4

CEC Knowledge and Skills Base for All Beginning Special Education Technology Specialists

Standard 1:	**Foundations**
Knowledge:	Concepts and issues related to the use of technology in education and other aspects of our society.
Skills:	Articulate a personal philosophy and goals for using technology in special education.
	Use technology-related terminology in written and oral communication.
	Describe legislative mandates and governmental regulations and their implications for technology in special education.
Standard 2:	**Development and Characteristics of Learners**
Knowledge:	Impact of technology at all stages of development on individuals with exceptional learning needs.
Skills:	None
Standard 3:	**Individual Learning Differences**
Knowledge:	Issues in diversity and in the use of technology.
Skills:	None
Standard 4:	**Instructional Strategies**
Knowledge:	None
Skills:	Identify and operate instructional and assistive hardware, software, and peripherals.
	Provide technology support to individuals with exceptional learning needs who are receiving instruction in general education settings.
	Arrange for demonstrations and trial periods with potential assistive or instructional technologies before making purchase decisions.
Standard 5:	**Learning Environments/Social Interaction**
Knowledge:	Procedures for the organization, management, and security of technology.
	Ergonomic principles to facilitate the use of technology.
Skills:	Evaluate features of technology systems.
	Use technology to foster social acceptance in inclusive settings.
	Identify the demands of technology on the individual with exceptional learning needs.
Standard 6:	**Language**
Knowledge:	None
Skills:	Use communication technologies to access information and resources electronically.
Standard 7:	**Instructional Planning**
Knowledge:	Procedures for evaluation of computer software and other technology materials for their potential application in special education.
	Funding sources and processes of acquisition of assistive technology devices and services.
	National, state, or provincial PK–12 technology standards.
Skills:	Assist the individual with exceptional learning needs in clarifying and prioritizing functional intervention goals regarding technology-based evaluation results.
	Identify elements of the curriculum for which technology applications are appropriate and ways they can be implemented.
	Identify and operate software that meets educational objectives for individuals with exceptional learning needs in a variety of educational environments.
	Design, fabricate, and install assistive technology materials and devices to meet the needs of individuals with exceptional learning needs.
	Provide consistent, structured training to individuals with exceptional learning needs to operate instructional and adaptive equipment and software until they have achieved mastery.

Verify proper implementation of mechanical and electrical safety practices in the assembly and integration of the technology to meet the needs of individuals with exceptional learning needs.

Develop and implement contingency plans in the event that assistive or instructional technology devices fail.

Develop specifications and/or drawings necessary for technology acquisitions.

Write proposals to obtain technology funds.

Standard 8:	**Assessment**
Knowledge:	Use of technology in the assessment, diagnosis, and evaluation of individuals with exceptional learning needs.
Skills:	Match characteristics of individuals with exceptional learning needs with technology product or software features.
	Use technology to collect, analyze, summarize, and report student performance data to aid instructional decision-making.
	Identify functional needs, screen for functional limitations and identify if the need for a comprehensive assistive or instructional technology evaluation exists.
	Monitor outcomes of technology-based interventions and reevaluate and adjust the system as needed.
	Assist the individual with exceptional learning needs in clarifying and prioritizing functional intervention goals regarding technology-based evaluation results.
	Work with team members to identify assistive and instructional technologies that can help individuals meet the demands placed upon them in their environments.
	Identify placement of devices and positioning of the individual to optimize the use of assistive or instructional technology.
	Examine alternative solutions prior to making assistive or instructional technology decisions.
	Make technology decisions based on a continuum of options ranging from no technology to high technology.
Standard 9:	**Professional and Ethical Practice**
Knowledge:	Equity, ethical, legal, and human issues related to technology use in special education.
	Organizations and publications relevant to the field of technology.
Skills:	Maintain ongoing professional development to acquire knowledge and skills about new developments in technology.
	Adhere to copyright laws about duplication and distribution of software and other copyrighted technology materials.
	Advocate for assistive or instructional technology on individual and system change levels.
	Participate in activities of professional organizations relevant to the field of technology.
Standard 10:	**Collaboration**
Knowledge:	Roles that related services personnel fulfill in providing technology services.
	Guidelines for referring individuals with exceptional learning needs to another professional.
Skills:	Conduct in-service training in applications of technology in special education.
	Refer team members and families to assistive and instructional technology resources.
	Collaborate with other team members in planning and implementing the use of assistive and adaptive devices.
	Instruct others in the operation of technology, maintenance, warranties, and troubleshooting techniques.

205

Source: Council for Exceptional Children (CEC). (in press). *What every special educator must know: Ethics, standards, and guidelines for special educators* (7th ed.). Arlington, VA: Author. Retrieved February 17, 2006, from http://www.cec.sped.org/ps/technology.doc

the same broad 21st-century skills articulated in the NETS standards, though the emphasis is on knowledge and skill sets specific to education professionals working with students with disabilities. While the term *technology specialist* is used with these standards, it may be argued that *all teachers* need these skills, given the IDEA mandate that AT must be considered in developing IEPs for students with developmental disabilities.

New Technology Roles for Education Professionals

The foregoing discussions bring into focus four current issues in the field of special education. First, there is a general awareness that an array of technology skills is needed, by all education professionals and by all students, in school settings and in the world of work, to be productive and to meet the needs of a 21st-century workforce. Second, professional groups have acknowledged the need to develop these skills by developing technology standards that should be integrated into pre K–16 educational systems. Third, existing standards are not currently being met either in teacher preparation programs or in public school settings. Fourth, a new paradigm for the preparation of education professionals is warranted (SEAT Center et al., 2006) to (a) develop a broad base of competent AT practitioners within school systems who work directly with children in the classroom and who are supported by (b) AT specialists, who have expertise in an array of devices and services and who work with teachers at the building level, and (c) AT leaders, who have skill sets enabling them to work across a school system (Peterson-Karlan, Wojcik, & Parette, 2005). Fundamentally, however, these AT practitioners, specialists, and leaders must be able to collaborate with general education professionals who themselves possess critical information age technology skills as well as some introductory knowledge of AT and UDL (Peterson-Karlan et al., 2005).

Lahm (2003) argued that AT specialists are needed to consult with teachers during the consideration process, assess students' specific needs, and teach students, teachers, parents, and other service providers to use targeted AT. Similarly, Ashton (2004) has noted the importance and effectiveness of providing a broad AT knowledge base to specialty teams within school districts who provide direct consultation to teachers and services to children. More recent thinking, particularly in light of the "funneling effect" that typically occurs in reliance on AT experts across school systems nationally (SEAT Center, 2004), is that four distinct levels of professional development are needed to ensure that capacity within schools is developed and that the intent of the IDEA mandate for AT consideration is fully realized.

First, pre-service programs must focus on developing general educators who are able to use identified accommodations for students with disabilities. These education professionals must be aware of the basic ideas of AT and UDL and must be able to solve problems, using available technology, to meet the needs of diverse learners (Peterson-Karlan et al., 2005).

Second, pre-service teacher education programs must develop special education professionals who are technically adequate in the use of IT and AT solutions in their classroom activities. This means they should be able to evaluate the needs of their students with disabilities, use information resources to identify potential AT solutions and support student progress in the curriculum, and apply AT interventions designed to meet student needs (Peterson-Karlan et al., 2005).

Third, AT specialists are needed who are prepared through graduate-level coursework, systematically designed professional development activities, or combinations of these two approaches. These specialists function at the case-specific level and collaborate with parents and other professionals, support development and delivery of AT services, train others in the use of AT solutions and tools, and lead teams in systematic delivery of AT services (Peterson-Karlan et al., 2005).

Fourth, the development of AT leaders is needed. These individuals function at the systemic level and are able to communicate district procedures and policies regarding assessment, acquisition, and implementation of AT, secure resources for funding, and influence district technology planning (Peterson-Karlan et al., 2005).

Implementing Professional Development

In the same ways that the convergence of technology development and information and communication tools has transformed the way both teachers and students prepare and learn, so too can this convergence transform the ways in which technologically proficient teachers are prepared and supported. Hybrid models of teacher preparation and professional development have been developed that make use of Web-based multimedia learning and knowledge assessment activities combined with direct experiential, performance-based learning with AT tools and strategies (Puckett, 2004; Wojcik et al., 2004). Such efforts can extend the reach of professional development from a few large, well-equipped teacher education programs and a proliferation of local and state professional development initiatives to a sustainable system of professional preparation. However, this will require research directed toward development and validation of an e-learning construct and service delivery model (Meyen et al., 2004).

Conclusion

Converging developments in ICT, IT, and AT, in the requirements for productive future citizens, in the abilities and experiences that information age learners bring to the context of their education, in increased curricular access by learners with developmental disabilities, and in expanded technology knowledge and skill requirements for educators have created the needs, opportunities, and resources to transform the integration of technology into the curriculum—a curriculum for learners in our schools as well as a curriculum for teacher preparation and professional development. Many of the aspects of this convergence are emerging and will require further research to refine their development or application or to fully validate their effectiveness (Hasselbring et al., n.d.; Maccini & Clavin-Magnon, 2005; Silver-Pacuilla et al., 2004; Sitko et al., 2005; Strangman & Dalton, 2005); development of appropriate constructs and models for preparing teachers and for professional development using ICT are also emerging (Meyen et al., 2004). Even so, technology-based solutions not only offer great promise but, when integrated into educational practices for learners with developmental disabilities, are effective as tools for curriculum access and implementation. Through technology integration the educational outcomes, quality of life, and post-school success in homes, jobs, and communities for these individuals can be significantly enhanced.

Glossary

Digital divide—Term that originated in the 1990s to describe the perceived gap between persons who have access to and the skills to use information and communication technology (ICT) and those who, for socioeconomic and/or geographical reasons, have limited or no access. There was a particular concern that ICT would exacerbate existing inequalities across geographic locations, age groups, gender, cultural, and/or economic status.

General curriculum—The overall plan for instruction adopted by a school or school system for students without disabilities, with the purpose of guiding instructional activities and providing consistency of expectations, content, methods, and outcomes.

Information and communication technology (ICT) literacy—The ability to use recent and emerging technologies such as computers, networking, audio, video, and other media and multimedia tools to learn and use 21st-century skills.

Instructional technology—The use of technology (computers, compact discs, interactive media, modems, satellites, teleconferencing, etc.) to support learning.

Media technologies—Tools, such as computers, CDs, DVDs, projection devices, digital audio and video recording or editing devices or software, used by teachers to prepare or present information in order to connect the learner to the instructional experience.

Millennial Generation—Individuals born between 1978 and 1982.

Net Generation—Used synonymously with Millenial Generation.

Productivity tools—Term used synonymously with "information and communication technologies," or those technologies that help us to communicate and interact with others, work, problem-solve, find information, and manage ourselves, our homes, and our lives more efficiently and effectively in a variety of home, school, work, and community settings.

Standards-related content—Modified content that relates to the concepts and ideas, but is different from standards-based content. Tasks are selected that meet the educational needs of learners with more-significant developmental disabilities but still represent the use of information, decision making, and digital tools.

Systems technology—Term used synonymously with "process technology" or systematic principles of instructional design and delivery, which include strategies, methods, and techniques.

Universal design—A concept or philosophy for designing and delivering products and services that are usable by people with the widest possible range of functional capabilities. Examples of universal design are curb cuts and captioning of television and movies.

Universally designed learning—Within the learning environment, flexible means of representing information, of expressing information, and of engaging students in the learning process.

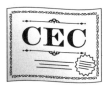

Knowledge and Skills for Entry-Level Special Education Teachers of Students With Developmental Disabilities Standards Addressed in This Chapter

Principle 1: Foundations

DD1K4   Trends and practices in the field of developmental disabilities.

Principle 4: Instructional Strategies

DD4S1   Use specialized teaching strategies matched to the need of the learner.

Principle 5: Learning Environments/Social Interaction

DD5S3   Use and maintain assistive technologies.

DD5S4   Structure the physical environment to provide optimal learning for individuals with developmental disabilities.

Principle 8: Assessment

DD8S1   Select, adapt, and use instructional assessment tools and methods to accommodate the abilities and needs of individuals with mental retardation and developmental disabilities.

Web Site Resources

Assistive Technology Industry Association (ATIA)

http://atia.org/

Host Web site for *assistive technology outcomes and benefits*—the only AT outcomes-focused journal in the United States.

Center for Applied Special Technology (CAST)

http://www.cast.org/

> Resources related to innovative, technology-based educational resources and strategies based on the principles of universal design for learning (UDL).

Family Center on Technology and Disability

http://www.fctd.info/summerInstitute/

> Resources designed to support organizations and programs that work with families of children and youth with disabilities. Information and services regarding assistive technologies, including discussion forums, a monthly newsletter, listing of AT organizations, AT success stories, fact sheets, and other helpful materials.

National Assistive Technology Research Institute (NATRI)

http://natri.uky.edu/

> Assistive technology (AT) research, theory and research into AT practice, and resources for improving delivery of AT services. Education professionals can share case studies of students who use AT.

National Center for Technology Innovation (NCTI)

http://www.nationaltechcenter.org/

> Facilitates learning opportunities for persons with disabilities by fostering technology innovation. Resources with particular emphasis on partnerships for the development of AT tools and applications by various stakeholders.

References

Alberto, P. A., & Troutman, A. C. (1999). *Applied behavior analysis for teachers* (5th ed.). Columbus, OH: Merrill/Prentice Hall.

Anderson, K. M., & Anderson, C. L. (2005). Integrating technology in standards-based instruction. In D. Edyburn, K. Higgins, & R. Boone (Eds.), *Handbook of special education technology research and practice* (pp. 521–544). Whitefish Bay, WI: Knowledge by Design.

Ashton, T. (2004). Assistive technology teams: A model for developing school district teams. *Journal of Special Education Technology, 19*(3), 47–49.

Becker, H. J., & Ravitz, J. (1999). The influence of computer and Internet use on teachers' pedagogical practices and perceptions. *Journal of Research on Computing in Education, 31,* 356–385.

Behrmann, M., & Jerome, M. K. (2002). Assistive technology for students with mild disabilities: Update 2002. *ERIC Digest E623,* Document No. EDO-EC-02-01.

Bergstahler, S. (2001). Bridging the digital divide in postsecondary education: Technology access for youth with disabilities. *Information Brief, 1*(2), 1–4.

Bergstahler, S. (2002, March). *Distance learning: Eliminating the digital divide.* Paper presented at the Society for Information Technology and Teacher Education International Conference, Nashville, TN.

Blackhurst, A. E. (1997). Perspectives on technology in special education. *Teaching Exceptional Children, 29*(5), 41–48.

Blackhurst, A. E. (2001). Designing technology professional development programs. In J. Woodward & L. Cuban (Eds.), *Technology, curriculum, and professional development: Adapting schools to meet the needs of students with disabilities* (pp. 138–186). Thousand Oaks, CA: Corwin.

Blackhurst, A. E. (2005). Historical perspective about technology applications for people with disabilities. In D. Edyburn, K. Higgins, & R. Boone (Eds.), *Handbook of special education technology research and practice* (pp. 3–29). Whitefish Bay, WI: Knowledge by Design.

Blau, A. (2002). Access isn't enough: Merely connecting people and computers won't close the digital divide. *American Libraries, 33*(6), 50–52.

Canadian Council on Social Development. (2002). *Focus on technology among persons with disabilities. CCSD's Information Sheet Number 7, 2002.* Retrieved February 9, 2005, from http://www.ccsd.ca/drip/research/dis7/

Carnine, D. W., Silbert, J., & Kameenui, E. J., (1990). *Direct instruction of reading* (2nd ed.). Columbus, OH: Merrill.

Carvin, A. (2000). Mind the gap: The digital divide as the civil rights issue of the new millennium. *Multimedia Schools, 7*(1), 56–59.

Center for Applied Special Technology. (n.d.). *UDL toolkits: Life cycle of plants (Grade 1).* Retrieved March 13, 2006, from http://www.cast.org/teachingeverystudent/

Child Trends Databank. (2003). *Home computer access and Internet use.* Retrieved February 26, 2006, from http://www.childtrendsdatabank.org/indicators/69HomeComputerUse.cfm

Cooper, K. B., & Victory, N. J. (2002). *A nation online: How Americans are expanding their use of the Internet.* Washington, DC: U.S. Department of Commerce.

Council for Exceptional Children (CEC). (in press). *What every special educator must know: Ethics, standards, and guidelines for special educators* (7th ed.). Arlington, VA: Author. Retrieved February 17, 2006, from http://www.cec.sped.org/ps/technology.doc

Cullen, R. (2001, August). *Addressing the digital divide.* Paper presented at the Conference of the Information and Foreign Languages Association (IFLA), Boston, MA. (ERIC Document Reproduction Service No. ED 459714).

Cushing, L. S., Clark, N. M., Carter, E. W., & Kennedy, C. H. (2005). Access to the general education curriculums for students with significant cognitive disabilities. *Teaching Exceptional Children, 38*(2), 6–13.

Davies, D., Stock, S., & Wehmeyer, M. L. (2001). Enhancing independent Internet access for individuals with mental retardation through the use of a specialized Web browser. *Education and Training in Mental Retardation and Developmental Disabilities, 36,* 107–113.

Davies, D., Stock, S., & Wehmeyer, M. L. (2002). Enhancing independent time management and personal scheduling for individuals with mental retardation through use of a palmtop visual and audio prompting system. *Mental Retardation, 40,* 358–365.

DeBell, M., & Chapman, C. (2004). Computer and Internet use by children and adolescents in 2001. *Education Statistics Quarterly, 5*(4). Retrieved February 4, 2005, from http://nces.ed.gov/programs/quarterly/vol_5/5_4/2_1.asp

Deshler, D. D., & Schumaker, J. J. (1986). Learning strategies: An instructional alternative for low-achieving adolescents. *Exceptional Children, 52,* 583–590.

Edyburn, D. L. (2000). Assistive technology and students with mild disabilities. *Focus on Exceptional Children, 32*(9), 1–24.

Edyburn, D. L. (2002). Remediation vs. compensation: A critical decision point in assistive technology consideration. *ConnSense Bulletin, 4*(3). Retrieved March 15, 2006, from http://www.connsensebulletin.com/edyburnv4n3.html

Fallows, D. (2004). *The Internet and daily life: Many Americans use the Internet in everyday activities, but traditional offline habits still dominate.* Washington, DC: Pew Internet & American Life Project.

Ford, A., Schnorr, R., Meyer, L., Davern, L., Black, J., & Dempsey, P. (1989). *The Syracuse community-referenced curriculum guide.* Baltimore: Brookes.

Friedman, M. (2004, March). *Assistive technology research and development collaborative on cognitive disabilities.* Paper presented at the 2004 CSUN Technology and Persons with Disabilities Conference, Northridge, CA. Retrieved February 9, 2005, from http://www.biausa.org/word.files.to.pdf/good.pdfs/CSUN2004finalused.pdf

Georgia Tech Research Corporation. (2004). *Accessibility in the analysis phase: Example user profiles.* Atlanta, GA: Information Technology Technical Assistance and Training Center. Retrieved February 9, 2005, from http://www.ittatc.org/technical/access-ucd/users_eg.php

Glor-Scheib, S., & Telthorster, H. (2006). Activate your student IEP team member using technology: How electronic portfolios can bring the student voice to life! *Teaching Exceptional Children Plus, 2*(3) Article 1. Retrieved March 4, 2006, from http://escholarship.bc.edu/education/tecplus/vol2/iss3/art1

Gorski, P. C. (2005). *Multicultural education and the Internet: Intersections and integrations* (2nd ed.). Boston: McGraw-Hill.

Guice, A. A., & McCoy, L. P. (2001, April). *The digital divide in Native American tribal schools: Two case studies.* Paper presented at the Annual Meeting of the American Educational Research Association, Seattle.

Hargittai, E. (2002). Second-level digital divide: Differences in people's online skills. *First Monday*, 7(4), 1–20.

Harris, K. R., & Graham, S. (1996). *Making the writing process work: Strategies for composition and self-regulation.* Cambridge, MA: Brookline.

Hasselbring, T. S., & Bausch, M. E. (2004, November). *Are AT knowledge and skills being developed at the pre-service level?* Paper presented at the annual meeting of the Teacher Education Division of the Council for Exceptional Children, Albuquerque, NM.

Hasselbring, T. S., & Bottge, B. A. (2000). Planning and implementing technology programs in inclusive settings. In J. D. Lindsey (Ed.), *Technology and exceptional individuals* (3rd ed., pp. 91–113). Austin, TX: PRO-ED.

Hasselbring, T. S., Lott, A. C., & Zydney, J. M. (n.d.). *Technology-supported math instruction for students with disabilities: Two decades of research and development.* Retrieved March 14, 2006, from http://www.techmatrix.org

Hendershot, G. (2001). *Internet use by people with disabilities grows at twice the rate of non-disabled, yet still lags significantly behind.* Retrieved February 4, 2005, from http://www.nod.org/content .cfm?id=682

Hinson, J., & Daniel, C. (2001, June). *Connecting across many divides: Digital, racial, and socio-economic.* Paper presented at the National Educational Computing Conference, Chicago.

Hitchcock, C. (2001). Balanced instructional support and challenge in universally designed learning environments. *Journal of Special Education Technology, 16*(4), 23–30.

Howe, N., & Strauss, W. (2000). *Millennials rising: The next great generation.* New York: Vintage Books, Random House.

Hughes, B., & Coyne, P. (1996, October). *Meeting the needs of 21st century literacy by using computers in family literacy circles.* Paper presented at the National Reading Research Conference on Literacy and Technology for the 21st Century, Boston.

Individuals with Disabilities Education Act of 1990, 20 U.S.C. §1400 *et seq.* (1990) (amended 1997).

Individuals with Disabilities Education Improvement Act of 2004, 118 Stat. 2647. (2004).

International ICT Literacy Panel (2002). *Digital transformation: A framework for ICT literacy.* Retrieved March 3, 2006, from http://www.ets.org/Media/Tests/Information_and_Communication_ Technology_Literacy/ictreport.pdf

International Society for Technology in Education (ISTE). (2006a). *ISTE/NCATE program standards.* Retrieved February 26, 2006, from http://www.cnets.iste.org/ncaten_overview.html

International Society for Technology in Education (ISTE). (2006b). *The National Educational Technology Standards Project.* Retrieved February 26, 2006, from http://www.cnets.iste.org

Jackson, V. L. (2003). *Technology and special education: Bridging the most recent digital divide.* (ERIC Document Reproduction Service No. ED 479685).

Kaiser Family Foundation. (1999). *Kids and media: The new millennium.* Menlo Park, CA: Author.

Kalyanpur, M., & Kirmani, M. H. (2005). Diversity and technology: Classroom implications of the digital divide. *Journal of Special Education Technology, 20*(4), 9–18.

Katsinas, S. G., & Moeck, P. (2002). The digital divide and rural community colleges: Problems and prospects. *Community College Journal of Research and Practice, 26,* 207–224.

Kaye, H. S. (2000). Disability and the digital divide. *Disability Statistics Abstract, 22,* 1–4.

King. T. W. (1999). *Assistive technology: Essential human factors.* Boston: Allyn & Bacon.

King-Sears, M. E. (2001). Three steps for gaining access to the general curriculum for learners with disabilities. *Intervention in School and Clinic, 37,* 67–78.

Lahm, E. A. (2003). Assistive technology specialists: Bringing knowledge of assistive technology to school districts. *Remedial and Special Education, 24,* 141–153.

Laughlin, J. (2006). *Student directed IEP meetings through PowerPoint presentations.* Retrieved March 4, 2006, from http://www.powerof2.org/teacher_vistas/interviews/jim

Lenhart, A., Horrigan, J., Rainie, L., Allen, K., Boyce, A., Madden, M., et al. (2003). *The ever-shifting Internet population: A new look at Internet access and the digital divide.* Washington, DC: Pew Internet and American Life Project. Retrieved February 8, 2005, from http://www .pewinternet.org/pdfs/PIP_Shifting_Net_Pop_Report.pdf

Leuchovious, D. (2006). *Student directed IEPs.* Retrieved March 4, 2006, from http://www.pacer .org/text/tatra/studentIEP.htm

Lewis, R. B. (1993). *Special education technology: Classroom applications.* Pacific Grove, CA: Brooks/Cole.

Litton, E. F. (2002, March). *Bridging the digital divide: A school's success story.* Paper presented at the Society for Information Technology and Teacher Education International Conference, Nashville, TN.

Maccini, P., & Clavin-Magnon, J. (2005). Mathematics and technology-based interventions. In D. Edyburn, K. Higgins, & R. Boone (Eds.), *Handbook of special education technology research and practice* (pp. 599–622). Whitefish Bay, WI: Knowledge by Design.

Malecki, E. J. (2003). Digital development in rural areas: Potentials and pitfalls. *Journal of Rural Studies, 19,* 201–214.

Marks, M. (2000). *Computer divide between white, African-American students narrows.* Retrieved February 26, 2006, from http://www.princeton.edu/pr/news/00/q2/0516-compute.htm

McDonnell, K., McLaughlin, M., & Morison, P. (1997). *Educating one and all: Students with disabilities and standards-based reform.* Washington, DC: National Academy Press.

McGregor, G., & Pachuski, P. (1996). Assistive technology in schools: Are teachers ready, able, and supported? *Journal of Special Education Technology, 13*(1), 4–15.

Menard-Warwick, J., & Dabach, D. B. (2002, April). *A digital divide? Class and gender in the computer practices of two Mexicano families.* Paper presented at the annual meeting of the American Educational Research Association, New Orleans.

Meyen, E. L., Aust, R., Gauch, J. M., Hinton, H. S., Isaacson, R. E., Smith, S., & Tee, M. Y. (2004). e-Learning: A programmatic research construct for the future. *Journal of Special Education Technology, 17*(3), 37–46.

Meyer, A., & Rose, D. H. (2000). Universal design for individual differences. *Educational Leadership, 58*(3), 39–43.

National Council of Teachers of Mathematics. (2003). *The use of technology in the learning and teaching of mathematics.* Retrieved March 8, 2006, from http://www.nctm.org/about/position_statements/

National Council of Teachers of Mathematics. (2005). *Computation calculators and common sense.* Retrieved March 8, 2006, from http://www.nctm.org/about/position_statements/

National Educational Technology Standards Projects. (2004). *Use of NETS by state.* Retrieved February 26, 2006, from http://cnets.iste.org/docs/States_using_NETS.pdf

National Educational Technology Standards Projects. (2005). *The NETS documents.* Retrieved February 24, 2006, from http://cnets.iste.org/getdocs.html#students

National Organization on Disability. (2001). *2000 NOD/Harris Survey on community participation* (Report No. 12076). New York: Harris Interactive.

National Telecommunications and Information Administration. (1995). *Falling Through the Net: A survey of the "have nots" in rural and urban America.* Retrieved May 12, 2005, from http://www.ntia.doc.gov/ntiahome/fallingthru.html

National Telecommunications and Information Administration. (2002). *A nation online: How Americans are expanding their use of the Internet.* Washington, DC: Author. Retrieved February 26, 2006, from http://www.ntia.doc.gov/ntiahome/dn/html/anationonline2.htm

Newby, T. J., Stepich, D. R., Lehman, J. D., & Russell, J. D. (2000). *Instructional technology for teaching and learning: Designing instruction, integrating computers, and using media* (2nd ed.). Upper Saddle River, NJ: Merrill/Prentice Hall.

No Child Left Behind Act of 2001, 20 U.S.C. 6301 *et seq.* (2002).

Parette, H. P. (2004, April). *Millennial children in a digital age: Assistive technology futures in special education.* Paper presented at the Council for Exceptional Children annual convention and expo, New Orleans.

Parette, H. P., & Brotherson, M. J. (2004). Family-centered and culturally responsive assistive technology decision making. *Infants and Young Children, 17,* 355–367.

Partnership for 21st Century Skills. (n.d.a). *Learning for the 21st century: A report and mile guide for 21st century skills.* Washington, DC: Author. Retrieved February 26, 2006, from http://www.21stcenturyskills.org/images/stories/otherdocs/P21-Report.pdf

Partnership for 21st Century Skills (n.d.b). *The road to 21st century learning: A policymaker's guide to 21st century skills.* Washington, DC: Author. Retrieved February 26, 2006, from http://www.21stcenturyskills.org/images/stories/otherdocs/P21_Policy_Paper.pdf

Pearson, T. (2001, November). *Falling behind: A technology crisis facing minority students*. Paper presented at the National Convention of the Association for Educational Communications and Technology, Atlanta.

Pearson, T., & Swain, C. (2001, March). *The digital divide in schools: We can make a difference*. Paper presented at the Society for Information Technology and Teacher Education International Conference, Nashville, TN.

Peterson-Karlan, G. R., & Parette, H. P. (2005a). Millennial students with mild disabilities and emerging assistive technology trends. *Journal of Special Education Technology, 20*(4), 27–38.

Peterson-Karlan, G., & Parette, P. (2005b, January). *Understanding technology use by adolescents with and without disabilities*. Paper presented at the Assistive Technology Industry Association 2005 Conference and Exhibition, Orlando, FL.

Peterson-Karlan, G. R., Wojcik, B. W., & Parette, H. P. (2005, November). *A comprehensive model for AT preparation*. Paper presented at the First Annual TAM-TED Conference, Portland, ME.

Puckett, K. S. (2004). Project ACCESS: Field-testing an assistive technology toolkit for students with mild disabilities. *Journal of Special Education Technology, 19*(2), 5–17.

Rose, D. H., Hasselbring, T. S., Stahl, S., & Zabala, J. (2005). Assistive technology and universal design for learning: Two sides of the same coin. In D. Edyburn, K. Higgins, & R. Boone (Eds.), *Handbook of special education technology research and practice* (pp. 507–518). Whitefish Bay, WI: Knowledge by Design.

Rose, D. H., & Meyer, A. (2002). *Teaching every student in the digital age: Universal design for learning*. Alexandria, VA: Association for Supervision and Curriculum Development.

Rosenthal, I. G. (1999). New teachers and technology: Are they prepared? *Technology and Learning, 19*(8), 22–24, 26–28.

Ryndak, D. L., & Alper, S. (2003). *Curriculum and instruction for students with significant disabilities in inclusive settings* (2nd ed.). Boston: Allyn & Bacon.

Shapiro, R. J., & Rohde, G. L. (2000). *Falling through the Net: Toward digital inclusion, a report on Americans' access to technology tools*. Washington, DC: U.S. Department of Commerce.

Shields, M. (2005, October 10). Study: Digital divide narrows. *Mediaweek*. Retrieved February 27, 2006, from http://www.mediaweek.com/mw/search/article_display.jsp?schema=&vnu_content_id=1001262975

Silver-Pacuilla, H. (2006). *Moving toward solutions: Assistive and learning technology for all students*. Washington, DC: National Center for Technology Innovation.

Silver-Pacuilla, H., Ruedel, K., & Mistrett, S. (2004). *A review of technology-based approaches for reading instruction: Tools for researchers and vendors*. Retrieved March 14, 2006, from http://www.techmatrix.org

Sitko, M. C., Laine, C. J., & Sitko, C. (2005). Writing tools: Technology and strategies for struggling writers. In D. Edyburn, K. Higgins, & R. Boone (Eds.), *Handbook of special education technology research and practice* (pp. 571–598). Whitefish Bay, WI: Knowledge by Design.

Sitlington, P. L. (1996). Transition to living: The neglected component of transition programming for individuals with learning disabilities. *Journal of Learning Disabilities, 29*(1), 31–39.

Sitlington, P. L., Clark, G. M., & Kolstoe, O. P. (2000). *Transition and education services for adolescents with disabilities* (3rd ed.). Boston: Allyn & Bacon.

Smith, R. O. (2000). Measuring assistive technology outcomes in education. *Diagnostique, 25*, 273–299.

Special Education Assistive Technology (SEAT) Center. (2004). *Day of visioning: Increasing access to assistive technology*. Normal, IL: Author. Retrieved February 26, 2006, from http://www.seat.ilstu.org/resources/Visioning2004/

Special Education Assistive Technology (SEAT) Center, National Center for Technology Innovation, and University of Kansas. (2006). *Assistive technology outcomes summit: Assistive technology and educational progress… Charting a new direction. Executive summary*. Retrieved March 20, 2006, from http://www.nationaltechcenter.org/documents/ExecutiveSummaryFinal.pdf

Strangman, N., & Dalton, B. (2005). Using technology to support struggling readers: A review of the research. In D. Edyburn, K. Higgins, & R. Boone (Eds.), *Handbook of special education technology research and practice* (pp. 545–569). Whitefish Bay, WI: Knowledge by Design.

Swain, C., & Pearson, T. (2003). Educators and technology standards: Influencing the digital divide. *Journal of Research on Technology in Education, 34*, 326–335.

Tapscott, D. (1998). *The rise of the Net generation: Growing up digital.* New York: McGraw Hill.

Test, D. W., Aspel, N. P., & Everson, J. M. (2006). *Transition methods for youth with disabilities.* Upper Saddle River, NJ: Pearson Merrill Prentice Hall.

Thompson, J. R., Bakken, J. P., Fulk, B. M., & Peterson-Karlan, G. (2005). *Using technology to improve the literacy skills of students with disabilities.* Retrieved January 3, 2005, from North Central Regional Education Laboratory Web site: http://www.ncrel.org/litweb/disability.pdf.

Thurlow, M. L. (2000). Standards-based reform and students with disabilities: Reflections on a decade of change. *Focus on Exceptional Children, 33*(3), 1–16.

U.S. Congress, Office of Technology Assessment. (1982). *Technology and handicapped people.* Washington, DC: U.S. Government Printing Office.

Wehmeyer, M. (2002). *Promoting the self-determination of students with severe disabilities. ERIC Digest* (ERIC Document Reproduction Service No. ED 470522).

Wehmeyer, M. L., Lattin, D., & Agran, M. (2001). Achieving access to the general curriculum for students with mental retardation: Curriculum decision-making model. *Education and Training in Mental Retardation and Developmental Disabilities, 36*, 327–342.

Wilhelm, T., Carmen, D., & Reynolds, M. (2002). *Connecting kids to technology: Challenges and opportunities.* Baltimore: Annie E. Casey Foundation. (ERIC Document Reproduction Service No. ED 467133).

Wojcik, B. W., Peterson-Karlan, G., Watts, E. H., & Parette, P. (2004). Assistive technology outcomes in a teacher education curriculum. *Assistive Technology Outcomes and Benefits, 1*, 21–32.

11

Instructional Planning for Students With Developmental Disabilities

Earle Knowlton

Summary

This chapter addresses long- and short-term instructional planning for students with developmental disabilities, beginning with an examination of the legal requirements related to planning for the instruction of students with developmental disabilities and the intent behind those requirements. A discussion of longitudinal planning considerations and techniques follows, with an introduction to "big picture" considerations such as maximum independence, the highest possible quality of life, and enhanced self-determination. With these principles of long-term planning as a backdrop, the text then discusses more-specific determinants of effective short-term or ongoing planning.

Learning Outcomes

After reading this chapter, you should be able to:

- Define the IDEIA-2004 provisions related to involvement and progress in the general education curriculum for students with developmental disabilities.

- Explain how consideration of and reflection on the "big picture" (e.g., ultimate quality of life) are crucial to both long- and short-term planning.

- Describe differentiated instruction in terms of its differences from individualized instruction and its implications for short-term instructional planning.

- Describe and exemplify content source dimensions for ongoing instructional planning.

Introduction

This chapter examines planning at two levels: longitudinal and ongoing. In longitudinal planning, the perspective presented is "big picture" in nature. For students with developmental disabilities it is crucial that education professionals engage in future planning on their behalf, often beginning at a very young age. The answers to two important questions help education professionals form this big picture: (a) What level of maximum independence for the student can our teaching strive for? and (b) What will the student's ultimate quality of life look like? (Knowlton, 1998).

As the big picture becomes clear and coherent to the team of individuals who collaborate in the development, implementation, and evaluation of the student's individualized education program (IEP), it becomes necessary for education professionals to engage in monthly, weekly, and daily planning in an ongoing, systematic way. Using the long-term plan, grounded in the student's IEP, as a framework, planning focuses on (a) *what* the student is learning (i.e., specific combinations of general education curriculum content, community-referenced knowledge and skills, and the student's annual goals as specified in the IEP); (b) *where* the student is learning, (i.e., the age-appropriate general education classroom, the special education resource room or learning center, various relevant community settings, and/or vocational settings); and (c) *how* the student is learning (i.e., teaching the student ways in which environmental demands can be met directly or circumvented and monitoring the student's progress).

A useful place to start this discussion is at the nexus of public policy and classroom practice: federal special education legislation. Although special education law speaks broadly of policies to integrate students with disabilities with their peers and to educate them appropriately and in concert with their civil rights, it has much to tell us specifically about the conduct of long- and short-term instructional planning.

What IDEIA-2004 Has To Say About Instructional Planning

On December 3, 2004, President George W. Bush signed into law the reauthorized Individuals With Disabilities Education Improvement Act of 2004 (IDEIA-2004; P.L. 108-466). Since the original federal mandate of a free, appropriate public education for students with disabilities in 1975 (Education for All Handicapped Children Act of 1975, P.L. 94-142), there have been many reauthorizations and amendments of the act, and some have had special significance. IDEIA-2004 ranks as one of the more significant amendments, in large part because of what it says about how we plan instruction. In comparison with the act's previous amendments (Individuals With Disabilities Education Act Amendments of 1997, P.L. 105-17, IDEA-1997), IDEIA-2004 maintains IDEA-1997's instructional planning emphasis on general education curriculum involvement and progress, but it is somewhat less prescriptive of the required content of the IEP and of the specific professionals who must engage in the development, implementation, and monitoring of the IEP. IDEIA-2004 also maintains the accountability role initiated in the federal No Child Left Behind Act of 2001 (NCLB, P.L. 107-110) and fulfilled by participation on the part of students with disabilities in district-wide and state assessments of the adequacy of their academic progress.

The IDEIA-2004 instructional planning language is largely contained within its IEP requirements. It establishes anew or reaffirms several best practices with regard to long- and short-term planning as standards against which the work of professional educators in local educational agencies will be judged. These planning standards and practices include: (a) the *involvement* of the student with developmental disabilities in the general education curriculum, (b) the student's *progress* in general education curriculum areas of study, and (c) the student's *functional* instructional needs that result from the developmental disability and that, in turn, affect general education curriculum involvement and progress.

The Student's Involvement in the General Education Curriculum

Instructional planning for the student with developmental disabilities assumes first that the local school district's standard curriculum (much, if not all, of it derived from state-specific curriculum standards in language arts, science, etc.) that is taught to typical students is the curriculum from which the student with developmental disabilities is entitled the opportunity to be taught (Wehmeyer, Sands, Knowlton, & Kozleski, 2002). This concept, closely tied to IDEIA-2004's principle of *zero reject* (Turnbull, Huerta, & Stowe, 2006), is an extremely important one for us to understand for instructional planning purposes. Ignorance of it produces undesirable professional practices fraught with misunderstanding: "We are required to teach algebra to a 17-year-old student with a significant cognitive impairment," for example.

Nowhere in IDEIA-2004 is it required, or even suggested, that the student, at all costs and without regard to cognitive and social/behavioral needs, must be taught with the standard curriculum. Instead, the zero-reject principle tells us that no student is to be *denied the opportunity* to receive an education that is free and appropriate to his or her needs. With regard to curriculum, this means that education professionals cannot reject out of hand the general education curriculum as a source (prominent or auxiliary) of instructional content for that student simply because of the nature and/or severity of his or her developmental disability.

Accordingly, educators of students with developmental disabilities are required to make what Turnbull and Turnbull (2000) call "rebuttable (refutable) presumptions" (p. 81) about what and where students are taught. Refutable presumptions are legal benefits of the doubt, if you will; education professionals *presume* that certain options for students with disabilities will be the most beneficial options until evidence convinces us otherwise. That is, until instructional data convincingly rebut, or refute, the presumed benefits of the less socially restrictive "what or where" option (Turnbull & Turnbull, 2000). It may be presumed, then, that unless or until compelling instructional data lead us to another conclusion, the general education curriculum is the source of the content taught to the student and general education environments comprise the settings in which this curriculum content is taught.

The Student's Progress in the General Education Curriculum

IDEIA-2004 requires that in addition to being educationally involved in the general education curriculum, the student also show progress, ideally in terms of the same general education curriculum evaluative measures used with students who do not have disabilities. Two specific, related legal requirements that have important implications for short- and long-term instructional planning exist to reflect the student's progress and the adequacy of this progress. The first is the IEP's progress-monitoring requirement, and the second is the alignment of IDEIA-2004 with the adequate yearly progress (AYP) requirement of NCLB.

Progress Monitoring

IDEIA-2004 includes specific requirements for keeping track of the student's progress toward attainment of IEP goals. The law requires each IEP to describe how the student's progress toward annual goals will be measured. Moreover, the IEP must include a description of when parents or guardians will receive periodic reports of their child's progress. Generally, progress reports should be no less frequent than those for students without disabilities (e.g., quarterly report cards) and probably should be more frequent in most cases (Knowlton, 2007).

Because professionals in the field of education have not always been particularly facile in effecting, let alone reporting, student progress, we have witnessed in recent years increasingly intensive federal policy measures designed to hold schools more accountable to parents and the public for the educational process of *all* students. The NCLB requires that district and state assessments be administered to all students, including those with disabilities, and that the resultant outcome data for all students be reported by districts in terms of data sets and subsets regarding student achievement progress. For students with disabilities, up to 1% of those with the most significant cognitive impairments are allowed to be assessed on the basis of alternate curriculum standards. Another cap of 2% has been allowed so that districts can identify "students with disabilities who need additional time and intensive instructions to meet standards" (U.S. Department of Education, 2005, p. 2). Unlike the 1% of students with the most significant cognitive impairments, who may be assessed against alternate curriculum standards, this group of students are assessed against the same standards as students without disabilities, though the standards may be modified.

Until the passage of NCLB, the IEP served as the single accountability vehicle for parents and guardians of students with disabilities, providing reports of the student's progress at least as frequently as for students without disabilities. Now, with the addition of performance data from district- and statewide assessments, the IEP's accountability mechanism vis-à-vis progress monitoring and reporting has been ratcheted up as well. Some of the better work in regard to progress monitoring has been produced by Vanderbilt University's faculty development project, the IRIS Center for Faculty Enhancement (IRIS Center, 2005), which provides teacher education faculty with training content and materials geared to general education teachers, school administrators, and other professionals to ensure that these professionals are well prepared to work with students who have disabilities and with their families. IRIS online materials include well-designed case studies in interactive formats enabling users to become familiar with best practices in year-end assessment and progress monitoring.

Whereas year-end assessment requires a *summative evaluation* of the student's growth from year to year, progress monitoring requires a *formative evaluation* of ongoing instructional effectiveness, thus allowing for adjustments in instructional plans and/or modifications in instructional delivery when necessary (IRIS Center, 2005).

No Child Left Behind Act AYP Requirements

Schools must demonstrate that students, including those with disabilities, are achieving in a manner that results in adequate annual progress. This provision of the NCLB has been fraught with controversy, mainly because states and local districts consider the federal rules that regulate the collection of assessment data and the grouping of students (including those with disabilities) into various data sets to be patently unfair. As of this writing, current U.S. Department of Education secretary Margaret Spellings has recently eased state and local consternation over this provision by announcing that the department will allow selected states to create customized data tracking systems that feature growth curves (U.S. Department of Education, 2005). This change will likely mean that districts could meet the law's AYP requirements by demonstrating growth in relation to students' previous achievement levels rather than in relation to absolute targets—though by 2014 NCLB continues to require that all students be achieving at grade level.

The Student's Instructional Needs in "Functional" Areas

Nearly lost in the shuffle of IDEIA's general education curriculum requirements are companion requirements that clearly acknowledge the fact that many students with disabilities need critical community-referenced skills that can afford them maximum independence and the highest possible quality of life (Knowlton, 1998), that is, the "functional" curriculum. The IDEIA-2004 regulations* call for the IEP's present performance levels to include not only those pertaining to academic achievement but also those addressing "functional performance" (Council for Exceptional Children [CEC], 2005).

As the IEP is developed, the IEP team must consider the student's "functional needs" in addition to his or her academic and developmental needs (CEC, 2005). Clearly, the team must examine the student's multifactored evaluation results and present levels of educational performance carefully in arriving at a determination of the student's functional needs. It is often helpful, however, for the team to look at a student's potential functional needs in terms of their dynamic relationship with the student's *developmental* needs. The term *developmental* is used specifically to refer to curriculum content that is part of a larger, research-based sequential framework in which there "is a walking-before-running premise" (Wehmeyer et al., 2002, p. 197). When developmental curriculum content is emphasized, it is presumed that a student's mastery of a target skill is predicated on mastery of one or more prerequisite skills. In turn, the target skill's mastery sets the stage for acquisition of the next skill in the sequence, and so on.

Unfortunately, many students with developmental disabilities experience cognitive difficulties, particularly in the areas of selective attention and working memory, that result in slower learning rates, ceilings in the complexity of skills that education professionals expect them to acquire, and problems with the transfer (generalization) of skills learned in one setting to other settings where those skills might be usefully applied (Cha & Merrill, 1994; Tomporowski & Tinsley, 1994; Zeaman & House, 1979; Zigler, 1999). A legacy of sorts has emerged during the past several decades, fueled by high-energy advocacy and frustrating post-secondary outcome data that have pointed to an overreliance on a developmental prerequisite emphasis in curricular and instructional practices, particularly in the 1950s and 1960s. In essence, teachers in worst-case scenarios marked time by force-feeding meaningless developmental tasks such as counting blocks (e.g., how can she count to 100 if she can't count to 10?) and the like, while often neglecting to teach skills that could serve to enhance independence and quality of life.

Figure 11.1 displays a relational way of thinking about and reflecting on the relationship between developmental and functional emphases in longitudinal curriculum planning.

Generally, the younger the student is, the more likely he or she is to need a set of skills that are developmentally sequenced. For example, single-utterance responses are taught before multiple-utterance responses in a discrete-trial approach to language training for a young child with autism (cf. Anderson, Avery, DiPietro, Edwards, & Christian, 1987). As the student ages, the emphasis becomes decidedly less developmental and more functional. The student with Asperger's syndrome, for example, is taught various social cue strategies without particular regard to developmental prerequisites (i.e., social "maturity") but with regard to the need to meet immediate social demands in the environment. The student might be taught specific ways to "read" and uncover what has been termed the "hidden curriculum" (Myles & Simpson, 2001, p. 279). It should be noted that it is rare that considerations of curricular emphasis are exclusively functional or developmental; planning for any one student should weigh the value of both emphases in enhancing independence and quality of life.

---

* As of this writing, IDEA's regulations are being finalized. The Council for Exceptional Children has developed "side-by-side" analyses of draft regulations with reference to various topics such as the IEP. These analyses are available at www.cec.org.

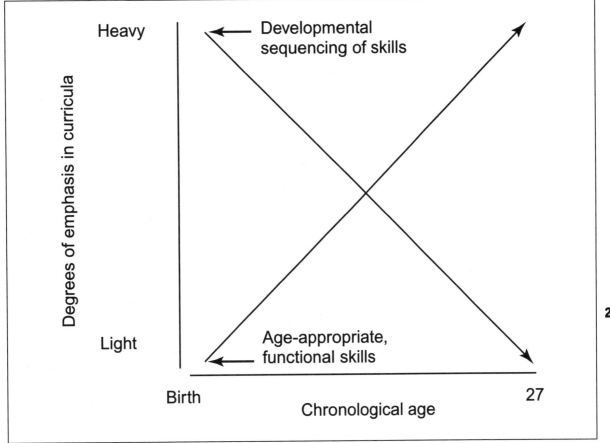

FIGURE 11.1. Relationship between developmental and functional curricular emphases for the student with a developmental disability. Source: Wehmeyer, M., Sands, D., Knowlton, H. E., & Kozleski, E. (2002). *Teaching students with mental retardation,* p. 197. Baltimore: Brookes. Reprinted with permission.

Recent evidence suggests a less prominent role for developmental theory in curriculum sequencing, even in academic areas such as expressive written language. Goldman, Hasselbring, and the Cognition and Technology Group at Vanderbilt University (1997) concluded that even high-functioning students with disabilities who were instructed with a planning focus on the written expression of ideas performed well ahead of what we would expect, given their difficulties with lower-level mechanics such as spelling and usage. Clearly some education professionals would wait for the mastery of so-called "prerequisites" in whatever areas they teach, thereby losing critically valuable time (Knowlton, 1998). A well-respected special educator recently remarked, "There's no such thing as 'pre'-anything in special education!" (S. Knowlton, personal communication, November 11, 2005).

Determining Long-Term Instructional Goals

When we set longitudinal goals for students with developmental disabilities, we make the obvious assumptions that the goals are attainable and that sufficient and accessible resources exist to achieve the goals. IDEA regards these resources and their manner of implementation as *special education and related services*. While it is not the intent of this chapter to focus on related services, with respect to special education per se, there is little left to question in the wording of the IDEIA definition "specially designed instruction that meets the unique needs of a student with a disability at no additional cost to parents" [20 U.S.C. 1402, § 602(16)]. IDEIA's regulations go on to clarify the definition's key phrase: "specially-designed instruction":

(3) Specially-designed instruction means adapting, as appropriate to the needs of an eligible child under this part, the content, methodology, or delivery of instruction—

(i) To address the unique needs of the child that result from the child's disability; and

(ii) To ensure access of the child to the general curriculum, so that he or she can meet the educational standards within the jurisdiction of the public agency that apply to all children. [20 U.S.C.1401, § 300.26(25)]

The student's progress as the result of specially designed instruction is predicated on how useful the long-term (annual) goal is as written. The author Lewis Carroll once wrote, "If you don't know where you are going, any road will take you there" (Carroll, 1999, p. 66). We must not lose sight of IDEIA's origins—i.e., P.L. 94-142—which came about because many of the people supposedly responsible for the education of students with developmental disabilities chose "any road." Education professionals must ask, "Do we know where we're going in the next year (and longer) with this student?" If the student's goal is written in a way that doesn't lend itself to clear implications for ongoing (short-term) instructional planning and to the assessment of progress, then the education professional is implicitly telling the student, the student's parents, and colleagues and employers that just about any old goal statement will do (Knowlton, 2007).

Useful annual goals are observable and measurable. Though it may be understood and agreed upon by all members of the team writing the student's IEP that we would want to increase the student's generative use of community-referenced vocabulary and to decrease his or her stereotypy, neither of these statements in its current form is measurable in ways that would result in monitoring and judgments of progress. To state goals so that the student's progress toward his or her goal is observable and measurable, we need to include information pertaining to (a) the time period in which we expect the goal to be attained (usually the school year or the calendar year); (b) the specific behavior(s) to be observed and measured (e.g., number of unprompted utterances in proper contexts of each of five words specific to partaking of the buffet); (c) under what conditions the behavior will occur (entering the buffet queue, entering the checkout queue); and (d) the level at which the behavior is to occur (100% usage of correct utterances in each queue) (Knowlton, 2007).

Making a goal measurable requires it to be written so that it will produce in our minds (and, importantly, in the minds of parents and others committed to the student's well-being) an image of the student performing the behavior that is explicated in the goal. Imagine that the student is about to enter the line leading to the buffet. In addition to the ways in which he or she should behave, what should the child be able to *say* to others in the line if the necessity arises? What might the child say to the server? To the checkout person? Thinking in terms of these images while developing goals will almost always result in the goals' being "observable." Observable behaviors are also measurable behaviors, and, similarly, observable goals are measurable goals.

Although IDEIA-2004 removed the requirement on IEPs for short-term objectives or benchmarks for most eligible students, it continues to be best practice to define short-term objectives or benchmarks by delineating the goal—that is, logically reducing the goal to observable, measurable parts. And, for students who will take alternate assessments in lieu of district- and statewide assessments, short-term objectives or benchmarks related to annual goals continue to be required (CEC, 2005).

The education professional can keep track of progress toward the IEP goal's explicit outcome by identifying mile markers, termed *benchmarks*, that can help monitor the student's progress from his or her present level of performance all the way through to the eventual attainment of the goal. Completing all the steps involved in independently cleaning out the refrigerator and disposing of perishables requires a few benchmarks along the way to achieving proficiency in that skill. The student may need first to reach a mile marker that signals that he or she is able to identify refuse and dispose of it properly with the help of physical, gestural, and verbal prompting from the education professional. We might notice our arrival at mile marker 2 when the student performs these tasks with only occasional verbal prompts and perhaps some key visual supports (see Jaime & Knowlton, in press). Passage of mile marker 3 occurs when we can supervise the student, providing prompts only as needed.

A more traditional form of goal analysis involves the use of short-term objectives. Short-term objectives are stated in the same way as goals are stated—they are micro-goals. Along the road toward attaining the goal, short-term objectives reflect successive approximations of (a) the behavior stated in the goal (e.g., uttering the first of five target vocabulary words), (b) the conditions stated in the goal (e.g., stated in any context before the target context), (c) the performance criteria stated in the goal (e.g., 70% of opportunities), or (d) various combinations of these.

Not only must IEP goals be measurable, but they must also be meaningful. A meaningful long-term goal responds to the needs, strengths, and circumstances expressed in the present levels of performance. The goal should logically derive from one or more areas addressed by the IEP's stated performance levels for the student. The goal needs to represent the team's best thinking in regard to general education and functional curriculum content at a grade/age level useful to the student. If the goal is to be meaningful, education professionals not only must be able to measure it, but also must be able to justify it as ultimately contributing to the student's maximum independence and highest possible quality of life (Knowlton, 1998; Wehmeyer et al., 2002).

We personalize the goal for the individual student in the context of the following important considerations, originally brought to the fore by Lou Brown and his colleagues at the University of Wisconsin: Does the goal derive logically from the student's present level of performance? Will the goal produce or enhance involvement and progress in the general education curriculum? Will the student's achievement of the goal result in her or his access to more home, school, and/or community environments? Do the student's family members regard the goal as a priority for intervention? Will it enhance the student's social status? Will it enhance the student's physical well-being? (Brown et al., 1985).

Remember to ask (and answer) these questions in your deliberations about the long-term goals to set for a student as you collaborate in the development of the student's IEP. In too many cases, an IEP does not contain any measurable goals. But it is often the case as well that goals may technically be observable and measurable but not necessarily meaningful. Best-practice IEP goals are both measurable and meaningful (Knowlton, 2007).

Factoring Independence, Quality of Life, and Self-Determination Into Long-Term Planning

Measurable and meaningful goals must be filtered through an individual student's relevant personal circumstances, such as age, gender, functional abilities, prognosis, personal-social network, past experiences, social-behavioral issues, and so on. This process is called curriculum personalization (Knowlton, 1998). With reference to a particular student, the IEP team needs to address three questions in order to adequately personalize his or her curriculum: What will maximum independence for this student ultimately look like? What will his or her lifestyle quality be at its most optimal level? To what degree will the student serve as a causal agent in the determination of his or her levels of independence and lifestyle quality (self-determination)?

Maximum Independence

It is probably the case that none of us truly is completely independent. As Covey (1989) suggests, it is more likely the case that all of us are *interpendent*. At a more lofty level of discourse, it is stimulating to consider absolute "independence" as unattainable in modern society; rather, people are capable of partial or *relative independence*. Accordingly, for our purposes, we will place the concept of independence in proper perspective and think of it in practical terms. Originally, Lou Brown and his associates (Brown et al., 1979) used the perspective of *functionality* in discussing independence; if the student cannot perform the skills that will respond to the demands of an environment, then, in order to access that particular environment, someone else will need to perform those skills in the student's stead. The degree to which education professionals can shift the preponderance of this responsiveness to environmental demands away from external supports and toward the individual is reflective of the amount of independence we should seek for that individual as part of long- and short-term instructional planning.

Using the "big-picture" perspective, a student's IEP team must carefully and reflectively consider three planning options regarding his or her ultimate independence and the role of any one long-term instructional goal in relation to independence. As an IEP team, members can decide to devote the special education/related services resources and the *time* necessary to teach the skills called for in the goal. Responding to environmental demands produced when accessing certain environments (e.g., a fitness center) may be of sufficient importance to the student and parents that it is critical that skills enabling the child to use weight machines and treadmills be taught.

The team might also determine for a variety of idiosyncratic reasons that it is an unwise use of resources and time to teach certain skills, that the student is better served if education professionals arrange to *circumvent* rather than meet head-on certain demands of the fitness center environments. Adjusting and fine-tuning the weight machine or treadmill might best be performed by a fitness center employee with whom arrangements would be made each time the student has a workout. Though most of the other fitness center clients would adjust the machines themselves, the "big picture" tells the team that there are other more important environments, sub-environments, and concomitant demands that merit instructional attention. These particular sub-environments (the weight machine and the treadmill) and their demands for performance (setting adjustments) can be handled by support people, thereby allowing the student to access the environment and its relevant sub-environments by circumventing their demands via support persons rather than meeting their demands head-on by performing newly acquired skills (Wehmeyer et al., 2002).

Quality of Life

Most of us, implicitly if not explicitly, hold to the belief that personal income and quality of life are positively correlated (Schalock & Verdugo-Alonzo, 2002). Wealthy people thus live high-quality lives and enjoy optimal lifestyle quality. However, there is evidence suggesting that, while others' perceptions or even objective measures of lifestyle quality for persons of wealth may be high, the individual's sense of personal well-being can often be unrelated to wealth (Parmenter & Donelly, 1997; Schalock & Verdugo-Alonzo, 2002).

Similarly, we may tread on thin ice when, as professionals, we assume that we can judge whether the quality of life for a person with developmental disabilities is satisfactory. Whether we should be making such judgments in the first place is largely open to question (cf. Bannerman, Sheldon, Sherman, & Harchik, 1990). Yet, as we engage in long- and short-term planning via the IEP process, we are often quick to impose our values and, indeed, our will, on individuals with disabilities and their family members without carefully examining whether these values are fitting, desirable, or advantageous. Such an imposition can have deleterious results. Numerous researchers have attempted to advance certain "core domains" of lifestyle quality (Schalock & Verdugo-Alonzo, 2002, p. 14). Among the more useful sets of core domains is Schalock's (2000), which, in abridged terms, includes (a) physical, emotional, and material well-being; (b) interpersonal relationships; (c) social inclusion; (d) civil rights; (e) personal development; and (f) a degree of self-determination. Given evidence suggesting the importance and value of self-perceived well-being in these areas as opposed to external judgments, by professionals and others, of "what is best" for the individual, we are well advised to be cognizant of the degree to which lifestyle quality can be self-determined (Wehmeyer et al., 2002).

Self-Determination

Advanced in the last decade principally by Michael Wehmeyer and his colleagues (Wehmeyer, 1998; Wehmeyer, Abery, Mithaug, Powers, & Stancliffe, 2003; Wehmeyer, Palmer, Agran, Mithaug, & Martin, 2000; see Chapter 6 for a more detailed discussion), self-determination in the context of instructional planning involves a progressive lifelong learning process for all of us, including people with developmental disabilities. Throughout the process, the planning emphasis "shifts from choice, self-awareness, and exploration to autonomy and self-sufficiency" (Wehmeyer et al., 2002, p. 234).

Wehmeyer et al. (2002) recommend that, for longitudinal instructional planning for students with developmental disabilities, special educators consider self-determination as an *augmentation* (Knowlton, 1998) of the student's curriculum—i.e., the superimposition of content onto an existing curriculum, such as the school district's standard general education curriculum, so that it promotes the student's long-term progress from simple choice making (e.g., selecting one of two vocabulary software programs to practice the use of community-reference words) through exploration and autonomy (e.g., providing the student with supports as he determines what steps must be taken to earn a driver's license in his state) to self-sufficiency (e.g., monitoring the student's completion of state and federal income tax forms). (Further detail will be provided to explain and exemplify curriculum augmentation as a curriculum personalization strategy later in this chapter.)

Short-Term Instructional Planning

Planning for Differentiated Instruction

Effective instructional planning for the short term (no longer than quarterly and more likely weekly to monthly) requires that the teacher differentially reflect on and adjust to the ongoing and often changing instructional needs of each student, using as a framework the longitudinal plans discussed in the first part of this chapter. This reflective process of ongoing planning teaching has been termed *differentiated instruction* (Gartin, Murdick, Imbeau, & Perner, 2002; Tomlinson, 2001; see Chapter 9 for a more detailed discussion). Tomlinson (2000) defined differentiated instruction as "a way of thinking about teaching and learning" (p. 6). This thinking has evolved significantly from the "individualized instruction" approach to short-term planning in which the education professional basically created and monitored instructional programs for each of his or her students.

Today, *all* education professionals, from those instructing college-bound honor students in physics to those who are responsible for what amount to self-contained classrooms for students with extensive instructional needs, must address widely diverse classes of students. Student variance is a given when there are two or more students. In response to wide classroom diversity, some teachers plan and teach on an individualized basis—providing what traditionally has been called individualized instruction. However, when we individualize our planning and instruction, we create "numerous mini classrooms" (Gartin et al., 2002, p. 9) of one student each, all of whom just happen to occupy the same physical space.

Differentiated instruction, on the other hand, involves teaching on the basis of personalized planning *and* inclusive education principles (Tomlinson, 2001). Schumm, Vaughn, and Leavell (1994) devised a simple model of instructional planning that assists teachers in determining how instruction for diverse groups of learners can be differentiated. Essentially, differentiated planning means that versions of the unit or topic of instruction, methods of instruction, and contexts of instruction (grouping, setting, etc.), as well as those doing the teaching (e.g., computer-based programs; cf. Wise, et al., in press) can be adapted by the teacher on the basis of individual learner characteristics. Such adaptations are made in light of (a) the specific part(s) of the curriculum content that will be learned by *some* students, (b) the specific part(s) of the curriculum content that will be learned by *most* students, and (c) the specific part(s) of the curriculum content that will be learned by *all* of the students in the class (Schumm et al., 1994).

To illustrate, consider the scenario of working with a classroom of 25 seventh-grade students in general social studies, 6 of these students with IEPs, 2 with developmental disabilities (autism and Down syndrome). The education professionals involved must address curriculum standards that call for a basic understanding on the part of all students of the three branches of government. The first cut identifies the content components that all 25 students will learn, the components that most will learn, and the components that only a few will learn. All students can learn the names of the three branches and a basic statement describing what each branch does. Most of the 25 students can examine Web-based materials such as, for example, news coverage of recent nominees to the U.S. Supreme Court. Most can write a report on the sequence of events that leads to the passage of legislation. Some students might present orally regarding the contributions of former presidents if they can partner with a peer-assistant who helps with the research. Two or three students might even create a Web site that could be used by other students in the class to assist them with selected content. In this manner, education professionals have differentiated the content, the instructional methods, the instructional contexts, and even the sources of instructional delivery for a garden-variety middle school social studies unit of instruction.

Content Sources for Ongoing Instructional Planning

Sources of differentiated planning and instruction are multidimensional. For students with developmental disabilities, education professionals consider three planning dimensions in terms of various combinations of two or perhaps all three of the dimensions. These three dimensions emerge as a function of longitudinal planning; specifically, ongoing instructional content is derived from (a) the student's annual IEP goals, (b) his or her involvement in the general education curriculum, and (c) the community referents, typically drawn from the city or town where the student attends school. Figure 11.2 depicts the interrelationship among these three instructional planning content dimensions.

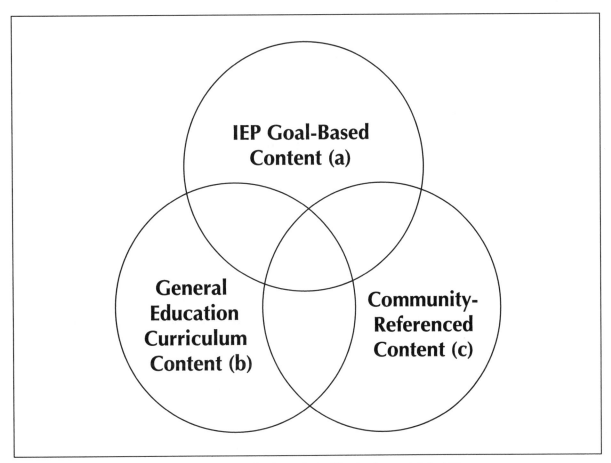

FIGURE 11.2. Relationship among content sources for the student with a developmental disability.

IEP Goal-Based Content

Usually, the student's IEP goals are the starting point for short-term planning. Best practice requires these goals to be individualized for the student on the basis of his or her strengths and needs, which are assessed and analyzed as part of the IDEIA-2004 multifactored evaluation requirements and regulatory procedures. However, it is neither necessary nor always advisable to devote the *entirety* of our instructional efforts exclusively to the student's IEP goals. That is, a student's IEP goals don't necessarily reflect *all* of his or her instructional targets; IEP goals are a necessary but not always sufficient marker of effective special education.

The IEP, is however, the primary source for ongoing instructional planning. The student's special educator and his or her classroom teachers begin short-term planning with each IEP goal, singularly or in logical combinations. For example, two specific goals for a 9-year-old student with Asperger's syndrome might involve reading comprehension and written language; these could be combined as an instructional unit is conceived in the area of literacy. As discussed earlier in the chapter, only students who are given alternate district-statewide assessments on the basis of alternate curriculum standards are *required* to have short-term objectives or benchmarks per IEP goal. However, effective ongoing planning will for the most part necessitate some sort of goal analysis process that yields smaller-scale benchmarks or more formalized objectives. In the literacy unit for the student with Asperger's syndrome, education professionals can use written language as a means to view and assess progress in comprehension as well as a targeted outcome in its own right (see Kucan & Beck, 1997). Education professionals can set a logical sequence of comprehension benchmarks in line with the IEP goal, using specific functional reading materials and/or typical comprehension components (e.g., vocabulary or factual recall) as guides.

General Education Curriculum Content

As discussed earlier in this chapter, IDEIA-2004 requires that education professionals involve the student with developmental disabilities in the general education curriculum and that they see to it that he or she shows progress in this curriculum. The planning can include both instruction geared toward such involvement and progress and instruction aimed exclusively toward other areas, such as the student's IEP goals and/or his or her specific community-referenced instructional needs.

Typically, education professionals would draw from either the same general education curricular standards that are applicable for students without disabilities or a subset of modified standards if available. In Kansas, for example, the special education unit of the state education department has developed what are called Extended Curricular Standards (Kansas State Department of Education, 2000). Under IDEIA-2004, students for whom reported assessment data will be taken from alternate assessments must be instructed from alternate standards as determined by their IEP teams. In addition, students who are administered the same assessments as students without disabilities but who require curriculum more relevant to their needs can also be instructed with content drawn from the extended standards (Susan Bashinski, personal communication, October 1, 2005). Unless explicitly prohibited by state law, which is unlikely, states that employ alternate curricular standards must require IEP teams to draw content from those curricula when the student takes alternate assessments, but there is no reason not to draw from alternate standards as appropriate for students who take standard assessments with or without accommodations.

Community-Referenced Content

The education professional might be interested in planning exclusively for the dimension of *community-referenced instruction*, which refers to any content and/or instructional practices that use community settings as contexts or applications of the curriculum or instruction. While *community-based instruction* refers exclusively to instruction conducted in actual community settings, *community-referenced instruction* serves as the broader term and can of course include classroom instruction so long as there is a community setting as the referent.

While the student's IEP goals may focus prominently on the community refer-ent, it is likely that some of his or her IEP goals are not community-referenced and that some of the community-referenced and community-based instruction planned for the student is not included within the IEP goals. Similarly, much of the cur-riculum that, for students with developmental disabilities, references one or more community settings is also the curriculum from which content for students without disabilities is drawn. Yet, for some students with developmental disabilities, educa-tion professionals might have social integrative experiences exclusively in mind when conducting community-referenced instruction. There may or may not be mention of such experiences in the student's IEP. Moreover, there may or may not be general education curriculum involvement. For example, Beck, Broers, Hogue, Shipstead, and Knowlton (1994) developed a "reverse mainstreaming" model, Community-Based Integrated Instruction (CBII), that features this level of flexibility. Essentially, CBII first identifies community referents in the general education curriculum for students without disabilities, then provides differentiated, community-based instruc-tion for these students and students with developmental disabilities in the relevant community settings.

Illustrations of Relevant Instructional Planning Source Dimensions

Using the Venn diagram shown in Figure 11.2 as a tool, education professionals can briefly exemplify each of four possible intercepts of these three source dimensions of instructional planning. Thus, while instructional planning could possibly be focused on a *single* dimension (i.e., IEP goals only, general education curriculum content only, community-referenced content only), best practices tend to combine these planning dimensions (e.g., IEP goals that reference the general education curriculum and/or community settings). Following are brief examples of such combinations.

Intercept 1 (abc). Jake is a 15-year-old student with Down syndrome. He is a highly verbal youngster with five older siblings—all male. They have made a considerable difference in his life with respect to his social and language development. Therefore Jake, a high school sophomore, functions fairly well socially and academically, though the content of his academic subjects is both adapted and augmented in order to fulfill goals he and his IEP team have developed (Knowlton, 1998).

Curricular adaptations for Jake are made with the support of the learning center special educator, who has taken each of his core subjects and adjusted their content to be applicable to relevant community settings and to meet his IEP goals. The special educator uses community referents for math, general science (applications of chemis-try and physics), and social studies (government, geography) to work with Jake in the learning center and as a co-teacher in some of his classes. In math, Jake has learned to determine sales tax on a calculator and how to adjust pizza recipes he makes at home according to the number of mouths to feed; in science, he has become the school's resident fireworks expert, and he knows how to determine the number of calories burned in 30 minutes of weightlifting at the local fitness center; in social studies he makes weekly reports on city council meetings and computer-generates local maps for his classmates—for a small fee.

The major augmentation to his curriculum was devised by the special educator to enhance Jake's self-determined behavior. The special educator, in collaboration with

Jake's parents, teachers, and siblings, has developed an ongoing self-determination contract (see Martin et al., 2003). As described in his IEP, Jake is given a work *plan* and a work *performance* record each morning by the special educator. The plan is basically a schedule, and the performance record adds specific class and homework assignments and other performance opportunities within major schedule items such as math class, science, etc. At the end of the day, one of Jake's parents or a sibling helps him *evaluate* his day by prompting him to answer yes/no questions about his performance (e.g., Enough time spent on assignment? Completed math problems?). At week's end, Jake and the special educator meet to examine the daily evaluations and *adjust* his plan as necessary (Martin et al., 2003). Though Jake is a unique kid, the fact that special education reflects a workable blend of IEP goals, general education content, and community-referenced instruction is not and should not be particularly unique.

Intercept 2 (ab). Elizabeth, 9 years old, has spastic cerebral palsy with quadriplegic involvement. She also exhibits a fairly significant cognitive impairment. Elizabeth cannot hold a pencil and therefore has always used a keyboard and mouse for class assignments that involve writing. Her program illustrates short-term instructional planning that takes into account her IEP goals and involvement in the general education curriculum. One of her IEP goals states that she will be able to type her name, street address, town, and zip code without prompts or assistance. Though she does not take alternate district-/statewide assessments, her IEP team will sometimes draw instructional content from her state's alternate curriculum standards. In written language, for example, there is an alternate standard titled "writing and expressive communication." One of its benchmarks states that the learner will use writing/expressive communication to convey important information. Among this benchmark's indicators is one pertaining to conveying personal information through written expression. Thus, Elizabeth's IEP goal and the general education curriculum are consonant with regard to written expression.

Intercept 3 (ac). An illustration of IEP-goal-related content that includes community referents involves Lydia, a 17-year-old student with significant cognitive and motor impairments. Throughout high school, her instruction has been drawn from a life-skills curriculum, and she has taken alternate assessments. Her IEP goals in recent years have centered on effectuating self-determined behavior through carefully constructed opportunities in which she acts as her own *causal agent* (Wehmeyer et al., 2000). Using selected community referents, as well as her home environment and sub-environments, Lydia receives teacher modeling, peer modeling, and teacher and peer prompting as she sets goals, takes goal-related actions, and makes adjustments to her goals and plans of action (Wehmeyer et al., 2000). For example, Lydia arranged for the purchase of an orthotic appliance that supports motor control in her hand so that she is better able to prepare simple meals at home independent of her mother and siblings.

Intercept 4 (bc). An example of community-referenced content that uses the general education curriculum involves Julian, who is 8 years old and has been diagnosed with pervasive developmental disorder. Julian's fourth-grade teacher works with the special educator to teach all of her students the basic mathematics skills involved in comparison shopping. Using the general education math curriculum standards as a guide, the classroom teacher has developed instruction around estimation, fractions, and decimals for the class. In addition, she has identified the local grocery store and the neighborhood convenience store as community referents. Digital photos were taken with permission of the store managers to allow all students to make price comparisons and shopping decisions in class; then in small groups the class shopped for selected items at each store. Julian's group purchased chocolate milk at the grocery store after estimating the relative amounts of money that would be left over if they had shopped at the convenience store versus the grocery store.

Conclusion

This chapter has attempted to advance the reader's thinking about long- and short-term planning for students with developmental disabilities. Sadly, some special education professionals and general classroom teachers still plan their instruction without taking into account one another's perspectives, let alone the options for collaborative assistance. Some plan only on a short-term basis, failing to see the big picture and to ask the big-picture questions as part of critical longitudinal planning. There continue to be teachers who cannot differentiate instruction for diverse groups of students, cannot think in terms of curricular augmentation and adaptations. Some are even unaware that students with developmental disabilities can be taught to be self-determined, to serve as their own causal agents.

We hope that the reader, having covered this chapter and studied the perspectives shared in this book, will not be one of those education professionals! We anticipate that readers will use at least one of the tools presented in this chapter beginning *tomorrow*—ask big-picture questions about lifestyle quality or the environments in which your student can fully meet environmental demands. Examine your students' educational programs to determine where they fit in the Venn diagram shown in Figure 11.2. Wherever these programs fit, are they working for the students? Could they work better? After all, those are the key questions that drive instructional planning.

Glossary

Circumvention of environmental demand—Teaching the student ways to get around an environmental demand if it is not plausible to attempt to teach the skills necessary to meet the demand.

Content-source dimensions of instructional planning—Sources of curriculum content generated from (a) IEP goals, (b) the general education curriculum, and (c) community referents.

Curricular personalization—Use of collaborative planning processes to tailor the intent of a longitudinal goal to the student's unique circumstances, such as age, gender, functional abilities, past experiences, personal-social network, etc.

Curriculum augmentation—Superimposition of content onto an existing curriculum, e.g., self-determination onto the general education curriculum.

Differentiated instruction—A way of thinking about teaching through the accommodation of classroom diversity. Instructional planning for instructional differentiation first divides content into components learned by all, most, and some of the students in the classroom, then manipulates methods, delivery agents, and contexts of instruction, thus differentiating it for a classroom of diverse learners.

Involvement and progress in the general education curriculum—IDEA's provision (in alignment with the No Child Left Behind Act) that all students should be involved with content drawn from their district's general education curriculum and that all students should make progress in that curriculum.

Rebuttable presumption—A refutable proposition that is assumed true until proven untrue.

Relative independence—The belief that in the present era no one is really independent in the absolute sense; rather, we are all interdependent.

Special education—Specially designed instruction that meets the unique needs of a student with a disability at no additional cost to parents.

Zero-reject—One of the more prominent principles of IDEA, requiring that all children and youth be provided the opportunity for an appropriate education.

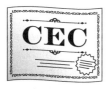

Knowledge and Skills for Entry-Level Special Education Teachers of Students With Developmental Disabilities Standards Addressed in This Chapter

Principle 7: Instructional Planning

DD7S1   Plan instruction for independent functional life skills relevant to the community, personal living, sexuality, and employment.

DD7S2   Plan and implement instruction for individuals with developmental disabilities that is both age-appropriate and ability-appropriate.

DD7S4   Design, implement, and evaluate specialized instructional programs for persons with developmental disabilities that enhance social participation across environments.

Web Site Resources

Council for Exceptional Children (CEC)—Analysis of Draft Regulations Regarding the Individualized Education Program (IEP).
http://www.cec.sped.org/cec_bn/side-by-sides.html

"Side-by-side" analyses of the federal Notice of Proposed Rule Making (proposed regulations to govern the implementation of IDEIA-2004) as compared with the older, current regulations that were based on IDEA-1997.

IRIS Faculty Enhancement Center
http://iris.peabody.vanderbilt.edu/gpm/cresource.htm

Resources that can enhance teachers' professional development. Several relevant instructional units, subsumed under the "Star Legacy Modules," as well as a variety of provocative case studies.

Kansas Extended Curricular Standards
http://www.kansped.org/ksde/assmts/ksalt/ksalt.html

Documents related to alternate assessment in Kansas, as well as the alternate curriculum standards that Kansas uses in the subject areas of reading, writing, mathematics, science, and social studies.

No Child Left Behind Act (Elementary and Secondary Education Act of 2001)
http://www.ed.gov/policy/elsec/leg/esea02/index.html

Not exactly riveting reading. However, the No Child Left Behind Act is perhaps the most controversial federal education law Congress has ever enacted. Of all of its supporters and critics, how many have actually read the law?

What Works Clearinghouse (WWC)
http://whatworks.ed.gov/

A product of the Institute of Education Sciences, U.S. Department of Education. Information on a wide range of topics related to teaching and learning. Numerous interventions that have been analyzed and evaluated with respect to their validity and utility.

References

Anderson, A., Avery, D., DiPietro, E., Edwards, G., & Christian, W. (1987). Intensive home-based early intervention with autistic children. *Education and Treatment of Children, 10*, 352–366.

Bannerman, D., Sheldon, J., Sherman, J., & Harchik, A. (1990). Balancing the right to habilitation with the right to personal liberties: The rights of people with developmental disabilities to eat too many doughnuts and take a nap. *Journal of Applied Behavior Analysis, 23*, 79–89.

Beck, J., Broers, J., Hogue, E., Shipstead, J., & Knowlton, H. E. (1994). Strategies for functional community-based instruction and inclusion for children with mental retardation. *Teaching Exceptional Children, 26*(2), 44–48.

Brown, L., Branston, M., Hamre-Nietupski, S., Pumpian, I., Certo, N., & Gruenwald, L. (1979). A strategy for developing chronological age-appropriate and functional curricular content for severely handicapped adolescents and young adults. *Journal of Special Education, 13*, 81–90.

Brown, L., Shiraga, B., Rogan, P., York, J., Zanella-Albright, K., McCarthy, E., & Loomis, R. (1985). The "why question" in educational programs for students who are severely intellectually disabled. In L. Brown, B. Shiraga, J. York, A. Udvari-Solner, K. Zanella-Albright, P. Rogan, et al. (Eds.), *Educational programs for students with severe intellectual disabilities* (Vol. 15, pp. 17–42). Madison, WI: Madison Metropolitan School District.

Carroll, L. (1999). *The annotated Alice: Alice's adventures in Wonderland and through the looking glass.* New York: Norton.

Cha, K., & Merrill, E. (1994). Facilitation and inhibition in visual selective attention processes of individuals with and without mental retardation. *American Journal on Mental Retardation, 98*, 594–600.

Council for Exceptional Children (2005, June). *Individualized Education Program (IEP) Draft Analysis.* Arlington, VA: Author.

Covey, S. (1989). *The seven habits of highly effective people.* New York: Simon & Schuster.

Education for All Handicapped Children Act of 1975, 20 U.S.C. § 1400 *et seq.* (1975).

Gartin, B., Murdick, N., Imbeau, M., & Perner, D. (2002). *How to use differentiated instruction with students with developmental disabilities in the general education classroom.* Arlington, VA: Council for Exceptional Children.

Goldman, S., Hasselbring, T., & the Cognition and Technology Group at Vanderbilt University (1997). Achieving meaningful mathematics literacy for students with learning disabilities. *Journal of Learning Disabilities, 30*, 198–208.

Individuals with Disabilities Education Act of 1990, 20 U.S.C. § 1400 *et seq.* (1990) (amended 1997).

Individuals with Disabilities Education Improvement Act of 2004, 118 Stat. 2647. (2004).

IRIS Faculty Enhancement Center. (2005). *Perspectives and Resources: Star Legacy Modules—Progress Monitoring.* Retrieved November 29, 2005, from http://iris.peabody.vanderbilt.edu/gpm/cresource.htm

Jaime, K., & Knowlton, H. E. (2007). Visual supports for students with cognitive and behavioral challenges. *Intervention in School and Clinic; 42*(5); 259–270.

Kansas State Department of Education (2000). *Extended curricular standards.* Retrieved November 29, 2005, from http://www.kansped.org/ksde/assmts/ksalt/ksalt.html

Knowlton, H. E. (1998). Considerations in the design of personalized curricular supports for students with developmental disabilities. *Education and Training in Mental Retardation/Developmental Disabilities, 33*, 95–107.

Knowlton, H. E. (2007). *Developing effective individualized education programs: A case based tutorial (CD-ROM).* Upper Saddle River, NJ: Merrill/Prentice Hall.

Kucan, L., & Beck, I. (1997). Thinking aloud and reading comprehension research: Inquiry, instruction, and social interaction. *Review of Educational Research, 67*, 271–299.

Martin, J., Mithaug, D., Cox, P., Peterson, L., Van Dycke, J., & Cash, M. (2003). Increasing self-determination: Teaching students to plan, work, evaluate, and adjust. *Exceptional Children, 69*, 431–447.

Myles, B., & Simpson, R. (2001). Understanding the hidden curriculum: An essential social skill for children and youth with Asperger syndrome. *Intervention in School and Clinic, 36*, 279–286.

No Child Left Behind Act of 2001, 20 U.S.C. 70 § 6301 *et seq.* (2002).

Parmenter, T., & Donelly, M. (1997). An analysis of the dimensions of quality of life. In R. I. Brown (Ed.), *Quality of life for people with disabilities: Models, research, and practice* (pp. 91–114). Cheltenham, UK: Stanley Thornes.

Schalock, R. (2000). Three decades of quality of life. In M. L. Wehmeyer & J. R. Patton (Eds.), *Mental retardation in the 21st century* (pp. 335–358). Austin, TX: PRO-ED.

Schalock, R., & Verdugo-Alonzo, M. A. (2002). *Handbook on quality of life for human service providers.* Washington, DC: American Association on Mental Retardation.

Schumm, J., Vaughn, S., & Leavell, A. (1994). Planning pyramid: A framework for planning diverse students' needs during content instruction. *Reading Teacher, 47,* 608–615.

Tomlinson, C. (2000). Reconcilable differences: Standards-based teaching and differentiation. *Educational Leadership, 58*(1), 6–11.

Tomlinson, C. (2001). *How to differentiate instruction in mixed-ability classrooms* (2nd ed.). Washington, DC: Association for Supervision and Curriculum Development.

Tomporowski, P., & Tinsley, V. (1994). Effects of target probability and memory demands on the vigilance of adults with and without mental retardation. *American Journal on Mental Retardation, 96,* 525–530.

Turnbull, H. R., Huerta, N., & Stowe, M. (2006). *The Individuals With Disabilities Education Act as amended in 2004.* Columbus, OH: Merrill/Prentice Hall.

Turnbull, H. R., & Turnbull, A. (2000). *Free appropriate public education* (6th ed.). Denver: Love.

U.S. Department of Education. (2005, November). *Secretary Spellings announces growth model pilot, addresses chief state school officers annual policy forum in Richmond.* Retrieved November 29, 2005, from http://www.ed.gov/news/pressreleases/2005/11/11182005.html

Wehmeyer, M. (1998). Self-determination and individuals with significant disabilities: Examining meanings and misinterpretations. *Journal of the Association for Persons With Severe Handicaps, 23,* 5–16.

Wehmeyer, M., Abery, B., Mithaug, D., Powers, L., & Stancliffe, R. (2003). *Theory in self-determination: Foundations for educational practice.* Springfield, IL: Thomas.

Wehmeyer, M., Palmer, S., Agran, M., Mithaug, D., & Martin, J. (2000). Promoting causal agency: The self-determined learning model of instruction. *Exceptional Children, 66,* 439–453.

Wehmeyer, M., Sands, D., Knowlton, H. E., & Kozleski, E. (2002). *Teaching students with mental retardation.* Baltimore: Brookes.

Wise, B., Cole, R., van Vuuren, S., Schwarz, S., Snyder, L., Ngampatipatpong, N., et al. (in press). Learning to read with a virtual tutor. In C. Kinzer & L. Verhoeven (Eds.), *Interactive literacy education.* Mahwah, NJ: Lawrence Erlbaum.

Zeaman, D., & House, B. J. (1979). A review of attention theory. In N. R. Ellis (Ed.), *Handbook of mental deficiency: Psychological theory and research* (2nd ed., pp. 63–120). Hillsdale, NJ: Lawrence Erlbaum.

Zigler, E. (1999). The individual with mental retardation as a whole person. In E. Zigler & D. Bennett-Gates (Eds.), *Personality development in individuals with mental retardation* (pp. 1–16). Cambridge, UK: Cambridge University Press.

12

Personalized Curriculum Development

Debra L. Shelden and Margaret P. Hutchins

Summary

This chapter provides an overview of a process for developing a personalized curriculum for learners with developmental disabilities. It presents existing models of curriculum development, with a discussion of their limitations, and briefly discusses underlying values and characteristics of effective curriculum. It then presents a recommended process for developing personalized curriculum—one that reflects those values and characteristics. That process begins with person-centered planning steps that lead to the development of a longitudinal vision statement, continues with a variety of assessments to identify educational priorities, and concludes with careful decision making about short-term and long-term priorities. The chapter closes with a discussion of the relationship of personalized curriculum to the general education curriculum.

Learning Outcomes

After reading this chapter, you should be able to:

- Identify existing models of curriculum development and describe their limitations for learners with developmental disabilities.

- Identify and describe the primary components of person-centered planning.

- Identify and describe the steps for using ecological inventories to generate a personalized curriculum.

- Describe the process for analyzing and organizing data to generate a longitudinal curriculum.

- Describe how access to the general education curriculum is addressed in personalized curriculum development.

Introduction

Curriculum is the term agreed upon by professional educators to describe the "what" that is taught to individuals participating in the educational process. It is understood that curriculum is the content component, in contrast to the methodology, or "how," component of the design and delivery of instructional programs. Therefore, because a curriculum specifies the target knowledge and skills that are the desired goals of an educational program, one should conceptualize the curriculum as a map or sequence of well-articulated learning objectives that lead to meaningful outcomes.

For learners who do not receive special education services, the curriculum that is specified is most often the result of one or more influences, such as federal mandates, state and local boards of education, textbooks, and professional organizations (Kauchak, Eggen, & Carter, 2002) and is usually referred to as the "general education curriculum" (Individuals with Disabilities Education Improvement Act of 2004). A general education curriculum is not created to meet students' individualized learning needs, but rather to delineate a series of educational objectives or standards that are considered to be socially valid for *most* learners participating in the public education system.

Access to the general education curriculum must also be provided for learners with developmental disabilities who receive special education services. However, these students are also entitled to an individualized education program (IEP) that designates curriculum modifications and enhancements by identifying specific annual goals that most effectively address the students' learning needs to achieve a wide array of desired educational outcomes. The individualization of the curriculum, which offers a focus on specific and unique learning objectives for each person with a developmental disability, can be designated a *personalized curriculum.*

It is important to emphasize that personalized curricula will vary dramatically across learners with developmental disabilities. The diversity among these learners in terms of strengths, support needs, values, and priorities suggests that the nature of the curriculum, and the balance among functional, academic, and social priorities, will be similarly diverse.

Historical Models of Curriculum Development

Since the time when professionals first attempted to focus on the learning needs of individuals with developmental disabilities, a variety of approaches for developing curriculum models have been utilized and cited. Wilcox and Bellamy (1982) offered a classification of curriculum models that included the *eliminative model, a developmental model,* and a *functional academics model.* More recently, a curricular approach that can be labeled as a *standards-based model* has evolved in general education. Finally, as early as 1976, an *ecological inventory* or "top down" curriculum model was initially introduced (Brown, et al., 1979) and was further supported by the dissemination of the McGill Action Planning System (MAPS) (Vandercook, York, & Forest, 1989), used to articulate desired educational outcomes. Eventually, professionals concerned with providing effective transition planning for individuals with disabilities adopted many of these earlier outcomes-based planning concepts and created a related model for developing curriculum that carries the label of *person-centered planning* (Miner & Bates, 2002). Each of these models will be described in the following sections.

Eliminative Model

The eliminative model (Wilcox & Bellamy, 1982) of curriculum development focuses on the belief that in order for an education professional to teach meaningful instructional or educational objectives, the student must be rid of interfering maladaptive or inappropriate behaviors. This model supports the concept that undesirable behaviors must be eliminated from a person's repertoire if he or she is to experience success in achieving additional instructional objectives. At one time, this approach may have been used to identify relevant educational interventions for persons with developmental disabilities. However, changing curricular trends over time and a more recent emphasis on functional behavior assessment and analysis (Ryan, Halsey, & Matthews,

2003; Shippen, Simpson, & Crites, 2003) have minimized the rationale for its adoption. In fact, support has increased for revealing the potential communicative intent of many less desirable behaviors exhibited by an individual. This development has highlighted the importance of fully exploring potential factors and explanations for maladaptive behaviors, which could include poor choices of instructional methods and/or curricular objectives. Rather than viewing adaptive behavior and instruction as discrete entities, the education professional should explore the relationship and interaction between curriculum and evidence of maladaptive behavior.

Developmental Model

The developmental model (Wilcox & Bellamy, 1982) supports the premise that the curriculum for an individual with developmental disabilities should be aligned with typical child development sequences. In other words, instructional content would be identified and selected on the basis of the identified deficits of an individual with a developmental disability, from resources that specify the developmental sequences of children without special needs. This approach appears to focus on the existing deficits of a learner with a disability and to support a type of "fix-it" model. Although the overlap in targeted curricula could be appropriate for young children with and without disabilities, the discrepancy between purported developmental deficits and the skills requisite for achieving adult life outcomes becomes greater as the learner matures. Over time this approach becomes limited and no longer serves as an adequate model as learners with developmental disabilities age, particularly since it lessens time spent on functional skills.

Functional Academic Model

The functional academic model (Wilcox & Bellamy, 1982) stems from the idea of providing instruction on the basic "reading, writing, and arithmetic" skills taught in general education. It was an early attempt to address the identification and selection of curricula that more closely represented the traditional academic world experienced by learners who did not have identified special needs. The approach supports the idea of approaching curriculum in applied and authentic contexts rather than in abstract and less meaningful ones. However, it, too, appears to be grounded in a "status quo" and "bottom-up" series of learning objectives that may not lead to meaningful adult outcomes in a timely fashion. This approach appears to accept assumptions regarding the need for respecting prerequisites and to adopt established curriculum sequences without completing more-thorough analyses of the outcomes and the diverse number of sequences of objectives that could lead to the accomplishment of individualized educational outcomes.

Standards-Based Model

The standards-based model emphasizes the acceptance of specified goals, standards, and indicators that represent measurable outcomes across all traditional academic areas for any learner. This approach forms the primary framework for many general education programs across the country. It is a committed attempt to provide consistency and equity in educational program content for all learners. However, these standards do not address every curricular domain, and no process exists for systematically evaluating and revising those standards that may need modification, enhancement, or an alternative interpretation in order to develop a personalized curriculum for individuals with developmental disabilities.

Ecological Inventory Model

The earliest ecological inventory model (Brown et al., 1979; Wilcox & Bellamy, 1982) supported the concept that in order to plan effectively for desired and meaningful outcomes as part of the educational process, education professionals should carefully analyze the environments, sub-environments, activities, and skills that define each outcome. Conceptualizing curricula from this "top-down" approach, in which sequences of objectives are specifically designed to meet a target outcome, **239** promotes the adaptation that is necessary in order to meet the individualized needs of the learner. Although learners may have similar desired outcomes, an ecological approach demands that (a) a more careful analysis be conducted with the criterion environments in which the learner will interact to validate the requisite skills for success and (b) unique and individualized factors be identified to personalize the curriculum with respect to assistive technology, learner maturation, and desired level of independence. This approach supports an IEP team's creating a *longitudinal vision* from which specific objectives can be identified and a personalized curriculum can be created. This approach is the focus of the remainder of this chapter.

The debate about what exemplifies appropriate curriculum for learners with developmental disabilities continues. Curricular focus for students with mild mental retardation has moved between a focus on life skills and a focus on remediation of academic skills (Bouck, 2004), while the curricular focus for students with severe disabilities has moved from a focus on functional skills to a focus on social skills and membership priorities (Dymond & Orelove, 2001). In the absence of sufficient research and the presence of continuing debate about what constitutes appropriate curriculum, the field should "balance [its] attention equally on academic, functional, and social skills, keeping in mind that the relative emphasis placed on each content area *depends on the needs of the individual child*" (Dymond & Orelove, 2001, p. 111, emphasis added).

Underlying Values and Characteristics of Effective Curricula

The process for developing a personalized curriculum discussed herewith assumes particular underlying values and characteristics. The following sections provide specific insights regarding each of these basic assumptions.

Values

First, we hold that the purposes of education for *all* learners—with and without disabilities—is to promote a high quality of life and prepare them for meaningful participation in their chosen communities. While the general education curriculum combined with individual and family supports and experiences may be sufficient for many learners, other learners will require more systematic curriculum planning to achieve these outcomes. The criterion of ultimate functioning (Brown, Nietupski, & Hamre-Nietupski, 1976) suggested a shift in the focus of curriculum design for learners with significant disabilities toward a more outcome-oriented approach that values community participation and interaction with individuals without disabilities. It also recognized that the nature of that participation will differ, depending not only on the individual learner but also on identified communities. Individualizing curriculum is the process of both identifying the meaningful and desired participation for an individual learner and mapping the learning that needs to occur in order for that learner to achieve the identified participation.

Second, individualized curriculum demands a respect for the unique culture of each family, which varies in terms of values, traditions, and beliefs (see Chapters 7 and 8 for a more detailed discussion of cultural issues). In relationship to curriculum development, important issues include family differences with respect to the construct and relative importance of independence and other dominant culture indicators of quality of life, interest in or valuing of future planning, and the meaning of equity (Harry, Rueda, & Kalyanpur, 1999). Professionals must strive for cultural reciprocity, which entails understanding their own culture as well as those of the families with whom they work (Kalyanpur & Harry, 1997).

Third, individualized curriculum should both respect and promote the learner's self-determination (see Chapter 6 for a more detailed discussion of self-determination). At times teachers may encounter a conflict between respecting family culture and respecting self-determination. However, self-determination can be viewed not only as an individual characteristic but also as a construct influenced by ecology (Abery & Stancliffe, 2003), a view that allows for cultural variance in how self-determination is addressed.

Characteristics

In addition to reflecting the values addressed above, appropriate curricula should also be (a) outcome-based, (b) longitudinal, (c) meaningful, (d) community-referenced, and (e) age-appropriate. An outcome-based curriculum is one that purposefully moves toward goals for the future. The personalized curriculum incorporates skills and activities necessary to reach the desired outcomes. Curricula must also be longitudinal and continuous, rather than episodic (Brown et al., 1976). Hence, a personalized curriculum will include both short-term and long-term priorities that promote movement toward desired outcomes. Activities and skills included in curricula must also be meaningful. This characteristic requires that we ask why we are including specific activities and skills in each personalized curriculum and what impact we expect those activities and skills to have on the learner's life. The community-referenced characteristic suggests that we look not simply to activities and skills of "typical" environments but also to those of the particular environments that the learner seeks to access. Finally, the curricula must be age-appropriate. Participation in the activities for peers of the same age will lead to more opportunities to develop relationships with those peers.

Process for Personalizing Curriculum

The process for personalizing curriculum has multiple components that involve various assessment procedures and careful decision making. Implementation of this process will vary. The essence of it, however, includes (a) developing a personal profile and a long-term vision for the learner, (b) conducting ecological inventories and additional assessments, and (c) identifying and organizing short-term and long-term educational priorities. This general process is commonly presented as a model for curriculum development for students with moderate and severe disabilities (Browder, 2001; Ryndak, 2003). We suggest, however, that the general process is appropriate for *all learners with developmental disabilities* (see Table 12.1). At its core, the process

TABLE 12.1
Summary of the Process for Personalized Curriculum Development

Step	Description of the Step	Who Is Involved?	How Is This Done?
Develop a personal profile	A summary of what is known about the learner, including relationships and strengths	Learner, learner's family, stakeholders identified by the learner and family, including friends and educational personnel	Guided team process Review of records
Formulate a vision statement	After discussing dreams, fears, preferences, generate a statement describing desired life in three to five years	Learner, learner's family, stakeholders identified by the learner and family, including friends and educational personnel	Guided team process Also may involve interview of learner and family and observation of learner
Conduct ecological inventories	Identify participation in current activities, environments, and activities in which participation is desired now and in the future, and identify skills needed to participate in those activities	Educational personnel, family, social validation source	Curriculum inventory checklists, observation, interview
Conduct additional assessments as needed	Gather more detailed data on skills and participation as required	Educational personnel, learner	Situational assessment tools
Develop a list of all priorities	Merge lists from family, learner, and ecological inventories on desired activities and skills still needed to facilitate participation in those activities	Educational personnel coordinates	
Prioritize	Differentiate between short-term and long-term priorities	Team	Guided team discussion

entails developing long-term goals, identifying what is needed to achieve those long-term goals, and then developing a plan to achieve them. While the level of detail required at different steps may vary according to individual differences, the same systematic planning process can be useful for all students.

Personal Profiles and Vision Statements

Well-crafted vision statements are critical to the curriculum development process. They represent the ultimate goal for a learner and hence give direction to the team and the curriculum. Vision statements should describe a life "worth working to achieve" (Miner & Bates, 2002, p. 16) and include desired outcomes in major life areas (e.g., home, community, work, relationships). In order to encourage forward-thinking and effective curriculum planning, vision statements must also be longitudinal, describing outcomes desired in three to five years.

Vision statements are typically developed through person-centered planning. Numerous person-centered planning guides and processes exist, including whole-life planning (Butterworth, Hagner, Heikkinen, DeMello, & McDonough, 1993), team environmental assessment mapping (Campbell, Campbell, & Brady, 1998), personal futures planning (Mount & Zwernik, 1988), essential lifestyle planning (Smull & Harrison, 1992), group action planning (Turnbull & Turnbull, 1996), and the McGill action planning system (Vandercook, et al., 1989). While the various processes differ in many ways, they each take direction from the learner and her or his family. The intent of person-centered planning is to generate both a vision for a learner's future and a series of actions that will facilitate movement toward that vision.

Personal Profiles

The person-centered planning component of personalizing curriculum should include a summary of what is known about the learner, a discussion of values, dreams, and fears, and the development of a long-term vision statement. While a review of the learner's records is useful and necessary for collecting data on the learner's present level of performance, additional information gathered through interviews or team meetings is also required. Miner and Bates (2002) suggest developing a personal profile that includes a pictorial representation and discussion of the learner's current relationships and community presence (settings used daily, weekly, and occasionally), a list of likes and dislikes, and a list of gifts and capacities. The result is a more holistic and positive summary of the learner than would typically be developed through a review of records only.

The following case study illustrates the key components of the personal profile developed for Rod, a 12-year-old boy with autism.

In preparing for Rod's IEP meeting, his teacher decided to work with his family to initiate a person-centered planning meeting. During that meeting, Rod's team discussed his relationships, community presence, strengths, and preferences prior to discussing his future. His relationship map showed that he has very close relationships with his immediate family and several of his teachers. He gets along well with and interacts often with his peers with disabilities at school, but rarely sees them outside of school. He has limited interactions with peers without disabilities at school. Relationships outside of family and school include families that are close to his own family, but he does not have individual relationships with members of those families. Rod is extremely active in his community. He and his family regularly access several recreational facilities, restaurants and coffeehouses, and libraries and museums. He is also now accessing those community environments with his classmates and teachers, though not frequently. When his team answered the question "Who is Rod?" they painted a picture of a boy who is loving, affectionate, and enthusiastic; has a good sense of humor; loves being physically active, particularly with swimming, roller skating, and bicycling; enjoys computers and drawing; likes watching movies but not listening to music; is a visual learner; responds well to structure; and does not like changes in his schedule or routine.

Envisioning the Future

After the profile of the learner has been developed, the process turns to the future. Issues about values, dreams and goals, fears and concerns, and priorities are discussed. Most person-centered planning team processes include guided questions to facilitate this discussion. Other curriculum development tools, such as *Choosing Outcomes and Accommodations for Children* (Giangreco, Cloninger, & Iverson, 1998), include a guide for interviewing families about these issues. Once data are collected from the learner, the family, and other stakeholders on values, dreams, and concerns, a longitudinal vision statement is developed and used to guide the rest of the curriculum development process.

The following approach was used by Rod's team in crafting a vision for his future.

> Rod's team discussed his future at great length. Family is highly valued in his home, and in the future everyone wants to maintain close relationships. However, everyone agreed that it is important for him to develop other relationships as well. His parents feel that shortly after leaving school, Rod should be prepared to move into his own apartment or house with friends. They also want him to be an active member of the community, including having a job. The entire team agreed that both the short-term and long-term future should include more varied relationships.

> His parents are adamant that Rod not live in a group home or work in a sheltered workshop. They also want his paid support to be as minimal and non-intrusive as possible. They hope that he will develop skills and supports to live in a supported living arrangement. In the short term, they want to strike a useful balance between a community-based curriculum and continuing academic and social development in general education classrooms. They would like for his typical day at school to include some time in a general education classroom, but one where he can be working on his own educational needs. Current priorities for the team included further developing communication, literacy, relationships, and self-management.

> Rod's team developed a six-year vision statement, expressing their hopes for his life upon reaching adulthood: Rod will continue to live with his family for a few years but will move into an apartment with roommates within a few years of leaving school. He will have a job that interests him. He'll be independent in most of his personal care skills, but he'll receive support from family, friends, or paid staff with shopping and budgeting. He'll be an active and safe member of his community and will have a full leisure life. He'll maintain close relationships with his family but will also have friends outside of his family.

Current and Future Skill Needs

Person-centered planning processes yield critical information for developing a personalized curriculum that addresses the values and hopes of individual learners and their families. For many students with developmental disabilities, however, the information gained is not sufficient to generate an effective curriculum. The curriculum development process is a series of assessments, from more-broad and less-direct assessments to specific and direct assessments (Browder, 2001). From this perspective, the development of a vision statement comes from an assessment of a family's values, beliefs, and hopes. Translating that vision into a concrete list of skills to include in a student's curriculum requires more specific information on the learner's current skills as well as the skill demands of future activities and settings.

Ecological Inventories of Current and Future Environments

As discussed above, ecological inventories are the evaluation of an individual's current and potential future environments in order to identify the activities and skills needed for that person to achieve his or her long-term vision. Ecological inventories should be conducted for current environments, activities, and skills in which the learner desires greater independence *and* for future environments, activities, and skills that constitute the long-term vision for the learner. The inventories ask three main assessment questions: (a) What is the learner's level of participation in current environments and activities? (b) What are the skill demands for greater participation in current environments and activities? and (c) What are the skills demands for participation in desired future environments and activities?

Originally, ecological inventory models focused on life-skills domains (community, domestic, leisure, and vocational). More recently, they have begun to include the academic domain as well, identifying school as a key environment in children's lives (Ryndak, 2003). Ecological inventories are conducted through observation and interview and include multiple data sources. The ecological inventory process (Brown et al., 1979) includes the following steps: (a) identify a domain, (b) identify natural environments in which the student is expected to participate within the domain, (c) select priority sub-environments within each identified environment, (d) identify activities that occur within each environment in which students are expected to participate, and (e) identify skills required to participate in activities. Ecological inventories of the general education curriculum include gathering data on curriculum content, activities, settings, and independent-functioning skills within a classroom, as well as the expected outcomes for the entire class (Ryndak, 2003).

An assessment of the learner's participation in current activities expands the personal profile developed through person-centered planning. Because direct assessment of all life skills is not feasible, this process typically begins with a family interview. The interviewee provides information on the student's current activities at home, in school, and in the community, as well as the level of independence that the student demonstrates in those activities. Several functional curriculum guides exist to facilitate the interview and data recording; among them are (a) *Syracuse Community-Referenced Curriculum Guide* (Ford et al., 1989); (b) *Choosing Outcomes and Accommodations for Children* (Giangrego et al., 1998); and (c) *Life Centered Career Education* (Brolin, 1997). These manuals include lists of activities and skills organized around major life activities and curriculum domains.

While it may be tempting to save time by sending a checklist home to be completed by a family member, a face-to-face interview yields richer data that will allow for more-effective curriculum development. Ryndak (2003) suggests also getting information from the family on desired components of the general education curriculum, including content knowledge, general skills (e.g., independent functioning) developed through partial participation, and functional activities within classroom activities. Finally, the interview concludes by asking the family to prioritize what they would like the student to learn, including both functional skills and general education components. Students may also be involved in identifying their current skills and their priorities.

The ecological inventory component also includes identifying skill demands of the desired future environments so that curricular objectives can be mapped longitudinally. Both interviewing and observing can be used to collect such data. Resources are identified to validate skills for particular activities. Scope and sequence charts from existing curriculum inventories (Ford et al., 1989) can be used as a starting place for understanding the expected skill demands for learners of various ages, but more detailed information about specific environments and activities will often be required. Useful tools for targeted activities include interviewing an individual who has knowledge of the demands of that environment and observing the activity.

An ecological inventory also typically includes a social validation component that entails identifying environments, sub-environments, and activities that are frequently engaged in by peers without disabilities and that are typically valued. Again, we must attend to family culture. Harry et al. (1999) discuss the potential cultural bias in identifying what is "typical," suggesting an *ecocultural analysis* approach to identifying priority activities in environments, as well as expected skill level. In an ecocultural approach, the comparative activities and skills are representative not of what is typical for most children but what is valued by and accessible to the particular learner and his or her family.

Rod's team accomplished this by using a process described in the following narrative.

> Many of Rod's environments and activities are reflected in his personal profile. His team was able to identify many of his general activities and skills during the team process. His teacher followed that with a more extensive interview of his mother. After providing data on his current activities and level of independence at home and in the community, Rod's mother identified the following as priorities: independence in his morning personal care routine, including using a picture schedule and self-monitoring; using a knife to cut food; making simple meals; washing dishes; independently crossing streets safely; using the community bus with an adult; paying cash for small purchases at the fitness center, fast-food restaurants, and the grocery store; and participating in community leisure activities with peers. Her general education curriculum priorities included engaging in cooperative activities with peers in general education classrooms, increasing verbal communication skills, increasing functional literacy skills, increasing functional math skills, and exploring career options in non-academic general education classrooms (e.g., computer class).
>
> On the basis of the identified priorities for Rod, his teacher asked additional questions to gather more specific information on several home, school, and community activities. In the domestic domain, she identified the home environment, including bathroom, kitchen, and living room. Priority activities in the bathroom included the morning routine (shower and wash hair, brush and floss teeth, and eventually shave), simple food preparation in the kitchen, and watching movies and interacting with

family and friends in the living room. Because the teacher was conducting the interview at Rod's home, she was able to look at these environments to assess skill demands. For instance, she noted that the kitchen had an electric stove and microwave and that the living room had both a VCR player and a DVD player. This provided her with more information about specific skills to target for Rod, and she was able to develop task analyses for further assessment and future instruction. Rod's teacher also conducted an ecological inventory of a computer class and an art class to identify curriculum content, course expectations, instructional strategies, and membership issues. In the computer class, she identified primary activities of creating Web pages and databases. Students in this class typically worked alone in a self-directed manner. Students used one model of computer throughout the classroom and several computer programs. In the art class, primary activities included drawing and painting. Student work was typically individual, but there was a good deal of socialization among students while they worked. The teacher provided one-to-one feedback and assistance. Finally, she observed priority activities in the community to assess skill demands in those settings for 10-year-olds (Rod's current age) and 13-year-olds (for longitudinal planning). At the coffeehouse frequented by Rod and his family, she noted through observation and interview the primary activities of ordering at a counter, eating, socializing, studying, and playing board games. While 10-year-olds would not typically be at the coffeehouse without adults, "young teens" sometimes came in together as groups. There was no paper menu available; it was on a chalkboard on the wall. There also appeared to be several items to order that were not on the menu but were visible in display cases. The coffeehouse took checks and cash but not credit or debit cards. Customers seated themselves, ordered at a counter, carried their own food to a table, and typically bussed their own tables. This information helped Rod's teacher again to identify skills that would contribute to his participation in this particular community environment.

Additional Assessments

Sometimes the personal profile and ecological inventory do not provide enough information to develop IEP objectives. In such cases, direct assessments should be used to collect additional information (Browder, 2001). Situational assessments are opportunities for the learner to engage in the targeted activity so that his or her performance on each component or skill of the activity can be assessed. The task analysis developed through ecological inventory is used to guide the assessment. The learner's level of independence and the type of assistance needed at each step are identified. Notes related to the learner's interest in and response to component skills can also be useful in designing future instruction.

Organizing the Personalized Curriculum

After ecological inventories and additional assessments have been completed, it is appropriate to organize and prepare the personalized curriculum. At this point, a personal profile and a long-term vision have already been developed. On the basis of the long-term vision, the learner's current participation in desired activities has been assessed, and the skill demands of desired current and future environments have been delineated. Then, a master list of priorities can be generated, and short- and long-term objectives can be identified.

The master list of priorities comes from multiple sources. First, priorities identified by the learner and the family during person-centered planning and other interviews are included. These priorities can be functional, social, or academic skills. Second, a *discrepancy analysis* is conducted to determine additional priorities. A discrepancy analysis compares the learner's current activities and skills to (a) the skill demands of his current activities and (b) the skill demands of his desired future activities. Differences are included as potential priorities on the master list.

Rod's teacher used the discrepancy analysis technique to identify priorities related to Rod's desire to frequent a coffeehouse, as described in the following narrative.

> Participating in the coffeehouse as a young teen typically involves scanning the chalkboard and displays for what is available, making an order, paying for the order with cash or check, finding a table, eating, socializing if seated with someone, and bussing the table. When with friends, young teens often play board games or bring their own handheld computer games to play. Rod currently attends the coffeehouse only with his family. His mother or father identifies several options for him to order, he points to something in the display case, and one of them places the order for him and pays for the purchase. Rod understands the notion of paying cash for items but does not yet discriminate between different bills or coins. Rod carries his own order to a table selected by one of his parents. They use time at the coffeehouse as an opportunity to address communication skills with him and encourage him to use his picture board while there. Rod busses his own dishes with a prompt from a parent. The discrepancy analysis leads Rod's teacher to note possible priorities of ordering without assistance, paying cash, and sitting at an available table. Additionally, she notes that participation in this setting in the long term might be enhanced if he is able to play some of the games common to the setting.

For many students the master list of priorities will be extensive. It is not reasonable to expect to provide instruction on every target skill at the same time. At this point, the team must make decisions about short-term and long-term priorities. Ryndak (2003) refers to this process as negotiation. First, she suggests simplifying the master list by removing any duplications and combining similar items. Second, the team reviews the list and decides which items are critical for the following year. Consideration should be given to learner, family, and school personnel opinions, as well as both the functional and the general education curriculum (Ryndak, 2003). Additional factors that can be taken into account include perceptions of the student's ability to learn the skill in an acceptable time frame, the age-appropriateness of the skill, whether learning the skill will enhance the learner's safety, whether it was noted as a high priority by the learner or the family, opportunities to utilize the skill across settings, and frequency of opportunities to utilize the skill (Renzaglia & Aveno, 1986). The team should also consider the relationship between short-term and long-term priorities. The question should be asked, "Are there skills that, if addressed in the short term, will facilitate learning on long-term priorities?" Finally, the team should attend to the long-term vision during this process. This requires them to ask, "Which priorities are most critical for movement toward the long-term vision?" Short-term priorities become the focus of instruction for the next year. Long-term priorities are not discarded; they are held for reconsideration in following years.

Once short-term and long-term priorities are identified, the curriculum can be further organized. First, anticipated outcomes for different priorities should be stated clearly. These outcomes are addressed by asking, "What level and type of participation is expected in a particular activity?" A priority for preparing simple meals may become "prepare simple microwave meals," "prepare simple no-cook meals that do not require cutting," "prepare five-step meals using microwave, electric oven, or no appliances," or any number of other possibilities. Data from ecological inventories will help with clarifying this information. A sequence of objectives can then be identified to reach the clarified outcomes. In cases where the individual learner's outcome corresponds directly to the general education curriculum, the sequence can be defined through the general education curriculum. For outcomes that do not correspond directly to general education standards, a sequence of meaningful and measurable instructional objectives is developed. Decisions about appropriate settings for instruction—including both general education and alternative settings—can then be made, based on the inventories of those settings.

The relationship between Rod's vision and the specific short-term objectives is illustrated in the following narrative.

Rod's curriculum includes priorities related to the coffeehouse. His clarified outcome is to utilize the coffeehouse with families and friends, independently ordering, paying with cash, sitting at a table identified by the person(s) he is with, and socializing while seated. In the short term, he will work on ordering independently while attending with his family. In subsequent years, paying cash with the dollar-up method and socialization with friends at the coffeehouse will be addressed. Rod also has a priority to explore computer-assisted design and graphic arts. His teacher will now work more closely with the computer teacher at his school to identify curricular adaptations within that class that can allow Rod to work on this priority.

Conclusion

A personalized curriculum is a map for an individual learner around which instruction and opportunities are organized. The intent of the personalized curriculum is to enable a learner to achieve his or her long-term vision in life. We cannot emphasize strongly enough that the curriculum is *based on the individual learner's needs*. It is not determined by an instructional setting or an educational placement. Decisions about instructional settings should be made on the basis of the vision for the student and the appropriateness of a setting for addressing the identified learning objectives for that year. We must also emphasize that teams do not need to make either-or decisions about the general education curriculum and an alternative curriculum. All students receiving special education services must have an individual curriculum. Individualized curricula will vary considerably with respect to the balance between general education priorities and alternative priorities. Even students progressing through the entire general education curriculum may have additional learning objectives related to self-determination, communication, and life skills. For many learners with developmental disabilities, the appropriate curriculum will be a blend of general education standards and individualized learning objectives. What is critical is that we base these decisions on the goals and needs of the individuals themselves.

Glossary

Curriculum sequence—A series of instructional objectives that lead to an educational outcome; the order in which skills are learned.

Developmental model—A curriculum model that focuses on aligning a learner's educational priorities with typical child development sequences of skill development.

Discrepancy analysis—Comparison of the learner's current activities and skills to skill demands of current and future environments and activities.

Ecocultural analysis—Ecological analysis that takes into consideration what is valued and accessible to the learner and his or her family.

Ecological inventory model—A curriculum model that emphasizes analysis of the environments, activities, and skills that constitute a learner's desired outcome.

Eliminative model—A curriculum model that focuses on decreasing or eliminating maladaptive behaviors.

Functional academics model—A curriculum model that focuses on basic academic skills applied in authentic contexts.

Longitudinal vision—The desired life outcomes for a learner, addressing all life domains and presented as a holistic and positive statement.

Personalized curriculum—Unique and specific objectives for an individual learner.

Standards-based model—A curriculum model that emphasizes specified goals, standards, and indicators across academic domains for all learners.

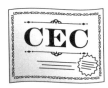

Knowledge and Skills for Entry-Level Special Education Teachers of Students With Developmental Disabilities Standards Addressed in This Chapter

Principle 4: Instructional Strategies

DD4K3   Specialized curriculum specifically designed to meet the needs of individuals with pervasive developmental disabilities, autism, and autism spectrum disorders.

Principle 7: Instructional Planning

DD7S1   Plan instruction for independent functional life skills relevant to the community, personal living, sexuality, and employment.

DD7S2   Plan and implement instruction for individuals with developmental disabilities that is both age-appropriate and ability-appropriate.

DD7S4   Design, implement, and evaluate specialized instructional programs for persons with developmental disabilities that enhance social participation across environments.

Web Site Resources

Curriculum Access for Students with Low-Incidence Disabilities
http://www.cast.org/publications/ncac/ncac_lowinc.html#toc

Universal design for learning and the curriculum development process for students with low-incidence disabilities.

Designing Personalized Learning for Every Student
http://www.urbanschools.org/publications/dpl_book.html

Sample curriculum planning tools, hosted by the National Institute for Urban School Improvement (NIUSI).

Person-Centered Planning Education Site
http://www.ilr.cornell.edu/edi/pcp/

Information on core person-centered planning practices, specific person-centered planning models, self-guided course, and links to additional resources.

References

Abery, B. H., & Stancliffe, R. J. (2003). Ecological theory of self-determination: Theoretical foundations. In M. L. Wehmeyer, B. H. Abery, D. E. Mithaug, & R. J. Stancliffe (Eds.), *Theory in self-determination: Foundation for educational practice* (pp. 24–42). Springfield, IL: Thomas.

Bouck, E. C. (2004). State of curriculum for secondary students with mild mental retardation. *Education and Training in Developmental Disabilities, 39*, 169–176.

Brolin, D. E. (1997). *Life centered career education: A competency-based approach* (5th ed.). Reston, VA: Council for Exceptional Children.

Browder, D. M. (2001). *Curriculum and assessment for students with moderate and severe disabilities.* New York: Guilford.

Brown, L., Branston, M. B., Hamre-Nietupski, S., Pumpian, I., Certo, N., & Grunewald, L. (1979). A strategy for developing chronological-age-appropriate and functional curricular content for severely handicapped adolescents and adults. *Journal of Special Education, 13*, 81–90.

Brown, L., Nietupski, J., & Hamre-Nietupski, S. (1976). Criterion of ultimate functioning. In M. A. Thomas (Ed.), *HEY, don't forget about me!* (pp. 2–15). Reston, VA: Council for Exceptional Children.

Butterworth, J., Hagner, D., Heikkinen, B., DeMello, S., & McDonough, K. (1993). *Whole life planning: A guide for organizers and facilitators.* Boston: Children's Hospital, Institute for Community Inclusion.

Campbell, P. C., Campbell, C. R., & Brady, M. P. (1998). Team environmental assessment mapping system: A method for selecting curriculum goals for students with disabilities. *Education and Training in Mental Retardation and Developmental Disabilities, 33*, 264–272.

Dymond, S. K., & Orelove, F. P. (2001). What constitutes effective curricula for students with severe disabilities? *Exceptionality, 9*, 109–122.

Ford, A. F., Schnorr, M. S., Meyer, L., Davern, L., Black, J., & Dempsey, P. (1989). *The Syracuse community-referenced curriculum guide for students with moderate and severe disabilities.* Baltimore: Brookes.

Giangreco, M. F., Cloninger, C. J., & Iverson, V. S. (1998). *Choosing outcomes and accommodations for children.* Baltimore: Brookes.

Harry, B., Rueda, R., & Kalyanpur, M. (1999). Cultural reciprocity in sociocultural perspective: Adapting the normalization principle for family collaboration. *Exceptional Children, 66*, 123–136.

Individuals with Disabilities Education Improvement Act of 2004, 118 stat. 2647. (2004).

Kalyanpur, M., & Harry, B. (1997). A posture of reciprocity: A practical approach to collaboration between professionals and parents of culturally diverse backgrounds. *Journal of Child and Family Studies, 6*, 485–509.

Kauchak, D., Eggen, P., & Carter, C. (2002). *Introduction to teaching: Becoming a professional.* Upper Saddle River, NJ: Merrill/Prentice Hall.

Miner, C., & Bates, P. (2002). Person-centered transition planning: Creating lifestyles of community inclusion and autonomy. In K. Storey, P. Bates, & D. Hunter (Eds.), *The road ahead: Transition to adult life for persons with disabilities* (pp. 7–24). St. Augustine, FL: Training Resource Network.

Mount, B., & Zwernik, K. (1988). *It's never too early, it's never too late: A booklet about personal-futures planning for persons with developmental disabilities, their families and friends, case managers, service providers, and advocates.* St. Paul, MN: St. Paul Metropolitan Council.

Renzaglia, A., & Aveno, A. (1986). *An individualized, functional curriculum assessment procedure for students with moderate to severe handicaps.* Charlottesville, VA: Curry School of Education, University of Virginia.

Ryan, L., Halsey, H. N., & Matthews, W. J. (2003). Using functional assessment to promote desirable student behavior in schools. *Teaching Exceptional Children, 35*(5), 8–15.

Ryndak, D. L. (2003). The curriculum content identification process: Rationale and overview. In D. L. Ryndak & S. Alper (Eds.), *Curriculum and instruction for students with significant disabilities in inclusive settings* (2nd ed., pp. 86–115). Boston, MA: Allyn & Bacon.

Shippen, M. E., Simpson, R. G., & Crites, S. A. (2003). A practical guide to Functional Behavior Assessment. *Teaching Exceptional Children, 35,* 36–45.

Smull, M., & Harrison, S. B. (1992). *Supporting people with severe reputations in the community.* Alexandria, VA: National Association of State Mental Retardation Program Directors.

Turnbull, A. P., & Turnbull, H. R. (1996). Group action planning as a strategy for providing comprehensive family support. In L. Kern-Koegel, R. Koegel, & G. Dunlap (Eds.), *Positive behavioral support: Including people with difficult behavior in the community* (pp. 99–114). Baltimore: Brookes.

Vandercook, T., York, J., & Forest, M. (1989). The McGill action planning system (MAPS): A strategy for building the vision. *Journal of the Association for the Severely Handicapped, 14,* 205–215.

Wilcox, B., & Bellamy, G. T. (1982). *Designing of high school programs for severely handicapped students.* Baltimore: Brookes.

13

Behavior Support Strategies for Learners With Developmental Disabilities

John J. Wheeler and David Dean Richey

Summary

This chapter provides an overview of *evidence-based* practices in the area of *positive behavior supports* designed to increase learning and lifestyle options for persons with developmental disabilities. The chapter includes a brief introductory examination of the conceptual models used to understand behavior, the origins of positive behavior supports, and ethical considerations in the design and delivery of positive behavior supports. Additional topics addressed are (a) collaboration with families and strategies for implementation, including antecedent management approaches, (b) functional behavior assessment, (c) design of behavior support plans, (d) behavior reduction strategies, and (e) development of self-determination skills in learners with developmental disabilities. The chapter provides a brief yet fundamental understanding of the theoretical framework of positive behavior supports and their application with learners with developmental disabilities.

Learning Outcomes

After reading this chapter, you should be able to:

- Understand the origins of positive behavior supports.

- Understand the ethical use of PBS procedures with learners with developmental disabilities.

- Understand the use of PBS with families.

- Describe the application of behavior support methods such as functional behavior assessment, antecedent management, development of behavior support plans, the teaching of replacement behaviors, and methods for promoting self-determination skills in learners with developmental disabilities.

Introduction

The passage of the 1997 amendments to the Individuals with Disabilities Education Act of 1990 (IDEA) brought increased attention to the need for understanding how to effectively deal with the problem of challenging behavior in school and classroom settings. Although problematic behavior is an age-old concern among teachers, it appears by all estimates to be on the rise in today's schools, and teachers continue to be confronted with challenging behaviors in their classrooms. Thus it is imperative that school personnel develop greater awareness and understanding of how to use positive behavior supports to address such behaviors proactively. Traditionally, consequences-based methods have been employed to suppress or control disruptive or noncompliant behavior in school environments. These approaches have used punitive consequences such as time out, response-cost, and in some instances corporal punishment. Unfortunately, these methods have not reliably reduced or eliminated problem behavior in the long term, nor have they been effective in teaching positive replacement behaviors or promoting self-determination skills in learners.

In response to these challenges, positive behavior supports (PBS) has emerged as the model of choice in developing proactive systems for understanding and ameliorating challenging behavior. PBS originated as an outgrowth of applied behavior analysis (ABA) and came to the fore in the early 1990s, when Horner and colleagues (1990) advocated for non-aversive methods of behavioral support for learners with severe disabilities. PBS is grounded in a philosophy of practice that is person-centered and aimed at improving quality of life for individuals. PBS uses evidence-based practices that have been empirically validated and that can be applied on three levels—individual, classroom, and schoolwide (Wheeler & Richey, 2005).

The PBS movement actually originated in the field of developmental disabilities. It is important to understand that positive behavior supports, although not designed exclusively for learners with developmental disabilities, have been important in the development and delivery of educational and habilitative treatment to persons with developmental disabilities within institutional settings since the 1950s and 1960s. Before that time, active treatment was rare, because many people believed that individuals with moderate and severe cognitive disabilities had minimal potential for learning meaningful skills. Research on the use of behavioral approaches for instruction of persons with developmental disabilities led to a transition from providing custodial care to active programs of teaching functional skills (Anderson & Freeman, 2000). Ultimately these methods were improved and expanded to school-age populations with the enactment of the Education for All Handicapped Children Act of 1975 (P.L. 94-142). In spite of the early application of behavioral approaches within special education, educational systems have been reluctant to embrace applied behavior analysis.

Origins of Positive Behavior Supports

In the behavioral model, behavior is viewed from a functional context and is measurable and observable. Behaviors serve a purpose or a function and have evolved as a direct result of one's individual learning history and interactions within his or her environments (Sulzer-Azaroff & Mayer, 1991). Behavioral procedures began to be used with persons with developmental disabilities in institutional settings with individuals with mental retardation in the early 1960s. Bijou (1963) was one of the first proponents of applied behavior analysis procedures such as functional analysis and systematic instruction for work with children with mental retardation. Behavior modification, as it was often referred to during this time, offered a ray of hope for teaching persons with mental retardation who had for so long been viewed as having limited potential. During this period numerous skill acquisition studies began to emerge, and Bijou (1970) advocated for the use of applied behavior analysis in educational settings. Bijou proposed that educators approach the interaction between environmental events and behavior from a scientific perspective, using observation and measurement as tools for gathering data. Bijou (1970) also proposed that educators consider the influence of environmental events on an individual's behavior, such as distant setting events, those biological, environmental, and social/interpersonal variables that pair with antecedent variables (triggers) to accompany severe and challenging forms of behavior. Bijou reinforced B. F. Skinner's view that the teacher serves as a facilitator of learning through careful arrangement of contingencies within the environment and the use of systematic instruction. These same elements are now called positive behavior supports.

Components of Positive Behavior Supports

PBS operates from a values base that strongly reinforces the importance of one's quality of life. Its intervention methods are behaviorally based, evidence-based, and non-aversive. Anderson and Freeman (2000) have identified three distinct elements in PBS: (a) it operates from a person-centered values base that is designed specifically for the needs of the individual and thus reflects socially valid goals and objectives that are meaningful given the individual's strengths and areas of need; (b) it ensures that the individuality of each person is preserved and therefore recognizes the need for flexibility in the provision of services and supports; and (c) it works toward meaningful outcomes that enhance overall quality of life for the individual, including participation in inclusive educational and community environments.

Positive behavior supports rely on the use of *functional behavior assessment* as a method of identifying variables that precipitate and perpetuate challenging behavior, including setting events and antecedent variables. Data obtained from the functional behavior assessment are used to construct plausible hypotheses about the function of these behaviors, the precipitating and/or maintaining variables, and the development of meaningful interventions. Functional behavior assessment is a comprehensive process that uses a variety of methods, including structured interviews with teachers, parents, and sometimes students; behavioral observation and recording of target behaviors, antecedents, and consequences; and sometimes functional analysis or actual manipulation of antecedent variables and consequences to ascertain their effects on behavior. The process should culminate in the following outcomes: (a) an operational definition of the target behavior, (b) identification of the conditions that are associated with occurrences/non-occurrences of the target behavior, (c) identification of consequences that are associated with the target behavior, (d) hypothesis statements about when and where the behavior occurs and the purpose or function of the behavior, and (e) data taken from direct observation that confirm the plausibility of the hypothesis (Sugai, Horner, & Sprague, 1999).

As previously noted, PBS and functional behavior assessment were largely introduced to schools through the passage of the 1997 amendments to the IDEA. This legislation mandated the use of functional behavior assessment and the design of a behavior intervention plan (BIP) for students who exhibited significant forms of challenging behavior, i.e., chronic and more severe. IDEA stipulates that the behavior intervention plan be developed from information derived from the functional behavior assessment, with the intent of ameliorating the problem behavior. One of the drawbacks of this legislation was that it failed to provide uniform guidelines for the components of functional behavior assessment and the behavior intervention plan. The mandate has served as a catalyst for the examination of how to address challenging behavior using proactive and preventive means of intervention, yet implementation within schools has been inconsistent. This result could be partly due to the lack of standard practices and policies in states and districts as well as in professional development practices among pre- and in-service professionals regarding use of PBS principles (Wheeler & Richey, 2005).

PBS represents a new technology designed to address the problems of challenging behavior within schools. The acceptance of this methodology among practitioners has been erratic (Anderson & Freeman, 2000), perhaps because of inconsistent training methods used in preparation programs for pre- and in-service teachers. Thomas (2004) has documented the absence of consistent training in teacher preparation programs as measured by competencies in positive behavior supports.

The number of research investigations of the use of positive behavior supports has increased since the passage of the 1997 amendments to IDEA. The efficacy and generalization of PBS practices have been demonstrated across learners of various ages, different types of disability, and multiple learning environments (Wheeler & Richey, 2005). Extant research shows that PBS provides a behavior-based intervention approach that can address and prevent challenging forms of behavior by enhancing the capacity of schools, teachers, families, and communities through skills building, the design of effective learning environments, and preventive and proactive evidence-based intervention practices.

PBS addresses challenging behaviors on three levels: school-wide, in individual classrooms, and with individual students. Generally, school-wide PBS is used as a prevention tool, reaching approximately 80% to 90% of learners in the school environment. PBS strategies at the classroom level are designed to improve classroom-wide behavior and offer proactive approaches to prevention and treatment of problem behavior. Classroom applications affect 5% to 15% of the student population. The final level of the PBS continuum of services provides specialized behavior supports for the small percentage of learners within the school population (1% to 2%) who display chronic and severe forms of challenging behavior. Functional behavior assessment and functional analysis are used at this level to identify antecedent and consequent events associated with the target behavior. The data obtained through the functional assessment process are then analyzed and employed in the design of the behavior intervention plan. Figure 13.1 illustrates the continuum of PBS services.

PBS represents a means of enhancing the capacity of schools, teachers, and families to engineer optimal learning environments that maximize positive learning

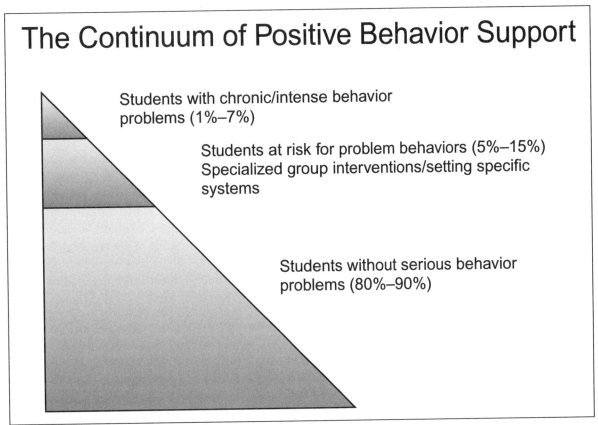

FIGURE 13.1. The continuum of positive behavior supports. Source: Sugai, G., et al. (2000). Applying positive behavior support and functional behavioral assessment in schools. *Journal of Positive Behavior Interventions, 2*(3), 131–143. Adapted with permission.

and behavioral outcomes for all students. Crone and Horner (2003) identified the basic assumptions of PBS and the merits of this intervention philosophy for school settings as follows: (a) all behavior is functional and challenging forms of behavior serve a function for learners who engage in such responses; (b) behavior is contextually relevant—that is, it is directly related to the environments within which a child functions, and (c) challenging behavior can be effectively changed, prevented, and eliminated through teaching appropriate replacement behaviors.

Ethical Considerations and Positive Behavior Supports

Ethics are the principles of conduct that govern individual professionals as well as their particular groups or disciplines. A professional knows the ethical codes and standards in his or her field and behaves accordingly. In a review of professional organizations in which education, special education, and in particular positive behavior support and challenging behavior are the central mission, Wheeler and Richey (2005) found that, while there are notable differences and occasional opposing beliefs, ethical codes and standards are largely compatible and encompass nine organizing themes.

First, as human beings, all children and youth have worth and dignity regardless of the nature or severity of their special needs or the form taken by their challenging behavior. Second, the behavior of children and youth always reflects a need. People respond out of need, and all behavior serves a function. Third, an understanding of the individual differences and uniqueness of children and youth, along with systematic and thoughtful management of learning environments, will prevent challenging behavior or diminish its impact. Fourth, the active participation of families as partners in all aspects of positive behavior, and in the ways best suited to them, is central to ethical practice. Fifth, family diversity should be taken into account in responding to challenging behavior. Sixth, while a full continuum of programs, services, and supports should be available for children who need positive behavior support, natural environments and inclusive settings are preferable, and interventions should have the goal of fostering inclusion. Seventh, self-discipline, independence, and self-determination are fostered through the application of naturally and logically occurring consequences to the extent possible, rather than through extraneous and contrived reward systems. Eighth, behavioral interventions should be positive and should not include corporal punishment or other punitive measures. Ninth, the actions taken by professionals to suppress undesirable behavior or to teach replacement and desired behavior should always reflect meaningfulness and functionality in daily life and should be aimed toward improving quality of life.

Partnerships With Families

The evolution of applied behavior analysis and positive behavior supports over the past decade has included changing views among professionals with regard to the parents and families of children and youth with special needs. A positive belief about parents and families as important, relevant participants with their children in a process of dynamic growth has replaced the old deficit or dysfunctional model of parents and families. Educators (in particular, special educators) who historically might have focused on the parents (especially mothers) are now more likely to approach the family as a unit and to understand the family from a systems perspective (Richey & Wheeler, 2000). As noted by Wheeler and Richey (2005), whereas historically, special education and related professionals

> might have seen parents as the recipients of training in content determined by the professionals and intended to foster generalization of behaviors into the home setting, now they are more likely to see themselves as in a partnership in which they learn, teach, and share. (p. 67)

Relating to families as collaborators and partners in all aspects of behavior support, including assessment, plan development, implementation of intervention, and ongoing evaluation of the effectiveness of the intervention has become an accepted part of recommended practice (Lucyshyn, Blumberg, & Kayser, 2000). Lucyshyn, Horner, Dunlap, Albin, and Ben (2002) stated that a collaborative partnership with families

> is defined as the establishment of a truly respectful, trusting, caring, and reciprocal relationship in which interventionists and family members believe in each other's ability to make important contributions to the support process; share their knowledge and expertise; and mutually influence the selection of goals, the design of behavior support plans, and the quality of family-practitioner interactions. (p. 12)

Substantial challenges do exist when professionals collaborate with families as partners in the planning and delivery of behavior support strategies. Following are four issues that may affect one's ability to partner with families to provide behavior supports.

1. Teachers and other professionals frequently lack sufficient content in their pre-service and in-service training, as well as in their accumulated experiences that deal with family systems theory, diversity and family functioning, the rationale for collaborating with families, and evidenced-based, practical methods and strategies for partnering with families.

2. Development of a trusting, caring, and reciprocal relationship requires not only willingness on the part of the professional but also frequently additional time and energy, as well as the understanding and support of supervisors and policy makers. That support, encouragement, and time may or may not be provided, or those in charge may take the view that relationships with families should be formal, focused on legal requirements, and minimal so as to avoid potential conflicts.

3. Collaborating with families can be "messy" and sometimes painful, particularly when responding to challenging and impeding behaviors of children. It is very important to determine how, when, and to what extent families wish to participate. It is also essential that education professionals be respectful of the developmental status of families and individuals and their family functions and interactions beyond behavior support planning and implementation. Effective communication skills in expressing one's point of view clearly and nonjudgmentally and in being a good listener are certainly central to success.

4. Expanding the context of intervention for challenging behavior beyond classrooms and/or clinical environments to include home and community settings may present special challenges for professionals throughout the process, in assessment, planning, implementation, and evaluation. Finding a fit between behavior support goals and strategies and the family context—the usual routines and activities of family life—requires that team members focus on a person-centered (Kincaid, 1996) planning approach, as opposed to focusing exclusively on educational goals and objectives.

In spite of these and other challenges to a professional's readiness and ability to partner with families, those who engage in the process experience substantial reward. Ultimately, the result can be the achievement of desired outcomes for children with challenging behavior and for their families.

Application of Behavior Support Methods

This section will explore the application of PBS strategies across learning environments with learners with developmental disabilities. One of the central features of positive behavior supports is the linkage between assessment and the development of behavior interventions that are relevant to the learner. PBS relies on functional behavior assessment to identify variables that precipitate and/or maintain challenging behavior. It is important that the functional behavior assessment be tied to the development of meaningful and individualized interventions.

Functional Behavior Assessment

FBA is a multi-step process that uses structured interviews with relevant stakeholders such as teachers, family members, and in some instances the student to identify the target behavior and specific antecedent and consequent variables associated with that behavior. Other components of the FBA process include behavioral observation of the learner in relevant environments and the use of scatter plot recording to gather frequency data on target behaviors within the context of times and days when the behaviors occur. This information leads to a more comprehensive understanding of the relationship between the target behavior and specific environmental events. For example, a child may engage in the target behavior frequently during specific time frames each day. These occurrences might be attributable to certain classes or activities that occur at these times. Scatter plot recording allows us to make these causal inferences by linking the occurrence of behaviors with specific events and time frames in the learner's daily schedule (Wheeler & Richey, 2005).

Sugai et al. (2000) identified five outcomes that should result from a functional behavior assessment: (a) the target behavior should be defined; (b) conditions that predict when the challenging behavior does and does not occur should be identified; (c) consequences that maintain the behavior should be identified; (d) hypothesis statements should be developed that provide insight concerning the function of the target behavior and the factors associated with its occurrence; and (e) direct-observation data that confirm the accuracy of the hypothesis statements should be gathered.

Antecedent Management Strategies

One of the most salient features of PBS is its emphasis on prevention through the identification and management of antecedents. Antecedents are actions that precede the problem behavior and serve as triggers for it. Related to antecedents are "setting events," which set the stage for the problem behavior to occur. Setting events may be (a) biological (thirst, hunger, fatigue, medication), (b) social (peer and other forms of social interactions), or (c) environmental (noise level, classroom density, instructional design and presentation, quality of physical environment). When such setting events are combined with a specific antecedent or trigger, problem behavior can occur (Wheeler & Richey, 2005).

Consider the following example: Bobby, a 9-year-old child with moderate mental retardation, feels unusually fatigued because of a head cold, but he remains at school. He is taking medication for the cold, which causes him to feel lethargic. When his teacher attempts to engage Bobby in a classroom assignment, he chooses not to complete the task and stares off into space. When the teacher prompts him again, Bobby yells at her to leave him alone. Here we see the effects of distant setting events combined with specific instructional antecedents on Bobby's behavior.

Antecedents related to problem behavior are often identified during the functional behavior assessment process through the tools of structured interviews, behavioral observation, and scatter plot recording. However, if plausible antecedent-behavior relationships cannot be identified, a structural analysis (Wacker et al., 1999), can provide a more in-depth analysis of the role of specific antecedents on behavior. The procedure involves the brief presentation of various antecedent stimuli such as forms of task demands (preferred versus nonpreferrred). A series of reversal designs (systematic presentation of tasks and removal of tasks) is typically used to validate experimentally the presence of a functional relationship between certain antecedents and occurrence of the target behavior (Wheeler & Richey, 2005).

Specific antecedent management strategies include modification of instructional practices (how instruction is delivered), modification of instructional task design (according to the strengths and challenges experienced by the learner), and modification of the classroom environment (including the physical layout). Since the teacher is responsible for facilitating learning for his or her students and must understand antecedent management to do so, it is imperative that he or she address how tasks are designed and how they are presented. The application of strategies proposed by Wheeler & Richey (2005) for use with learners with developmental disabilities could serve to prevent or minimize the frequency of challenging behaviors in the classroom.

Task Design

The first strategy in this area is to ensure that *tasks are relevant* to the learner—age-appropriate, developmentally appropriate, and socially valid, and functional for the needs of the learner. For children with developmental disabilities this has been a recurring problem. Too often learners with developmental disabilities are given assignments that are neither functional nor age-appropriate, which can lead to boredom on the part of the individual and subsequent problem behavior.

The second strategy is to *match tasks* to the abilities of the learner. All tasks should be modified for the needs and skill level of the learner. Tasks that are too difficult can trigger challenging behavior.

The third strategy is to *vary activities*. Variety is important for maintaining the student's interest and avoiding boredom and frustration, which are often precursors to behavior problems.

The fourth strategy is to establish *individual and classroom schedules*. Schedules help students with developmental disabilities to remain engaged with the task, to know what to expect next, and to manage their own behavior. Schedules can take various forms (written, symbol, photo, object).

Task Presentation

Task presentation is also an important part of managing instructional antecedents and designing instruction for students with developmental disabilities. Wheeler and Richey (2005) have recommended some strategies:

First, teachers should use *clear and consistent cues*. Appropriate instructional cues are vitally important to successful instruction and meaningful learning outcomes. Cues should be designed with the individual learner in mind; for students with developmental disabilities visual and/or gestural cues can facilitate acquisition and compensate for the student's language and communication challenges.

Second, teachers should use *embedded cues*. Embedded cues are prompts provided within the task that help the learner to complete the task with minimal assistance. They provide a mechanism for promoting greater degrees of student independence and less reliance on the teacher for assistance. They also promote generalization or "skill transfer" for the student and build performance fluency (the ability of the student to repeat the task rapidly with minimal errors).

Third, teachers should use *interspersed requesting* in the delivery of tasks, alternating high-demand activities (less preferred by the students) with low-demand activities (more preferred) as a way of sustaining task engagement in students with developmental disabilities.

Fourth, teachers should employ *systematic instruction*. Historically, systematic instruction is perhaps the most well studied element of instruction of students with developmental disabilities (Snell & Brown, 2006). This strategy incorporates prompt hierarchies and error correction procedures, with the goal of facilitating errorless learning.

Development of Behavior Support Plans

The functional behavior assessment process should yield sufficient insight and data for the development of a behavior support plan (BSP). Critical to the development of the BSP is an understanding of the function(s) of the target behavior and hypotheses concerning the behavior, such as the relationship of specific antecedents and consequences to the behavior of concern (A—antecedents or triggers; B—behavior; C—consequences). As stated earlier, the majority of children will not need either a full functional behavior assessment or a behavior support plan. These tools are most useful for the few students with chronic behaviors that impede their own educational progress or the learning of others. IDEA 1997 uses the term *impeding behavior*, which it defines as externalizing behaviors (such as self-injury, verbal abuse, or property destruction), internalizing behaviors (such as physical or social withdrawal, depression, passivity, resistance, social or physical isolation, or noncompliance), manifestations of biological or neurological conditions (such as obsessions, compulsions, stereotypy, or irresistible impulses), or disruptive behaviors (such as annoying, confrontational, defiant, and/or truant activities) (Turnbull & Turnbull, 2000).

Positive behavior support plans should include both prevention methods or antecedent management strategies that serve to eliminate or minimize triggers that result in the target behavior and replacement behaviors that are incompatible with the target behavior. A replacement behavior is a behavior that (a) serves the same function; (b) is taught through direct instruction to the learner; and (c) facilitates access to the same functional outcome for the student, thus making the behavior efficient in meeting the individual's needs (Scott & Nelson, 1999).

Once a replacement behavior has been identified, the next step in the process is operationalizing the plan. Questions to consider in this phase of the process include:

(a) Are the goals of the BSP socially valid and functionally relevant to the learner?

(b) What current skills does the student have that will assist in the implementation of the BSP?

(c) How do parents and family members feel about the intervention?

(d) Will there be a home/school partnership to facilitate the acquisition of replacement behaviors?

(e) Are professionals and paraprofessionals adequately trained and prepared to implement the plan?

(f) Is there an instructional plan for teaching replacement skills?

(g) Can the environment be engineered to provide more support of the student during this process?

(h) What are the formal and informal supports available to the student that will enhance the probability of success in the training of replacement skills?

Quality of Life, Self-Determination, and Behavior Support Strategies

While it may sound simplistic, the overriding and most meaningful rationale for providing behavior support strategies to persons with developmental disabilities is to improve the quality of their lives. The case may be made that historically, given the focus on short-term behavior change and highly measurable outcomes, attention to quality of life as a goal and outcome has been insufficiently addressed (Wehmeyer, Baker, Blumberg, & Harrison, 2004). Anderson and Freeman (2000) have described the positive behavior support movement as having three prominent features: a focus on person-centered values, recognition of individual needs and flexibility to accommodate them, and meaningful outcomes that enhance the quality of life of individuals, including participation in inclusive educational and community settings.

Schalock (2000) defined quality of life as "a concept that reflects a person's desired conditions of living related to eight core dimensions of one's life: emotional well-being, interpersonal relationships, material well-being, personal development, physical well-being, self-determination, social inclusion, and rights" (p. 121). Over the past decade, the concept of quality of life has been addressed as an outcome that may be assessed and measured through the use of both personal appraisal (asking an individual how satisfied he or she is with aspects of life) and functional assessment (Schalock, 2000). Before we address the self-determination component of quality of life, it is important to acknowledge the place of social validity in the process of providing supports and services to persons with developmental disabilities. *Social validity* refers to the meaningfulness and validity of objectives and goals of intervention for the lives of the persons for which they are intended (Wheeler and Richey, 2005). The connections among social validity, quality of life, and self-determination are evident. Carpenter, Bloom, and Boat (1999) suggest that, in the effort to provide special education services that are socially valid and that improve quality of life, education professionals keep in mind the following four goals: to enhance self-esteem, to produce high levels of self-determination, to increase empowerment, and to promote joy in the lives of students.

As one important dimension of quality of life, the promotion of self-determination for persons with developmental delays has gained increasing attention in the professional literature. While self-determination has been defined in various ways, a consensus definition has been provided by Field, Martin, Ward, and Wehmeyer (1998):

> Self-determination is a combination of skills, knowledge, and beliefs that enable a person to engage in goal-directed, self-regulated, autonomous behavior. An understanding of one's strengths and limitations together with a belief in oneself as capable and effective are essential to self-determination. When acting on the basis of these skills and attitudes, individuals have greater ability to take control of their lives and assume the role of successful adults. (p. 3)

According to Wehmeyer (1999) self-determination comprises four components: autonomous functioning, self-regulation, psychological empowerment (i.e., believing that one can exert control over areas important to him or her), and self-realization. Wehmeyer and Schalock (2001) concluded that increased emphasis on quality of life and self-determination may become more important in educational environments for all children and youth, and in turn may better promote integration between general and special education. In a study of adults with mental retardation, Wehmeyer and Schwartz (1998) found that people who were more self-determined reported a higher quality of life, and the researchers concluded that self-determination should continue to be advanced as a central feature of intervention for adults with mental retardation and developmental disabilities.

What the reader may conclude is that, in the process of planning, implementing, and evaluating behavior support strategies for learners with developmental disabilities, attention to the impacts of intervention on quality of life and the fostering of self-determination are of fundamental importance. It is important not only to include quality of life and self-determination as measurable, quantifiable outcomes of intervention, but also to take into account the effects of a collaborative approach among home, school, and community (Brotherson, Cook, Cunconan-Lahr, & Wehmeyer, 1995) on assessment and planning as well as on the teaching of self-determination. While the inclusion of self-determination as an important component of curriculum and teaching strategies in special education is relatively recent, numerous resources are now available to assist in assessing students' self-determination and in selecting and applying curricula (Browder et al., 2001).

Conclusion

This chapter represents a brief overview of positive behavior supports and their application with students with developmental disabilities. Many questions remain concerning the application of PBS in educational and learning environments for these learners, among them: Will PBS evolve into a unified approach among educators in the treatment of challenging behavior? If so, how? Will consensus be reached on the use of ethical procedures in the delivery of PBS supports and services to learners with developmental disabilities? The use of positive behavior supports holds great promise for enrichment of learning environments for children with developmental disabilities in school and classroom settings. The authors encourage readers to consult the rich array of resources that are available on PBS and to consider the adoption of these evidence-based practices for learners with developmental disabilities.

Glossary

Antecedent—A stimulus that precedes a behavior (often referred to as a trigger for problem behavior).

Applied behavior analysis—The scientific study of human behavior in certain settings.

Consequence—An immediate consequence or event following a behavior that strengthens, reduces, or has no effect on the behavior.

Evidence-based practices—Practices that have been identified through empirical inquiry as having a measure of success in addressing a specific issue in the area of positive behavior supports.

Family diversity—Cultural differences in and among families.

Function—The purpose of a behavior, such as to gain social or tangible reinforcement, to modify or control sensory input, or to escape an aversive condition.

Functional behavior assessment—The systematic assessment of challenging behavior and the antecedents and consequences that elicit and/or maintain these responses in persons with developmental disabilities.

1997 Amendments to IDEA—Mandated the use of functional behavior assessment and behavioral intervention plans to address challenging behavior in children with chronic forms of problem behavior.

Positive behavior supports—Practices aimed at teaching positive alternative responses and dedicated to improving the quality of life of individuals with developmental disabilities who engage in challenging forms of behavior.

Quality of life—A concept that reflects an individual's desired conditions of living across eight major areas: (a) emotional well-being, (b) personal development, (c) physical well-being, (d) self-determination, (e) social inclusion, (f) rights, (g) interpersonal relationships, and (h) material well-being.

Social validity—The degree to which interventions are found socially acceptable and personally relevant to the individuals for whom they are intended.

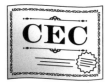

Knowledge and Skills for Entry-Level Special Education Teachers of Students With Developmental Disabilities Standards Addressed in This Chapter

Principle 1: Foundations

    DD1K5   Theories of behavior problems of individuals with developmental disabilities.

Principle 4: Instructional Strategies

    DD4K2   Evidence-based practices for teaching individuals with pervasive developmental disabilities, autism, and autism spectrum disorders.

Principle 8: Assessment

    DD8K2   Environmental assessment conditions that promote maximum performance of individuals with developmental disabilities.

Web Site Resources

Center for Effective Collaboration and Practice

http://www.air.org/cecp

> Offers a wealth of information pertaining to the use of positive behavior supports in the classroom.

Positive Behavioral Interventions and Supports

http://www.pbis.org

> Link to the Office of Special Education Programs on Positive Behavior Interventions and Supports.

References

Anderson, C. M., & Freeman, K. A. (2000). Positive behavior support: Expanding the application of applied behavior analysis. *Behavior Analyst, 23,* 85–94.

Bijou, S. W. (1963). Theory and research in mental (developmental) retardation. *Psychological Record, 13,* 95–110.

Bijou, S. W. (1970). What psychology has to offer education now. *Journal of Applied Behavior Analysis, 3,* 65–71.

Brotherson, M. J., Cook, C. C., Cunconan-Lahr, R., & Wehmeyer, M. L. (1995). Policy supporting self-determination in the environments of children with disabilities. *Education and Training in Mental Retardation and Developmental Disabilities, 30,* 3–14.

Browder, D. M., Wood, W. M., Test, D. W., Karvonen, M., & Algozzine, B. (2001). Reviewing resources on self-determination: A map for teachers of children with disabilities. *Remedial and Special Education, 22,* 233–244.

Carpenter, C. D., Bloom, L. A., & Boat, M. B. (1999). Guidelines for special educators: Achieving socially valid outcomes. *Intervention in School and Clinic, 34,* 143–149.

Crone, D. A., & Horner, R. H. (2003). *Building positive behavior support systems in schools.* New York: Guilford.

Education for All Handicapped Children Act of 1975, 20 U.S.C. § 1400 *et seq.* (1975).

Field, S., Martin, J. E., Miller, R., Ward, M., & Wehmeyer, M. L. (1998). *A practical guide to teaching self-determination.* Reston, VA: Council for Exceptional Children.

Horner, R. H., Dunlap, G., Koegal, R. L., Carr, E. G., Sailor, W., Anderson, J., et al. (1990). Toward a technology of "nonaversive" behavioral support. *Journal of the Association for Persons with Severe Handicaps, 15,* 125–132.

Individuals with Disabilities Education Act of 1990, 20 U.S.C. § 1400 *et seq.* (1990) (amended 1997).

Kincaid, D. (1996). Person-centered planning. In L. K. Koegel, R. L. Koegel, & G. Dunlap (Eds.), *Positive behavioral support: Including people with difficult behavior in the community*. Baltimore: Brookes.

Lucyshyn, J. M., Blumberg, E. R., & Kayser, A. T. (2000). Improving the quality of support to families of children with severe behavior problems in the first decade of the new millennium. *Journal of Positive Behavior Interventions, 2*, 113–115.

Lucyshyn, J. M., Horner, R. H., Dunlap, G., Albin, R. W., & Ben, K. R. (2002). Positive behavior support with families. In J. M. Lucyshyn, G. Dunlap, & R. Albin (Eds.), *Families and positive behavior support: Addressing problem behavior in family contexts* (pp. 3–43). Baltimore: Brookes.

Richey, D. D., & Wheeler, J. J. (2000). *Inclusive early childhood education*. Albany: Delmar.

Schalock, R. L. (2000). Three decades of quality of life. *Focus on Autism and Other Developmental Disorders, 15*, 116–127.

Scott, T. M., & Nelson, C. M. (1999). Using functional behavioral assessment to develop effective intervention plans: Practical classroom applications. *Journal of Positive Behavioral Interventions, 1*, 242–251.

Snell, M. E., & Brown, F. (2006). *Instruction of students with severe disabilities*. Upper Saddle River, NJ: Pearson Merrill Prentice-Hall.

Sugai, G., Horner, R. H., Dunlap, G., Hieneman, M., Lewis, T. J., Nelson, C. M., et al. (2000). Applying positive behavior support and functional behavior assessment in schools. *Journal of Positive Behavior Interventions, 2*(3), 131–143.

Sugai, G., Horner, R. H., & Sprague, J. (1999). Functional-assessment-based behavior support planning: Research to practice research. *Behavioral Disorders, 24*, 253–257.

Sulzer-Azaroff, B., & Mayer, G. R. (1991). *Behavior analysis for lasting change*. Fort Worth, TX: Harcourt Brace.

Thomas, R. A. (2004). *An analysis of university-based methods and practices for training school personnel in positive behavior interventions and supports*. Unpublished doctoral dissertation, Tennessee Technological University, Cookeville.

Turnbull, A. P., & Turnbull, H. R. (2000). Achieving "rich" lifestyles. *Journal of Positive Behavior Interventions, 1*, 252–255.

Wacker, D. P., Cooper, L. J., Peck, S. M., Derby, K. M., & Berg, W. (1999). Community-based functional assessment. In A. C. Repp & R. H. Horner (Eds.), *Functional analysis of problem behavior* (pp. 32–56). Belmont, CA: Wadsworth.

Wehmeyer, M. L. (1999). A functional model of self-determination: Describing development and implementing instruction. *Focus on Autism and Other Developmental Disabilities, 14*, 53–61.

Wehmeyer, M. L., Baker, D. J., Blumberg, R., & Harrison, R. (2004). Self-determination and student involvement in functional assessment: Innovative practices. *Journal of Positive Behavior Interventions, 6*, 29–36.

Wehmeyer, M. L., & Schalock, R. L. (2001). Self-determination and quality of life: Implications for special education services and supports. *Focus on Exceptional Children, 33*(8), 1–16.

Wehmeyer, M. L., & Schwartz, M. (1998). The relationship between self-determination and quality of life for adults with mental retardation. *Education and Training in Mental Retardation and Developmental Disabilities, 33*, 3–12.

Wheeler, J. J., & Richey, D. D. (2005). *Behavior management: Principles and practices of positive behavior supports*. Columbus, OH: Merrill/Prentice Hall.

14

Grouping Arrangements and Delivery of Instruction for Students With Developmental Disabilities

Dennis D. Munk and Toni Van Laarhoven

Summary

This chapter describes research on grouping arrangements and delivery of instruction to students with developmental disabilities, presenting a concise summary of early research on group instruction, as well as a more detailed description of studies published since 1995. The differences in the purpose and content of studies from these two periods are remarkable: Early studies established the viability of group (versus individual) instruction and demonstrated elements of effective instruction. More recent studies have expanded the focus of group instruction to include delivery to blended groups, by peers or video modeling, in the general education classroom. The practice of including students with developmental disabilities in general education classrooms has stimulated research on models for delivering effective instruction in a group arrangement. To date, embedded instruction and CWPT—classwide peer tutoring—(with modifications) have proven promising models for inclusive classrooms.

A common thread throughout both the early and the more recent research is the use of systematic, effective instructional procedures, regardless of the grouping arrangement. The success of group instruction is dependent on the use of effective prompting, error correction, and reinforcement procedures. Peers who deliver instruction must be adequately prepared if the group instruction is to be effective not only for the group members with disabilities, but also for their peers without disabilities. Indeed, ineffective instruction may result not only in minimal skill acquisition but also in a negative disposition of classmates toward working in groups with their peers with disabilities. Thus much is at stake, and practitioners must take the time necessary to provide training to peers who will deliver instruction.

The use of technology within group arrangements is beginning to emerge as a viable option for instructing students with developmental disabilities in regular classroom settings. Although research on video modeling and computer-assisted instruction is typically conducted with students in one-to-one formats, the potential exists for those media to be used as effective tools for delivering instructional trials to students within the structure of daily routines. With technology usage increasing dramatically in educational settings and teachers becoming more proficient at using technology, we predict that technology-delivered instruction will continue to be studied and integrated into classroom activities for students with developmental disabilities.

Future research should extend our knowledge of instructing students with and without disabilities in blended groups, expand the types of curriculum to include complex, multi-step tasks that require more peer interaction, and investigate the role of technology in enhancing student performance.

Learning Outcomes

After reading this chapter, you should be able to:

- Describe various models for instructing students with developmental disabilities in homogeneous and blended groups.

- Compare and contrast grouping arrangements for instructing a student with mild, moderate, or severe disabilities on academic, functional, or social skills.

- Contrast the relative benefits of group instruction delivered by the instructor, peers, or video.

- Generate a checklist for planning, implementing, and evaluating instruction in a group arrangement.

- Plan a lesson that involves instruction in a group arrangement.

Introduction

Our knowledge of how best to instruct students with developmental disabilities in group arrangements has increased considerably over the past 25 years. Before the late 1970s individualized instruction was perceived as optimal for working with students with moderate to severe disabilities, primarily because of the perception that the intensive, highly systematic instruction that had been proven effective could not be delivered in a group arrangement. This assumption was challenged in the late 1970s (e.g., Storm & Willis, 1978) as researchers began investigating group instruction as a more efficient format for instructing multiple students, and suggested potential benefits such as increases in student motivation, incidental learning, and generalization across persons, settings, and materials (Brown, Holvoet, Guess, & Mulligan, 1980).

It may be said that research on group instruction has paralleled that in the larger field of educating and supporting individuals with disabilities in that the focus has evolved from establishing the necessary elements of effective instruction to providing such instruction in the general education classroom, and presented by technology or mediated by peers. We begin with an account of early research that established the efficacy and specific features of effective group instruction and move on to address more recent research, which has not only contributed to our understanding of how to structure group instruction but also expanded the contexts in which it can occur.

Previous definitions of group instruction (e.g., Munk, Van Laarhoven, Goodman, & Repp, 1998) have assumed that a small number (2–5) of students are receiving teacher-directed instruction at the same time. Such definitions emphasize that students are receiving largely the same systematic instruction they might receive individually, but in a group arrangement. Our definition of group instruction expands the parameters to include models or arrangements in which students with disabilities receive individualized, embedded instruction within the routine of the general education classroom, as well as those in which students and peers serve as tutors and tutees in dyads within a larger group of students. Our rationale is that as more students with developmental disabilities are included in general education classrooms, educators require strategies for instructing those students within a larger, blended group.

Early Research
in Group Instruction

Several early studies sought to establish group instruction as a viable format for students with developmental disabilities by comparing the effects of individual and group instruction on learners with moderate to severe disabilities. In cases where similar effects were observed for both types of instruction, group instruction was perceived to be more efficient since it produced the same benefits for more students within the same amount of instructional time. Early studies suggested that group instruction (a) was more efficient than individual instruction (Bourland, Jablonski, & Lockhart, 1988; Fink & Sandall, 1978; Kamps, Walker, Maher, & Rotholz, 1992; Westling, Ferrell, & Swenson, 1982), (b) promoted generalization of skills (Oliver & Scott, 1981), and (c) promoted incidental learning among group members (Gast, Wolery, Morris, Doyle, & Meyer, 1990; Oliver, 1983; Orelove, 1982). In a study comparing effects for different types of tasks, Alberto, Jobes, Sizemore, and Duran (1980) reported that individual instruction was more effective than group instruction for teaching multi-step tasks.

Several studies investigated the scope of curriculum that could be taught to students with moderate to severe disabilities in a group-instruction format. Group instruction has been effective for teaching (a) functional academics (e.g., discriminating words or numbers; Bourland et al., 1988; Karsh & Repp, 1992; Oliver & Scott, 1981; Westling et al., 1982), (b) daily living skills (e.g., identifying household items; Kamps, Dugan, Leonard, & Daoust, 1994), (c) social skills (e.g., questioning; Wildman, Wildman, & Kelly, 1986), and (d) language skills (e.g., manual signs; Faw, Reid, Schepis, Fitzgerald, & Welty, 1981). The type of response required of students in the above studies was most often a discrete motoric response such as pointing, touching, or handing an object to another person. When students possessed the necessary language skills, they were required to provide a vocal response.

Early research also revealed different models or approaches for structuring group instruction (e.g., Collins, Gast, Ault, & Wolery, 1991; Reid & Favell, 1984). Before initiating instruction the practitioner must determine how instruction will be delivered to each member of the group and how students will be expected to respond. Students may be instructed sequentially, or one at a time. In the *sequential model* the instructor provides direct instruction to each person while other members of the group observe and wait for their turn (e.g., Alberto et al., 1980). Potential benefits of the sequential model are that each student receives the instructor's full attention and that incidental learning may occur as students observe other group members responding to instruction. A potential limitation of the sequential model is that each student will experience some waiting time during instruction, and an opportunity exists for interfering behavior to occur if students are not observing the process at all times. An alternative designed to increase engagement by all group members is the *concurrent-sequential model* (Karsh & Repp, 1992; Repp & Karsh, 1992), in which some instruction is delivered to all group members concurrently (simultaneously) and they are expected to respond in unison. Concurrent responding requires that all students have their set of materials to which they can respond. In this model, some instruction is also delivered sequentially, especially if the task is more complex or if individual students need more instruction to "catch up" to the others and participate in concurrent instruction. Concurrent instruction involves a unison response from the group, which is best facilitated by use of a signal (e.g., finger snap, or hand drop, "Ready, point").

Students with developmental disabilities will receive the most benefit from group instruction when they possess prerequisite skills for effective participation. Early research identified prerequisite skills such as sitting quietly while waiting for a turn, maintaining eye contact, following simple instructions, and imitating simple responses (Gast et al., 1990; Karsh and Repp, 1992; Oliver & Scott, 1981; Storm & Willis, 1978). In the *tandem, individual-to-group model* (Reid & Favell, 1984), learners receive individual instruction on prerequisite skills until they can meet the criteria necessary to join the group.

A common element of all early studies was the use of effective, systematic instruction. Clearly, practitioners must have knowledge and skill in the areas of prompting hierarchies (e.g., system of least-to-most prompts), time-delay prompting procedures (e.g., constant time delay), error correction procedures (e.g, model-test sequence), and reinforcement strategies (e.g., verbal praise). Though explicit description of these procedures is beyond the scope of this chapter, interested readers are encouraged to review the original sources summarized here or to consult one of several texts on effective instructional procedures (Snell & Brown, 2006; Westling & Fox, 2004).

In their 1998 review, Munk et al. concluded that the basic questions regarding the efficacy and critical features of group instruction had, for the most part, been answered. The authors suggested that future research should focus on delivery of instruction to blended groups of learners, potentially in the general education classroom.

Recent Research in Group Instruction

Since 1995, the focus of research on group instruction for students with developmental disabilities has expanded to include effectiveness in blended groups, and when delivered by peers or video.

Instruction for Blended Groups

The practice of educating students with developmental disabilities in the regular classroom has sparked research interest in effective instructional strategies for that setting. While research has reported positive outcomes for these students (e.g., Hunt & Goetz, 1997), general and special educators often struggle to identify effective instructional procedures for the regular classroom setting (Harrower, 1999; McDonnell, 1998), and students with severe disabilities may receive too few instructional trials (Schuster, Hemmeter, & Ault, 2001). For students with moderate to severe disabilities, that challenge may be greater in that they require more exposure and practice on specific skills than is provided in the general education classroom, even when modifications and accommodations are made. Group instruction in this scenario may involve providing individualized instruction to a student in the context of the regular classroom while his or her peers are also engaged in instruction or transition activities. Or, instruction may involve working with students with and without disabilities who are blended in a group. In the remainder of this section we will describe research on methods for instructing students with developmental disabilities in blended groups in general education classrooms and special settings.

Teacher-Delivered Embedded Instruction

Several studies have investigated the effects of embedded instruction, in which instruction for individual students is delivered within the ongoing routine of the classroom. The procedures (e.g., systematic prompting, error correction) used during embedded instruction are similar or identical to those used in massed trials; the unique aspect of embedded instruction is that it is scheduled to occur during natural breaks in the regular classroom routine, such as during transitions between activities or during breaks (McDonnell, Johnson, Polychronis, & Riesen, 2002). Embedded instruction allows students with developmental disabilities to participate in the regular classroom instruction, and also to receive intensive individualized instruction without having to leave the classroom grouping. Johnson and McDonnell (2004) used embedded instruction to teach three students with moderate to severe disabilities to identify sight words, manually sign "help," or identify the greater of two numbers. General educators delivered the embedded instruction during breaks in their instruction to the rest of the class. Results indicated that two of the three students met the criterion (100% correct) for their skill, while the third peaked at 60% despite additional procedures to facilitate correct responding. The participating general educators reported high levels of satisfaction with the embedded instruction. Embedded instruction has also been used to teach students' ages 13–14, with moderate cognitive disabilities and autism to read vocabulary words or verbally define key vocabulary words (Riesen, McDonnell, Johnson, Polychronis, & Jameson, 2003). Paraprofessionals delivered the embedded instruction in the regular classroom and alternated between simultaneous and constant time-delay prompting procedures. In simultaneous prompting, the instructor pairs the controlling prompt with the discriminative stimulus, as is also the case for constant time delay. Rather than gradually fading the controlling prompt, as is done with time-delay procedures, the instructor first tests the student's ability to respond correctly before providing any prompting. The controlling prompts are then delivered during the instructional sequence. Results of the study indicated that two of the three students met criterion (100% correct) for their skill under both prompting conditions, while one did so only with simultaneous prompting. In addition, naturalistic probes conducted within the classroom with various materials revealed that the students generalized their skills to the novel materials. McDonnell et al. (2002) taught four students, ages 13–15, with moderate disabilities to read 15 cooking/nutrition symbols, provide definitions for 15 health-related terms, or define 15 computer-repeated terms, using embedded instruction in general education classrooms. Paraprofessionals delivered the embedded instruction, which resulted in all of the students achieving criterion of 100% correct in 2.8–4.6 trials per word. A follow-up assessment two weeks after the completion of the instruction indicated that the students had maintained these skills.

Finally, in a study conducted in an advanced high school English class, two students with moderate disabilities were taught related facts about punctuation and grammar as well as unrelated social studies facts by two general educators using embedded instruction (Collins, Hall, Branson, & Holder, 1999). Results indicated that students acquired the skills in an average of 10 trials, with more-difficult facts taking longer or not being acquired. Although the general educators were satisfied with the instructional procedures and believed they were easily administered within the context of a class, they felt that teaching some of the unrelated facts (social studies facts in the English class) seemed somewhat awkward.

In sum, research has shown embedded instruction to be an effective approach for instructing students with moderate to severe disabilities, including autism, within the routine of the general education classroom. It is important to note that all the instruction described in the above studies included features of effective instruction, including systematic prompting, error correction, and reinforcement for correct responses. Instruction was delivered by general educators and by paraprofessionals, who reported high levels of satisfaction with the procedure.

Peer-Delivered Embedded Instruction

Research has also been conducted to determine if peers can effectively implement systematic instructional procedures to improve social interactions of individuals with developmental disabilities within the context of daily routines (DiSalvo & Oswald, 2002). Similar to embedded instruction, in which the teaching assistant or general educators embed instructional trials, several researchers have taught peers to present instructional trials to individuals with disabilities to improve social skills. Within the last 10 years, examples of these peer-mediated or "peer-training" instructional approaches have included the use of peer networks (Garrison-Harrell & Kamps, 1997) and/or pivotal response training (Pierce & Schreibman, 1997).

Garrison-Harrell and Kamps (1997) defined peer networks as groups of individuals who demonstrate an interest and understanding of individuals with disabilities and have an impact on their lives by creating a support system that promotes a positive social environment. In their study, three students with autism who were included in first-grade classrooms were targeted for intervention. Five typical peers in each child's classroom were provided with instruction on social skills interventions and asked to implement these strategies during identified academic sessions (e.g., reading, lunch, language arts, recess). Each network of peers received eight 30-minute social skills training interventions on topics such as initiating and responding, conversing, sharing, giving instructions, and saying "nice" things. During the training, the experimenter modeled the social skills, and then the peers engaged in role-play situations and were given feedback. Peers were also taught how to use the target students' communication systems. The three students with autism were taught to use the augmentative communication systems during one-on-one instructional sessions and also attended two of the social skills training sessions with their peer network. Peers delivered instruction or interacted socially with target students in identified academic settings, and results indicated that the peer network intervention (including augmentative communication training) increased the frequency and duration of peer interactions across three settings for all three students. In addition, communicative vocal behavior, use of augmentative communication systems with untrained peers, and positive peer nominations increased for all three students across most settings.

In a similar study, Pierce and Schreibman (1997) embedded social skills instruction delivered by peers in an elementary school setting. In this investigation, two children with autism (ages 7 and 8) and eight typical peers (four peers per child—three trained and one untrained for generalization purposes) participated. Three of the four peers for each target child were given individual instruction on how to provide social skills instruction during recess periods. The trained peers were given manuals and instructions on the following: (a) getting attention, (b) giving choices, (c) varying toys, (d) modeling social behavior, (e) reinforcing attempts, (f) encouraging conversation (requesting that the child ask for a toy before giving it to them), (g) extending conversation (asking questions), (h) taking turns, (i) narrating play, and (j) teaching responsivity to multiple cues ("Do you want the small green ball?"). Trained peers delivered prompting procedures in a one-to-one format with the target child during recess. New peers were systematically trained and introduced as the children with autism began engaging in more social behavior with the trained peers. Results indicated that children with autism engaged in high levels of interactions, initiations, varied toy play, and language use. They also increased language usage in both frequency and quality (longer sentences). Generalization of social behaviors occurred across settings, stimuli, and untrained peers. Although training peers to deliver embedded instructional trials within ongoing classroom routines is an effective practice, research has indicated that teachers must continue to monitor, prompt, and reinforce the attempts of peers in order to maintain improvements in student responding (DiSalvo & Oswald, 2002).

Classwide Peer-Delivered Instruction

Researchers have also investigated the effects of an instructional arrangement involving entire classrooms of students delivering instruction to one another in the context of the general education classroom. *Classwide peer tutoring (CWPT)* has been demonstrated effective for teaching students without disabilities (Greenwood, 1991) and those with mild disabilities (e.g., Harper, Mallette, Maheady, Parkes, & Moore, 1993). In CWPT, a classroom of students is divided into teams of two, with each member taking turns as both tutor and tutee. The tutoring teams may also meet in a larger group of multiple teams for instruction. Before beginning instruction, students are provided with training on how to present the instructional materials, prompt responses, correct errors, deliver reinforcement, and record data. CWPT is designed to maximize the number of observable responses a student can make during instruction, and its use has recently been extended to students with developmental disabilities. Studies involving blended groups are described here, while those involving homogeneous groups of students with disabilities will be described in a later section. Mortweet and colleagues (1999) implemented CWPT in two general education classrooms, each consisting of 25 students without disabilities and 2 students (ages 8–10) with mild cognitive disabilities. The 4 students with disabilities were randomly assigned with peers without disabilities to tutoring teams and to larger tutoring groups. The effects of CWPT versus teacher-led instruction for spelling were assessed through spelling tests. Results indicated that the students with disabilities achieved higher test scores and were engaged a greater amount of time in the CWPT condition. The students averaged over 82% on the spelling tests, while their peers without disabilities averaged 83%, and the gains from the pretest to posttest were more significant for students with disabilities. Additionally, the participating teachers reported that the CWPT model resulted in greater acceptance of the students with mild cognitive disabilities by their peers. Peer responses indicated that 95% liked the CWPT model, and 81% said that their peers with disabilities performed better than they had thought they would.

Researchers have investigated "peer learning" arrangements that require blended groups of students to have "roles" other than "tutee" or "tutor" to deliver instructional content. Using a modified model of CWPT that involved three students per tutoring group, McDonnell, Mathot-Buckner, Thorson, and Fister (2001) investigated the effects of the group instructional procedure with three students with moderate to severe disabilities, ages 13–15, and three of their peers without disabilities who served as groupmates. The traditional CWPT model was modified to include not only the tutor and the tutee but also an observer, whose role was to support the student with a disability in providing the instruction to the tutee, observing the response, and providing either error correction or reinforcement. Tasks for the three students with disabilities were linked to the general education class in which the instruction would take place. Student 1 participated in a pre-algebra class and was instructed by peer tutors on converting percentages to decimals and using a calculator to determine percentages. Student 2 participated in a regular physical education class and was instructed on basic basketball skills such as dribbling and shooting a foul shot. Student 3 participated in a regular history class and received instruction on artifacts of Utah history, such as the Conestoga wagon. Results for the tutoring model included (a) significant increases in academic engagement (e.g., engaging in verbal behavior related to the task) and (b) decreases in competing behaviors (e.g., disrupting the class) for the students with disabilities and their groupmates without disabilities. Content-related posttests given weekly indicated that participating in the tutoring model had not affected scores for one of the peers without disabilities but had resulted in increased scores for the other peers. Posttest scores for the students with disabilities were as follows: Student 1— 71% (40–100), Student 2—33% (0–57), and Student 3—68% (57–100).

In a study involving a similar instructional model, McDonnell, Thorson, Allen, & Mathot-Buckner (2000) created three different peer-learning triads that comprised three students (one student with severe disabilities and two classmates) to teach each other spelling words. Students within the triads each spelled words (word wizard), presented words (word conjurer), provided feedback to the speller (word keeper), and checked accuracy (word keeper and conjurer). All switched roles during the course of the instructional procedure. Spelling accuracy was assessed during weekly spelling tests. Results indicated that the peer learning arrangement led to improved spelling accuracy for students with severe disabilities and did not negatively affect accuracy of peers. It also led to improved rates of academic engagement and slight reduction for rates of competing behavior for five of six students.

In another example of how peers can be utilized to deliver instruction, Garfinkle and Schwartz (2002) conducted research on increasing the social interactions of students with disabilities by providing peer imitation procedures within the context of blended small-group instruction in an integrated preschool setting. In this instructional sequence, the teacher selected a "leader" to demonstrate how to use materials. Each child had a turn to present materials. The teacher waited until all students were simultaneously imitating the leader before moving to the next child. Results indicated an increase in peer imitation during small group and results generalized to free-play situations. However, social interactions had minimal increases. The teachers who participated in the investigation found the procedure to be easily implemented and important.

Teacher-Directed Instruction with Blended Groups

Another practice often found in general education classrooms is teacher-directed small-group instruction for students with and without disabilities. Small-group instruction is typically conducted with students who have similar skill levels and are working on similar tasks. However, providing homogeneous small-group instruction can be problematic when students with cognitive disabilities are included in general education settings. Some researchers have investigated the use of small-group instruction with groups of students who have different skill levels and are working on different tasks (Fickel, Schuster, & Collins, 1998; Parker & Schuster, 2002). Fickel et al. and Parker and Schuster investigated the effectiveness of teaching varied tasks to blended groups of students, using different stimuli within the context of a typical school day. Both of these investigations were conducted in a pull-out manner (e.g., the groups of students were taught in a setting other than the classroom) and had small groups that were composed of individuals with cognitive disabilities and their typical peers.

Fickel et al. (1998) conducted their study in a middle school with 4 students who were between the ages of 13 and 15 and had varying abilities. Three of the students attended a self-contained program at the school (1 mild, 1 moderate, 1 severe), and one peer buddy was a general education student. Sessions were conducted in the school cafeteria, and the experimenters used simultaneous prompting and presented trials to students in a sequential format. Each student had different tasks and stimulus materials that included naming states, naming the sum of simple addition problems, manually signing names of pictures, and naming national flags. Three to four sets of stimuli per student were used throughout the study. Results indicated that all students acquired their targeted stimuli within 39 sessions, maintained most of the skills for up to 35 days (2 students did not maintain all stimuli), and generalized behaviors across settings and materials. The researchers also assessed observational learning for the learners, and 3 students acquired information that was unknown to them before training (manual signs and states). The researchers indicated that providing corrective feedback during the daily probe sessions may have facilitated observational learning and also mentioned that providing more trials to students with significant needs during group instruction would enhance their learning.

Parker and Schuster (2002) conducted a similar study with a group of high school students (ages 15–19) that included 2 students with cognitive disabilities (1 mild, 1 moderate) and 2 students without disabilities who were selected from the peer tutoring group. The teacher used a simultaneous prompting procedure and instructive feedback strategies to teach students different tasks, including reading sets of grocery words and occupational words, defining prefixes, and identifying elements on the periodic table. The instructive feedback stimuli were related to the targeted stimuli (e.g., What does this occupation do?) and were presented following instructional trials. Results indicated that all students met criterion on each set of stimuli and that 3 of the 4 students were able to maintain their skills with 93% to 100% accuracy for a period of three months. Students also generalized their skills to other settings and materials (with the exception of 2 students who did not have high generalizations scores on two out of their three sets of stimulus materials). The researchers also found that observational learning did occur for 3 of the 4 students but not as high as reported in other studies. The authors believe it resulted from the use of different tasks and stimuli and that the students with cognitive disabilities had a more difficult time learning the higher-order skills. They also found that 3 of the 4 students acquired some of the instructive feedback given for the targeted stimuli. The researchers indicated that although the simultaneous prompting procedure was effective, they felt that too many probe errors occurred, and they suggested that probes be conducted every second or third session rather than every day. They also indicated that students with more-severe disabilities might perform better if given many more trials during small-group instruction.

In addition to teaching academic skills in blended groups, several researchers have taught social skills within the context of inclusive classrooms. However, because not all students require social skills training, researchers have investigated grouping patterns that would allow for students with disabilities to be taught social skills alongside their peers. Gonzalez-Lopez and Kamps (1997) did so by bringing typical peers into a self-contained classroom to receive training, while Simpson, Langone, and Ayres (2004) taught social skills to individual students with disabilities by using computer-based applications and then having them practice their skills in small groups in an integrated classroom.

Gonzalez-Lopez and Kamps (1997) taught social skills to small, blended groups of students in an elementary school. A total of 4 children with autism and 12 of their typical peers (6 kindergartners and 6 first graders) participated in the study. Before the social skills training, the experimenters provided information about disabilities and training in basic behavior-management procedures to the typical peers (e.g., prompting, reinforcing, and ignoring). Social skills training was then provided in a small-group format and consisted of direct instruction using training scripts to teach greetings, imitation/following simple instructions, sharing/taking turns, and asking for help/requesting things. The groups were composed of 1 child with autism and 3 typical peers and were led by the teacher in the special education classroom. Following social skills instruction, the students were allowed to engage in free play activities and the effects of the training were monitored. Teachers then reinforced interactions of students during the free play situation with a star chart. The social skills instruction did improve interactions, but the introduction of the reinforcement system greatly increased interactions.

Social skills have also been taught through the use of technology. In a study conducted by Simpson et al. (2004), 4 students with autism were taught social skills through computer-assisted instruction and later practiced the skills with their peers during small-group activities in the classroom. In this grouping arrangement, the students with disabilities were taught individually and then practiced the skills in group activities. The researchers presented participants with anchored instruction (videos of typical peers in real situations) on the computer, followed by answering questions on the computer, and generalization of skills to typical small-group classroom activities. The students were taught skills such as sharing, following teacher directions, and greetings. Each subject interacted with the computer-based program for 30 minutes a day independently in a special education classroom (with the teacher present to provide some prompting for navigation through the materials). They then practiced the skills within the context of a small-group activity in inclusive classrooms and were given at least four opportunities to use learned social skills (three times a day within each small-group activity). These included reading, math, and arts/crafts. The results indicated that all students increased unprompted engagement in the social skills. Although not really addressed in text, use of the technology required staff presence to assist participants in using the computer program. No data were collected on maintenance or non-trained settings (videos were of small-group activities). However, the use of technology may become an efficient way to provide instructional opportunities to individuals with disabilities in inclusive settings.

Instruction for Groups of Students With Disabilities

Research on instructing groups of students with disabilities has progressed to include classwide peer tutoring, social skills instruction, and teacher-directed group instruction. The term *homogeneous* will be used to describe groups that include only students with disabilities, although the level of disabilities among the group members may vary.

Classwide Peer Tutoring With Homogeneous Groups

Classwide peer tutoring (CWPT) was described earlier in studies involving blended groups, and this model has also been investigated for instruction of groups of students in which all have disabilities. CWPT was implemented in a special education classroom with 5 students, ages 7–9, with moderate cognitive disabilities (Utley, Reddy, Delquadri, Greenwood, & Bowman, 2001). Using flash cards, the randomly paired tutor teams instructed each other on health and safety topics such as body parts and their functions, poisons, drugs and their effects, and dangerous situations. Effects for the CWPT model were compared with those for traditional instruction on the percentage of correct answers on posttests for each topic area. Results revealed a mean correct of 92% and 94% (range of 82–100) for the CWPT conditions, as compared to a mean of 7% (range of 0–12) under traditional instruction. The positive results for CWPT were evidenced across all of the topic areas, and the participating teachers reported high levels of satisfaction, as did the participating students, who expressed particular satisfaction with belonging to a team. Butler (1999) investigated the effects of CWPT on sight word reading by 10 students with mild to moderate cognitive disabilities in a fourth-and-fifth-grade special education classroom. The students' reading abilities varied from K.6 to 3.3, and individualized materials were used for the instruction. A unique feature of this study was a group "Tutor Huddle" (Butler, p. 424) before the CWPT in which the tutors practiced words they might be presenting to a tutee with a higher level of reading ability. Results after 38 sessions of CWPT revealed that students mastered 55%–79% of the words presented. All students progressed approximately one grade level in sight word reading. The author reported that the students enjoyed the CWPT model and self-initiated its use for spelling and math.

Together, the above studies suggest that CWPT can be used successfully for students with mild to moderate cognitive disabilities. Students with moderate disabilities may need additional training to prepare them for the tutor's role.

Social Skills Instruction for Homogeneous Groups

As stated previously, social skills are important for functioning in everyday situations and are therefore frequently targeted for instruction for individuals with developmental disabilities. Although social skills are frequently high educational priorities, it may be more difficult for educators to provide such instruction to students with disabilities within the context of a typical school day, particularly when students are placed in inclusive classrooms. In some cases, providing social skills instruction in after-school or non-education environments is suggested. Two studies that provided social skills instruction in community environments have been described in the literature.

In the study reported by Barry et al. (2003), 4 high-functioning elementary-age students (ages 6–9) with autism were taught greetings, conversation, and play skills followed by play sessions with typical peers. The sessions included specific social scripts for greeting, conversation, and play interactions, role play and active practice of the skills, practice in an unstructured social activity (e.g., snack), followed by two 5-minute play sessions with typically developing peers, a show-and-tell-time, and presentation or "reports" to parents demonstrating the skills they had learned.

As in the studies by Pierce and Schreibman (1997) and Gonzalez-Lopez and Kamps (1997), peers in the Barry et al. (2003) study were given instruction on ways to interact with children with autism. Seven typical peers (4 males and 3 females, ages 7–9) participated and received a two-hour peer education session describing autism and other pervasive developmental disorders as well as strategies for helping individuals with autism (e.g., combining nonverbal cues with verbal information, ignoring inappropriate comments or repetitive behaviors, and suggesting changes in topic). They then role-played the strategies to be used. Peers were taught to wait at least 30 seconds to allow the student with autism to initiate interaction and to wait an additional 30 seconds to allow the student with autism to initiate further conversation or play. Two typical peers attended each assessment session. Results indicated that the group instruction improved greetings and play skills, with more variable improvements with conversation skills. Children with autism reported increased feelings of social support from classmates, but parents indicated that they noticed improvements only in greeting skills in non-clinic settings.

In a community-based social skills group conducted by Webb, Miller, Pierce, Strawser, and Jones (2004), 10 boys with developmental disabilities between the ages of 12 and 17 attended a community-based program twice a week for social skills instruction. The researchers used the SCORE Skills strategy to work on five social skills (share ideas, compliment others, offer help or encouragement, recommend changes nicely, and exercise self-control) and embedded body language expectations (voice sound, facial expression, and eye contact) throughout the sessions. Instruction was presented through discussion, modeling, partner role-playing practice, and an application activity. Results indicated that all boys made significant gains on social skills that were tested with a role-play assessment. Consumer satisfaction was high for both parents and participants.

Small-Group Direct Instruction With Homogeneous Groups

Although more and more students with disabilities are being educated in general education settings, self-contained classrooms still exist, and researchers have investigated different ways to teach academic skills to students within small-group structures. For example, Singleton, Schuster, and Ault (1995) and Johnson, Schuster, and Bell (1996) investigated the use of simultaneous prompting for teaching students discrete tasks within small homogeneous groups. In addition, small-group structures have been used to teach discrete tasks to preschool students using a discrete trial format (Taubman et al., 2001) and to elementary-age students through the use of video technology (Norman, Collins, & Schuster, 2001). In most cases, instructional trials have been structured with sequential presentations (Johnson et al., 1996; Norman et al., 2001; Singleton et al., 1995) or a combination of concurrent and sequential presentations (Taubman et al., 2001).

In the study conducted by Singleton and colleagues (1995), 2 male students, ages 7 and 11, with moderate disabilities were taught to verbally label eight photographs of community signs each through the use of simultaneous prompting. In addition, non-target information was presented through instructive feedback (e.g., descriptions of what the signs meant). Results indicated that simultaneous prompting was effective in teaching the students their targeted signs. Students maintained these effects for two weeks and generalized results to community environments. In addition, students acquired, maintained, and generalized some of their own non-target information (e.g., the meaning of the signs) as well as some target and non-target information presented to their peer during observational learning.

In another study, Johnson and colleagues (1996) compared the effectiveness of simultaneous prompting with and without error correction to teach science vocabulary to 5 students (ages 16 and 17) with mild disabilities (2 with mild MR and 3 with LD). All instructional sessions were presented in a large-group format with 11 students in a resource room science class, but data were collected on only the 5 target students. All students learned to read science vocabulary words; simultaneous prompting with error correction was more efficient for 3 of the 5 subjects and 4 of the 5 students made fewer errors. During the probes, error correction was basically saying, "No. This word is _____. Say _____." No feedback was given during probes conducted with the simultaneous-prompt-alone condition when there was an incorrect response or no response. Words that were mastered in both conditions were maintained and generalized equally well under both conditions. Researchers found that instructive feedback (the teacher reading the definition of each word following a choral response on vocabulary) did very little to improve students' ability to define vocabulary words.

Using a discrete trial instructional approach, Taubman and colleagues (2001) used a combination of sequential and choral responding as well as overlapping instruction to teach 8 preschoolers with autism and other developmental disabilities song activities, pre-math, and language activities. The overlapping instructional trials involved presenting a new trial to a new student as the previous student was completing the instructional trial. Results indicated an increase in mean percentage of correct responding across task areas. The researchers indicated that they liked the overlapping instruction because it allowed for an inter-trial interval and could allow for observational learning if a student was having difficulty with the task or having behavioral issues. They hypothesized that the overlapping trials reduced demand-related challenging behavior and allowed for individualization while reducing "wait" time.

Norman and colleagues (2001) used video technology to teach self-help skills to 3 elementary students with moderate disabilities in a small-group format. Students were taught to clean sunglasses, put on a wristwatch, and zip a jacket using video modeling and video prompting with a constant time-delay procedure. Students sat at a kidney-shaped table in the back of a self-contained classroom and watched video sequences on a TV that was placed on the table. The students watched a video segment of the entire task, then watched individual steps, and then were asked to try the step in the task analysis (as the tape was paused by the instructor). This was done in a sequential small-group instructional format, and the student who went first was changed across sessions. Only one student needed additional one-to-one trials for the first task. Results indicated that the video prompting procedure was effective and all students learned the self-help skills, maintained their skills, and generalized their skills to novel instructors/materials. The researchers indicated that the drawbacks for conducting instruction within this format were that the teacher had to operate the technology (start/stop/fast-forward/rewind) and be present to provide error correction and to reinforce students. The students also had a group criterion and some may have learned the task faster. However, they also indicated that the group format and use of technology decreased the need for the teacher to provide repeated models for each participant, the tapes could also be used to assist with maintenance of skills, and the students may have made more gains within the group as a result of watching their peers perform the skills.

Table 14.1 presents an overview of the recent studies described in this chapter.

 CASE STUDY

The following case study describes the planning and design of instruction for two students with severe disabilities in a general education classroom.

Mikaela and Sam, both age 8, attend a regular third-grade classroom, where they are instructed and supported by Mrs. Ochoa, the third-grade teacher, Mr. Barry, the special educator, and Mrs. Keeney, the paraprofessional. Since the beginning of the school year, the team has met three times per week to discuss how best to provide instruction to Mikaela and Sam in the regular classroom. Their concern is that the students may not be receiving enough practice (i.e., trials) on important skills targeted by their IEP goals and objectives. A second concern relates to the amount of interaction that peers initiate with Mikaela and Sam. At first, several students seemed to go out of their way to interact; however, it is now mid-October and the rest of the class seems to be too engaged in their group work to interact with them. Mrs. Ochoa and Mr. Barry agree that a model or strategy for involving Mikaela and Sam in group instruction could provide them with more practice on important skills and facilitate more interaction with their peers. With this goal in mind, the teachers consult the professional literature and identify a model, Classwide Peer

TABLE 14.1

Overview of Research (1995–Present) on Small-Group Instruction for Students With Developmental Disabilities

Topic Area	How Delivered	Instructional Format and Critical Components	Research Supports Use With Students With:	Research Supports Use to Teach These Skills:	Research Suggests These Strengths:	Research Suggests These Potential Limitations:
Instructing groups of students with disabilities	Teacher-directed instruction	Sequential presentation in small groups (e.g., Johnson et al., 1996; Parker & Schuster, 1995) Features: Systematic instruction (e.g., simultaneous prompting), with teacher delivering trials to students one at a time	Mild MR and learning disabilities (Johnson et al., 1996) Moderate MR (Parker & Schuster, 1995)	Read science vocabulary words Name photographs of community signs	Observational learning of other students' stimulus materials May also learn additional information if "instructive feedback" (e.g., defining words) is also presented during instructional trials	Students in group must pay attention to others if observational learning is to occur (reference) Sequential presentation could result in "wait time" and increase likelihood of behavioral challenges (Repp & Karsh, 1992)
		Concurrent, sequential, and overlapping presentations in small groups (Taubman et al., 2001) Features: Systematic instruction (discrete trial) presented with all students responding simultaneously for concurrent (e.g., action songs), sequentially (each student takes turn), or overlapping (present trial to next student as one student is completing trial)	Preschool students with autism or other developmental disabilities (Taubman et al., 2001)	Perform actions to songs Placing items sequentially in containers and/or counting aloud (e.g., pre-math) State or sign names of pictures/objects or point to named items	Observational learning Overlapping presentation can provide an intertrial interval and can also reduce demand-related challenging behavior by moving to next child and coming back	Required more staff (e.g., instructional assistants) to provide additional error correction and prompting during the lesson
		Community-based or outpatient social skills groups (Barry et al., 2003; Webb et al., 2004) Features: Involves demonstration/modeling of social skills, role-playing activities, and some form of application or practice activity Barry et al. (2003) also used social scripts and had two typical peers present during brief play assessment conditions	High-functioning individuals with autism spectrum disorder, ages 12–17 (Webb et al., 2004) or 6–9 (Barry et al., 2003)	Sharing ideas, complimenting others, offering help or encouragement, recommending changes nicely, and exercising self-control (adolescents) Greetings, conversation and play skills	Can provide social skills instruction in an alternative setting to overcome logistical problems in school settings	Maintenance and generalization of skills may be difficult

(continues)

TABLE 14.1 (Continued)

Topic Area	How Delivered	Instructional Format and Critical Components	Research Supports Use With Students With:	Research Supports Use to Teach These Skills:	Research Suggests These Strengths:	Research Suggests These Potential Limitations:
	Peer-delivered instruction	Classwide peer tutoring (Utley et al., 2001) Features: Students form tutoring/tutee teams, provide prompting, error correction, and reinforcement; may include third student to support peer with a disability in tutor role	Moderate MR (Utley et al., 2001) Mild to moderate MR (Butler, 1999)	State facts and definitions for health and safety topics Read sight words	High levels of engagement and opportunity to respond	Has been evaluated with only discrete responses, and not multi-step tasks
	Technology delivered instruction	Video technology presented through constant time delay in a small group setting Features: Video scenes depicting entire tasks (e.g., self-help skills) followed by step-by-step video segments for students to watch and follow as they engage in task	Elementary students with moderate disabilities	Cleaning sunglasses, putting on a wrist watch, zipping a jacket	Decreased need for teacher to provide repeated models Tapes could be used to assist with maintenance of skills Having students view videos and practice skills in a group setting may have increased the number of models	Teacher had to operate the technology and frequent starting, stopping, rewinding, could be challenging Presenting instruction in a group format required a group criterion and may have prevented some students from moving more quickly through instruction
Instructing blended groups of students with and without disabilities	Teacher-directed instruction	Embedded instruction (McDonnell et al., 2002, and others) Features: Systematic prompting, error correction, and reinforcement in massed trials within natural breaks in classroom routine	Moderate to severe MR (McDonnell et al., 2002) Moderate MR and autism (Riesen et al., 2003; Collins et al., 1999)	Discriminate sight words or symbols Manual signs Identifying the greater of two numbers State factual information related to grammar & punctuation or social studies facts	Can be implemented in the general education classroom Can be implemented by teachers or paraprofessionals	Has been evaluated with only discrete responses, not multi-step tasks
		Sequential presentation in small blended groups (Fickel et al., 1998; Parker & Schuster, 2002) Features: Systematic instruction (e.g., simultaneous prompting) with teacher delivering trials to students one at a time	Mild and moderate MR high school students (Parker & Schuster, 2002) Mild, moderate, and severe MR middle school students (Fickel et al., 1998)	Reading grocery and occupational words Defining prefixes (gen. ed.) Identifying elements on the periodic table (gen. ed.) Naming states from outline shape	Able to teach different tasks with different stimuli to meet educational objectives of each student Observational learning of other students' stimulus materials	Needed to provide additional trials for students with moderate and severe MR Difficult for students with more severe disabilities to acquire higher order skills presented to higher-functioning students

Type	Features	Population	Target skills	Benefits	Limitations
Peer-delivered instruction	Peer-mediated with instructional trials embedded within ongoing routine (Garfinkle & Schwartz, 2002; Garrison-Harrell & Kamps, 1997; Pierce & Schreibman, 1997) Features: Peer Imitation in small groups (Garfinkle & Schwartz, 2002); peer networks/peer training (Garrison-Harrell & Kamps, 1997; Pierce & Schreibman, 1997)	Preschoolers with autism and developmental delays (Garfinkle & Schwartz, 2002) Elementary students with autism (Garrison-Harrell & Kamps, 1997; Pierce & Schreibman, 1997)	Social skills and language skills such as: Interactions, initiations, toy play, language, peer imitation, use of augmentative communication systems Naming sum of simple addition problems Signing names of pictures Naming national flags	Social behaviors and language can increase with peer implementation Provides support for students with disabilities in blended classrooms May also teach additional information if "instructive feedback" (e.g., defining words) is also presented during instructional trials	Requires ongoing prompting and reinforcement of student and peer attempts (DiSalvo & Oswald, 2002) Social skills often do not transfer to unknown peers or settings
Peer-delivered instruction	Classwide peer tutoring (Mortweet et al., 1999) Features: Students form tutoring/tutee teams, provide prompting, error correction, and reinforcement; may include third student to support peer with a disability in tutor role Partner learning (McDonnell et al., 2000) Features: Modified CWPT model includes group practice with materials before moving to tutor/tutee dyads; students maintain individual folders with flash cards and a progress chart	Mild MR (Mortweet et al., 1999) Severe MR (McDonnell et al., 2000) Mild to moderate MR (Butler, 1999)	Spelling words	High levels of engagement and opportunity to respond Students with disabilities can serve as tutors	Has been evaluated with only discrete responses, and not multi-step tasks Students with more severe disabilities require more assistance in reading words for peers
Technology-delivered instruction	Computer-based video instruction followed by peer practice (Simpson et al., 2004) Features: Students individually view video samples on computer, answer questions presented on the computer, and practice skills within small group activities in the classroom	Elementary-aged children with autism (Simpson et al., 2004)	Sharing, following teacher directions, greetings	Skills transferred to settings that were depicted on videos and had an increase in unprompted social skills in small-group activities within the classroom	May require technological skills of the teacher Students may need assistance operating computer

Tutoring (CWPT), for structuring peer-delivered instruction in blended groups that include students with severe disabilities (McDonnell et al., 2001, 2000). CWPT involves the development of peer teams and can be implemented classwide, while also allowing for individualization of the skills and materials for students with severe disabilities. McDonnell and colleagues (2000, 2001) modified CWPT to add a third student to the typical tutor/tutee pairing. This third team member, the observer, provides support to the student with a disability. The presence of the observer will allow Mikaela and Sam to participate as both tutor and tutee. An additional modification to the original CWPT model involves the use of different tasks for students with disabilities. This innovation will allow Mikaela and Sam to work on specific skills from their IEPs that are related, but not identical to, the skills addressed in the tutoring for peers without disabilities.

Following the procedures described by McDonnell et al. (2000, 2001), Mrs. Ochoa and Mr. Barry identify a specific skill—reading sight words—that both Mikaela and Sam have been working on through individual instruction. The teachers agree that instruction on sight word reading could occur when the rest of the class is working on the weekly vocabulary words that are linked to their novel studies. Instruction on vocabulary words involves giving the students the list of words, reading them aloud one time, and then having the students write the definitions. The students then practice reading each word and verbally stating the definition. To prepare for the peer tutoring, the teachers begin preparing the word lists for Mikaela and Sam, and for the rest of the class.

Next, Mrs. Ochoa reviews her class list, identifies high-achieving, average-achieving, and low-achieving students in reading (especially vocabulary tasks), and selects one high-achieving and one low-achieving student each to be groupmates with Mikaela and Sam. The next several class periods are spent preparing the entire class for classwide peer tutoring, including Sam and Mikaela and their groupmates. Students are taught to present a card with a word and say, "Read this word and say what it means." They are instructed to listen carefully to the definition to decide if the tutee has provided the correct response, and to provide either a correction that involves saying the word or reading the definition, or say "That's right" for correct responses. Sam and Mikaela are required only to say the word, and therefore their word lists are longer than those of their classmates.

The groups that include Mikaela and Sam receive special training on how to work as the observer in the group. The observer's duties include checking the accuracy of the tutee's response and providing verbal praise for a correct response. The observer can also assist the tutor with the presentation of the word to be read/defined, and in providing error correction if needed. Although all of the team members rotate through all of the roles, Sam and Mikaela will obviously receive significant support from their peers in the observer role.

Mrs. Ochoa and Mr. Barry are aware that the model of CWPT they are implementing has not been researched with sight word reading for students with severe disabilities; therefore, they plan to carefully monitor the progress of Mikaela, Sam, and their groupmates by recording correct and incorrect responses each time instruction occurs. These data will be used to measure Mikaela and Sam's progress on their IEP goals for reading sight words. In addition, the teachers plan to observe peer interactions with Mikaela and Sam both during the group instruction and at other times of the day. Hopefully, group instruction will result not only in academic progress but also in the fostering of social interactions throughout the day.

Glossary

Classwide Peer Tutoring (CWPT)—An instructional arrangement that groups all students in a classroom into dyads. Each student in the pair takes turn being either the tutor or the tutee and the students deliver instructional trials to each other, provide error correction, deliver reinforcement, and collect data.

Concurrent-sequential model—A model in which instruction is delivered to all students in a group and they are expected to respond in unison. This is followed by individual trials for some members of the group.

Embedded instruction—An instructional procedure for delivering instructional trials to learners within the ongoing schedule of the classroom.

Incidental learning—Acquisition of information that was not directly targeted for instruction but was presented within the instructional context (e.g., students learn to read sight words that were presented to a peer during group instruction).

Sequential or intrasequential model—A model in which instruction is delivered to each member of a group in a sequential fashion. Each member of the group receives several turns during a typical lesson and must wait for his or her turn.

Tandem, individual-to-group model—A grouping model that involves having learners initially receive one-to-one instruction and then systematically adding students to the group.

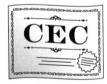

Knowledge and Skills for Entry-Level Special Education Teachers of Students With Developmental Disabilities Standards Addressed in This Chapter

Principle 1: Foundations

DD1K4   Trends and practices in the field of developmental disabilities.

Principle 5: Learning Environments/Social Interaction

DD5S5   Plan instruction for individuals with developmental disabilities in a variety of placement settings.

Principle 7: Instructional Planning

DD7S1   Plan instruction for independent functional life skills relevant to the community, personal living, sexuality, and employment.

Web Site Resources

CAST—Teaching Every Student (TES)

http://www.cast.org/teachingeverystudent

Information on instructional methods such as peer-delivered instruction. Menu of tools and activities for instructing blended classes of learners with and without disabilities.

CAST—Universal Design for Living

http://www.cast.org

Nonprofit organization that conducts and promotes research on improving learning opportunities for all individuals, including those with disabilities, through innovation in instructional methods. Focuses primarily on technological advances in universal instructional design.

Council for Exceptional Children (CEC)
http://www.cec.sped.org

> Information regarding governmental policies, professional standards, and the latest news and updates in the special education field.

Division on Developmental Disabilities for the Council for Exceptional Children
http://www.dddcec.org

> Information on many issues related to the field of developmental disabilities. Search archives for articles pertaining to instruction of learners with developmental disabilities.

References

Alberto, P., Jobes, N., Sizemore, A., & Duran, D. (1980). A comparison of individual and group instruction across response tasks. *Journal of the Association for Persons With Severe Handicaps, 5*, 285–293.

Barry, T. D., Klinger, L. G., Lee, J. M., Palardy, N., Gilmore, T., & Bodin, S. D. (2003). Examining the effectiveness of an outpatient clinic-based social skills group for high-functioning children with autism. *Journal of Autism and Developmental Disorders, 33*, 685–701.

Bourland, G., Jablonski, E. M., & Lockhart, D. L. (1988). Multiple-behavior comparisons of group and individual instruction of persons with mental retardation. *Mental Retardation, 26*, 39–46.

Brown, F., Holvoet, J., Guess, D., & Mulligan, M. (1980). The Individualized Curriculum Sequencing Model (III): Small group instruction. *Journal of the Association for Persons with Severe Handicaps, 5*, 352–367.

Butler, F. M. (1999). Reading partners: Students can help each other learn to read. *Education and Treatment of Children, 22*, 415–426.

Collins, B. C., Gast, D. L., Ault, M. J., & Wolery, M. (1991). Small-group instruction: Guidelines for teachers of students with moderate to severe handicaps. *Education and Training in Mental Retardation, 26*, 18–32.

Collins, B. C., Hall, M., Branson, T. A., & Holder, M. (1999). Acquisition of related and unrelated factual information delivered by a teacher within an inclusive classroom. *Journal of Behavioral Education, 9*, 223–237.

DiSalvo, C. A., & Oswald, D. P. (2002). Peer-mediated interventions to increase the social interaction of children with autism: Consideration of peer expectancies. *Focus on Autism and Other Developmental Disabilities, 17*, 198–207.

Faw, G. D., Reid, D. H., Schepis, M. M., Fitzgerald, J. R., & Welty, P. A. (1981). Involving institutional staff in the development and maintenance of sign language skills with profoundly retarded persons. *Journal of Applied Behavior Analysis, 14*, 411–423.

Fickel, K. M., Schuster, J. W., & Collins, B. C. (1998). Teaching different tasks using different stimuli in a heterogeneous small group. *Journal of Behavioral Education, 8*, 219–244.

Fink, W. T., & Sandall, S. R. (1978). One-to-one vs. group academic instruction with handicapped and nonhandicapped preschool children. *Mental Retardation, 16*, 236–240.

Garfinkle, A. N., & Schwartz, I. S. (2002). Peer imitation: Increasing social interactions in children with autism and other developmental disabilities in inclusive preschool classrooms. *Topics in Early Childhood Special Education, 22*(1), 26–38.

Garrison-Harrell, L., & Kamps, D. (1997). The effects of peer networks on social-communicative behaviors for students with autism. *Focus on Autism and Other Developmental Disabilities, 12*, 241–254.

Gast, D. L., Wolery, M., Morris, L. L., Doyle, P. M., & Meyer, L. L. (1990). Teaching sight word reading in a group instructional arrangement using constant time delay. *Exceptionality, 1*, 81–96.

Gonzalez-Lopez, A., & Kamps, D. M. (1997). Social skills training to increase social interactions between children with autism and their typical peers. *Focus on Autism and Other Developmental Disabilities, 12*, 2–14.

Greenwood, C. R. (1991). Longitudinal analysis of time, engagement, and achievement in at-risk versus non-risk students. *Exceptional Children, 57* (4), 521–535.

Harper, G. F., Mallette, B., Maheady, L., Parkes, V., & Moore, J. (1993). Retention and generalization of spelling words acquired using a peer-mediated instructional procedure by children with mild handicapping conditions. *Journal of Behavioral Education, 3*, 25–38.

Harrower, J. (1999). Educational inclusion of children with severe disabilities. *Journal of Positive Behavioral Interventions, 1*, 215–230.

Hunt, P., & Goetz, L. (1997). Research on inclusive educational programs, practices, and outcomes for students with severe disabilities. *Journal of Special Education, 31*, 3–29.

Johnson, J. W., & McDonnell, J. (2004). An exploratory study of the implementation of embedded instruction by general educators with students with disabilities. *Education and Treatment of Children, 27*, 46–63.

Johnson, P., Schuster, J., & Bell, J. K. (1996). Comparison of simultaneous prompting with and without error correction in teaching science vocabulary words to high school students with mild disabilities. *Journal of Behavioral Education, 6*, 437–458.

Kamps, D., Walker, D., Maher, J., & Rotholz, D. (1992). Validation of small group instruction for students with autism and developmental disabilities. *Journal of Autism and Developmental Disorders, 22*, 277–293.

Kamps, D. M., Dugan, E. P., Leonard, B. R., & Daoust, P. M. (1994). Enhanced small group instruction using choral responding and student interactions for children with autism and developmental disabilities. *American Journal on Mental Retardation, 99*, 60–73.

Karsh, K. G., & Repp, A. C. (1992). The Task Demonstration Model: A concurrent model for teaching students with severe disabilities. *Exceptional Children, 59*, 54–67.

McDonnell, J. (1998). Instruction for students with severe disabilities in general education settings. *Education and Training in Mental Retardation and Developmental Disabilities, 33*, 199–215.

McDonnell, J., Johnson, J. W., Polychronis, S., & Riesen, T. (2002). Effects of embedded instruction on students with moderate disabilities enrolled in general education classes. *Education and Training in Mental Retardation and Developmental Disabilities, 37*, 363–377.

McDonnell, J., Mathot-Buckner, C., Thorson, N., & Fister, S. (2001). Supporting the inclusion of students with moderate to severe disabilities in junior high school general education classes: The effects of classwide peer tutoring, multi-element curriculum, and accommodations. *Education and Treatment of Children, 24*, 141–160.

McDonnell, J., Thorson, N., Allen, C., & Mathot-Buckner, C. (2000). The effects of partner learning during spelling for students with severe disabilities and their peers. *Journal of Behavioral Education, 10*, 107–121.

Mortweet, S. L., Utley, C. A., Walker, D., Dawson, H. L., Delquadri, J. C., Reddy, S. S., et al. (1999). Teaching children with mild mental retardation in inclusive classrooms. *Exceptional Children, 65*, 524–536.

Munk, D. D., Van Laarhoven, T., Goodman, S., & Repp, A. C. (1998). Small-group direct instruction for students with moderate to severe disabilities. In A. Hilton & R. Ringlaben (Eds.), *Best and promising practices in developmental disabilities* (pp. 127–138). Austin, TX: PRO-ED.

Norman, J. M., Collins, B. C., & Schuster, J. W. (2001). Using an instructional package including video technology to teach self-help skills to elementary students with mental disabilities. *Journal of Special Education Technology, 16*, 5–18.

Oliver, P. (1983). Effects of teaching different tasks in group vs. individual training formats with severely handicapped individuals. *Journal of the Association for Persons With Severe Handicaps, 8*, 79–91.

Oliver, P. R., & Scott, T. L. (1981). Group versus individual training in establishing generalization of language skills with severely handicapped individuals. *Mental Retardation, 19*, 285–289.

Orelove, F. P. (1982). Acquisition of incidental learning in moderately and severely handicapped adults. *Education and Training of the Mentally Retarded, 17*, 131–136.

Parker, M., & Schuster, J. W. (2002). Effectiveness of simultaneous prompting on the acquisition of observational and instructive feedback stimuli when teaching a heterogeneous group of high school students. *Education and Training in Mental Retardation and Developmental Disabilities, 37*, 89–104.

Pierce, K., & Schreibman, L. (1997). Using peer trainers to promote social behavior in autism: Are they effective at enhancing multiple social modalities? *Focus on Autism and Other Developmental Disabilities, 12,* 207–218.

Reid, D. H., & Favell, J. E. (1984). Group instruction with persons who have severe disabilities: A critical review. *Journal of the Association for Persons With Severe Handicaps, 9,* 167–177.

Repp, A. C., & Karsh, K. G. (1992). An analysis of a group teaching procedure for persons with developmental disabilities. *Journal of Applied Behavior Analysis, 25,* 701–712.

Riesen, T., McDonnell, J., Johnson, J. W., Polychronis, S., & Jameson, M. (2003). A comparison of constant time delay and simultaneous prompting within embedded instruction in general education classes with students with moderate to severe disabilities. *Journal of Behavioral Education, 12,* 241–259.

Schuster, J. W., Hemmeter, M. L., & Ault, M. J. (2001). Instruction of students with moderate to severe disabilities in elementary classrooms. *Early Childhood Research Quarterly, 16,* 329–341.

Simpson, A., Langone, J., & Ayres, K. M. (2004). Embedded video and computer-based instruction to improve social skills for students with autism. *Education and Training in Developmental Disabilities, 39,* 240–252.

Singleton, K. C., Schuster, J. W., & Ault, M. J. (1995). Simultaneous prompting in a small group instructional arrangement. *Education and Training in Mental Retardation and Developmental Disabilities, 30,* 218–230.

Snell, M. E., & Brown, F. (Eds.). (2006). *Instruction of students with severe disabilities* (6th ed.). Upper Saddle River, NJ: Prentice Hall.

Storm, R. H., & Willis, J. H. (1978). Small-group training as an alternative to individual programs for profoundly retarded persons. *American Journal of Mental Deficiency, 83,* 283–288.

Taubman, M., Brierly, S., Wishner, J., Baker, D., McEachin, J., & Leaf, R. B. (2001). The effectiveness of a group discrete trial instructional approach for preschoolers with developmental disabilities. *Research in Developmental Disabilities, 22,* 205–219.

Utley, C. A., Reddy, S. S., Delquadri, J. C., Greenwood, C. R., & Bowman, V. (2001). Classwide peer tutoring: An effective teaching procedure for facilitating the acquisition of health education and safety facts with students with developmental disabilities. *Education and Treatment of Children, 24,* 1–27.

Webb, B. J., Miller, S. P., Pierce, T. B., Strawser, S., & Jones, W. P. (2004). Effects of social skill instruction for high-functioning adolescents with autism spectrum disorders. *Focus on Autism and Other Developmental Disabilities, 19*(1), 53–62.

Westling, D. L., Ferrell, K., & Swenson, K. (1982). Intraclassroom comparison of two arrangements for teaching profoundly mentally retarded children. *American Journal on Mental Deficiency, 86,* 601–608.

Westling, D. L., & Fox, L. (2004). *Teaching students with severe disabilities* (3rd ed.). Upper Saddle River, NJ: Prentice Hall.

Wildman, B. G., Wildman, H. E., & Kelly, W. J. (1986). Group conversational skills training and social validation with mentally retarded adults. *Applied Research in Mental Retardation, 1,* 443–458.

SECTION 5

LEARNING ENVIRONMENTS AND SOCIAL INTERACTIONS

15

Facilitating Social Relationships and Friendships in School Settings

MaryAnn Demchak

Summary

Having friends and belonging is important for all individuals. Friends provide emotional support, companionship, nurturing, and a sense of security. This chapter discusses research-based strategies for facilitating social relationships and friendships, including (a) minimizing the potential negative influence of adults, particularly paraprofessionals, in educational settings, (b) facilitating positive attitudes, (c) implementing peer buddy programs, (d) encouraging involvement in extracurricular and non-instructional activities, (e) engaging in conversations, and (f) implementing friendship circles.

Learning Outcomes

After reading this chapter, you should be able to:

- Distinguish between social relationships and friendships.

- Identify the importance of social relationships and friendships between students with and without disabilities.

- Identify and implement strategies for facilitating social relationships and friendships.

Introduction

Developing social relationships, friendships, and membership in social groups is important for all individuals. *Social relationships* are interactions between children that can be short term or long term and can take various forms that can be positive or negative. Relationships also can vary in terms of intensity, from brief, minimal contact to more-intense, lasting interactions. Viewing relationships along a continuum can lead one to friendships at the positive end of the continuum. *Friendships* are close, positive social relationships that are typically intense and mutually reciprocal between individuals. Friendships can take a variety of active and passive roles (e.g., verbal communication, physical interaction, playing together) (Lee, Yoo, & Bak, 2003). *Membership in a social group* is about belonging to and being accepted by a group or a larger social network (Erwin & Guintini, 2000; Schwartz, 2000). Individuals can be members of small groups, classrooms, schools, or outside-school activities (Schwartz, 2000). Having friends and belonging are important for all individuals, including those with developmental disabilities. Friends provide emotional support, companionship, nurturing, and a sense of security.

Friendships for students with disabilities are viewed as important by parents (Ivey, 2004; Overton & Rausch, 2002), general education teachers (Hamre-Nietupski, Hendrickson, Nietupski, & Shokoshi-Yekta, 1994), and special educators (Hamre-Nietupski,

Hendrickson, Nietupski, & Sasso, 1993). Friendship development, a quality-of-life issue, can be facilitated by both educators and parents (Geisthardt, Brotherson, & Cook, 2002).

Unfortunately, individuals with developmental disabilities, especially those that are more severe, often have fewer relationships and friends than do individuals without disabilities. However, friendships between individuals with disabilities and individuals without disabilities are possible and can be beneficial to both groups.

Strategies for Facilitating Social Relationships and Friendships

For social relationships and friendships to develop between students with disabilities and those without disabilities, it is typically necessary for educators and parents to implement various strategies that encourage or facilitate such interactions. Hall and Strickett (2002) found that regardless of setting, strategies to facilitate peer relationships between students with and without disabilities are needed to promote positive interactions during unstructured school times. Similarly, Carter, Hughes, Guth, and Copeland (2005) found that without actions to facilitate social connections between peers with and without disabilities, it is unlikely that frequent interactions will occur. Regardless of educational setting and amount of physical integration, it is important that educators implement evidenced-based strategies to bring about peer interactions (Carter et al., 2005; Hall & Strickett, 2002).

Minimizing the Potential Negative Influence of Adults/Paraprofessionals

Using paraprofessionals to facilitate the inclusion of students with disabilities in general education classes is a widespread practice. Although an often-cited reason for inclusion of students with disabilities, especially severe disabilities, is that they will reap social benefits, the paraprofessionals who are hired to assist are not typically provided with any training or guidance for the task, and sometimes their presence can actually interfere with social interactions between peers with and without disabilities (Giangreco, Edelman, Luiselli, & MacFarland, 1997).

In a survey of middle school students regarding friendships with peers with severe disabilities, the students themselves reported that the presence of paraprofessionals interfered with their interactions with the peers with disabilities (Han & Chadsey, 2004). Adults can interfere with peer interactions in a preschool setting as well. Harper and McCluskey (2003) examined child–child interactions in an inclusive preschool setting. They found that after an adult initiated an interaction with a child, the child was less likely to initiate an interaction with a peer and more likely to initiate another interaction with the adult. These researchers also found that peer-initiated interactions increased the likelihood that a child would subsequently initiate an interaction with a peer.

One specific aspect of paraprofessional involvement that can interfere with peer interactions is the paraprofessional's physical proximity to the student with disabilities. Giangreco and Broer (2005) found that paraprofessionals reported spending about 86% of their time within three feet of their assigned student(s) with disabilities. Giangreco and Broer highlighted the atypical nature of this adult proximity for most students in schools in the United States. It is not difficult to expect that such proximity would influence peer interactions and social relationships. Giangreco and Doyle (2002) recommend exploring alternatives to paraprofessional proximity by using natural supports such as peers and using a paraprofessional as a classroom assistant rather than strictly as a one-on-one aide.

Other paraprofessional actions and practices can also interfere with interactions and the ultimate development of relationships. Giangreco et al. (1997) observed that paraprofessionals regularly separate students with disabilities from the class (e.g., leaving for special classes such as art and music earlier than the rest of the group, sitting away from the class or on the fringe of a group). One very simple strategy to address this issue is to determine whether such isolating practices are necessary (Is it necessary to leave early for the special session? Is it necessary for the student with disabilities to accompany the paraprofessional on an errand to the workroom?). Giangreco et al. also recommend that qualified teachers (general and special educators) as well as support personnel (e.g., related services personnel as necessary) plan classroom activities that are designed to physically and programmatically include students with disabilities rather than inadvertently isolating them in the classroom.

Perhaps most important of all, paraprofessionals must receive specific training on how to facilitate peer interactions. Causton-Theoharis and Malmgren (2005a, 2005b) provide recommendations for paraprofessional training with the purpose of facilitating peer interactions. The training protocol for this investigation (Causton-Theoharis & Malmgren, 2005b) comprised (a) enhancing perspective through the use of a *circles of friends* activity (described later), (b) establishing the importance of peer interaction through discussion questions and written material, (c) clarifying the paraprofessional's role in facilitating interactions by brainstorming sessions, and (d) increasing the paraprofessional's knowledge base by directly teaching facilitation strategies (e.g., modeling, highlighting similarities between students, identifying student strengths, direct teaching of interaction skills, partnering students). This intervention package resulted in an increase in the facilitating behaviors of the paraprofessionals and a corresponding and substantial increase in student-to-student interactions. The results highlight the importance of providing training to paraprofessionals regarding the importance of and strategies for facilitating peer interactions.

Facilitating Positive Attitudes

Bunch and Valeo (2004) discuss the importance of *social learning theory* and *social referencing theory* as related to peer attitudes toward students with disabilities. Social learning theory asserts that an individual learns by observing and imitating those around him, while social referencing theory states that known and trusted authority figures guide or influence an individual's actions. The tenets of these theories have direct implications for interactions, relationships, and friendships between peers with and without disabilities. For example, the manner in which an adult (e.g., a teacher or paraprofessional) interacts with a student with disabilities can subsequently influence how peers view and interact with that student. Thus, if the adult interacts in a positive, accepting manner, peers are more likely to do so. The adult might be viewed as a known and trusted authority figure (i.e., social referencing theory) as well as a person who models specific actions that the peers can observe and imitate (i.e., social learning theory).

Broer, Doyle, and Giangreco (2005) surveyed young adults identified as having mild to moderate intellectual disabilities regarding their perspectives on paraprofessional support. One particular finding of this study relevant to attitudes and social learning and social referencing theories is the negative associations pertaining to the perception of the "paraprofessional as mothering." Having a "mother" present (even in the form of a paraprofessional) can obviously interfere with interactions. However, the attitude conveyed by an adult acting in a "mothering" role can also influence peer interactions, in that peers may imitate these actions (i.e., social learning theory) and thus interact with the student with disabilities in a less than desirable way.

Another occurrence that can influence how peers view students with disabilities relates to involvement in conversations. It is not unusual for peers to engage the paraprofessional, or any other adult who is present, in a conversation rather than directing comments or questions directly to the student with disabilities (Causton-Theoharis & Malmgren, 2005a). For example, when getting ready to go to lunch, a peer may ask the adult, "Is Susie going outside after she eats?" In another situation, a peer might comment to the adult, "I don't think Jeff likes _____" (a statement based on Jeff's affect which shows dislike). If the adult answers for the student with disabilities, the message that might inadvertently be conveyed is that the student cannot communicate or cannot understand what is being said. Rather than responding for the student with disabilities when such interactions occur, the adult should redirect the peer to ask the question or make the comment to the student. The adult can model how to communicate with the student and, if necessary, help the peer to interpret the response of the student with disabilities. Modeling such behavior can facilitate a positive attitude toward the student with disabilities and can encourage such interactions in the future.

Implementing Peer Buddy Programs

Peer buddy programs can be implemented at any age. They are frequently structured so that general education students ("buddies") receive academic credit for spending at least one period a day with a peer in a special education class, as well as learning about various types of disabilities, instructional techniques, and ideas for including peers with disabilities in routine school activities (Hughes et al., 1999). Hughes et al. (2001) suggest that peer buddies can accompany peers with disabilities to general education classes, help peers with disabilities be involved in ongoing high school routines, assist in the community or at job sites, and provide friendship. These types of interactions between peers with and without disabilities result in benefits to both groups of students (Fisher, 1999; Peck, Donaldson, & Pezzoli, 1990; Pottie & Sumarah, 2004).

Hughes et al. (1999) suggest the following steps for implementation of a peer buddy program in a high school setting:

1. Add a one-credit course for the program to the school's curriculum.

2. Recruit peer buddies through announcements, posters, newsletter articles, and presentations to classes or at club meetings.

3. Screen volunteers and match them to a special education class.

4. Train the peer buddies by modeling communication skills and prompting strategies, and provide feedback and reinforcers, as well as information about the concept of "people first," disability awareness, and strategies for responding to inappropriate behavior.

5. Establish expectations regarding attendance and participation and evaluate progress.

6. Invite the peer buddies to interact at lunch, establish a peer buddy club for ongoing support for the peer buddies, and provide for feedback sessions.

7. Establish an advisory board with representation from the peer buddies, students with disabilities, parents of both groups, general education and special education teachers, administrators, and guidance counselors.

Hughes et al. (2001) followed such a process to extend the findings of earlier studies with a focus on attitudes and benefits identified by the participants, perceptions of interactions, and suggestions for implementing such programs. They found that the peer buddies reported having positive attitudes and experiencing personal growth in interpersonal skills, friendships, knowledge and awareness of individuals with disabilities, strategies for interactions, and comfort when interacting with people with disabilities. Peer buddies reported spending their time both in helping peers with disabilities to learn new skills and in befriending, socially interacting with, and participating in recreational activities with their peers identified as having disabilities. The peer buddies also suggested publicizing and advocating for involvement of peers in earlier grades.

Goldstein and English (1995) discussed a peer buddy training program for teaching preschoolers to be peer buddies. Similar to Hughes et al. (1999), Goldstein and English began the training process by providing information about communication skills, disability awareness, friendship concepts, and what it means to be a buddy. This general training was followed by teaching the peers three buddy skills: STAY, PLAY, and TALK. That is, the peers were taught to stay close by the child with a disability; to play with that child by joining in his or her activity, bringing a toy to the child, or suggesting an activity; and to talk to and respond to communicative attempts by the child. Initially an adult is present to facilitate implementation throughout the day and to provide support by prompting the students as necessary. Goldstein and English reported that peers who have participated in this training are more likely to choose their buddies for other play activities in addition to those that were specifically taught.

Encouraging Involvement in Extracurricular Activities and Non-Instructional Activities

In a survey of middle school students, the most commonly cited factor for peers without disabilities not having friends with severe disabilities was the lack of opportunity to interact with peers with severe disabilities (Han & Chadsey, 2004). The survey respondents (i.e., typically developing students) also reported that sports activities were the most common activities they did with their peers without disabilities. Thus, one implication of these survey results is that involving students with severe disabilities in sports activities or adapted sports activities could provide greater opportunities for peers with and without disabilities to interact with one another. However, it is likely that modifications will be needed to allow for meaningful participation. The suggestions provided by Block (2000) for physical education classes have been applied by Ohtake (2004) for meaningful inclusion in team sports. Block provides strategies for modifying instruction, curricula, group games, and sports, as well as strategies for facilitating social acceptance. Ohtake stresses the importance of students' participating in the *essential part of the game or sport*, which is defined as "the core meaning of a sport and contributes to getting scores or defending one's team from being scored on" (p. 23). Providing modifications that allow a student with disabilities to participate in the essential part of the game or sport can facilitate the student's being viewed as a valued, contributing member of the game or team.

Carter, Hughes, Copeland, and Breen (2001) reported that if opportunities for contact between students with disabilities and students without disabilities are expanded (e.g., extracurricular activities), it can result in high school students' having a greater willingness to interact with their peers who have severe disabilities. When students spend time together outside of school in extracurricular activities, mutual interests can result, which can facilitate interactions and closer relationships.

Engaging in Conversations

Han and Chadsey (2004) reported that peers without disabilities indicated that the major activity done with their friends with severe disabilities was "talking." Carter et al. (2005) found that peer buddies and students with intellectual disabilities engaged in various conversational topics that were related to the school location where the exchange took place. That is, topics depended upon the location of the conversation: in general education settings topics focused on academics, in the gym conversation focused on greetings and the ongoing activities, and in cafeterias, hallways, and special education classrooms, the topics were varied and included both academic and social subjects.

Han and Chadsey (2004) and Carter et al. (2005) suggested that social interaction interventions should address conversational topics and skills. Opportunities for interaction must be structured and planned; otherwise, interactions are not likely to occur between students with and without disabilities, even when they are in close proximity to one another (Mu, Siegel, & Allinder, 2000). Additionally, Mu and colleagues found that the students with severe disabilities were more likely to assume passive roles when compared to their peers without disabilities. The students with disabilities were more likely to be on the receiving end of interactions (i.e., assistance, instruction, criticism, joking) rather than on the "providing" end (i.e., instruction, assistance, criticism, joking). That is, the students with disabilities received more social interactions than they initiated.

Students with disabilities should be taught how to initiate and engage in conversations. At the same time, peers without disabilities need to be taught how to communicate with their peers with disabilities who may have limited communication skills or use augmentative/alternative communication options (Han & Chadsey, 2004). The findings of Carter et al. (2005) indicate that it would also be important to target conversational topics that are relevant to the setting. For example, Hughes et al. (2000) taught participants to prompt themselves to use conversation starters from communication books to increase the number of topics discussed and to decrease inappropriate initiations.

It is important not only to teach conversational skills but also to structure situations in such a manner that social interactions are likely to occur. Hughes, Carter, Hughes, Bradford, and Copeland (2002) investigated the effects of *instructional* versus *non-instructional roles* on the social interactions of high school students. They found that when the general education students were assigned a non-instructional role (e.g., playing board games, completing jigsaw puzzles, drawing, looking at photographs or magazines) rather than an instructional role (e.g., assisting with an academic task or a job skill), the students with disabilities initiated more interactions. In that situation the interactions between the two groups of students were also more likely to cover a wider range of conversational topics and to be social exchanges (e.g., joking, discussing social events) during non-instructional roles as compared to instructional roles.

Thus, not only is it necessary to teach socially relevant conversational skills, but it is also important to provide structured opportunities for such skills to be used with peers in non-instructional situations. A variety of resources are available that highlight strategies for teaching communication skills (Beukelman & Mirenda, 2005; Downing, 2005). Expanding conversational topics and skills and opportunities for using these skills can result in increased interactions, which can lead to enhanced social relationships and friendships.

Implementing Friendship Circles

Friendship circles, also known as circles of friends, circles of support, peer networks, and peer-supported committees, are a structured strategy to review the importance of friendships and relationships in everyone's lives and to generate ideas for facilitating a relationship with a vulnerable person. These types of support networks center on the needs of a particular person. For example, Hunt, Alwell, Farron-Davis, and Goetz (1996) investigated the effectiveness of child-specific support "clubs" for 3 elementary-age children with significant physical and intellectual disabilities. Their intervention package consisted of providing information about the students who needed support (e.g., how to communicate with them, information about any adaptive equipment), identifying and using various media for interactive exchanges (e.g., voice-output communication devices, interactive computer activities, toys and games), as well as ongoing facilitation and support by educational staff. These support networks led to increases in (a) reciprocal interactions between the peers with and without disabilities and (b) interactions initiated by the students targeted for support. Additionally, it was reported that the focus students received fewer interactions involving assistance from paraprofessionals. Qualitative data indicated that peers without disabilities identified themselves as friends of the focus students, a finding supported by feedback from teachers. These results indicated that structured support networks lead to more-balanced interactions occurring between the students with and without disabilities and that friendships can develop.

Haring and Breen (1992) investigated the effects of a peer support network on (a) the social interactions of students with disabilities and (b) peer satisfaction, attitude, and friendship development. Two junior high school students who were identified as having moderate and severe disabilities were the focus students. The peer support network "package" consisted of recruiting volunteers and explaining the network, why a network was being implemented, and how and when the network would be put into practice. Implementation of the peer support network resulted in increases in the quality and quantity of interactions as well as promoting the development of friendships.

A frequently recommended *circles of friends* process is discussed by O'Brien and Forest (1989), who propose the following steps for implementing this process:

1. Discuss the importance of friendships and relationships in everyone's life.

2. Provide students with four concentric circles and ask them to identify the important relationships in their lives.

3. In the inner circle, ask them to put the names of those individuals to whom they are closest (e.g., those they love the most, those with whom they share their secrets).

4. In the second circle, ask them to list those people they really like, but not quite as much as those in the first circle (i.e., those with whom they do *not* share their secrets).

5. In the third circle, ask them to identify those individuals with whom they like to do things because of the groups to which they belong (e.g., sports teams, clubs, dance groups, scouts).

6. In the fourth, or outermost, circle ask them to list those people who are paid to be in their lives (e.g., doctor, dentist, teachers, coaches; see sample in Figure 15.1).

7. After the students have completed each circle, ask them to share their responses if they are willing. After discussing the circles of

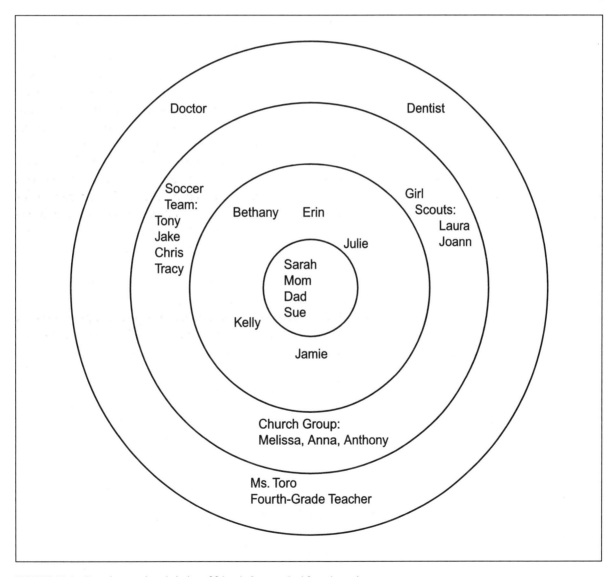

FIGURE 15.1. Sample completed circles of friends for a typical fourth grader.

several volunteers, show the class the circles of an individual who has very few relationships (e.g., only family members in the inner circle, perhaps no one in Circles 2 and 3, and numerous service providers in Circle 4; see sample in Figure 15.2).

8. Ask the students to discuss (a) how they would feel and (b) how they would act if their circles looked like those of someone with few relationships. List their responses on chart paper so that a record is made of their reactions.

9. Explain to the class that the circles of a classmate with a disability may not look very different from that of the hypothetical individual with few relationships. Ask them what they could do to change that situation. Again, log their responses on chart paper so that a record of possible strategies exists to provide ideas.

10. Ask the class if there is anyone who would like to become part of the circles of the classmate with a disability. Be sure that the class members know that not everyone has to volunteer. List the names of those who are interested.

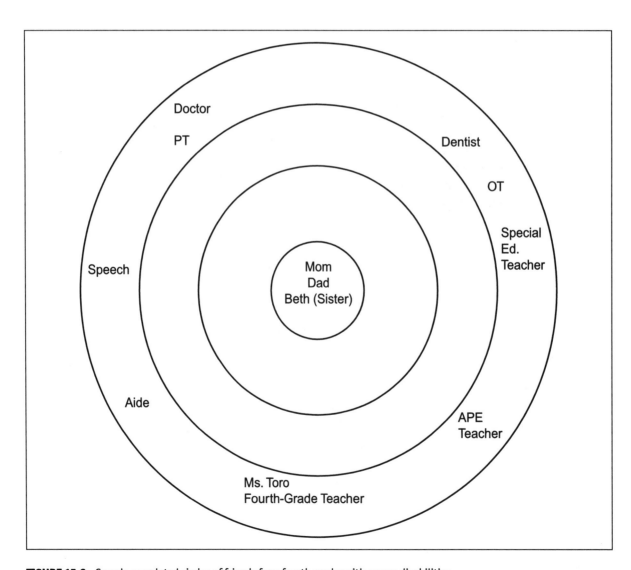

FIGURE 15.2. Sample completed circles of friends for a fourth grader with severe disabilities.

11. Hold regular weekly meetings with this classmate's newly developed circle of friends to help them brainstorm ways of interacting and being friends. The student with a disability should be involved in these ongoing meetings and have input regarding the suggested strategies, since he or she is the focus of the circle. It may be necessary for various communication approaches to be used to ensure this participation (e.g., augmentative/alternative communication).

Miller, Cooke, Test, and White (2003) investigated the use of the circles of friends process on the social interactions of three students with mild disabilities. Following a class activity that employed the approach outlined above, students were asked to volunteer to be part of friendship circles. One of these participants was an 11-year-old boy identified as having a mild developmental disability. The students in this friendship circle met initially to discuss the purpose and responsibilities of participating, to name their friendship circle, to discuss friendship characteristics, and to discuss times when they had demonstrated friendship. Subsequent once-a-week 30-minute meetings focused on strengths, concerns, and suggestions based on the previous week's interactions. The results showed that the friendship circle was effective in increasing appropriate interactions at lunch for this participant and also resulted in friendly play at recess (an unstructured portion of the school day). Anecdotal data provided by the teacher indicated that the students in the friendship circle appeared to be the target student's friends and others also began to assist and include him. The teacher also reported that at recess the student made friends with students from other classes.

Regardless of the approach followed for friendships circles or support networks, such a process can be an effective way of facilitating the development of social relationships and friendships between peers with and without disabilities. The adult(s) acting as facilitator(s) for a circle of friends should encourage the group to develop strategies that focus on various types of interactions. It is essential to remember that a circle of friends is an ongoing process that requires follow-through by meeting on a regular basis with an adult facilitator to solve problems and to review activities. Friendship circles will not be effective if they are structured as a one-time activity intended as a quick fix. When completed correctly and facilitated as an ongoing process, however, peer support networks can be effective in encouraging social relationships and friendships (Haring & Breen, 1992; Hunt et al., 1996; Kamps, Potucek, Lopez, Kravits, & Kemmerer, 1997; Miller et al., 2003).

Conclusion

Implementing strategies such as those discussed in this chapter can facilitate the development of social relationships and friendships between students with and without disabilities. It is important to remember that simply being present with peers is insufficient for the formation of relationships and friendships. Opportunities for interactions and the encouragement of positive social relationships can be first steps toward the development of meaningful friendships. However, specific strategies need to be implemented to encourage interactions that can lead to social relationships and meaningful friendships. Although school staff can implement such strategies, they cannot guarantee to any family that friendships will result. However, the strategies discussed here do have a research base that shows they are effective. Ultimately, relationships and friendships can lead to a greater sense of membership and belonging to a larger social network.

Glossary

Circles of friends—Specific strategy proposed by O'Brien and Forest (1989) that uses four concentric circles and related discussion to explore the support within one's life and to develop friendship and support strategies for a target individual.

Essential part of a game or sport—"The core meaning of a sport and contributes to getting scores or defending one's team from being scored on" (Ohtake, 2004, p. 23).

Friendship circles—Also known as circles of friends, circles of support, peer networks, and peer-supported committees. Friendship circles is a structured strategy to review the importance of friendships and relationships in everyone's life and to generate ideas for facilitating a relationship with a vulnerable person.

Friendships—Close, positive social relationships that are typically intense and mutually reciprocal between individuals.

Instructional roles—Interactions between students with and without disabilities that focus on the peer without a disability assisting the individual with a disability to complete an academic task, job skill, etc.

Membership—Belonging to and being accepted by a group or larger social network.

Non-instructional roles—Interactions between students with and without disabilities that focus on social and leisure activities such as looking at or reading magazines, completing jigsaw puzzles, drawing or coloring, playing board games, looking at photographs, etc.

Paraprofessional proximity—The physical closeness or distance maintained by a paraprofessional when providing instructional or social support for a student with a disability.

Peer buddy program—Program in which general education students ("buddies") receive academic credit for spending at least one period a day with a peer in a special education class, as well as learning about various types of disabilities, instructional techniques, and ideas for including peers with disabilities in routine school activities (Hughes et al., 1999).

Social learning theory—An individual learns by observing and imitating those around him.

Social referencing theory—Known, trusted authority figures guide or influence an individual's actions.

Social relationships—Interactions between children that can be short term or long term and can take various forms that can be positive or negative.

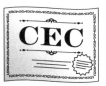

Knowledge and Skills for Entry-Level Special Education Teachers of Students With Developmental Disabilities Standards Addressed in This Chapter

Principle 4: Instructional Strategies

DD4K2   Evidence-based practices for teaching individuals with pervasive developmental disabilities, autism, and autism spectrum disorders.

Principle 5: Learning Environments/Social Interaction

DD5S4   Structure the physical environment to provide optimal learning for individuals with developmental disabilities.

Principle 7: Instructional Planning

DD7S4   Design, implement, and evaluate specialized instructional programs for persons with developmental disabilities that enhance social participation across environments.

Web Site Resources

Community Works
http://www.communityworks.info/articles/friendship.htm

> Focuses on circle of friends and provides information regarding the importance of friendships for persons with disabilities.

Friends and Relationships
http://www.mycitymyplace.com/friends.htm

> Recommendations for developing friendships, along with numerous links to other sites where persons with disabilities can develop friendships with others.

Importance of Friendships Between People With and Without Mental Retardation
http://www.thearc.org/faqs/friend.html

> Maintained by the ARC. Q&A format regarding a range of issues related to friendships for persons with mental retardation.

Person-Centered Planning and Friendships
http://www.beachcenter.org/?act=view&type=General%20Topic&id=8

> Several articles pertaining to friendships, archived at the Beach Center on Disability at the University of Kansas.

References

Beukelman, D. R., & Mirenda, P. (2005). *Augmentative and alternative communication: Supporting children and adults with complex communication needs* (3rd ed.). Baltimore: Brookes.

Block, M. E. (2000). *A teacher's guide to including students with disabilities in general physical education* (2nd ed.). Baltimore: Brookes.

Broer, S. M., Doyle, M. B., & Giangreco, M. F. (2005). Perspectives of students with intellectual disabilities about their experiences with paraprofessional support. *Exceptional Children, 71,* 415–430.

Bunch, G., & Valeo, A. (2004). Student attitudes toward peers with disabilities in inclusive and special education schools. *Disability and Society, 19,* 61–76.

Carter, E. W., Hughes, C., Copeland, S. R., & Breen, C. (2001). Differences between high school students who do and do not volunteer to participate in a peer interaction program. *Journal of the Association for Persons With Severe Handicaps, 26,* 229–239.

Carter, E. W., Hughes, C., Guth, C. B., & Copeland, S. R. (2005). Factors influencing social interaction among high school students with intellectual disabilities and their general education peers. *American Journal on Mental Retardation, 110,* 366–377.

Causton-Theoharis, J., & Malmgren, K. (2005a). Building bridges: Strategies to help paraprofessionals promote peer interaction. *TEACHING Exceptional Children, 37*(6), 18–24.

Causton-Theoharis, J. N., & Malmgren, K. W. (2005b). Increasing peer interactions for students with severe disabilities via paraprofessional training. *Exceptional Children, 71,* 431–444.

Downing, J. E. (2005). *Teaching communication skills to students with severe disabilities* (2nd ed.). Baltimore: Brookes.

Erwin, E. J., & Guintini, M. (2000). Inclusion and classroom membership in early childhood. *International Journal of Disability, Development, and Education, 47,* 237–257.

Fisher, D. (1999). According to their peers: Inclusion as high school students see it. *Mental Retardation, 37,* 458–467.

Geisthardt, C. L., Brotherson, M. J., & Cook, C. C. (2002). Friendships of children with disabilities in the home environment. *Education and Training in Mental Retardation and Developmental Disabilities, 37,* 235–252.

Giangreco, M. F., & Broer, S. M. (2005). Questionable utilization of paraprofessionals in inclusive schools: Are we addressing symptoms or causes? *Focus on Autism and Other Developmental Disabilities, 20,* 10–26.

Giangreco, M. F., & Doyle, M. B. (2002). Students with disabilities and paraprofessional supports: Benefits, balance, and band-aids. *Focus on Exceptional Children, 34*(7), 1–12.

Giangreco, M. F., Edelman, S. F., Luiselli, T. E., & MacFarland, S. Z. C. (1997). Helping or hovering? Effects of instructional assistant proximity on students with disabilities. *Exceptional Children, 64,* 7–18.

Goldstein, H., & English, K. (1995). Use of peers as change agents in communicative interactions with preschoolers with disabilities. *Preventing School Failure, 39*(4), 16–20.

Hall, L. J., & Strickett, T. (2002). Peer relationships of preadolescent students with disabilities who attend a separate school. *Education and Training in Mental Retardation and Developmental Disabilities, 37,* 399–409.

Hamre-Nietupski, S., Hendrickson, J., Nietupski, J., & Sasso, G. (1993). Perceptions of teachers of students with moderate, severe, or profound disabilities on facilitating friendships with nondisabled peers. *Education and Training in Mental Retardation, 28,* 111–127.

Hamre-Nietupski, S., Hendrickson, J., Nietupski, J., & Shokoshi-Yekta, M. (1994). Regular educators' perceptions of facilitating friendships of students with moderate, severe, or profound disabilities with nondisabled peers. *Education and Training in Mental Retardation and Developmental Disabilities, 29,* 102–117.

Han, K. G., & Chadsey, J. G. (2004). The influence of gender patterns and grade level on friendship expectations of middle school students toward peers with severe disabilities. *Focus on Autism and Other Developmental Disabilities, 19,* 205–214.

Haring, T. G., & Breen, C. G. (1992). A peer-mediated social network intervention to enhance the social integration of persons with moderate and severe disabilities. *Journal of Applied Behavior Analysis, 25,* 319–333.

Harper, L. V., & McCluskey, K. S. (2003). Teacher-child and child-child interactions in inclusive preschool settings: Do adults inhibit peer interactions? *Early Childhood Research Quarterly, 18,* 163–184.

Hughes, C., Carter, E. W., Hughes, T., Bradford, E., & Copeland, S. R. (2002). Effects of instructional versus non-instructional roles on the social interactions of high school students. *Education and Training in Mental Retardation and Developmental Disabilities, 37,* 146–162.

Hughes, C., Copeland, S. R., Guth, C., Rung, L. L., Hwang, B., Kleeb, G., et al. (2001). General education students' perspectives on their involvement in a high school peer buddy program. *Education and Training in Mental Retardation and Developmental Disabilities, 36,* 343–356.

Hughes, C., Guth, C., Hall, S., Presley, J., Dye, M., & Byers, C. (1999). "They are my best friends": Peer buddies promote inclusion in high school. *TEACHING Exceptional Children, 31*(5), 32–37.

Hughes, C., Rung, L. L., Wehmeyer, M. L., Agran, M., Copeland, S. R., & Hwang, B. (2000). Self-prompted communication book use to increase social interaction among high school students. *Journal of the Association for Persons With Severe Handicaps, 25,* 153–166.

Hunt, P., Alwell, M., Farron-Davis, F., & Goetz, L. (1996). Creating socially supportive environments for fully included students who experience multiple disabilities. *Journal of the Association for Persons With Severe Handicaps, 21,* 53–71.

Ivey, J. K. (2004). What do parents expect? A study of likelihood and importance issues for children with autism spectrum disorders. *Focus on Autism and Other Developmental Disabilities, 19,* 27–33.

Kamps, D. M., Potucek, J., Lopez, A. G., Kravits, T., & Kemmerer, K. (1997). The use of peer networks across multiple settings to improve social interaction for students with autism. *Journal of Behavioral Education, 7,* 335–357.

Lee, S., Yoo, S., & Bak, S. (2003). Characteristics of friendships between children with and without mild disabilities. *Education and Training in Developmental Disabilities, 38,* 157–166.

Miller, M. C., Cooke, N. L., Test, D. W., & White, R. (2003). Effects of friendship circles on the social interactions of elementary age students with mild disabilities. *Journal of Behavioral Education, 12,* 167–184.

Mu, K., Siegel, E. B., & Allinder, R. M. (2000). Peer interactions and sociometric status of high school students with moderate or severe disabilities in general education classrooms. *Journal of the Association for Persons With Severe Handicaps, 25*, 142–152.

O'Brien, J., & Forest, M. (1989). *Action for inclusion: How to improve schools by welcoming children with special needs into regular classrooms.* Toronto: Inclusion Press.

Ohtake, Y. (2004). Meaningful inclusion of all students in team sports. *TEACHING Exceptional Children, 37*(2), 22–27.

Overton, S., & Rausch, J. L. (2002). Peer relationships as support for children with disabilities: An analysis of mothers' goals and indicators for friendship. *Focus on Autism and Other Developmental Disabilities, 17*, 11–29.

Peck, C. A., Donaldson, J., & Pezzoli, M. (1990). Some benefits nonhandicapped adolescents perceive for themselves from their social relationships with peers who have severe handicaps. *Journal of the Association for Persons With Severe Handicaps, 15*, 241–249.

Pottie, C., & Sumarah, J. (2004). Friendships between persons with and without developmental disabilities. *Mental Retardation, 42*, 55–66.

Schwartz, I. S. (2000). Standing on the shoulders of giants: Looking ahead to facilitating membership and relationships for children with disabilities. *Topics in Early Childhood Special Education, 20*, 123–128.

16

Transition Practices for Persons With Developmental Disabilities

Dianne Zager, James Brown, Pamela H. Stenhjem, and Arthur Maloney

Summary

Transitional service components related to independent living continue to pose concerns in terms of definition of services, limited career choices, racial prejudice, limited community participation, and the pervasive isolation of individuals with cognitive and developmental disabilities. While transitional services are a vital part of the Individuals with Disabilities Education Improvement Act of 2004 (IDEIA) legislation, many individuals who are eligible and in need of transitional services are continuing a disappointing pattern of limited participation in post-secondary programs. Given such results, renewed efforts have been made to create new initiatives and broader perspectives in approaching all constituencies to achieve better access to information, more-comprehensive assessment practices, and greater participation by the entire community in addressing these concerns.

Responses to this problem have included more emphasis on a student-centered approach to the planning and delivery of services coupled with enhanced community linkages so that individuals are directly involved in their own choices and have increased opportunities for successful community participation. Accomplishing this goal of greater self-determination, community participation, and independence will require an emphasis by educators on earlier interventions to promote self-advocacy, a more sophisticated appreciation of assistive technology (AT) services, better community outreach, and a heightened sensitivity to the magnified challenges posed for students from under-resourced communities. Disproportionality, lack of cultural awareness, and a persistent failure in establishing meaningful school–family partnerships continue to be major concerns in providing an acceptable level of transitional services to minority youngsters.

The No Child Left Behind Act of 2001 has further complicated the already formidable and necessary task of having the schools provide effective integration of transitional experiences with the existing curriculum. One of the more-effective devices to address transitional issues for students with developmental disabilities is a renewed commitment to service learning, with its emphasis on active participation, sufficient reflection regarding clarity of goals, and authentic learning placements outside the classroom. Through an integration of service learning into the substance of the individualized education program (IEP), a host of promising opportunities emerges that provide for a broader array of career choices, a synergistic development of school–community relationships, and a greater confidence that students with disabilities will make the connections necessary for long-term success.

One promising model for collaborative partnerships is Minnesota's Community Transition Interagency Committees (CTICs), which have played a vital role in creating transitional programming. This program addresses the needs of students for community and curricular integration while mobilizing the civic and business communities to long-term commitments based on respectful, substantive, and life-sustaining opportunities for young adults with disabilities. What remains clear is that more efforts need to be directed at the formidable obstacles, which have produced perennially disappointing results nationally for transitional programs. With fewer than one in three students currently employed after leaving high school

* The authors appreciate the assistance of Patricia Merrill, communications coordinator, University of Minnesota Institute on Community Integration, in the literature search for the preparation of this chapter.

and a 36% drop-out rate among students with disabilities, more resources must be devoted to addressing student-centered delivery systems, a broader array of experiential school-to-work opportunities, and a significant educational effort to engage racial and socioeconomic issues, the potential for assisted technology, and the creation of effective community partnerships.

Learning Outcomes

After reading this chapter, you should be able to:

- Identify strategies that promote successful transitions for individuals with developmental disabilities.

- Recognize safe, equitable, positive, and supportive learning environments in which diversities are valued.

- Understand the components of teaching self-advocacy and self-determination to enhance transition.

- Review model career/vocational programs for individuals with developmental disabilities.

- Engage in collaboration among professionals and families to plan transition to adulthood that encourages full community participation.

Introduction

Preparing students with mental retardation and developmental disabilities for meaningful employment has been a perennial challenge for special educators—one that remains a pressing issue. Transition preparation received a good deal of attention in the 1980s and early 1990s, but in the past few years, only a limited number of research studies have been supported, and fewer innovative programs have been publicized, leaving one to wonder why special educators haven't accomplished more. Despite promising figures showing a substantial increase in supported employment in the 1990s (Parent, Kregel, & Johnson, 1996), a more recent study by Wehman, Targett, West, and Kregel (2005) showed that people with severe disabilities constituted only a very small segment of all people with mental retardation placed in nationally supported programs (Smith & Philippen, 2005). Certo et al. (2003) reported that adults with disabilities had no better employment rates than they did 20 years earlier.

To counter the limited attention given to this area and to challenge the field with a call to action, this chapter examines research-based and emerging best practices in employment preparation for persons with developmental disabilities. Specifically, it presents an overview of transition service components related to independent living and community partners, futures-based planning, outcome-oriented secondary program options, and community linkages for persons with developmental disabilities. Essential school-to-work opportunities are discussed, with emphasis on self-advocacy and self-determination. While most of the information presented here is supported by research, some promising practices that are emerging are also included for consideration.

Student-Centered Transition Planning

To maximize the benefits of transition services in terms of student outcomes, the nature of individual students and their vocational preferences must be considered. Neubert (2003) noted that transition-related programming should be based on the needs, preferences, and interests of students with disabilities. A student-centered approach to the planning and delivery of transition support services requires that transition-related service providers understand and address students' needs, interests, and preferences with regard to prospective educational, vocational, and post-school environments. Neubert also noted that such information is crucial in efforts to effectively provide the transition services mandated in the Individuals with Disabilities Education Act Amendments of 1997.

This focus on the student-centered aspect of transition planning is supported by Sowers, McLean, and Owens (2002), who noted that a paradigm shift from professional to customer-directed services should be used to improve persistent high unemployment rates for individuals with developmental disabilities. Sowers et al. proposed that such efforts would enable individuals with developmental disabilities to: (a) make informed choices and better direct their employment processes, (b) select from a wider array of career choices available within their communities, (c) receive and integrate meaningful advice and support, (d) define their career goals, (e) utilize budgets that support their individual career goals and paths, (f) access appropriate services supported by their funding resources, and (g) directly communicate with their service providers.

Neubert (2000) suggested that transition practices for individuals with significant disabilities focus on three key assessment phases: (a) initial assessment upon entrance into transition programs, (b) ongoing assessment during training, and (c) analysis and communication of assessment results among employers and service providers. Kerka (2003) identified eight characteristics of effective programs for learners who require intensive transition programming. Such characteristics may be adapted by persons seeking to effectively address the transition needs of students with developmental disabilities within a holistic approach that includes individual students' social, academic, and career-related transition needs. An effective program will: (a) assure the presence of caring, knowledgeable adults in order to help establish a setting in which youth feel that they are receiving attention in a climate of trust and support, (b) provide a sense of community in order to encourage a sense of belonging, (c) use an assets approach that focuses on the resources possessed by youth, rather than on their deficits, (d) demonstrate respect for youth and treat them as adults—noting that a perceived sense of disrespect from peers and adults often results in feelings of alienation and marginalization, (e) maintain realistic yet high expectations for academic achievement and responsible behavior, (f) provide a holistic, comprehensive, multidimensional curriculum that responds to student needs, interests, and learning styles, (g) provide authentic, engaging learning experiences that connect school and work in meaningful ways, and (h) provide long-term support and follow-up services that seek to develop relationships so that young people will not feel that they will be abandoned.

Using Self-Determination to Enhance Transition

The concept of student-centered transition enhancement approaches is related to the concept of self-determination and reflects the belief that all individuals have the right to influence the directions pursued within their own lives. *Self-determination* has been defined as encompassing concepts such as free will, civil and human rights, freedom of choice, independence, personal agency, self-direction, and individual responsibility (National Research and Training Center, 2002).

Enhancing self-determination has been shown to improve the likelihood of a successful transition to adulthood (Wehmeyer & Schwartz, 1997). Self-determination does not, however, emerge successfully simply from being offered the opportunity to direct one's life. Individuals do not become effective users of self-determination simply because they have the necessary knowledge and skills; they also need to function in a context that is conducive to self-determination (Deci & Ryan, 2000). Wehmeyer, Kelchner, and Richards (1996) operationally defined self-determination as the creation of situations in which individuals are enabled to utilize knowledge and understanding of their personal characteristics, strengths, and limitations. This is a useful goal for individuals with developmental disabilities. In order to foster self-determination development, Wehmeyer et al. (1996) suggested that attention be given to (a) choice making, (b) exploration of possibilities, (c) reasonable risk taking, (d) problem solving, (e) self-advocacy, (f) development of self-esteem, (g) goal setting and planning, and (h) awareness and understanding of one's abilities and disabilities.

It is unjustifiable that youth and their families be held solely responsible for developing self-determination of youth with disabilities. Bremer, Kachgal, and Schoeller (2003) hold that the creation and maintenance of environments that will develop and maintain self-determination are also the responsibility of educators, employers, and institutions. Transition-enhancement initiatives should be provided in supportive environments to facilitate collaborative efforts between special education programs and career and technical education (CTE) programs. The following section addresses issues associated with CTE programs that serve persons with developmental disabilities.

Enhancing Career Paths for Persons With Developmental Disabilities

Persons with developmental disabilities face numerous barriers to employment, career development, and work-based learning (National Council on Disability, 2000). Unemployment after leaving school continues to be at unacceptably high levels for young adults with developmental disabilities (Blackorby & Wagner, 1996). Some initiatives that have been developed to address these issues employ comprehensive strategies that focus on enhancing both career growth and stability.

In support of such efforts, advocates for the enhancement of employment for persons with developmental disabilities are encouraged to review the following information from the Texas Council for Developmental Disabilities (2004). The Texas Council has posted an Internet Web page that contains a position statement affirming key issues related to the employment of persons with disabilities. The document is based on the assumption that people with developmental disabilities have the right to job training, employment at competitive wages, and career growth as lifelong learners. The Texas Council promotes (a) open employment opportunities, (b) lack of discrimination, and (c) lack of segregation. Also encouraged is the use of employment to (a) gain entry into the community, (b) instill a sense of being valued, and (c) receive wages and job benefits. These outcomes have been shown to be related to increased levels of independence and freedom from public support systems. The council's position statement concludes with the following list of affirmations:

1. Students with developmental disabilities should receive a sound foundation in their public school education from which to transition to a career path after graduation. Secondary education must provide a range of courses in career education (e.g., vocational skills, career and technology education, preparation for entry into postsecondary education, and community employment opportunities).

2. People with disabilities have the right to self-determination and choice in their career path, career goals, job placement or self-employment options, retention, advancement, and retirement rights.

3. People with disabilities should have access to an array of individualized, flexible, and coordinated support services, including assistive technology and natural supports, as long as necessary to obtain and maintain employment.

4. The employment needs of people with disabilities should be effectively addressed by a collaborative effort between businesses, professional organizations, and state and local governments.

5. All entities involved in statewide employment initiatives should disseminate information about civil rights laws that protect people with disabilities, about resources to support people with disabilities in the workplace, and about the tangible benefits that accompany employment of people with disabilities in the workforce. (p. 1)

These statements strongly support the belief that special educators should maintain, develop, and/or enhance effective working relationships with other educators and agency personnel who are involved in the career development of individuals. Their expertise and support are crucial to the effective career development of youth and young adults with developmental disabilities. In fact, there is strong evidence that career and technical education programs play a meaningful role in the reduction of drop-out rates of a wide range of at-risk learners, such as those with disabilities (Wonacott, 2002). Wonacott concluded that work-based learning opportunities offered primarily by CTE programs tend to have positive effects on a wide range of students' educational, attitudinal, and employment outcomes. To paraphrase Wonacott, special educators are encouraged to seek out ways for CTE programs to engage students with developmental disabilities in CTE's work-based learning opportunities and to increase engagement in learning among students with disabilities, both in schools and in out-of-school settings.

Assistive Technology (AT)

As mentioned earlier by the Texas Council for Developmental Disabilities (2004), persons with developmental disabilities should have access to the benefits of AT. Parette and McMahan (2002) noted that AT includes both devices and services. Parette and McMahan used the AT device definition provided by the IDEA Amendments of 1997:

> any item, piece of equipment, or product system . . . that is used to increase, maintain, or improve the functional capabilities of children with disabilities" (20 U.S.C. 1401[25]). Examples include: simple communication boards, sophisticated electronic communication devices, mobility aids, adapted keyboards for computers, and magnification devices or adapted computer screens. (p. 56)

Parette and McMahan (2002) used the following definition for an AT service: "any service that directly assists an individual with a disability in the selection, acquisition, or use of an assistive technology device (20 U.S.C. 1401[25]). Examples include physical therapy, occupational therapy, and speech therapy" (p. 56). They proposed four key questions that special education team members should ask family members regarding AT.

First, what are the family's expectations regarding the youth's independence? This can be analyzed by determining the following: (a) Will the AT be used in community settings outside the home? (b) What skills or commitment will be required of others in the community for the youth to be able to successfully use the assistive device? and (c) Does the family want the youth to perform routine tasks or do other family members expect to do daily tasks for that person?

Second, to what extent does the family want the youth to be accepted by others? This question is related to the tendency for families to be concerned that AT devices may draw attention to students or otherwise stigmatize them. Families with cultural or linguistic backgrounds that place high priority on the value of acceptance and blending into communities may be averse to using devices that attract attention. The following points may provide insight into these concerns: (a) some factors preclude using the AT outside the home, (b) AT may make an individual more self-conscious, and (c) other people may influence the feelings of parents and their children (Parette & McMahan, 2002).

Third, what are the family's expectations regarding the immediacy of the benefits of AT? If this issue is not considered and AT devices subsequently fail to live up to expectations, the AT devices may be abandoned prematurely. Several questions should be considered: (a) What will the AT device do for the recipient? (b) What actual benefits can be expected? (c) To what extent will benefits be immediate? (d) What training will be required to use the device(s) effectively? (e) How will the device(s) be paid for? (f) How often will the device(s) be used? (g) Will the user need assistance? and (h) If so, who will provide that assistance? (Parette & McMahan, 2002).

Fourth, what are the family's resource commitments for the implementation of AT devices? This becomes a crucial consideration when resource demands exceed the levels that families can, or will, commit to the AT devices. A family may be unwilling to use an AT device at home for any of a number of reasons. For example, AT devices may have undesirable effects on users, on home environments, or on other family members. These concerns illustrate the necessity of understanding a wide variety of factors that can influence the outcomes of the use of AT devices in school, home, and community settings for children (Parette & McMahan, 2002).

Once the preceding contextual issues have been adequately analyzed, myriad questions arise regarding the selection and implementation of actual AT devices and support services for children. Cormier (2001) has suggested that the development of an action plan can help to maximize the effectiveness of efforts to use AT. Such a plan would include information about (a) what equipment needs to be ordered, (b) what training will be needed, (c) who will conduct the training, (d) who will be a part of the training, and (e) what timeline for implementation is necessary.

The selection of AT devices is an important and potentially complex process, and an adequate evaluation of the range of devices is beyond the scope of this chapter. Chapters 10 and 20 offer more-specific AT content and recommendations. Readers are also encouraged to explore the many other sources of information that are available. For example, Cormier (2001) recommended the following Web sites, all of which contain information specifically related to the evaluation of AT resources:

1. Closing the Gap (includes a searchable database). http://www.closingthegap.com

2. National Center for Research on Evaluations, Standards, and Testing. http://www.cse.ucla.edu

3. Learning Disabilities and Attention Deficit Disorder Assessments. http://www.iser.com/steps.html

4. Trace Research and Development Center, University of Wisconsin. http://www.trace.wisc.edu/

5. Wisconsin Assistive Technology Initiative. http://www.wati.org

6. LD OnLine. http://www.ldonline.org

7. Assessing Assistive Technology Needs of Children with Disabilities article. http://www.nasdse.com/AAATE%20Paper.html

Those seeking additional resources will find extensive listings at the Web sites noted above, as well as in traditional library reference libraries and through Web-based search engines. Internet-based sources of information are likely to be much more up-to-date than printed resource materials.

Independent Living and Community Participation

Independent living is not only a philosophy; it is also a civil rights movement, aiming to ensure that individuals with developmental disabilities have access to the same rights, privileges, and choices that society at large enjoys. Full and equal participation in the community is the ultimate outcome of effective transition programs. The independent-living movement and philosophy are based on the belief that individuals with disabilities are the experts on their own lives, that they are qualified to participate meaningfully in determining what they need, and that they can successfully create solutions for situations.

The independent-living movement began in 1972 in Berkeley, California, when Ed Roberts, a University of California student with a severe disability, wanted the right to make his own decisions, have control over his life, and live more independently. Along with other students with disabilities, he founded the Physically Disabled Students' Program (PDSP), a holistic program that provided comprehensive services at a central location. This program fueled the creation of what is now known as Centers for Independent Living (CILs). Today there are hundreds of CILs across the United States that operate according to the same philosophy as the original PDSP.

Item	Rehabilitation Paradigm	Independent-Living Paradigm
Definition of problem	Physical impairment/lack of vocational skill	Dependence on professionals, relatives, etc.
Locus of problem	In individual	In environment
Solution to problem	Professional intervention by physician, physical therapist, occupational therapist, vocational rehab counselor, etc.	Peer counseling, advocacy self-help, consumer control, removal of barriers
Social role	Patient/client	Consumer

FIGURE 16.1. Comparison of Rehabilitation and Independent-Living Paradigms. Source: De Jong, G. (1979). Independent living: From social movement to analytic paradigm. *Archives of Physical Medicine and Rehabilitation, 60,* 435–446. Adapted with permission.

Gerben DeJong (1979) expanded the definition of independent living by creating the Independent Living (IL) model (see Figure 16.1). In this model, problems stem from environmental causes, including the rehabilitation process and the physical and social control mechanisms within society as a whole. Advocacy, peer counseling, self-help, consumer control, and barrier removal are trademarks of the IL paradigm.

Defining Community Participation

Community participation means full access to and involvement in all aspects of community life. It means having a voice and participating directly in decision making about issues that affect everyone in a community. Community participation provides opportunities to contribute individual strengths, time, and talents that directly affect the community where a person works, lives, and enjoys life. The National Organization on Disability (NOD, 2001) reported that people with disabilities spend significantly less time outside the home, in socializing and other activities, than people without disabilities. They tend to feel more isolated and participate in fewer community activities than their non-disabled counterparts. NOD suggests a number of venues for participation in the community that can strengthen involvement by individuals with disabilities (see Figure 16.2).

Youth With Disabilities and Self-Determination

The terms *self-determination* and *empowerment* are often used interchangeably within the disability-rights and independent-living movements. For youth with disabilities, the development of strong self-determination skills is essential for community participation and independence. According to Schalock (1996), self-determination is one of eight core principles that contribute to quality of life: (a) emotional well-being, (b) interpersonal relationships, (c) material well-being, (d) personal development, (e) physical well-being, (f) self-determination, (g) social inclusion, and (h) rights.

Social	Accessible and inclusive opportunities to become involved in community sports leagues, neighborhood watch programs, volunteering, etc.
Religious	Inclusive places of worship that provide physical, mental, and emotional access, a welcoming environment, respect for values and contributions individuals with disabilities can make
Political	Accessible voting locations, opportunities to volunteer, running for office
Emergency Preparedness	Development of community guidelines for assisting and evacuating individuals with disabilities during emergencies, universally designed protocols that address all disability categories
Economic	Access to a variety of employment opportunities, paying taxes, contributing through monetary giving, etc.

FIGURE 16.2. Venues for community participation by individuals with disabilities.

Schalock suggests that once an individual's basic needs are met, his or her life is further enhanced by the addition of community integration and participatory decision making. Wehmeyer and Schalock (2001) state that self-determination behavior has four essential characteristics—it is autonomous, self-regulated, psychologically empowered, and self-realized.

Barriers

Although research has identified components of best practice when planning for life after high school, individuals with disabilities continue to face significant barriers to success. A national survey conducted by the Harris Poll on behalf of the National Organization on Disability (Taylor, 2000) identifies social isolation and reduced community participation as critical issues. Although people with disabilities would like to be more involved in their communities, many feel their participation is not welcomed by community organizations. Compared to their non-disabled peers, individuals with disabilities responded with much higher rates of dissatisfaction regarding their level of community involvement and significantly higher rates of feeling isolated and left out of community activities. Many respondents reported that they were never invited to express their opinions on community issues. Reasons given for minimal involvement in their community included lack of encouragement by community organizations (54%), lack of income (53%), and lack of awareness about existing opportunities for involvement (46%). People without disabilities were substantially less likely to provide these same answers.

Connecting Independence, Community Participation, and Self-Determination

Community participation, independence, and self-determination form the foundation for successful community integration. Beginning in early childhood, youth with disabilities should be encouraged and supported to be good self-advocates.

Self-determination skills are essential for self-advocacy and for involvement in community activities. Youth with disabilities experience the same basic developmental needs and desires as their peers without disabilities, including the need and desire for friendships and personal relationships, involvement in recreational activities, success in academics and a career, and independence as an adult. Early self-awareness coupled with strong support and encouragement from family and professionals creates the building blocks for independence later in life.

Addressing Diversity in Special Education

Three specific issues arise when addressing the needs of students with disabilities from diverse socioeconomic and ethnic minority backgrounds who are also receiving special education services: the influence of poverty, overrepresentation of minority populations, and lack of cultural understanding and skill on the part of staff members who are providing services.

Outcomes for minority youth receiving special education are more likely to include school failure, school dropout, drug abuse, unemployment, academic failure, and increased incarceration rates (Duncan & Brooks-Gunn, 2000; Hughes et al., 2004; Hughes, Stenhjem, & Newkirk, in press; U.S. Department of Labor, 2002; Vartanian & Gleason, 1999). American Indian, Hispanic, and African American youth are more likely than their white or Asian American peers to attend schools that have limited resources and are located in impoverished neighborhoods (Annie E. Casey Foundation, 2003; Losen & Orfield, 2002).

The Influence of Poverty

Poverty creates numerous barriers to quality learning and successful outcomes for minority youth (Rylance, 1998). Affluent, same-age peers typically attain higher academic performance (Duncan & Brooks-Gunn, 2000; Eamon, 2001), and the dropout rate for impoverished youth is six times higher than that for youth from the top socioeconomic categories (Swanson, 2003). Seventy-nine percent of white students are expected to graduate from high school, compared to 33%, 36%, and 50% of American Indian, Hispanic, and African American students, respectively (Proctor & Dalaker, 2001). Poverty rates for whites are one third those of Hispanics, African Americans, American Indians, Alaska Natives, Asian Americans, and Pacific Islanders. These figures are strong evidence of the correlation between race and poverty.

Minority youth living in poverty are at much greater risk for exposure to unhealthy circumstances such as substance abuse, mental health problems, antisocial behavior, and involvement with the correctional system (Duncan, Duncan, & Strycker, 2002; Eamon, 2001). They are much less likely to volunteer, become actively involved in their communities, or participate in organized sports, extracurricular activities, or community groups. Learning through one-on-one mentoring and instruction is much less frequent among minority youth (Hughes et al., 2004; Ross & Roberts, 1999). Living in poverty has a negative effect on emotional development, resulting in high levels of anxiety, aggressiveness, hyperactivity, low self-esteem, lack of self-confidence, and poor peer acceptance (Checchi & Pravettoni, 2003; Ross & Roberts, 1999; Wilson & Portes, 1975). These factors represent critical need areas that affect post–high school outcomes for high-poverty minority youth with disabilities.

Overrepresentation of Minority Populations

The term *disproportionality* refers to problems resulting from situations in which students are misdiagnosed as disabled and placed in special education programs that they do not need (Meyers & Stenhjem, 2005). Researchers are now trying to better understand how conceptual, cultural, historical, and systemic issues interact to create imbalance (Patton, 1998). In addition to poverty, two other key issues are school cultures that are unsupportive with respect to issues of race, culture, and class (Hilliard, 2001; Steele, 1997) and definitions of disability and difference (Artiles & Trent, 1994).

Unsupportive school culture, stemming from the lack of cultural competence by school staff and administration, results from discriminatory policies, a deficiency of reciprocal and meaningful partnerships between families and schools, and inappropriate referral, assessment, evaluation, and placement in special education. The way disability is defined can also lead to significant differences in practice. If students learn differently from their peers, they may be labeled as having a learning disability, though in reality such learning differences may simply be a reflection of their culture. Although 35% of school-age children in the United States come from minority groups, cultural diversity is still seen as "different" or as a "deviance" from the dominant, white, middle-class culture. Under the No Child Left Behind Act of 2001, all children are held to high expectations for achievement and are required to take standardized tests in order to graduate—tests that are rarely culturally sensitive. Today approximately 1 in 10 students is referred for special education services, a figure that reflects a 35% increase in children served by IDEA over the last decade. Students of color are more often labeled as having a disability than their white same-age peers because of our schools' inability to separate social and cultural differences from disability issues (Meyers & Stenhjem, 2005).

Racism

Lack of understanding about how racism affects the lives of young adults can interfere with development of long-lasting relationships and resolution of long-term issues. Biased views about youth from racial minority backgrounds may influence the perspectives as well as the expectations of educators and affect those students' access to equal opportunities in school, extracurricular activities, and employment. According to the Poverty and Race Research Action Council (2004), entitlement, self-identity, and homework supervision issues tend to adversely affect young adults living in poverty (Figure 16.3).

Agencies that work with youth from minority ethnic backgrounds are affected by racial prejudice and bias as well. Rutstein (2001) observed:

Entitlement	A sense of entitlement is, on average, class-based. Parents living in poverty tend to have jobs without authority or autonomy, contributing to low self-worth and value. This assessment can be passed on to children through a tendency not to encourage them to negotiate and advocate for what they need, to instruct by giving directions rather than through dialogue, and to instill a fatalistic sense of what is possible both in and out of school.
Self-Concept	Poverty often results in a poorly developed sense of self that is formed early in life and reinforced every day at home. Although teachers may often be unaware of their own racial bias and prejudice, their expectations for racial-minority students may be lower than those for young people who come from more-affluent homes.
Homework Supervision	Supervision of homework often varies by social class. Parents in lower-income brackets tend to help their children through direct instruction, resulting in completion of homework but no skill development. Parents from lower socioeconomic classes may not possess the subject knowledge to ask helpful questions of their children.

FIGURE 16.3. Issues affecting minority youth living in poverty.

> Racism was not only promulgated by well-meaning teachers, but in the textbooks as well. . . . Writers of these books didn't try to prove scientifically . . . that people of color didn't matter in the scheme of things, that they were inherently inferior. The mere absence of any mention of black, Asian American, Native American and Latin American people's meaningful accomplishments reinforced the established notion that only whites were responsible, creative, intelligent and worthy of leadership. It is important to note that, in the main, today's political, judicial, economic, educational and religious leaders were exposed to these white-is-best indoctrinated teachers and textbooks when they went to school. (p. 23)

A Call to Action

High-poverty minority youth with disabilities are at a significant disadvantage in post–high school education, training, employment, and successful life outcomes. Jan Richter (2003), of Connect for Kids, noted in an interview that poverty is an accumulation of a great many very small deprivations. When asked what one thing would make the most difference for youth if it was changed, Turkheimer (cited in Richter, 2003) suggested improving the living conditions and circumstances of families living in poverty by removing the conditions that are typically present.

It is clear that educators need to monitor processes for referral of high-poverty minority youth to special education services. Staff and administrators must be trained to understand the implications of race combined with high poverty for a young person's performance and behavior in school. Finally, support systems, health care, affordable and decent housing, early childhood education services, and alternative programs, such as summer school and after-school programs, must be greatly improved. Legislation for the disability community, as well as for high-poverty minority communities, must overlap and complement each other in order to address the multiple issues and barriers that exist at the intersection of these two groups of people.

Service Learning

In its report titled *Learning in Deed: The Power of Service-Learning for American Schools*, the National Commission on Service-Learning defines *service learning* as an approach that brings together community service with academic study to enrich learning, teach civic responsibility, and strengthen communities through teaching and learning (Fiske, 2001). According to Fiske, the Corporation for National and Community Service (CNCS, Figure 16.4) includes the following components in its framework for service learning: (a) learning through active participation, (b) structured time for reflection, (c) skills and knowledge used in real-life situations, (d) learning beyond the classroom, and (e) a sense of caring for others. The connection between classroom content and personal development often links service learning to school and college courses, but it is also frequently used by community organizations. Service learning benefits participants in a variety of ways, among them development of social skills, participation in social, recreational, and career development opportunities, and a connection to and learning more about community resources. According to Fiske, service learning also encourages problem solving, higher-order thinking, and teamwork skills.

In general, authentic service learning experiences have some common characteristics including articulated and authentic learning goals, a response to genuine community needs, youth decision making, and analytical reflection. Service learning is more powerful when it includes positive, meaningful, and real contexts from which to learn; cooperative rather than competitive experiences; skill development related to teamwork, community involvement, and citizenship; complex problems in intricate settings, as opposed to simple problems in isolation; problem solving using knowledge and understanding of the specific community context and challenges; and powerful opportunities for development of critical-thinking skills.

Service learning is likely to be personally meaningful to participants because it takes place in the community, addresses a community issue or problem, and includes

---

- Service projects have clear educational goals that require the application of concepts, content, and skills from the academic disciplines and involve students in constructing their own knowledge.
- Projects engage students in challenging cognitive and developmental tasks.
- Teachers use assessment to enhance student learning and to document and evaluate how well they have met standards.
- Service tasks have clear goals, meet genuine community needs, and have significant consequences.
- Teachers use formative and summative evaluation in a systematic evaluation.
- Students have a voice in selecting, designing, implementing, and evaluating their service project.
- Diversity is valued and demonstrated by participants, practice, and outcomes.
- Service projects foster communication, interaction, and partnerships with the community.
- Students are prepared for all aspects of their work.
- Students reflect before, during, and after service. Reflection encourages critical thinking and is a central force in the design and fulfillment of curricular objectives.
- Multiple methods acknowledge, celebrate, and validate students' service work.

FIGURE 16.4. Essential elements of service learning.

hands-on and immediate learning. It is also likely to produce emotional consequences, challenge values as well as ideas, and support social, emotional, and cognitive learning and development (Eyler & Giles, 1999).

Inclusion of opportunities for service learning in both secondary and postsecondary academic settings expanded greatly in the 1990s. By 1999 almost one third of public schools (including close to half of all high schools) included service learning as part of their curriculum (Fiske, 2001). One reason for this growth is the immediate and powerful impact of service learning on young people and their personal development (Eyler & Giles, 1999). This link often provides a springboard for educational organizations to build strong partnerships with community-based organizations.

Students With Disabilities and Service Learning

Students with disabilities face many challenges after high school. Enrollment in post-secondary education programs among such students is significantly lower than that for the general population. Bureau of Labor data indicate that only 30.9% of individuals with disabilities aged 18–24 were employed, compared to 84.7% of those without disabilities (Houtenville & Daly, 2003). The National Longitudinal Transition Study found that 36% of students with disabilities drop out of high school and nearly 80% of those who are incarcerated are dropouts (Blackorby & Wagner, 1996). It was also reported that 46% of youth with a disability in corrections had a diagnosed learning disability and 45% had a diagnosed emotional disturbance.

Involvement of students with disabilities in integrated, high-quality service learning can change their own and others' perceptions of what youth with disabilities are capable of contributing. It can also build skills needed for employment and increase school and community engagement. A major goal of accessing the general education curriculum is the acquisition of a standard diploma. One challenge facing educators is the integration of transition experiences within the general curriculum. Yet academic achievement is now emphasized by the No Child Left Behind Act of 2001. Service learning provides a way to simultaneously meet academic, nonacademic, and transition requirements. While some examples of service learning are tied to special education, the strategy is underutilized and unfamiliar to many professionals who work with students with disabilities.

Service learning should be included in the goals and objectives of the individualized education program (IEP) because it provides meaningful life and career experiences, development of job skills, applied academics, and a hands-on method for students to identify their likes, dislikes, strengths, and need for accommodations. Service learning projects can be created and implemented in such a way as to meet many of the national standards for education. Educators should consider linking inclusive service learning activities to the evidence of learning required for each state's alternate educational assessment, as stated in the IDEA Amendments of 1997 (Kleinert et al., 2004). Schools can collaborate with an existing service learning project or develop their own projects in the school or the community, making connections with organizations such as local churches, elder-care facilities, and recreation centers.

Interagency Collaboration: A Proactive Model

In 1987 the State of Minnesota passed legislation mandating the formation of Community Transition Interagency Committees (CTICs). The intent of the legislation was to ensure that schools, community service providers, and families would work collaboratively to improve transition services for youth with disabilities, ages 14–21. The mandate was unfunded, which required CTICs to depend upon in-kind contributions from committee partners to do their work. Today, there are still more than 70 active CTICs.

CTICs have gone beyond the mandate to form collaborative partnerships, with a diverse membership that includes paraprofessionals, community-based transition program staff, centers for independent living, and local business owners. Most importantly, CTICs have taken an active role in recruiting and maintaining the involvement of youth with disabilities and their family members as formal members of the committee. They have developed and implemented a variety of resources and training opportunities, including resource guides, informational booklets, resource fairs, training on transition and related services, community, recreational, and independent living programs, and partnerships with local and state employers. CTICs have been a vital component in creating transition systems with integrity, respect, and proactive methodologies that address the real needs of youth with disabilities and their families. Legislation legitimated the need for essential partners to work together rather than separately. Experience, dedication, and positive outcomes have replaced legislation as the key motivators for continuing to work together. Even today, members of CTICs report that the best and most relevant information on transition planning is acquired through working in concert with other CTIC members toward the shared goal of improving transition services for youth with disabilities.

Conclusion

Proactive, youth-driven planning is critical to successful outcomes for youth with disabilities as they leave high school and enter adult life. Transition programming is a comprehensive, holistic planning process that must take into account the entire spectrum of an individual's life. In addition to mandated transition planning requirements through the Individuals with Disabilities Act of 1990 and IDEA Amendments of 2004, a number of other elements can enhance youths' skills, abilities, and outcomes, among them cultural competence, involvement in service learning activities, active community involvement, and independent living. A best-practice model of coordination has been presented to provide an illustration of effective collaboration.

Glossary

Assistive technology (AT)—Any item, piece of equipment, or product system used to increase, maintain, or improve the functional capabilities of disabled children. The term may also describe a specific service that assists a disabled person in the selection, acquisition, or use of an assistive technology device.

Disproportionality—Problems resulting from situations in which students from low socioeconomic backgrounds are misdiagnosed as disabled and placed in special education programs that are not appropriate to their circumstances or abilities.

Independent living—A philosophy that subscribes to the idea that disabled individuals are the experts on their own lives and choices. An active civil rights movement ensures that disabled persons have access to the same rights and opportunities enjoyed by society at large.

Self-determination—Encompasses concepts such as free will, civil and human rights, freedom of choice, independence, personal agency, self-direction, and individual responsibility.

Service learning—A procedural approach that joins community service with curricular study to enrich understanding, teach civic responsibility, and strengthen communities through teaching and learning.

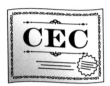

Knowledge and Skills for Entry-Level Special Education Teachers of Students With Developmental Disabilities Standards Addressed in This Chapter

Principle 1: Foundations

DD1K4   Trends and practices in the field of developmental disabilities.

Principle 2: Development and Characteristics of Learners

DD2K4   Factors that influence overrepresentation of culturally/linguistically diverse individuals.

Principle 7: Instructional Planning

DD7K1   Model career/vocational transition programs for individuals with developmental disabilities, including career/vocational transition.

DD7S1   Plan instruction for independent functional life skills relevant to the community, personal living, sexuality, and employment.

Principle 10: Collaboration

DD10K1   Services, networks, and organizations for individuals with developmental disabilities.

DD10S1   Collaborate with team members to plan transition to adulthood that encourages full community participation.

Web Site Resources

Disabilities Studies and Services Center

http://www.dssc.org/

> Programs that meet the unique information, technical assistance, training, and research needs of professionals and that serve to improve the lives of infants, toddlers, children, youth, and adults with disabilities and their families. DSSC administers the National Information Center for Children and Youth with Disabilities (NICHCY), the Federal Resource Center for Special Education (FRC), the Comprehensive School Reform Demonstration (CSRD) Alignment Study, and the Family Center on Technology and Disability. DSSC is a partner in the National Collaborative on Workforce and Disability for Youth (NCWD/Y) and runs the Healthy & Ready to Work (HRTW) National Center.

Indiana Institute on Disability and Community: Transition From School to Adult Life

http://www.iidc.indiana.edu/cclc/transition1.htm

> Sections focus on a number of pertinent topics.

National Business and Disability Council

http://www.nbdc.com/

> Web site claiming that it is the leading national corporate resource for hiring, working with, and marketing to people with disabilities. Seeks to integrate people with disabilities

into the workplace with companies seeking to reach them in the consumer marketplace. Provides links to numerous Web-based resources, newsletters, and cost-free access to résumé posting for job searchers with disabilities.

National Center for Secondary Education and Transition
http://ici1.umn.edu/ncset/

A wide variety of disability support–related resources. Four of the sections focus on upcoming conferences, national standards, resources related to IDEA, and a component developed by and for teens with disabilities.

National Centers for Career and Technical Education
http://www.nccte.org/

Partners of the National Centers for Career and Technical Education. Web site, http://www.nccte.org:8765/query.html?qt=disability, accesses numerous disability-related publications.

Parent Advocacy for Coalition for Educational Rights
http://www.pacer.org/tatra/tatra.htm

Web site's component titled "Technical Assistance on Transition and the Rehabilitation Act" is a valuable resource for parents and educators alike.

Wisconsin Department of Public Instruction: Transition Services for Students With Disabilities
http://dpi.wi.gov/sped/transition.html

A department of public instruction (DPI) state discretionary project that offers a comprehensive approach to providing transition services in the state of Wisconsin. Useful information on such topics as assistive technology and transition issues, as well as links to other useful transition-related Web sites.

References

Annie E. Casey Foundation. (2003). *Kids count pocket guide—American Indian youth: State level measures of child well-being from the 2000 Census.* Retrieved November 22, 2004, from http://www.aecf.org/kidscount/pubs/american_indian_pocket_guide_2004.pdf

Artiles, A. J., & Trent, S. C. (1994). Overrepresentation of minority students in special education: A continuing debate. *Journal of Special Education, 27,* 410–437.

Blackorby, J., & Wagner, M. (1996). Longitudinal outcomes for youth with disabilities: Findings from the National Longitudinal Study. *Exceptional Children, 62,* 399–419.

Bremer, C. D., Kachgal, M., & Schoeller, K. (2003). *Self-determination: Supporting successful transition.* Retrieved November 15, 2005, from http://ncset.org/publications/printsource.asp?id=962

Certo, N. J., Mautz, D., Pumpian, I., Smallery, K., Wade, H., Noyes, D., Luecking, R., Wechsler, L., & Batterman, N. (2003). A review and discussion of a model for seamless transition to adulthood. *Education and Training in Developmental Disabilities, 38,* 3–17.

Checchi, D., & Pravettoni, G. (2003). *Self-esteem and educational attainment* (Working paper). Milan: Università degli Studi di Milano, Dipartimento di Economia Politica e Aziendale. Retrieved November 30, 2004, from http://www.economia.unimi.it/pubb/wp169.pdf

Cormier, C. (2001). *Points to consider for an assistive technology evaluation.* ConnSENSE Bulletin. Retrieved November 15, 2005, from http://www.connsensebulletin.com/cormiernov2.html

Deci, E. L., & Ryan, R. M. (2000). The "what" and "why" of goal pursuits: Human need and the self-determination of behavior. *Psychological Inquiry, 11,* 227–268.

DeJong, G. (1979). Independent living: From social movement to analytic paradigm. *Archives of Physical Medicine and Rehabilitation, 60,* 435–446.

Duncan, G. J., & Brooks-Gunn, J. (2000). Family poverty, welfare reform, and child development. *Child Development, 71,* 188–196.

Duncan, S. C., Duncan, T. E., & Strycker, L. A. (2002). A multilevel analysis of neighborhood context and youth alcohol and drug problems. *Prevention Science, 3,* 125–133.

Eamon, M. K. (2001). Poverty, parenting, peer, and neighborhood influences on young adolescent antisocial behavior. *Journal of Social Services Research, 28,* 1–23.

Eyler, J., & Giles, D. (1999). *Where's the learning in service-learning?* San Francisco: Jossey-Bass.

Fiske, E. B. (2001). *Learning in deed: The power of service-learning for American schools.* Battle Creek, MI: W. K. Kellogg Foundation.

Hilliard, A. G. (2001). Race, identity, hegemony, and education: What do we need to know now? In W. H. Watkins, J. H. Lewis, & V. Chou (Eds.), *Race and education: The roles of history and society in educating African American students* (pp. 7–25). Needham Heights, MA: Allyn & Bacon.

Houtonville, A. J., & Daly, M. C. (2003). Employment declines among people with disabilities. In D. C. Stapleton & R. V. Burkhauser (Eds.), *The decline of employment of people with disabilities: A policy puzzle* (pp. 87–124). Kalamazoo, MI: Updike Institute.

Hughes, C., Stenhjem, P., & Newkirk, R. (in press). *The influence of poverty on minority youth in special education.* Minneapolis: National Center on Secondary Education and Transition, University of Minnesota.

Hughes, C., Wehby, J. H., Carter, E. W., Plank, D., Wilson, L., Johnson, S., et al. (2004). Summer activities of youth with high-incidence disabilities from high-poverty backgrounds. *Career Development for Exceptional Individuals, 27,* 27–42.

Individuals with Disabilities Education Act of 1990, 20 U.S.C. § 1400 *et seq.* (1990) (amended 1997).

Individuals with Disabilities Education Improvement Act of 2004, 118 Stat. 2647. (2004).

Kerka, S. (2003). Alternatives for at-risk and out-of-school youth. *ERIC Digest, 248.* (EDO-CE-03-248). Retrieved May 10, 2005, from www.cete.org/acve/docs/dig248.pdf

Kleinert, H., McGregor, V., Durbin, M., Blandford, T., Jones, K., Owens, J., et al. (2004). Service-learning opportunities that include students with moderate and severe disabilities. *Teaching Exceptional Children, 37*(2), 28–34.

Losen, D. J., & Orfield, G. (2002). *Racial inequality in special education.* Cambridge, MA: Harvard Education Press.

Meyers, G., & Stenhjem, P. (2005). *The relationship between poverty and overrepresentation of minority students in special education* (Issue brief). Minneapolis: National Center on Secondary Education and Transition.

National Council on Disability. (2000). *Transition and post-school outcomes for youth with disabilities: Closing the gaps to postsecondary education and employment.* Washington, DC: Author.

National Organization on Disability. (2001). *Barriers to community participation.* Excerpt from the 2000 NOD/Harris Survey on Community Participation. Retrieved May 15, 2005, from http://www.nod.org/index.cfm?fuseaction=page.viewPage&pageID=1430&nodeID=1&FeatureID=119&redirected=1&CFID=1879720&CFTOKEN=5721503

National Research and Training Center. (2002). *Self-determination framework for people with psychiatric disabilities.* Chicago: Author. Retrieved July 18, 2002, from http://www.psych.uic.edu/UICNRTC/sdframework.pdf

Neubert, D. A. (2000). *Transition assessment practices for students ages 18–21 with significant disabilities* (OCO Fact Sheet 3). College Park: On-Campus Outreach, Department of Special Education, University of Maryland. Retrieved May 20, 2005, from www.education.umn.edu/oco

Neubert, D. A. (2003). The role of assessment in the transition to adult life process for students with disabilities. *Exceptionality, 11*(2), 63–75.

No Child Left Behind Act of 2001, 20 U.S.C. 6301 *et seq.* (2002).

Parent, W., Kregel, J., & Johnson, A. (1996). Consumer satisfaction: A survey of individuals with disabilities who receive supported employment services. *Focus on Autism and Other Developmental Disabilities, 11,* 207–221.

Parette, P., & McMahan, G. A. (2002). What should we expect from assistive technology? *Teaching Exceptional Children, 35*(1), 56–61.

Patton, J. M. (1998). The disproportionate representation of African Americans in special education: Looking behind the curtain for understanding and solutions. *Journal of Special Education, 32*(1), 25–31.

Poverty and Race Research Action Council. (2004). Schools and the achievement gap: A symposium. *Poverty and Race, 13*(5), 1–2, 7–10.

Proctor, B. D., & Dalaker, J. (2001). *Poverty in the United States: 2001* (U.S. Census Bureau, Current Population Reports, P60-219). Washington, DC: U.S. Government Printing Office.

Richter, J. (2003). *New thinking on children, poverty, and IQ.* Retrieved November 15, 2005, from http://www.connectforkids.org/node/516?tn=lc/ra

Ross, D. P., & Roberts, P. (1999). *Income and child well-being: A new perspective on the poverty debate.* Retrieved November 30, 2004, from http://www.ccsd.ca/pubs/inckids/

Rumberger, R. W., & Larson, K. A. (1998). Student mobility and the increased risk of high school dropout. *American Journal of Education, 107,* 1–35.

Rutstein, N. (2001). *The racial conditioning of our children: Ending psychological genocide in schools.* Albion, MI: National Resource Center for the Healing of Racism.

Rylance, B. J. (1998). Predictors of post–high school employment for youth identified as severely emotionally disturbed. *Journal of Special Education, 32,* 184–192.

Schalock, R. L. (1996). Reconsidering the conceptualization and measurement of quality of life. In R. L. Schalock (Ed.), *Quality of life: Conceptualization and measurement* (pp. 123–139). Washington, DC: American Association on Mental Retardation.

Skinner, R., & Chapman, C. (1999). *Service-learning and community service in K–12 public schools. Statistics in Brief.* Retrieved November 21, 2005, from http://nces.ed.gov/pubs99/1999043.pdf

Smith, M. D., & Phillipen, L. R. (2005). Community integration and supported employment. In D. Zager (Ed.), *Autism spectrum disorders: Identification, education, and treatment* (pp. 493–514). Mahwah, NJ: Erlbaum.

Sowers, J., McLean, D., & Owens, C. (2002). Self-directed employment for people with development disabilities: Issues, characteristics, and illustrations. *Journal of Disability Policy Studies, 13*(2), 97–104.

Steele, C. M. (1997). A threat in the air: How stereotypes shape intellectual identity and performance. *American Psychologist, 52,* 613–629.

Swanson, C. B. (2003). *Who graduates? Who doesn't? A statistical portrait of public high school graduation, Class of 2001.* Washington, DC: Urban Institute.

Taylor, H. (2000). *Many people with disabilities feel isolated, left out of their communities, and would like to participate more.* Harris Poll, #34. July 5, 2000. Retrieved May 15, 2005, from http://www.harrisinteractive.com/harris_poll/ index.asp?PID=97

Texas Council for Developmental Disabilities. (2004). *Employment: Position statement.* Retrieved May 20, 2005, from www.txddc.state.tx.us/council/position/employ.asp

U.S. Department of Labor. (2002). *Report on the youth labor force.* Washington, DC: Author.

Vartanian, T. P., & Gleason, P. M. (1999). Do neighborhood conditions affect school dropout and college graduation rates? *Journal of Socio-Economics, 28,* 21–41.

Wehman, P., Targett, P., West, M., & Kregel, J. (2005). Productive work and employment for persons with traumatic brain injury: What have we learned after years? *Journal of Head Trauma Rehabilitation, 20,* 115–127.

Wehmeyer, M., Kelchner, K., & Richards, S. (1996). Essential characteristics of self-determination behavior in individuals with mental retardation. *American Journal on Mental Retardation, 100,* 632–642.

Wehmeyer, M., & Schwartz, M. (1997). Self-determination and positive adult outcomes: A follow-up study of youth with mental retardation or learning disabilities. *Exceptional Children, 63,* 245–255.

Wehmeyer, M. L., & Schalock, R. (2001). Self-determination and quality of life: Implications for special education services and supports. *Focus on Exceptional Children, 33*(8), 1–16.

Wilson, K. L., & Portes, A. (1975). The educational attainment process: Results from a national sample. *American Journal of Sociology, 81,* 343–363.

Wonacott, M. E. (2002). Dropouts and career and technical education. *ERIC Clearinghouse on Adult, Career, and Vocational Education, 23,* 1–2. Retrieved May 21, 2005, from www.cete.org/acve/docs/mr00038.pdf

SECTION 6

COMMUNICATION

17

Using Technology to Enhance and Augment Communication of Persons With Developmental Disabilities

Ann R. Beck

Summary

This chapter reviews what is known regarding children's attitudes toward their peers with developmental disabilities that result in complex communication needs and the use of augmentative and alternative communication (AAC). The chapter also discusses factors that do and do not appear to influence peers' attitudes, as well as an intervention program designed to alter peers' attitudes toward children who use AAC. Implications for intervention targeted at altering attitudes are examined. Additionally, the chapter defines characteristics of beginning communicators and reviews evidenced-based suggestions for when AAC interventions should be initiated for beginning communicators, the responses that should be taught first, how the environment should be modified or adapted, strategies for teaching comprehension and production skills, and the types of technology that should be considered for beginning communicators with developmental disabilities.

Learning Outcomes

After reading this chapter, you should be able to:

- Understand definitions pertaining to AAC systems.

- Understand the importance of peer attitudes toward children with developmental disabilities who use AAC.

- Design interventions targeted at increasing positive attitudes toward children who use AAC.

- Define the characteristics of a beginning communicator.

- Recognize when AAC interventions should be initiated with beginning communicators and demonstrate knowledge of behaviors to be taught and strategies for teaching those behaviors.

Introduction

Approximately 2 million people in the United States who have complex communication needs rely on *augmentative and alternative communication (AAC) systems*, and in the schools, between 0.3% and 1% of children use AAC systems (Glennen & Decoste, 1997). The most common causes of complex communication needs in children are autism, cerebral palsy, mental retardation, and developmental apraxia of speech (Beukelman & Mirenda, 1998). Beukelman and Mirenda indicate that while the etiologies of communication disorders vary, children who use AAC all have the unifying characteristic of being unable to communicate functionally using natural skills and therefore requiring the use of assistive technology, specifically AAC.

According to the American Speech-Language-Hearing Association (ASHA, 2002), "AAC is, foremost, a set of procedures and processes by which an individual's communication skills (i.e., production as well as comprehension) can be maximized for functional and effective communication" (p. 98). That AAC is a set of procedures and processes emphasizes the fact that it should be viewed not as a single component or device but rather as a set of components or an overall system for communicating.

ASHA (2002) further describes AAC as either supplementing or replacing natural speech with aided and/or unaided symbols. An *aided symbol* is one that requires some type of transmission device (e.g., a picture, a communication board, an electronic voice-output device), and an *unaided symbol* is one that requires nothing in addition to the body to produce it (e.g., speech, gestures, signs). Other terms defined by ASHA include strategies, which are ways in which symbols can be communicated most effectively and efficiently, and techniques, which are methods of transmitting messages.

Communicative Competence

For children to utilize AAC systems optimally, they must develop *communicative competence*, or "the quality of being functionally adequate in daily communication or of having sufficient knowledge, judgment, and skills to communicate" (Light, 1989, p. 138). Communicative competence might best be thought of as a "socially constructed concept, rather than a 'dispositional' characteristic of individuals" (Peck, 1989, p. 12). Peck indicates that such a viewpoint underscores the transactional nature of the development of children's communicative competence and thereby the importance of the child's environment. Elements of a child's communicative environment that play critical roles in development are the partners with whom the child communicates and the attitudes and interaction styles of those partners. Therefore, best practices indicate that when implementing AAC systems with children who have complex communication needs, educators must take into account not only which AAC components and intervention strategies are most appropriate for a given child but also the knowledge, skills, and attitudes of the communication partners in the child's environment (Beukelman & Mirenda, 1998).

Attitudes

Attitudes have been defined as "a psychological tendency that is expressed by evaluating a particular entity with some degree of favor or disfavor" (Eagly & Chaiken, 1993, p. 1). In this discussion, the "entity" is a child with complex communication needs who possesses stimuli that elicit evaluative responses from his or her peers. Three-factor theories of attitude indicate that evaluative responding can be done on an emotional basis, a behavioral basis, and/or a cognitive basis (Eagly & Chaiken, 1993). Emotional responding is determined by the feelings the child elicits in his or her peers. The behavioral aspect deals with how peers act, or intend to act, toward the child who uses AAC. The cognitive aspect consists of the ideas or thoughts that peers have about the child with complex communication needs. Evaluative responding on the basis of any or all of these components can cause attitudes to be more or less positive.

Two-factor theories of attitude have also been proposed, in which attitudinal responses are the results of immediate, automatically activated affective responses and of controlled, deliberative, cognitive processes (Fazio, 1990; Reeder, 1993). Behavioral reactions may then be an outcome of the combination of emotional and cognitive evaluations. In a two-factor framework, attitudinal reactions to a child who uses AAC would first involve immediate emotional responses to the child. These affective responses might then be altered by controlled cognitive evaluations of the child that considered such variables as the cause of the disability, the type and severity of the disability, and how the disability influenced a child's ability to perform certain tasks. The outcome of emotional and cognitive evaluations would be key determinants of peers' behavioral responses toward the child who used AAC.

Attitudes, however, should not be thought of as synonymous with behaviors. Other variables, such as motivational incentives and cultural norms, also influence behaviors. Despite the fact that attitudes and behaviors can differ, the importance of stated attitudes should not be minimized. Hymel (1986) indicated that people typically try to maintain consistency between their attitudes and their observed behaviors. Indeed, Hymel found that grade-school children's previous attitudes about a peer influenced the way they interpreted that peer's behavior. If a child was liked, then peers tended to credit the child for positive behaviors performed and not to blame him or her for negative behaviors performed. When children viewed the behavior of peers they did not like, however, this positive bias was not apparent. Hymel stated that "such interpretive bias . . . operates in the service of maintaining affectively congruent perceptions of others" (p. 438). This interpretive bias results in a cycle in which, once a child is disliked, the interpretation of subsequent behaviors continues to "perpetuate negative attitudes toward that child" (p. 439).

In addition, strong social pressure exists for people to act in a manner consistent with their expressed attitudes. Most people will seek to interact with others who hold attitudes similar to their own so that they are encouraged, if not actually forced, to act in a manner consistent with their attitudes (Kraus, 1995). Furthermore, according to Kraus, not only will attitudes influence with whom individuals choose to interact, but they will also influence the situations that people choose to enter. Kraus concludes that the process of influencing situations that individuals elect to enter is perhaps "one of the most powerful ways in which attitudes influence behavior" (p. 71).

Children's Attitudes Toward AAC

A series of experiments has been conducted to investigate the dimensions and determinants of children's attitudes toward their peers who use AAC (Beck, Bock, Thompson, Bowman, & Robbins, 2006; Beck, Bock, Thompson, & Kosuwan, 2002; Beck & Dennis, 1996; Beck, Fritz, Keller, & Dennis, 2000; Beck, Kingsbury, Neff, & Dennis, 2000; Blockberger, Armstrong, O'Connor, & Freeman, 1993; Dudek, Beck, & Thompson, 2006; Lilienfeld & Alant, 2002). All of the studies on children's attitudes that are cited above and that will be reviewed in this chapter were well-designed group studies in which participants were randomly assigned to conditions. Schlosser and Raghavendra (2003) proposed two hierarchies for ranking the certainty of evidence from efficacy research in AAC. One of these was for research with participants who were not disabled. Well-designed group studies using random assignment were ranked relatively high in this hierarchy. Evidence from the studies of children's attitudes reviewed in this chapter can therefore be regarded as having a fairly high degree of certainty.

Factors That Influence Children's Attitudes Toward Peers Who Use AAC

Children's Gender, Age, and Familiarity With Children With Disabilities

A consistent finding has been that the self-reported attitudes of girls toward a peer who uses AAC are more positive than are those of boys (Beck et al., 2002; Beck & Dennis, 1996; Beck, Fritz, et al., 2000; Beck, Kingsbury, et al., 2000; Blockberger et al., 1993; Dudek et al., 2006; press; Lilienfeld & Alant, 2002). Another consistent finding has been that children who are familiar with children who have disabilities tend to report more-positive attitudes toward a peer who uses AAC than do children who are not familiar with children with disabilities (Beck & Dennis, 1996; Beck, Fritz, et al., 2000; Beck, Kingsbury, et al., 2000; Blockberger et al., 1993).

The positive influence of familiarity, however, was tempered by the results of a two-part study conducted by Beck, Fritz, et al. (2000). In the first part, a reliable and valid scale for assessing children's attitudes toward peers who use AAC (the Assessment of Attitudes Toward AAC, or the AATAAC) was developed. The participants in this study were children in grades 1, 3, and 5 who were not familiar with children with disabilities. The second part investigated attitudes of children in grades 1, 3, and 5 who were familiar with children with disabilities toward peers who use AAC. In the first part, no developmental trends in attitude were found across age groups. Developmental trends were, however, apparent in attitudes for children in the second part. The younger children were more positive toward a peer who used AAC than were the older children.

Additionally, Beck, Fritz, et al. (2000) reported a significant grade-by-gender interaction. The positive nature of boys' attitude scores fell consistently across grade levels, and that of girls' dipped from grades 1 to 3 and rose again in grade 5. While previous researchers had concluded that boys' attitudes were not as influenced by exposure to children with disabilities as were girls' attitudes (Beck & Dennis, 1996), Beck, Fritz, et al. (2000) suggested that the attitudes of boys who were exposed to children with disabilities actually became more negative across grade levels.

Length of Augmented Message

Beck, Kingsbury, et al. (2000) conducted a study aimed at determining how the length of a message influenced the attitudes of children in grades 3 and 5 toward children who use AAC. Half of their participants in both grades were familiar with children with disabilities, and half were not. Their results indicated that phrase length had little influence on the reported attitudes of children who were familiar with children with disabilities. For the children who were unfamiliar with children with disabilities, however, those who heard the long message reported more-positive attitudes toward children who use AAC than did those who heard the short message. These findings were true for children in both grade 3 and grade 5.

Presence or Absence of Voice Output

Lilienfeld and Alant (2002) found that the attitudes of children who were unfamiliar with peers with severe disabilities and who were in grades 6 and 7 (i.e., ages 11 through 13) were positively influenced by the presence of voice output. The attitudes of participants who watched a video of a peer communicating with another peer using an electronic AAC device with voice output were more positive than those of participants who watched the same video with the voice output edited out.

Factors That Do Not Influence Children's Attitudes Toward Peers Who Use AAC

Type of AAC Technique

The influence of AAC technique type on children's attitudes has been investigated in several studies (i.e., Beck et al., 2002; Beck & Dennis, 1996; Beck, Fritz, et al., 2000; Blockberger et al., 1993; Dudek et al., 2006). No study found that children's attitudes toward their peers who use AAC were influenced by the type of AAC techniques investigated (i.e., unaided, non-electronic communication board, digitized voice-output device, synthesized voice-output device, static screen device, or dynamic screen device). Additionally, Beck et al. (2002) documented that how responsive a child was when using an AAC device (i.e., responding immediately and needing no prompts versus delayed responding that necessitated prompts) did not influence other children's attitudes toward the child who used AAC.

Type of Vocabulary Programmed on a Device

Beck et al. (2006) investigated the influence of formal versus informal vocabulary on children's attitudes toward their peers who use AAC. Children with complex communication needs who are preliterate often depend upon another person to choose their words for them. Typically this person is an adult. Various clinicians have emphasized the importance of selecting vocabulary for a child that sounds like his or her peers rather than like the adults in his or her environment (Beukelman & Mirenda, 1998; Downing, 1999). While this is a clinically logical suggestion, the results of Beck et al.'s study found no influence of informal, childlike vocabulary over formal, adultlike vocabulary on peers' attitudes.

Summary of Attitude Studies and Implications for Intervention

From the cumulative research to date, variables that have been found to influence children's attitudes toward peers who use AAC are primarily ones that are intrinsic to the children (i.e., gender, age, level of familiarity). Variables that are specific to the child who uses AAC (i.e., type of device used, vocabulary programmed on device, responsiveness of the child) do not appear to influence peers' attitudes toward the child.

Cognitive social psychologists indicate that young children tend to have global emotional responses of great intensity to people and events in their life (Weiner & Graham, 1984). As their cognitive skills develop, children become more capable of differentiating their emotional responses, and the overall intensity of a single emotional reaction decreases. Weiner and Graham found that by the mean age of 10.4 years, children had attained sufficient cognitive levels to consider causes and attributional cues that would allow them to mediate their emotional responses. The findings of the attitude studies reviewed herein suggest that grade-school-age children's attitudinal reactions toward peers who use AAC are based primarily on emotions derived from past experience and on dispositional characteristics of the children themselves rather than on children's ongoing cognitive evaluations of the attributional characteristics of each individual child who uses AAC.

The findings of two studies (Beck, Kingsbury, et al., 2000; Lilienfeld & Alant, 2002) appear, at first, to contradict the idea that children's attitudes tend not to be influenced by attributional characteristics of the child who uses AAC and/or his or her AAC system. In Beck, Kingsbury, et al.'s (2000) study, children who were unfamiliar with children with disabilities were more positive toward a child who communicated with augmented messages of two to four words in length as compared to a child who communicated with augmented messages one word in length. Similarly, in Lilienfeld and Alant's (2002) study, children who were unfamiliar with peers with severe disabilities reported more-positive attitudes toward a peer when he communicated with voice output than when he communicated without it.

Beck, Kingsbury, et al. (2000) indicated that while their participants appeared to have the cognitive levels needed to consider attributional cues, the level of familiarity with children with disabilities was also a critical factor. They speculated that children who have little-to-no experience with peers with disabilities might not have the same preconceived notions concerning children who use AAC as would be held by children who are familiar with children with disabilities. Children who are unfamiliar with peers who have disabilities (e.g., the unfamiliar peers in both Beck, Kingsbury, et al., 2002 and Lilienfeld & Alant, 2002) therefore might react to a child who uses AAC without the same emotional responses experienced by the familiar children. A less intense or more neutral emotional reaction could allow children to make greater use of cognitively processed information. Additionally, Lilienfeld and Alant's (2002) participants were of middle-school age. Older children are likely to possess more-developed cognitive skills than children in grade school, a factor that could also aid their cognitive processing of specific characteristics of a peer who used AAC.

Children's attitudes toward their peers who use AAC appear to be driven primarily by their emotional reactions based on dispositional factors (e.g., gender, age) and experience with children with complex communication needs. By later- to middle grade-school age, children might be able to utilize cognitive evaluations to alter their attitudes, unless their emotional responses have been strengthened by interactions with children who use AAC. These statements emphasize the importance of planning and implementing inclusionary activities that allow children to understand and respect individual differences and to increase the positive nature of their emotional reactions to children who use AAC. The evidence also suggests that educators need to be especially attentive to boys' attitudes and how they are influenced by various inclusion experiences.

Another implication of the research on children's attitudes is that programming two- to four-word phrases on a voice-output device might be a factor that could increase the positive nature of children's attitudes during initial interactions with a peer who uses AAC (Beck, Kingsbury, et al., 2000; Lilienfeld & Alant, 2002). Additionally, Beck et al. (2006) indicate that, while informal vocabulary terms were not found to result in more-positive attitudes than formal terms, decisions regarding the type of vocabulary that is included on a child's AAC device should be made carefully, with input from both the child who uses AAC and his or her peers. Educators must also conduct careful follow-up evaluations of peers' reactions to the type of vocabulary being communicated by a child who uses AAC to ensure that the child's AAC system is improving the quantity and quality of the child's social interactions rather than creating unintentional barriers for that child.

Final implications for intervention suggested by the data on children's attitudes are that type of AAC technology used by a child (Beck et al., 2002; Beck & Dennis, 1996; Beck, Fritz, et al., 2000; Blockberger et al., 1993; Dudek et al., 2006) and whether or not a child needs occasional prompts to access the desired message (Beck et al., 2002) do not appear to influence peers' attitudes. The good news in this for educators is that no particular type of AAC technique seems to be favored by communication partners over another. As long as a child can use an AAC technique to communicate competently, even if it takes a few prompts to do so, that child's initial acceptance should not be influenced by whether he or she is using a communication board or a high-tech voice-output AAC device.

An Intervention to Alter Children's Attitudes

The majority of studies regarding children's attitudes toward their peers who use AAC have aimed to investigate the determinants and dimensions of children's attitudes. Only one study to date (Beck & Fritz-Verticchio, 2003) has investigated the effectiveness of an intervention program designed to alter children's attitudes toward their peers who use AAC. Beck and Fritz-Verticchio reported that when children are introduced to peers who use AAC, a first step educators often take is to inform children about what AAC is, why a child would use it, and what to expect when a child does use it. Educators might do this by simply telling children about AAC through verbal descriptions and videotapes, or they might design activities that allow children to role-play being nonspeaking.

Beck and Fritz-Verticchio (2003) investigated which approach—provision of information regarding AAC in combination with a role-playing experience or provision of information alone—was more effective in increasing children's positive attitudes toward peers who use AAC. Because, as they reasoned, educators would be most likely to use informational techniques when first introducing a child with complex communication needs to his or her peers, their participants were children who were not familiar with children with disabilities and included equal numbers of boys and girls in grades 2, 4, and 6. Results indicated that the attitudes of the oldest children were more influenced by the role-playing experience than were those of the younger children and that boys' attitudes were more positively influenced by role-playing than were girls'.

For educators, the implications of Beck and Fritz-Verticchio's (2003) findings are that when introducing a child with complex communication to his or her peers, including opportunities for hands-on experiences simulating being nonspeaking as well as descriptions of AAC in informational sessions would be more likely to predispose peers to have positive attitudes toward the child who used AAC than would information sessions where only passive descriptions (e.g., verbal descriptions and explanations, videos) were provided. This appears to be especially true for older grade-school-aged children and for boys.

Despite the positive findings of their research, Beck and Fritz-Verticchio (2003) stated that "given the unique communication modes used by children who use AAC, the possibility exists that in addition to general information about AAC and an experience role-playing being nonspeaking, peers would need explicit instructions on how to communicate with children who use AAC in order to engage in appropriate social interactions with them" (p. 57). Examples of behaviors that could be taught to communication partners to increase the appropriateness of social interactions with early intentional communicators are (a) using expectant pauses to encourage initiations, (b) recognizing a peer's behavior as an attempt at communication and interpreting the intent of that behavior, and (c) reacting to the interpreted intent of the behavior in an appropriate manner (Siegel & Cress, 2002).

Enhancing Beginning Communicators' Use of AAC Systems

Who Are Beginning Communicators?

According to Beukelman and Mirenda (1998), a *beginning communicator* who is a candidate for AAC can be a person of any age range "with one or more developmental disabilities such as cerebral palsy, autism, dual sensory impairments, mental retardation, or developmental apraxia of speech" (p. 265). Beukelman and Mirenda add that beginning communicators rely primarily on nonsymbolic modes of communication (e.g., gestures, eye gaze, body language) and are just learning to use unaided symbols, non-electronic communication displays, or simple technology to communicate basic messages for participation and communication. Romski, Sevcik, Hyatt, and Cheslock (2002) stated that while the ages and etiologies of beginning communicators vary, "it is likely that beginning communicators have disabilities that have been present since birth because these individuals may have encountered difficulty with spoken communication from the onset of development" (p. 5).

When Should AAC Be Initiated?

In the past, the implementation of AAC systems with children with developmental disabilities was often delayed. Several primary reasons existed for this delay. One reason was that it was believed that certain cognitive prerequisites (e.g., evidence of object permanence, means–ends, cause–effect) had to be developed before a child could benefit from AAC. Assessments were then focused on determining a child's eligibility for AAC interventions based on whether or not he or she had developed these skills (Beukelman & Mirenda, 1998).

Research has not supported the belief that cognitive prerequisites for AAC use exist. Indeed, the appropriate use of AAC in naturalistic environments has been found to help a child develop some of the cognitive prerequisites that were once thought to be necessary before AAC could be implemented (Siegel & Cress, 2002). Best practice for AAC assessments today does not seek to determine a child's eligibility for AAC interventions, but rather to determine how best to utilize the child's existing behaviors to increase communication skills. As Romski et al. (2002) state, "The task . . . is not determining eligibility for AAC but rather ascertaining where along the communication continuum an individual will begin the AAC intervention process" (p. 1).

Another reason the implementation of AAC systems was often delayed in the past was the belief that use of AAC systems would impede the development of natural speech skills. Millar, Light, and Schlosser (2000; as cited in Schlosser, 2003) completed a synthesis of research efforts regarding the effects of AAC on the development of natural speech. Twenty-four studies met their criteria for inclusion and had evidence that was at a suggestive level of certainty. Most of the studies used participants who had mental retardation or autism. The results of their review suggest that the natural speech skills of most of the participants actually improved after AAC interventions were implemented.

Today it is widely acknowledged that early intervention for severe communication disorders, such as might be characteristic of children with motor impairments, Down syndrome, and autism, is critical (Siegel & Cress, 2002). It is in the first years of life that communication skills are developed and that children learn that they can have an effect on their environment through the use of intentional communication. If children are not given the opportunity to exert some control over their environment, they may learn a sense of helplessness that will be detrimental to their overall development (Borysenko, 1987). For children with developmental disabilities resulting in complex communication needs, the timely introduction of AAC systems can help prevent helplessness from developing. As Siegel and Cress indicate, "specialized AAC techniques are necessary to enhance early communication and AAC strategies can be viewed as part of a continuum that can benefit diverse learners" (p. 26).

What Responses Should Be Taught

Teaching Requesting and Rejecting

A review of the literature indicates that typically developing children first use their prelinguistic acts to reject, request, and comment (Sigafoos, Drasgow, & Schlosser, 2003). Sigafoos et al. state, however, that children with developmental delays who are beginning communicators often do not develop all the communicative functions that their typically developing peers do. Indeed, beginning communicators who do not speak often use their prelinguistic behaviors to protest or reject and to request objects and actions, but not to comment. An evidence-based implication, then, is that educators should teach beginning communicators appropriate methods of rejecting and requesting before teaching other communicative functions.

The first step in teaching appropriate rejecting and requesting to a child with developmental disabilities who is a beginning communicator is to assess the behaviors the child currently uses to convey these communicative intents and the conditions under which the child uses them (Sigafoos et al., 2003). Existing behaviors should then be shaped into more-appropriate communicative behaviors that would serve the same function. An example of teaching appropriate rejecting would be that if a child strikes out to indicate that he wants to quit an activity, that child could instead be taught to activate a simple switch programmed with the message "I'm all done." An example of teaching an appropriate request would be if a child grabbed items that he wanted during an art activity, a picture of "want" could be used to block his access to the item. When the child touched the picture of "want," the educator could say "Oh, you want _____" as she handed the desired object to the child.

The above examples demonstrate several important, empirically supported procedures for teaching rejecting and requesting. First, these behaviors should be taught in the natural environment when the child is motivated to produce them. In teaching requesting, this can be done by identifying items that are reinforcing to the child and by then modifying the child's environment to encourage the child to request those reinforcing items. Several ways to structure this are to block a child's access to a desired object, interrupt a behavior chain, omit a needed object when setting up a preferred activity, delay assistance, and present a wrong item (Sigafoos & Mirenda, 2002). In teaching rejecting, the educator can present nonpreferred items to the child or can take advantage of times when the child spontaneously rejects items or events.

All instructional opportunities for teaching rejecting and requesting must end with the child producing the desired response, even if the educator must prompt the response (Sigafoos et al., 2003). Additionally, Sigafoos et al. indicate that during early stages of teaching, each appropriate request response should be reinforced immediately, while the old response is ignored or extinguished. Similarly, each new appropriate rejecting behavior should be negatively reinforced (i.e., whatever the child is rejecting should be removed or discontinued).

Another intervention approach that is used to teach children with autism and with other developmental disabilities to initiate requests is the *Picture Exchange Communication System* (PECS; Bondy & Frost, 1994). PECS has been supported by a large body of anecdotal literature (Mirenda, 2001) as well as by several controlled empirical investigations (Charlop-Christy, Carpenter, Le, LeBlanc, & Kellet, 2002; Hanley, 2003). Before initiating PECS, a reinforcer inventory must be conducted for the child. Once items that are reinforcing for a child are identified, pictures of those items are created. The PECS protocol, as specified by Bondy and Frost (1994), consists of six training phases that begin with Phase 1, teaching a child to exchange a picture for a tangible positive reinforcer, in which two interventionists are required. One, the communication partner, sits at the table across from the child; the other is behind the child. The picture of the desired item is on the table between the communication partner and the child. The item is either held by the communication partner or placed behind the picture, closer to the communication partner than to the child. No verbal prompts are given to the child. If the child initiates an inappropriate request (i.e., anything other than picking up the picture and releasing it into the communication partner's outstretched hand) or does not initiate any request, the interventionist who is behind the child physically prompts the child to produce the picture exchange. The communication partner then says, "You want _____" and gives the desired item to the child. PECS Phase 2 builds persistence in communication by requiring the child to travel some limited distance to get the picture and to exchange it with the communication partner, who eventually turns away from the child so that the child has to get his or her attention in order to complete the exchange. Phase 3 requires the child to discriminate between two or more pictures. Phases 4 through 6 progressively teach the child to build sentences using a sentence strip beginning with "I want," to respond to direct questioning, and to comment.

Teaching Other Communication Functions

Light, Parsons, and Drager (2002) indicate that while requesting and rejecting allow a child with developmental disabilities to communicate wants and needs, which is one of the purposes of communicative interactions, three other purposes also exist (developing social closeness, exchanging information, and fulfilling social etiquette routines). Social closeness is a communicative function that typically developing infants learn early when they use their vocalizations to draw caretakers into contact with them and to maintain that contact. Light et al. believe that social closeness is a critical communicative function for children who use AAC that allows them to develop meaningful relationships with other people. They state, however, that it is often overlooked by educators and other interventionists. One simple suggestion that these authors offer to improve the social closeness aspect of aided communication is to reduce the gaze-shifting demands made on a child with developmental disabilities by making sure that the partner, the activity, and the AAC system are all close to each other.

Evidence-based practice suggests that communicative functions of requesting and rejecting should be the first communicative functions taught to children with developmental disabilities who are beginning communicators. Educators, however, need to be sure that intervention programs do not stop with simply teaching requesting and rejecting skills that allow a child to express his or her basic needs and wants. Children with complex communication needs also should be provided with AAC system components and support that enable them to develop skills for fulfilling all the purposes of communication.

Supporting Comprehension

Environmental supports that have been empirically validated for use with children with developmental disabilities and that are likely to be implemented with children who use AAC are visual schedules (Bopp, Brown, & Mirenda, 2004). Visual schedules support the comprehension of language by clarifying the "sequence of activities, steps, or rules that apply to specific individuals and routines" (Bopp et al., 2004, p. 14). Visual schedules can take a number of forms, from object boxes to picture boards to more-complex calendar schedules. Regardless of the form taken, the primary purpose of visual strategies is to allow a child to better understand and predict upcoming activities, so that problem behaviors are reduced and the child's independence is increased (Bopp et al. 2004).

Depending on the individual, visual schedules might be needed to help the child transition between activities or within activities. A child might also have difficulty understanding the overall rules for functioning within a specific context. In this case, a visual schedule can be created to specify the rules for that context (Bopp et al., 2004). Bopp et al. indicate that a functional assessment can assist in identifying the specific type of visual schedule that would be most helpful for an individual child.

Interventions to Promote Children's Production and Comprehension Skills

AAC is defined by ASHA (2002) as a way of maximizing an individual's production and comprehension of language. The majority of AAC interventions, however, are focused on increasing a person's production skills (Harris & Reichle, 2004). Two aided AAC intervention approaches have been designed to teach production while simultaneously enhancing comprehension: Aided Language Stimulation (ALS; Goossens', Crain, & Elder, 1992) and System for Augmenting Language (SAL; Romski & Sevcik, 1996). Both of these intervention approaches teach children with complex communication needs to use their AAC systems functionally within natural environments, and both involve facilitators modeling the use of AAC systems (Harwood, Warren, & Yoder, 2002). In ALS the facilitator highlights a desired symbol by either touching it or using a flashlight cue while also speaking the corresponding word or message. The children are then prompted to produce the message. Similarly, in SAL the facilitator models the use of a graphic means of communication. In SAL, however, a voice-output communication aid (VOCA) is always used and the voice output that occurs when a symbol label is selected is considered a critical element of the intervention (Romski & Sevcik, 1996). Additionally, SAL does not uses explicit prompts for production but encourages production through modeling (Harwood et al., 2002).

The use of ALS has been supported primarily by anecdotal reports and case studies (Harwood et al., 2002) and by one single-subject multiple-probe experiment (Harris & Reichle, 2004). The use of SAL was supported by a 2-year longitudinal study of 13 children and youth with moderate to severe mental retardation (Romski & Sevcik, 1996). As Harwood et al. (2002) point out, however, the ability to generalize these results is restricted because of the small number of participants. Both ALS and SAL deserve further study as intervention procedures that "have the potential for teaching the meanings behind graphic symbols while simultaneously promoting functional communication and language development" (Harwood et al., p. 83).

Use of Technology

One question many educators have when planning AAC interventions for children **343** with developmental disabilities who are beginning communicators concerns the type of technology that should be employed. Romski et al. (2002) reported that manual signs and simple communication boards were the primary AAC modes cited in the general AAC literature as being used with beginning communicators. They speculated that this was true because of the belief that "beginning communicators could not benefit from using more sophisticated technologies" (p. 15).

Contrary to this belief, Romski et al. (2002) argued that beginning communicators could benefit from the use of electronic VOCAs. In an earlier longitudinal study, Romski and Sevcik (1996) successfully taught beginning communicators with moderate or severe developmental disabilities to communicate using VOCAs programmed with abstract symbols. Additionally, Mirenda, Wilt, and Carson (2000) did a 5-year retrospective study of 170 students with autism who had received either VOCAs or computer and software technologies. They determined that for these students, both types of technology appeared to support participation in education, "especially in the areas of writing, expressive communication, and social interaction with peers" (p. 13). Further support for the use of VOCAs was found by Schepis, Reid, Behrmann, and Sutton (1998), who conducted a single-subject study in which they evaluated the effects of a VOCA on the communicative behaviors of young children with autism. Their results indicated that the use of a VOCA was effective in increasing communicative interactions for the children in their study.

Sigafoos et al. (2003) indicated that there does not appear to be one AAC mode or system that can be recommended as best for beginning communicators. They reported that some experts have argued for the advantage of manual signs over other forms of technology because the production of some signs is a fairly simple motoric response that can be easily prompted by educators and because signs are portable. The disadvantage of signs, however, is that they are less likely to be understood by unfamiliar communication partners than are aided AAC components such as pictures and VOCAs. Sigafoos et al. stated that determining the best mode of communication may include consideration of factors such as cost, acquisition, generalization, maintenance, and the personal preference of the child who will be using AAC and his or her family.

The results of an alternating-treatment single-subject design conducted by Stoner, Bock, and Beck (2004) support the importance of considering individual preference and performance. Their study compared the ability of 6 preschool students with developmental delays and no functional communication system to learn to use and to generalize the use of PECS and a VOCA. Stoner et al. used the PECS teaching protocol, as specified by Bondy and Frost (1994), to teach each child a set of five desired items using either picture exchange or activation of a VOCA. Within a relatively short time frame, all of Stoner et al.'s participants learned to initiate a request spontaneously using both a VOCA and pictures and showed some evidence of maintaining these behaviors during generalization probes in the classroom.

The results of Stoner et al.'s (2004) generalization probes, however, indicated that while all children learned to use both a VOCA and a picture exchange to some degree, 5 of them appeared to have a preference for one type of communication modality over the other. This finding emphasizes the importance of considering the individual child and of remembering that all communicators use more than one way to express themselves. Children appear to be able to learn at least two functional modes of communication at the same time. Teaching a child several means of communication, then, allows the child to select from an array of options when given the opportunity to choose how to express himself or herself. It also allows interventionists to offer a child a means of communication that might be more advantageous than another means in a specific situation.

Light, Drager, and Nemser (2004) also stressed the importance of considering the child's preferences. They indicated that "it seems reasonable to argue that early intervention is more likely to be effective if AAC systems are highly appealing to young children with complex communication needs" (p. 137). They stated further, however, that the aided AAC systems that are currently available do not seem to hold strong appeal either for children who have complex communication needs or for their typically developing peers. By comparing the design of AAC devices with popular toys, these authors created a list of design features, such as color, materials, shape, size and weight, movement and actions, sounds and voices, lights, and themes, that could be altered to increase children's interest in AAC devices. They also suggested that if children are allowed to have input into the appearance and configuration of their AAC systems, their overall sense of empowerment, ownership of their AAC system, and motivation to use AAC can be increased.

Conclusion

Utilizing AAC to enhance the communication of children with developmental disabilities entails much more than simply deciding upon a piece of technology and teaching children to use it to express their wants and needs. Best practices indicate that AAC should be viewed as a set of processes and procedures, or as an entire system of communication, that is taught within the child's natural environment. Research-based evidence suggests that there is no one best AAC technology mode for all children. The preferences, skills, and needs of each child and his or her family must be considered when deciding upon the various components of an AAC system for that child. For all children with complex communication needs, however, AAC interventions should be started as early in life as possible to give the children every opportunity available to learn to communicate and to exert appropriate control over their environment. Furthermore, the children who will serve as communication partners must be educated to not only accept but also respect individual differences. Only when all people learn such acceptance and respect and attitudinal barriers no longer exist can the appropriate use of technology result in the goal of full inclusion in life for individuals who use AAC.

Glossary

Aided symbol—One that requires some type of transmission device (e.g., a picture, a communication board, an electronic voice-output device) in addition to the communicator's body.

Attitudes—"A psychological tendency that is expressed by evaluating a particular entity with some degree of favor or disfavor" (Eagly & Chaiken, 1993, p. 1).

Augmentative and alternative communication (AAC)—"AAC is, foremost, a set of procedures and processes by which an individual's communication skills (i.e., production as well as comprehension) can be maximized for functional and effective communication" (ASHA, 2002, p. 98).

Augmentative and alternative communication system—An integrated group of components, including the symbols, aids, strategies, and techniques used by individuals to enhance communication. The system serves to supplement any gestural, spoken, and/or written communication abilities (ASHA, 1991, p. 10).

Beginning communicator—A candidate for AAC of any age range "with one or more developmental disabilities such as cerebral palsy, autism, dual sensory impairments, mental retardation, or developmental apraxia of speech" who relies primarily on nonsymbolic modes of communication (Beukelman & Mirenda, 1998, p. 265).

Communicative competence—"The quality of being functionally adequate in daily communication or of having sufficient knowledge, judgment, and skills to communicate" (Light, 1989, p. 138).

Strategies—Ways symbols can be communicated most effectively and efficiently (ASHA, 2002, p. 98).

Techniques—Methods of transmitting augmented messages (ASHA, 2002, p. 98).

Unaided symbol—One that requires nothing in addition to the body to produce (e.g., speech, gestures, signs; ASHA, 2002, p. 98).

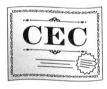

Knowledge and Skills for Entry-Level Special Education Teachers of Students With Developmental Disabilities Standards Addressed in This Chapter

Principle 4: Instructional Strategies
DD4K1   Specialized materials for individuals with developmental disabilities.

Principle 5: Learning Environments/Social Interaction
DD5S4   Structure the physical environment to provide optimal learning for individuals with developmental disabilities.

Principle 6: Language
DD6S1   Plan instruction on the use of alternative and augmentative communication systems.

Web Site Resources

AAC Intervention.Com
http://aacintervention.com/#AAC

Helpful tips about implementing AAC with children who are nonspeaking, as well as information about creating overlays for early intervention.

AAC Rehabilitation Engineering Research Centers (RERC)
http://www.aac-rerc.com/

Information about AAC funding and research, as well as links to vendor Web sites and universities.

Assistive Technology Resources for Children and Adults With Special Needs
http://www.closingthegap.com/

Information on AT hardware and software and on current issues concerning AAC and AT.

International Society for Augmentative and Alternative Communication (ISAAC)
http://www.isaac-online.org/

Links to AAC resources, publications, events, and conferences.

References

American Speech-Language-Hearing Association. (1991). Report: Augmentative and alternative communication. *ASHA, 33* (Suppl. 5), 9–12.

American Speech-Language-Hearing Association. (2002). Augmentative and alternative communication: Knowledge and skills for service delivery. *ASHA* (Suppl. 22), 97–106.

Beck, A., Bock, S., Thompson, J. R., Bowman, L., & Robbins, S. (2006). Is awesome really awesome? How the inclusion of information terms on an AAC device influences children's attitudes towards peers who use AAC. *Research in Developmental Disabilities, 27,* 56–69.

Beck, A., Bock, S., Thompson, J., & Kosuwan, K. (2002). The influence of communicative competence and AAC technique on children's attitudes toward a peer who uses AAC. *Augmentative and Alternative Communication, 18,* 217–227.

Beck, A., & Dennis, M. (1996). Attitudes of children toward a similar-aged child who uses augmentative communication. *Augmentative and Alternative Communication, 12,* 78–87.

Beck, A., Fritz, H., Keller, A., & Dennis, M. (2000). Attitudes of school-aged children toward their peers who use AAC. *Augmentative and Alternative Communication, 16,* 13–26.

Beck, A., & Fritz-Verticchio, H. (2003). The influence of information and role-playing experiences on children's attitudes toward peers who use AAC. *American Journal of Speech-Language Pathology, 12,* 51–60.

Beck, A., Kingsbury, K., Neff, A., & Dennis, M. (2000). The influence of length of augmented message on children's attitudes toward peers who use AAC. *Augmentative and Alternative Communication, 16,* 239–249.

Beukelman, D., & Mirenda, P. (1998). *Augmentative and alternative communication: Management of severe communication disorders in children and adults* (2nd ed.). Baltimore: Brookes.

Blockberger, S., Armstrong, R., O'Connor, A., & Freeman, R. (1993). Children's attitudes toward a nonspeaking child using various augmentative and alternative communication techniques. *Augmentative and Alternative Communication, 9,* 243–250.

Bondy, A., & Frost, L. (1994). The Picture Exchange Communication System. *Focus on Autistic Behavior, 9,* 1–9.

Bopp, K., Brown, K., & Mirenda, P. (2004). Speech-language pathologists' roles in the delivery of positive behavior support for individuals with developmental disabilities. *American Journal of Speech-Language Pathology, 13,* 5–19.

Borysenko, J. (1987). *Minding the body, mending the mind.* New York: Bantam.

Charlop-Christy, M., Carpenter, M., Le, L., LeBlanc, L., & Kellet, K. (2002). Using the Picture Exchange Communication System (PECS) with children with autism: Assessment of PECS acquisition, speech, social-communicative behavior, and problem behavior. *Journal of Applied Behavior Analysis, 35,* 213–231.

Downing, J. (1999). *Teaching communication skills to students with severe disabilities.* Baltimore: Brookes.

Dudek, K., Beck, A., & Thompson, J. (2006). The influence of AAC device type, dynamic vs. static screen, on peer attitudes. *Journal of Special Education Technology, 21,* 17–27.

Eagly, A., & Chaiken, S. (1993). *The psychology of attitudes.* Fort Worth: Harcourt Brace Jovanovich College Publishers.

Fazio, R. (1990). Multiple processes by which attitudes guide behaviors: The MODE model as an integrated framework. In L. Berkowitz (Ed.), *Advances in experimental social psychology* (Vol. 23, pp. 75–108). New York: Academic Press.

Glennen, S., & DeCoste, D. (1997). *Handbook of augmentative and alternative communication.* San Diego, CA: Singular.

Goossens', C., Crain, S., & Elder, R. (1992). *Engineering the preschool environment for interactive, symbolic communication.* Birmingham, AL: Southeast Augmentative Communication Conference Publications.

Hanley, L. (2003). *Teaching the Picture Exchange Communication System: The learning and generalization of functional communication.* Unpublished master's thesis, Illinois State University, Normal, Illinois.

Harris, M., & Reichle, J. (2004). The impact of aided language stimulation on symbol comprehension and production in children with moderate cognitive disabilities. *American Journal of Speech-Language Pathology, 13,* 155–167.

Harwood, K., Warren, S., & Yoder, P. (2002). The importance of responsivity in developing contingent exchanges with beginning communicators. In J. Reichle, D. Beukelman, & J. Light (Eds.), *Exemplary practices for beginning communicators: Implications for AAC* (pp. 59–95). Baltimore: Brookes.

Hymel, S. (1986). Interpretations of peer behavior: Affective bias in childhood and adolescence. *Child Development, 57,* 431–445.

Kraus, S. (1995). Attitudes and the prediction of behavior: A meta-analysis of the empirical literature. *Personality and Social Psychology Bulletin, 21,* 58–75.

Light, J. (1989). Toward a definition of communicative competence for individuals using augmentative and alternative communication systems. *Augmentative and Alternative Communication, 5,* 137–144.

Light, J., Drager, K., & Nemser, J. (2004). Enhancing the appeal of AAC technologies for young children: Lessons from toy manufacturers. *Augmentative and Alternative Communication, 20,* 137–149.

Light, J., Parsons, A., & Drager, K. (2002). There's more to life than cookies. In J. Reichle, D. Beukelman, & J. Light (Eds.), *Exemplary practices for beginning communicators: Implications for AAC* (pp. 187–218). Baltimore: Brookes.

Lilienfeld, M., & Alant, E. (2002). Attitudes of children toward an unfamiliar peer using an AAC device with and without voice output. *Augmentative and Alternative Communication, 18,* 91–101.

Mirenda, P. (2001). Autism, augmentative communication, and assistive technology: What do we really know? *Focus on Autism and Other Developmental Disabilities, 16,* 141–151.

Mirenda, P., Wilt, D., & Carson, P. (2000). A retrospective analysis of technology use patterns of students with autism over a five-year period. *Journal of Special Education Technology, 15,* 5–16.

Peck, C. (1989). Assessment of social communicative competence: Evaluating environments. *Seminars in Speech and Language, 10,* 1–15.

Reeder, G. (1993). Trait-behavior relations and dispositional inference. *Personality and Social Psychology Bulletin, 19,* 586–593.

Romski, M., & Sevcik, R. (1996). *Breaking the speech barrier: Language development through augmented means.* Baltimore: Brookes.

Romski, M., Sevcik, R., Hyatt, A., & Cheslock, M. (2002). A continuum of AAC language intervention strategies for beginning communicators. In J. Reichle, D. Beukelman, & J. Light (Eds.), *Exemplary practices for beginning communicators: Implications for AAC* (pp. 1–23). Baltimore: Brookes.

Schepis, M., Reid, D., Behrmann, M., & Sutton, K. (1998). Increasing communicative interactions of young children with autism using a voice output communication aid and naturalistic teaching. *Journal of Applied Behavior Analysis, 31,* 561–578.

Schlosser, R. (2003). Effects of AAC on natural speech development. In R. Schlosser (Ed.), *The efficacy of augmentative and alternative communication: Toward evidence-based practice* (pp. 403–425). Amsterdam: Academic Press.

Schlosser, R., & Raghavendra, P. (2003). Toward evidence-based practice in AAC. In R. Schlosser (Ed.), *The efficacy of augmentative and alternative communication: Toward evidence-based practice* (pp. 259–297). Amsterdam: Academic Press.

Siegel, E., & Cress, C. (2002). Overview of the emergence of early AAC behaviors. In J. Reichle, D. Beukelman, & J. Light (Eds.), *Exemplary practices for beginning communicators: Implications for AAC* (pp. 25–57). Baltimore: Brookes.

Sigafoos, J., Drasgow, E., & Schlosser, R. (2003). Strategies for beginning communicators. In R. Schlosser (Ed.), *The efficacy of augmentative and alternative communication: Toward evidence-based practice* (pp. 323–346). Amsterdam: Academic Press.

Sigafoos, J., & Mirenda, P. (2002). Strengthening communicative behaviors for gaining access to desired items and activities. In J. Reichle, D. Beukelman, & J. Light (Eds.), *Exemplary practices for beginning communicators: Implications for AAC* (pp. 123–156). Baltimore: Brookes.

Stoner, J., Bock, S., & Beck, A. (2004). *A comparison of high and low technology methods for increasing functional communication.* Poster session presented at Conference on Developmental Disabilities, Las Vegas, Nevada.

Weiner, B., & Graham, S. (1984). An attributional approach to emotional development. In C. Izard, J. Kagan, & R. Zajonc (Eds.), *Emotions, cognition, and behavior* (pp. 167–191). Cambridge, UK: Cambridge University Press.

18

Language and ASD:

The Impact on the Classroom

Julia B. Stoner

Summary

This chapter presents an overview of communication of children with autism spectrum disorder (ASD), describes specific, effective interventions that have been supported by research, describes the difficulty children with ASD experience with horizontal transitions, provides a framework to facilitate transitions, and provides guidelines for communicating with parents of children with ASD. Children with ASD represent a heterogeneous population, which includes a wide variety of communication abilities and deficits. The interventions described here are supported by empirical research, but it should be noted that they are not implemented in isolation. Children with ASD require a comprehensive behavioral and instructional program, tailored to the needs of the individual child and addressing all areas of deficits, including communication. Knowledge and implementation of effective classroom strategies that target communication, one of the core deficits of ASD, are essential when educating children with ASD.

Learning Outcomes

After reading this chapter, you should be able to:

- Understand definitions of language comprehension, language production, and pragmatic language.

- Understand the effect of ASD on communication skills.

- Describe research-based interventions for each of the three areas of communication: language comprehension, language production, and pragmatic language.

- Understand the difficulty that children with ASD experience with horizontal transitions.

- Identify effective interventions that assist with transitions.

- Understand the heightened need for communication with parents of children with ASD.

- Identify effective means of communicating with parents of children with ASD.

Autism Spectrum Disorder and Communication

The number of children with ASD who are served in special education has increased significantly in recent years. It is important to note that the prevalence rate of ASD is now estimated to be 1 out of every 166 children. This increase is not occurring across all disabilities. Prevalence estimates, based on data supplied by the Office of Special Education (OSE), are *underestimates* because of reporting inconsistencies across states and lack of reporting of those children with ASD who are not receiving special education services (Newschaffer, Falb, & Gurney, 2005). The field of special education has been significantly affected in terms of training educators and providing services.

ASD is a complicated disorder, and the adage "When you know *one* child with autism, you know *one* child with autism" is appropriate. Wide heterogeneity exists among the cognitive, behavioral, and communication skills of children with ASD (see Chap 5 for a specific description of the disorders that fall under the autism spectrum). Inappropriate behavior is frequently noted—but there is a strong interrelationship between communication deficits and behavior. Numerous studies have reported that as many as 75% to 80% of behavior problems may have a communicative function and that improvements in communication skills result in decreased behavior problems (Derby et al., 1992; Iwata & Pace, 1994; Matson, Benavidez, Compton, Paclawskyj, & Baglio, 1996). Consequently, communication deficits seen in children with ASD are not treated separately from behavioral and instructional issues. Since much of the "maladaptive" behavior in children with ASD is viewed as communicative, many interventions assess the functions of the maladaptive behavior (Frea, Koegel, & Koegel, 1993). Once the function of the behavior is determined, intervention focuses on providing the student with communication that has the same function as the inappropriate behavior. Therefore, it is essential that special educators understand behavioral interventions as well as effective communication strategies.

All aspects of communication, both language comprehension and language production, are affected by ASD. Language skills of children with ASD have been described as heterogeneous, and the variability is significant (Kuder, 2003). Approximately 50% of children with ASD will never communicate through verbal means (Prizant, 1983). Others will have the ability to speak and may evidence only minor characteristics of ASD in their speech production, such as unusual prosody. Some children will have significant difficulty with the comprehension of auditory language and may be assisted with visual supports, while others may evidence mild difficulty with language comprehension. The pragmatic component of language, which encompasses how individuals interact with others, is consistently impaired, although at varying levels. Even with the wide variance of abilities among individuals with ASD, there are certain impairments that are common.

The *Diagnostic and Statistical Manual of Mental Disorders* (DSM-IV; American Psychiatric Association, 1994) and the *International Classification of Mental and Behavioral Disorders* (ICD-10; World Health Organization, 1993) specify that a diagnosis of autism must include impairments in social interaction, repetitive patterns of behaviors, interests, and activities, and communication impairments. The communication impairments are frequently described as *qualitative* in nature (Kuder, 2003). At its most basic, this term implies that the communication of children with ASD is not simply delayed but is substantially *different* from that of typically developing children.

Communication is a dynamic process involving three primary components: (a) language comprehension, or receptive language, (b) language production, or expressive language, and (c) pragmatic language, or language use. When an individual has adequate skills in all these areas, that individual is perceived as a competent communicator, one who (a) can intentionally communicate, both verbally and nonverbally, a message, (b) can repair that message if it is misunderstood by a listener, (c) can use language in various social settings, and (d) is also an effective listener capable of maintaining the ebb and flow of communication (Kuder, 2003). Competent communication is dynamic, complex, and necessary for independence. Children with ASD can have difficulty with each of the three components of language.

This chapter describes each of the language components, identifies the difficulties children with autism experience in each of these areas, and reviews some effective interventions. It is important to understand that while each of these components can be discussed separately, they are all interrelated, with one component affecting the others. The wide variance of language skills of children under the autism spectrum makes it imperative that the classroom teacher understand each individual student's strengths and areas of difficulty, implement interventions based on the individual student's needs, and continually assess the effectiveness of the interventions, making adjustments as necessary.

The National Academy of Science (NAS) created a subcommittee, the National Research Council (NRC), to identify educational practices that effectively serve young children with ASD. The committee reported that both comprehensive programs and individually based interventions can be effective (National Research Council, 2001). Additionally, the committee identified program components that were common to effective interventions: (a) early intervention, (b) intense intervention, (c) active involvement of families, (d) staff training, (e) use of a highly systematic curriculum, (f) establishment of a highly supportive environment, (g) provision of individual intervention, and (h) support of transition services. These guidelines are offered before discussion of specific interventions because they reinforce the need for a comprehensive education program for children with ASD.

Prelinguistic Language Development and ASD

Abnormalities in language development are often the major reason parents seek medical help (DeGiacomo & Fombonne, 1998; Rogers & DiLalla, 1990). Some young children evidence abnormalities in prelinguistic language development. The development of joint attention, joint reference, and joint action is established before 12 months of age. This critical development lays the foundation for the infant to engage in an exchange with another individual, to share information, and it is the basis for social communication. Numerous research studies have indicated that the frequency of prelinguistic intentional communication predicts later language levels in children with disabilities (Mundy, Kasari, Sigman, & Ruskin, 1995; Smith & von Tetzchner, 1986; Yoder & Warren, 1999).

Joint attention means that the infant can follow movements of the caregiver, attend to utterances addressed to her or him, respond to pointing by the caregiver, and engage in pointing and showing an object to a caregiver. The development of joint attention is crucial to the ability to name and establish a topic for a conversation, or a communicative exchange (Owens, 2001).

Joint reference occurs when two individuals share a common focus on an object or person. For example, if an adult points out a "dog" to a child and names the animal, joint reference has occurred if the child and the adult are focusing on the dog. Children learn new words best through joint reference, which requires the child to be simultaneously engaging in joint attention (Carpenter & Tomasello, 2000).

Joint action occurs when the infant and caregiver participate in routine behaviors that allow the infant to experience language in a structured manner. An example of joint action is game playing, such as peekaboo or patty-cake. These actions have been described as "the most crucial infant learning and participating experiences" (Owens, 2001, p. 187).

For typically developing children, the prelinguistic skills of joint attention, joint reference, and joint action set the stage for more-advanced language learning. Gesture development incorporates the prelinguistic skills of joint attention and joint reference. The development of gestures occurs at approximately 7 months of age and indicates an internal motivation to communicate. Gestures are social in nature, since they involve pointing and showing an object to another individual. Gestures also have an internal motivational base and are correlated with the emergence of naming (Koegel, 2000).

Children with ASD show a lack of or a reduced number of gestures, or produce primitive gestures. Numerous researchers have reported a lack of gestures such as pointing, giving, showing, or using eye gaze to signal communication (Koegel, 2000; Stone, Ousley, Yoder, Hogan, & Hepburn, 1997; Wetherby, Yonclass, & Bryan, 1989) in children with ASD. Primitive, presymbolic gestures may be used predominantly by children with ASD. These include pulling, pushing, or leading someone to a desired object or place (Wetherby, Prizant, & Schuler, 2000). Children with cognitive disabilities or hearing impairments may use gestures to augment communication or compensate for language deficits. Children with ASD who do not employ gestures will not have this compensation ability.

Interventions That Facilitate Prelinguistic Skills

There has not been a large body of work that has focused on improving prelinguistic skills of children with ASD, primarily because children with autism are often not identified until the age of 2 or 3 years. Much of the research focusing on intervention to improve prelinguistic skills has involved children with developmental delays, who may or may not have autistic characteristics (Koegel, 2000). Yoder and Warren (1999, 2001) have described an intervention, Prelinguistic Milieu Teaching (PMT), that targets prelinguistic intentional communication for children with developmental delays. Their work on early communication and language intervention is based on three premises: (a) an individual's ability to communicate effectively will affect his or her success in school, work, and social relationships; (b) the earlier the intervention takes place, the better; and (c) the quantity and quality of input that the child receives from the environment is critically important (Warren & Yoder, 1996).

PMT targets two types of gestures: proto-imperatives and proto-declaratives. Proto-imperatives are gestures that signal another individual to get a desired object or engage in a desired action. For example, if a child points to an object that he or she desires and wants another individual to get it, he or she is using a proto-imperative. Proto-declaratives occur when a child uses an object to gain the attention of another individual. An example would be if a child picks up a toy and shows it to another individual. PMT attempts to increase the probability of these gestures occurring.

Specifically, play routines, such as peekaboo, were established in the Yoder and Warren (1999) study. During peekaboo, the trainer would withhold his or her participation after three turns and wait for the child to initiate a resumption of the activity, using a proto-imperative. If the child initiated a request for resumption using an appropriate proto-imperative, the trainer would verbally reinforce that behavior and continue with the game playing. If the child did not initiate a request, the trainer would then say, "Look at me" and wait for the child to respond. If the child looked at the trainer, the trainer verbally reinforced the child's proto-imperative and resumed the game. If the child did not respond at all, the trainer would continue the game, in an attempt to maintain a positive milieu environment (Yoder & Warren, 1999).

Yoder and Warren (1999) also addressed proto-declaratives once proto-imperatives were used more frequently. The trainer once again used a routine to establish joint attention on either an experience or an object. The trainer demonstrated proto-declaratives and established the child's need to draw the trainer's attention to an object or another focus of interest. The trainer then withdrew attention from the child occasionally and waited for the child to use proto-declaratives to regain the attention. Results from the Yoder and Warren studies (1999, 2000) indicated improvement and generalization of the use of proto-imperatives and proto-declaratives for these children with developmental delays. Intervention on prelinguistic language is an area that begs for additional research, especially since these skills appear to lay the foundation for future language learning (Koegel, 2000).

Recommendations for the Classroom

The foregoing considerations suggest a number of classroom strategies for the education professional:

1. For young children, use play-based activities that offer a high degree of repetitive behavior. Pair language with that behavior and involve the child in joint attention, joint reference, and joint action.

2. Use songs, rhymes, or any other language-based activities that are paired with action to assist the child in developing an understanding of the function of language.

3. Reinforce evidence of joint attention, joint action, and joint reference. If the child is not engaged during a joint action game, stop the action, wait for the child to look at you, and then continue the action.

Language Comprehension and ASD

Language comprehension, or receptive language, has been defined as responding nonverbally to the verbal stimuli of others (Lovaas, 2003; Sundberg & Partington, 1998). An assessment of receptive language is usually completed using standardized receptive language instruments, such as the *Peabody Picture Vocabulary Test* (PPVT) or the *Receptive One-Word Vocabulary Test* (ROWVT). These assessments require the student to point to pictures that are named by the evaluator. Other informal assessment procedures may include noting how well the child follows single-step commands and whether the child demonstrates the ability to follow complex commands. Yet these traditional assessments present difficulties for children with ASD. Most of them require the child's cooperation, and many do not measure pragmatic aspects of language, which is the prime area of deficit for children with ASD. Therefore, traditional assessments of language comprehension may have limited use. Informal assessment, which focuses on nonlinguistic response strategies, understanding of conventional meanings, and comprehension of vocabulary, sentences, and discourse, may provide a more complete picture of the child's comprehension of language (Wetherby & Prizant, 1992).

In typically developing children, receptive language, or language comprehension, develops prior to expressive language skills, although there is no agreement on how long receptive skills exceed expressive skills (Owens, 2001). Children with ASD may not follow this typical developmental pattern, may have higher expressive language skills than receptive skills (Bartak, Rutter, & Cox, 1977), or may have no difference in language comprehension and language production skills (Jarrold, Boucher, & Russell, 1997). A recent study by Chan, Cheung, Leung, Cheung, and Cheung (2005) indicated significant heterogeneity in the language impairments of children with ASD. An assessment of both language comprehension and language production abilities of 46 Chinese children with ASD indicated that 63% had significant language deficits. Of those 63%, 21% had typical language comprehension ability and significant language production deficits and 42% had difficulty with both language production and language comprehension. Once again, it is important that professionals working with children with ASD understand the *individual* language abilities of the student and recognize the heterogeneity among this population.

Interventions That Facilitate Language Comprehension

Children with ASD frequently evidence severely disrupted language comprehension abilities (Koegel, 2000; Lovaas, 1987). Individuals with autism have reported difficulty "attending to, modulating, or understanding auditory input" (Hodgdon, 2003, p. 13). Little empirical evidence exists of effective interventions that target language comprehension alone (Gillum & Camarata, 2004). Effective interventions that facilitate language comprehension also focus on facilitating desired behavior.

Visual supports have become standard practice in intervention programs designed for children with ASD (Odom et al., 2003). Visual supports are "visual cues that may prompt or remind children to engage in behavior or prepare them for another activity" (p. 171). The primary goal of visual supports is to enhance student understanding. Information that is received through the auditory channel is transient information, which can be difficult to process and remember because it is presented quickly and is not permanent (Hodgdon, 2003).

People in our society use visual supports frequently in all types of situations. Lists, calendars, and daily planners are examples of visual supports that education professionals may use regularly. Visual supports are helpful because they give a concrete form of information and act as a reminder to engage in a certain behavior.

Children with ASD have difficulty in situations where they must shift and reestablish their attention. Visual supports are permanent and can offer stable information that children can attend to repeatedly. In addition, a typical classroom environment is noisy, full of activity, and presents numerous sources of distraction. Typically developing children often have difficulty attending to the necessary information from the teacher while blocking out background noises, and that task can be especially difficult for children with ASD. Therefore, visual supports offer necessary information through vision, are nontransient, and diminish the need to rely solely on auditory information (Hodgdon, 2003).

Examples of visual supports used with children with autism are schedules, task analyses, calendars, and daily planners. They are developed individually, according to the student's literacy skills and level of comprehension. Effective visual supports are those that are easily recognizable and understood by the student and by those individuals with whom the student interacts. Dettmer, Simpson, Myles, and Ganz (2000) reported successful use of visual supports to assist with transitions across activities in the classroom. Numerous researchers have reported effective use of visual supports during instruction of a specific skill (Gines, Schweitzer, Queen-Autry, & Carthon, 1990; Krantz & McClannahan, 1993, 1998; Martin, Mithaug, & Frazier, 1992; Newman, et al., 1995; Vaughn & Horner, 1995).

Visual supports are not difficult to implement in the classroom. In a single-subject design study, Johnston, Nelson, Evans, and Palazolo (2003) successfully used visual supports to facilitate preschool children's entrance into play activities. The preschool staff was questioned about the implementation of the supports and responded that it was appropriate and important, and 89% reported no difficulty in incorporating the visual support into the classroom routine. Effective implementation of visual supports requires knowledge of each student's abilities, knowledge of the student's needs, and time to design and produce visual strategies for the classroom.

Recommendations for the Classroom

The foregoing considerations suggest a number of classroom strategies for the education professional:

1. Develop a schedule of the day's activities and post it on the student's desk or close to him or her. Then refer to the schedule throughout the day's activities.

2. Whenever there is a change in the day's activities, such as an assembly or a field trip, change the visual schedule to reflect the change *before* it occurs.

3. When teaching a task, use a pictured task analysis and present the student with a means of visually moving from one task to the next. For example, when the child is finished with a component of the task, have the child place the picture in a "finished" envelope. An excellent resource for visual supports is *Visual Strategies for Improving Communication* by Hodgdon (2003).

Language Production and ASD

Children with ASD evidence wide variability in language production (Wetherby, Prizant, & Schuler, 2000). The majority of children with ASD will have a significant delay in language expression or be nonspeaking (Chan et al., 2005). Estimates of the proportion of children with ASD who will not develop functional, verbal communication range from 50% to 35% (Mesibov, Adams, & Klinger, 1997; Prizant, 1983; Rutter, 1978; Volkmar et al., 1994). Children with ASD who do have verbal skills may demonstrate echolalia, telegraphic speech, idiosyncratic speech, pronoun reversals, inflexible and ritualistic language, and deficits of prosodic performance (Chan et al., 2005; Kuder, 2003; Paul, Augustyn, Klin, & Volkmar, 2005). These characteristics once again demonstrate the *qualitative* difference in language production of children with ASD.

Typically developing children demonstrate growth in language production that is highly predictable (Kuder, 2003). Children begin babbling, move into vocal play, develop jargon, and finally produce single words by approximately 1 year of age. Some children with ASD follow this typical development sequence until a regression of language skills occurs, usually between the ages of 18 and 24 months (Tuchman & Rapin, 1997). Estimates of children with ASD who experience regression range from 10% to 50% (Hoshino et al., 1987; Tuchman & Rapin, 1997). Of those children who do experience regression, loss of all language production ability is estimated to occur in 20% to 40% (Goldberg et al., 2003). The wide variability of deficits in language expression highlights the necessity of tailoring intervention to the individual child with ASD.

Language Production and Effective Intervention

Numerous researchers have concluded that early intervention is preferred and that effective intervention procedures meet certain criteria (Goldstein, 2002; Koegel, 2000). **357** If intervention is begun before the age of 5 and systematically contains certain effective components, estimates of children diagnosed with ASD who learn to communicate verbally increase to 85% to 90% (Koegel, 2000; McGee, Daly, & Jacobs, 1994). Koegel (2000) delineates the following components of effective early intervention: (a) following the child's lead, (b) capitalizing on the child's motivation to respond, and (c) providing frequent opportunities for responding in natural environments. These components have been effective with nonspeaking children with ASD as well as with those who are speaking but have delayed language production (Koegel, Koegel, & Surratt, 1992).

Goldstein (2002) reviewed 60 empirical studies that evaluated speech and language interventions with children with ASD over the past 20 years. Studies that incorporated sign language, discrete trial training, and milieu teaching reported improved communicative performance with children with ASD. Goldstein summarized that many questions need to be answered when attempting to ascertain effective communication intervention but concluded that children who are nonverbal require more-specific intervention and progress more slowly. Children who have some language production skills and can imitate speech respond to a wide variety of interventions.

In his review of empirical studies, Goldstein (2002) reported that approaches using total communication had positive results for teaching both receptive and expressive vocabulary. Most studies paired speech with sign language, which appeared to be more effective than the use of sign language alone. The studies did not focus on teaching sign language but instead used sign language in conjunction with speech to teach vocabulary. Goldstein suggests that sign language was an effective intervention because it is less transient than speech and is easier to prompt than verbal production.

Goldstein (2002) reviewed 12 studies that attempted to teach language comprehension and/or production using discrete trial training formats. Discrete trial training has been effective in laying the foundation to teach children with autism discriminative performances but has failed to show much promise with generalization outside training sessions. The studies reviewed used a variety of discrete trial formats with differential reinforcement and correction procedures. Goldstein summarized these studies as positive, since they focused on teaching more-sophisticated language and improved the generalization of the learned language skills.

Milieu language teaching, a group of procedures that capitalize on the student's interests in his or her natural environment, is used primarily to teach requesting and employs imitation, mand-model, or time-delay procedures to facilitate responses (Goldstein, 2002). Goldstein contends that there is no compelling evidence that milieu teaching procedures are clearly more effective than discrete trial. Indeed, the procedures employed with both milieu teaching and discrete trial training are similar, and both have reported positive results.

The use of alternative and augmentative communication (AAC) with individuals with disabilities was discussed in chapter 17. Several studies have reported the use of picture-based AAC systems to facilitate and increase speech production with children with ASD (Mirenda & Erickson, 2000; Romski & Sevcik, 1996). One of the most widely used forms of AAC for children with autism is the *Picture Exchange Communication System* (PECS; Bondy & Frost, 2002), which was described in detail in Chapter 17. Numerous studies have reported an increase in spontaneous speech during utilization of PECS with children with autism (Bondy & Frost, 1994, 1995, 2001; Charlop-Christy, Carpenter, Le, LeBlanc, & Kellet, 2002; Ganz & Simpson, 2004). It has been the author's experience that parents often are hesitant about the use of PECS because they fear that PECS will inhibit speech development. Current research suggests that PECS does not inhibit speech production and in fact may actually facilitate it.

Recommendations for the Classroom

The foregoing considerations suggest a number of classroom strategies for the education professional:

1. Work closely with the speech-language pathologist on interventions that are tailored for the student. Consistent intervention should be provided in the classroom.

2. Provide numerous opportunities throughout the day for the student to engage in language production. Language production should be reinforced by honoring the child's communication attempts.

3. Communicate frequently with parents, suggesting strategies for them to implement in the home, listening to their experiences, and advising them on how they can better communicate with the student.

Language Use and ASD

The pragmatic or social use of language is an area of significant impairment for children with ASD (Kuder, 2003). It has been described as "the one area that is pathognomic of the syndrome itself" (Twachtman-Cullen, 2000, p. 239), has been identified as the single most defining feature of autism (Kanner, 1943), and has been viewed as the most "handicapping feature as well" (Rogers, 2000, p. 399). Effective use of language is a complex and multifaceted process. For individuals to use language well they must have the knowledge of the rules that govern language use, know when to apply them, have the ability to comprehend language that is directed to them, and produce language so that their listener can understand them.

In a typically developing child, the development and use of gestures is one of the first indications of pragmatic development. Gestures indicate knowledge of a topic *and* a listener. As previously discussed, gesture development is often absent or primitive in children with ASD. Other indications of pragmatic growth are the use of prosody to communicate functions. For example, if a child says "cookie" with a rising intonation, that child is requesting. If "cookie" is said with a flat affect, then the child may be simply naming the item. Lack of prosody is characteristic of children with ASD, and this lack affects their pragmatic ability (Paul et al., 2005). Additional characteristics such as impairment in maintaining eye gaze, lack of expression of affect, and difficulty with topic initiation, maintenance, and termination are other pragmatic deficits that children with ASD may evidence (Frea, 1995; Kuder, 2003).

Children with ASD who are considered high functioning may have age-appropriate language production and language comprehension skills but poor pragmatic abilities. It is often difficult to assess such children formally, since standardized scores don't capture their pragmatic impairment (Twachtman-Cullen, 2000). Comprehensive assessment of the social-pragmatic use of language is difficult to obtain unless behavioral assessments are completed within home, school, and community settings (Koegel, Koegel, & Smith, 1997). Consequently, children with ASD who do not exhibit language delays or speech deficits, and therefore may not be assessed further, may still have significant difficulties with pragmatic language or social deficits (Lord, 2000).

Interventions That Facilitate the Pragmatic-Social Use of Language

Chapter 5 delineates several interventions that have been used to increase the social skills of children with ASD. These include Social Stories™ (Gray Center for Social Learning and Understanding, 2000–2005), power cards, cartooning, and Stop Observe Deliberate Act (SODA; Andrews & Mason, 1991). Rogers (2000) reviewed numerous interventions (visual cueing, pivotal response training, peer mediation, peer tutoring, self-management techniques, video-modeling techniques, and direct instruction) that were designed to facilitate socialization in children with ASD and concluded that children with ASD are responsive to many interventions that target social interactions with typical peers and adults. Additionally, there is some evidence that interventions resulting in increases in socialization skills of verbal children with ASD also increased language skills. Increases have been noted in the area of frequency and use of novel language constructions. Decreases in inappropriate behavior have also been reported (Koegel & Frea, 1993; Krantz & McClannahan, 1993; Lee & Odom, 1996; Stahmer, 1995; Thorp, Stahmer, & Schriebman, 1995).

All effective strategies that increased social skills, and thus affected the use of language, whether symbolic or nonsymbolic, involved using peers that were typically developing. When only adults were involved in interventions, spontaneous generalization to peer interactions did not occur (Rogers, 2000). Consequently, social interaction with typically developing peers should be a primary goal and needs to be actively targeted (Frea, 1995).

Recommendations for the Classroom

The foregoing considerations suggest a number of classroom strategies for the education professional:

1. Provide effective interventions that are age-appropriate, such as Social Stories[TM] or power cards.
2. Involve typically developing peers during interventions that target pragmatic language. Use of peers will increase generalizations and promote social interaction.
3. Be creative, and develop social groups around a specific activity that is interesting to the child with ASD. Typically developing peers should be encouraged and reinforced to engage in these activities.

Transitions and ASD

Transition planning is critical for all children (Polloway, Patton, & Serna, 2001), and it is imperative for children with ASD. Transitions that are unpredictable, and even those that are predictable, can cause confusion and anxiety in individuals with ASD (Earles, Carlson, & Bock, 1998). Two types of transitions, vertical and horizontal, have been discussed in the literature (Kagan, 1992; Polloway et al., 2001).

Vertical transitions are predictable, developmental, and experienced by all students. Examples of vertical transitions include transitions from early-intervention programs to preschool, yearly grade changes, and the major transition from school to adult life. Planning for vertical transitions is essential, since ineffective or unsuccessful transition planning can result in negative effects on both the social and the academic progress of students (Adreon & Stella, 2001; Kagan & Neuman, 1998). Indeed, vertical transitions have received most of the focus in the professional literature (Rosenkotter, Whaley, Hains, & Pierce, 2001).

Horizontal transitions, which are more likely to affect students in classrooms, refer to movements of students from one situation to another, occur on a daily or weekly basis, are individual and specific, and are not as predictable as vertical transitions (Polloway et al., 2001). Examples of horizontal transitions include going from home to school, moving between activities or classes, and encountering unfamiliar settings, such as an office visit to a doctor or dentist. For children with ASD, horizontal transitions can be especially challenging and stressful, resulting in stereotypical or aggressive behaviors. Therefore planning and devising strategies for horizontal transitions is critical (Adreon & Stella, 2001; Dettmer et al., 2000).

Strategies to Facilitate Transitions

Numerous studies in the existing literature offer effective intervention practices using visual strategies to facilitate transitions for children with ASD (e.g., Dettmer et al., 2000; Hodgdon, 2003). A recent study by Stoner, Angell, House, and Bock (in press) detailed a strategy that parents of young children with autism have utilized successfully during horizontal and vertical transitions.

The identify–observe–explore strategy that parents described as aiding transitions with their children involves three steps: (a) identifying transitions before they occur, (b) allowing children time to observe new situations, and (c) giving children opportunities to explore the new environments (Stoner et al., 2007). The classroom teacher can implement the identify–observe–explore strategy before a new transition. For example, if library visits are to be initiated, the teacher may identify this as a difficult transition for the child with autism. Consequently, the child could be given an opportunity to observe the library, as well as to explore the library when no other demands, such as checking out books, are made. The child then has the opportunity to be prepared for this horizontal transition. Once the day arrives for the library visit, the strategy has been implemented and the child may transition with greater ease. Incorporating a picture schedule before the visit would also be valuable in easing the transition process. This strategy involves identifying the child's needs and planning supports before the transition occurs, which is consistent with best practices reported by several researchers (e.g., Adreon & Stella, 2001; Feinberg & Vacca, 2000).

Recommendations for the Classroom

The foregoing considerations suggest a number of classroom strategies for the education professional:

1. Allow the student time to observe and explore the environment where new transitions will occur. This is especially valuable at the beginning of the school year. The student and his or her family should be invited to the classroom before school starts. Meet the student at the door, walk him or her to the room, show the student his or her desk, allow him or her to explore the classroom. If the student's anxiety is high, the education professional should repeat these steps as many times as possible to facilitate the transition.

2. Communicate with parents and obtain their input on how they handle transitions with their child. They may have highly effective procedures in place that can be implemented in the classroom.

3. Identify transitions that are difficult for the student, and provide visual strategies for all transitions, especially those difficult ones. Allow the student time to observe and explore the new environment.

Communication With Parents of Children With ASD

Perhaps the foremost need of parents of children with ASD regarding interaction with education professionals is communication. Communication between home and school has been repeatedly identified by parents as a concern (Feinberg & Vacca, 2000; Lake

& Billingsley, 2000; Stoner et al., 2005; Stoner et al., 2007). When a child has a pervasive communication disorder, as is the case with children with ASD, this need is compounded and heightened.

When parents of typically developing children want to monitor their children at school, such as understanding the events of a school day, identifying problems at school, or learning about the types of activities their children are engaging in, they simply ask their children. If typically developing children report difficulties, parents can address them. Parents of children with ASD do not have the "typical" parent-to-child avenue of communication available to them.

Consequently parents of children with ASD report monitoring the behavior of their child, saying their child's behavior is a reliable indicator of how things are going in the classroom. Parents notice instances of inappropriate behavior and surmise that these changes may arise from difficulties at school (Stoner et al., 2005). When this occurs, it is imperative that open and honest communication take place. Education professionals must address the communication needs of parents, must not dismiss their concerns, and must continue to offer avenues to monitor their child's education. Research has indicated that communication between parents and teachers is more frequent in the primary grades (Starr, Foy, & Cramer, 2001), but communication should not diminish in either quality or frequency as children move on to middle and high school.

A lack of communication and collaboration between parents and education professionals has historically been an area of weakness for many programs that serve students with ASD. Numerous studies have emphasized the importance of acknowledging parental expertise on their children, respecting parents' opinions, and incorporating their suggestions into school-based practices used with children with ASD (e.g., Feinberg & Vacca, 2000; Lovitt, 1999; Starr et al., 2001). When surveyed or interviewed, parents have repeatedly named communication as an area of concern (Defur, Todd-Allen, & Getzel, 2001; Kohler,1999; Lake & Billingsley, 2000; Stoner et al., 2005; Stoner et al., 2007).

Facilitating Communication Between Home and School

Communication between home and school can be facilitated through communication notebooks that travel between home and school, phone calls, e-mail messages, and informal conversations whenever possible. It is especially imperative to communicate with parents to report positive situations or events. Many times classroom teachers contact parents only when negative situations arise. Frequent communication that addresses the positives as well as any problems will facilitate the parent–school relationship.

An effective strategy that has been reported by parents of younger children with ASD is sending a picture communication tool home each day (Stoner et al., 2005). This communication tool can employ pictures that describe the day's activities and identify who the student played with, what the student ate for lunch, and so forth, as well as providing an overview of the student's behavior. The classroom teacher can make numerous copies of these communication sheets, tailored for the individual child, copy them, and simply circle the appropriate picture each day. The child can also become involved by either pointing to the picture or using the pictures to facilitate verbal communication about his or her day with the parent.

Listening to parents, acknowledging the experience that parents have acquired by interacting with their children, and incorporating parental suggestions into the educational program are essential. Parents have reported instances when their knowledge of their child has been either ignored or dismissed. When this happens, action-oriented parents report that they monitor their child's education program more intensely and frequently (Stoner et al., 2005). Effective programming for children with ASD requires communication between parents and professionals and encourages parental involvement.

Recommendations for the Classroom

The foregoing considerations suggest a number of classroom strategies for the education professional:

1. Recognize the heightened need for communication between parents and school. This is especially important if the student is nonspeaking.
2. Utilize communication notebooks, e-mails, and frequent informal contacts. This will address the parents' need to know what their child is experiencing throughout the day.
3. Use pictures that describe who the student has been playing with, what the student has been doing, and how the student has been behaving. These communication tools should be sent home daily and involve the student in their use.

Conclusion

Understanding the communication difficulties of the child with ASD requires knowledge of all aspects of the child's language. Knowledge of the individual child's strengths and difficulties is the first step in facilitating and increasing the child's communication abilities. Language comprehension, language production, and pragmatic language skills can all be affected by ASD. However, children's communication deficits exhibit a great deal of heterogeneity, and no single intervention is effective with all children with ASD. Knowledge of effective interventions, correct implementation of the interventions, diligent communication, and partnerships with families can assist the classroom teacher in enhancing communication for the student with ASD.

Glossary

Augmentative and alternative communication (AAC)—Methods, devices, and techniques that are used to either supplement or substitute for spoken communication.

Competent communicator—One who (a) can intentionally communicate, both verbally and nonverbally, a message; (b) can repair that message if it is misunderstood by a listener; (c) can use language in various social settings; and (d) can be an effective listener, capable of maintaining the ebb and flow of communication.

Expressive language—The language a person is able to produce. This term, used synonymously with language production, usually refers to speech, though it includes written expressive language and the use of AAC.

Horizontal transitions—Movements of students from one situation to another, which occur on a daily or weekly basis, are individual and specific, and are not as predictable as vertical transitions. Examples are going to therapy, moving from one room to the other, practicing fire drills, etc.

Joint action—Occurs when the infant and caregiver participate in routine behaviors that allow the infant to experience language in a structured manner.

Joint attention—Occurs when two people are attending to one object or event simultaneously.

Joint referent—Occurs when two individuals share a common focus on an object or person.

Language comprehension—Also called receptive language. Ability to respond nonverbally to the verbal stimuli of others.

Language production—Also called expressive language. The ability to produce language, usually through verbal output. However, written language, use of AAC, or sign language are also forms of language production.

Pragmatic language—Also called language use. Ability to use language in different settings and for different purposes.

Prelinguistic communication—Communication by the infant that precedes verbal language production. Examples are communication that signals discomfort, establishes closeness, or attains a desirable object.

Primitive gestures—Gestures that develop first in typically developing children and may be the primary gesture development of children with autism. An example of a primitive gesture is pulling a person toward a desired object.

Proto-declaratives—The intentional use of an object to get the attention of another person.

Proto-imperatives—An intentional gesture that signals another individual to get a desired object.

Qualitative language disorder—Language that is substantially different from that of typically developing children. An example would be a child who can recite the alphabet but cannot tell you his name.

Quantitative language disorder—Language that develops in a typical sequence but is delayed.

Receptive language—The language a person can comprehend; used synonymously with language comprehension.

Visual supports—Picture or symbol systems designed to enhance language comprehension. Examples are schedules, task analyses, and calendars.

Vertical transitions—Movements of students from one situation to another that are predictable, developmental, and experienced by all students. Examples are changing grades, changing schools, and changing teachers yearly.

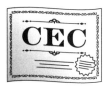

Knowledge and Skills for Entry-Level Special Education Teachers of Students With Developmental Disabilities Standards Addressed in This Chapter

Principle 1: Foundations

DD1K4 Trends and practices in the field of developmental disabilities.

Principle 2: Development and Characteristics of Learners

DD2K3 Identification of significant core deficit areas for individuals with pervasive developmental disabilities, autism, and autism spectrum disorders.

Principle 4: Instructional Strategies

DD4K2 Evidence-based practices for teaching individuals with pervasive developmental disabilities, autism, and autism spectrum disorder.

Principle 5: Learning Environments/Social Interaction

DD5S4 Structure the physical environment to provide optional learning environments for individuals with developmental disabilities.

Principle 6: Language

DD6S2 Use pragmatic language instruction to facilitate ongoing social skills instruction.

Web Site Resources

American Speech-Language-Hearing Association

www.asha.org/public/speech/disorders/Augmentative-and-Alternative.htm

> Information on augmentative and alternative communication (AAC), including a broad overview of AAC, professionals involved in planning for AAC, and the role of the family.

Autism Society of America

www.autism-society.org/site/PageServer

> Multidisciplinary and family Web site containing basic information about autism.

Center for Autism and Related Disabilities

www.card.ufl.edu/

> Link to visual supports, plus examples and tips for creating visual supports for use in different environments.

National Institute for Mental Health

www.nimh.nih.gov/healthinformation/autismmenu.cfm

> Definitions, signs and symptoms, treatments, and accessing local help.

References

Adreon, D., & Stella, J. (2001). Transition to middle and high school: Increasing the success of students with Asperger syndrome. *Intervention in School and Clinic, 36,* 266–271.

American Psychiatric Association. (1994). *Diagnostic and statistical manual of mental disorders (DSM-IV)* (4th ed.). Washington, DC: Author.

Andrews J. F., & Mason, J. M. (1991). Strategy usage among deaf and hearing readers. *Exceptional Children, 57,* 536–545.

Bartak, L., Rutter, M., & Cox, A. (1977). A comparative study of infantile autism and specific developmental receptive language disorder: II. Discriminant function analysis. *Journal of Autism and Childhood Schizophrenia, 7,* 383–396.

Bondy, A., & Frost, L. (1994). The Picture Exchange Communication System. *Focus on Autistic Behavior, 9,* 1–9.

Bondy, A., & Frost, L. (1995). Educational approaches in preschool: Behavior techniques in a public school setting. In E. Schopler & G. Mesibov (Eds.), *Learning and cognition in autism* (pp. 311–333). New York: Plenum

Bondy, A. S., & Frost, L. (2001). The Picture Exchange Communication System. *Behavior Modification, 25,* 725–744.

Bondy, A. S., & Frost, L. (2002). *A picture's worth: PECS and other visual communication strategies in autism.* Bethesda, MD: Woodbine House.

Carpenter, M., & Tomasello, M. (2000). Joint attention, cultural learning, and language acquisition. In A. M. Wetherby & B. M. Prizant (Eds.), *Autism spectrum disorders: A transactional developmental perspective* (pp. 31–54). Baltimore: Brookes.

Chan, A. S., Cheung, J., Leung, W. W. M., Cheung, R., & Cheung, M. (2005). Verbal expression and comprehension deficits in young children with autism. *Focus on Autism and Other Developmental Disabilities, 20,* 117–124.

Charlop-Christy, M., Carpenter, M., Le, L., LeBlanc, L., & Kellet, K. (2002). Using the Picture Exchange Communication System (PECS) with children with autism: Assessment of PECS acquisition, speech, social-communicative behavior, and problem behavior. *Journal of Applied Behavior Analysis, 35,* 213–231.

Defur, S. H., Todd-Allen, M., & Getzel, E. E. (2001). Parent participation in the transition planning process. *Career Development for Exceptional Individuals, 24,* 19–36.

DeGiacomo, A., & Fombonne, E. (1998). Parental recognition of abnormalities in autism. *European Child and Adolescent Psychiatry, 7*(3), 131–136.

Derby, K. M., Wacker, D. P., Saso, G., Steege, M., Northup, J., Cigrand, K., & Asmus, J. (1992). Brief functional assessment techniques to evaluate aberrant behavior in an outpatient setting: A summary of 79 cases. *Journal of Applied Behavior Analysis, 25,* 713–721.

Dettmer, S., Simpson, R. L., Myles, B. S., & Ganz, J. B. (2000). The use of visual supports to facilitate transitions of students with autism. *Focus on Autism and Other Developmental Disabilities, 15,* 163–169.

Earles, T. L., Carlson, J. K., & Bock, S. J. (1998). Instructional strategies to facilitate successful learning outcomes for students with autism. In R. L. Simpson & B. S. Myles (Eds.), *Educating children and youth with autism* (pp. 75–77). Austin, TX: PRO-ED.

Feinberg, E., & Vacca, J. (2000). The drama and trauma of creating policies on autism: Critical issues to consider in the new millennium. *Focus on Autism and Other Developmental Disabilities, 15,* 130–138.

Frea, W. D. (1995). Social-communicative skills in higher-functioning children with autism. In R. L. Koegel & L. K. Koegel (Eds.), *Teaching children with autism* (pp. 53–66). Baltimore: Brookes.

Frea, W. D., Koegel, R. L., & Koegel, L. K. (1993). *Understanding why problem behaviors occur: A guide for assisting parents in assessing causes of behavior and designing treatment plans.* Santa Barbara: University of California at Santa Barbara.

Ganz, J., & Simpson, R. L. (2004). Effects on communicative requesting and speech development of the Picture Exchange Communication System in children with characteristics of autism. *Journal of Autism and Developmental Disorders, 34,* 395–409.

Gillum, H., & Camarata, S. (2004). Importance of treatment efficacy research on language comprehension in MR/DD research. *Mental Retardation and Developmental Disabilities Research Reviews, 10,* 201–207.

Gines, D. J., Schweitzer, J. R., Queen-Autry, T., & Carthon, P. (1990). Use of color-coded food photographs for meal planning by adults with mental retardation. *Mental Retardation, 28,* 189–190.

Goldberg, W. A., Osann, K., Filipek, P. A., Laulhere, T., Jarvis, K., Modahl, C., Flodman, P., & Spence, M. A. (2003). Language and other regression: Assessment and timing. *Journal of Autism and Developmental Disorders, 33,* 607–616.

Goldstein, H. (2002). Communication intervention for children with autism: A review of treatment efficacy. *Journal of Autism and Developmental Disorders, 32,* 373–396.

Gray Center for Social Learning and Understanding. (2002–2005). *Social Stories*[TM]. Retrieved May 16, 2005, from http://www.thegraycenter.org/Social_Stories.htm

Hodgdon, L. A. (2003). *Visual strategies for improving communication: Vol. 1. Practical supports for school and home.* Troy, MI: Quirk Roberts.

Hoshino, Y., Kaneko, M., Yashima, Y., Kumashiro, H., Volkmar, F. R., & Cohen, D. J. (1987). Clinical features of autistic children with setback course in their infancy. *Japanese Journal of Psychiatry and Neurology, 41,* 237–245.

Iwata, B. A., & Pace, G. M. (1994). The functions of self-injurious behavior: An experimental-epidemiological analysis. *Journal of Applied Behavior Analysis, 27,* 215–241.

Jarrold, C., Boucher, J., & Russell, J. (1997). Language profiles in children with autism. *Journal of Autism and Developmental Disorders, 21,* 281–290.

Johnston, S., Nelson, C., Evans, J., & Palazolo, K. (2003). The use of visual supports in teaching young children with autism spectrum disorder to initiate interactions. *AAC: Augmentative and Alternative Communication, 19,* 86–104.

Kagan, S. L. (1992). The strategic importance of linkages and the transition between early childhood programs and early elementary school. In *Sticking together: Strengthening linkages and the transition between early childhood education and early elementary school* (National Policy Forum). Washington, DC: U.S. Department of Education.

Kagan, S. L., & Neuman, M. J. (1998). Lessons from three decades of transition research. *Elementary School Journal, 98,* 365–379.

Kanner, L. (1943). Autistic disturbances of affective content. *Nervous Child, 2,* 217–250.

Koegel, L. K. (2000). Interventions to facilitate communication in autism. *Journal of Autism and Developmental Disorders, 30,* 383–391.

Koegel, L. K., Koegel, R. L., & Smith, A. (1997). Variables related to differences in standardized test outcomes for children with autism. *Journal of Autism and Developmental Disorders, 27,* 233–240.

Koegel, R. L., & Frea, W. D. (1993). Treatment of social behavior in autism through the modification of pivotal social skills. *Journal of Applied Behavior Analysis, 26,* 369–377.

Koegel, R. L., Koegel, L. K., & Surratt, A. (1992). Language intervention and disruptive behavior in preschool children with autism. *Journal of Autism and Developmental Disorders, 22,* 141–153.

Kohler, F. W. (1999). Examining the services received by young children with autism and their families: A survey of parent responses. *Focus on Autism and Other Developmental Disabilities, 14,* 150–158.

Kuder, S. J. (2003). *Teaching students with language and communication disabilities* (2nd ed.). Boston: Allyn & Bacon.

Krantz, P. J., & McClannahan, L. E. (1993). Teaching children with autism to initiate to peers: Effects of a script-fading procedure. *Journal of Applied Behavior Analysis, 26,* 121–132.

Krantz, P. J., & McClannahan, L. E. (1998). Social interaction skills for children with autism: A script-fading procedure for beginning readers. *Journal of Applied Behavior Analysis, 31,* 191–202.

Lake, J., & Billingsley, B. (2000). An analysis of factors that contribute to parent-school conflict in special education. *Remedial and Special Education, 21,* 240–252.

Lee, S., & Odom, S. L. (1996). The relationship between stereotypic behavior and peer social interaction for children with severe disabilities. *Journal of the Association for Persons With Severe Handicaps, 21,* 88–95.

Lord, C. (2000). Commentary: Achievements and future directions for intervention research in communication and autism spectrum disorders. *Journal of Autism and Developmental Disorders, 30,* 393–398.

Lovaas, O. I. (1987). Behavioral treatment and normal educational and intellectual functioning in young autistic children. *Journal of Consulting and Clinical Psychology, 55,* 3–9.

Lovaas, O. I. (2003). *Teaching individuals with developmental delays: Basic intervention techniques.* Austin, TX: PRO-ED.

Lovitt, T. C. (1999). Parents of youth with disabilities: Their perceptions of school programs. *Remedial and Special Education, 20,* 134–143.

Martin, J. E., Mithaug, D. E., & Frazier, E. S. (1992). Effects of picture referencing on PVC chair, love seat, and settee assemblies by students with mental retardation. *Research in Developmental Disabilities, 13,* 267–286.

Matson, J. L., Benavidez, D. A., Compton, L. S., Paclawskyj, T., & Baglio, C. S. (1996). Behavioral treatment of autistic persons: A review of research from 1980 to the present. *Research in Developmental Disabilities, 17,* 433–465.

McGee, G. G., Daly, T., & Jacobs, H. A. (1994). The Walden school. In S. L. Odom and J. S. Handleman (Eds.), *Preschool education programs for children with autism* (pp. 127–162). Austin, TX: PRO-ED.

Mesibov, G. B., Adams, L. W., & Klinger, L. G. (1997). *Autism: Understanding the disorder.* New York: Plenum Press.

Mirenda, P., & Erickson, K. A. (2000). Augmentative communication and literacy. In A. M. Wetherby & B. M. Prizant (Eds.), *Autism spectrum disorder: A transactional approach* (pp. 333–369). Baltimore: Brookes.

Mundy, P., Kasari, C., Sigman, M., & Ruskin, E. (1995). Nonverbal communication and early language acquisition in children with Down syndrome and in typically developing children. *Journal of Speech and Hearing Research, 38,* 157–167.

National Research Council. (2001). *Educating children with autism.* Washington, DC: National Academy Press.

Newman, B., Buffington, D. M., O'Grady, M. A., McDonald, M. E., Poulson, C. L., & Hemmes, N. S. (1995). Self-management of schedule following in three teenagers with autism. *Behavioural Disorders, 20,* 190–196.

Newschaffer, C. J., Falb, M. D., & Gurney, J. G. (2005). National autism prevalence trends from United States special education data. *Pediatrics, 115,* 277–282.

Odom, S. L., Brown, W. H., Frey, T., Karasu, N., Smith-Canter, L. L., & Strain, P. S. (2003). Evidence-based practices for young children with autism: Contributions for single-subject design research. *Focus on Autism and Other Developmental Disabilities, 18,* 166–175.

Owens, R. E. (2001). *Language development* (5th ed.). Boston: Allyn & Bacon.

Paul, R., Augustyn, A., Klin, A., & Volkmar, F. (2005). Perception and production of prosody by speakers with autism spectrum disorders. *Journal of Autism and Developmental Disorders, 35,* 205–220.

Polloway, E. A., Patton, J. R., & Serna, L. (2001). *Strategies for teaching learners with special needs.* Upper Saddle River, NJ: Merrill/Prentice Hall.

Prizant, B. (1983). Language acquisition and communicative behavior in autism: Toward an understanding of the "whole" of it. *Journal of Speech and Hearing Disorders, 48,* 296–307.

Rogers, S. J. (2000). Interventions that facilitate socialization in children with autism. *Journal of Autism and Developmental Disorders, 30,* 399–409.

Rogers, S. J., & DiLalla, D. L. (1990). Domains of the Childhood Autism Rating Scale: Relevance for diagnosis and treatment. *Journal of Autism and Developmental Disorders, 24,* 115–128.

Romski, M., & Sevcik, R. (1996). *Breaking the speech barrier: Language development through augmented means.* Baltimore: Brookes.

Rosenkotter, S. E., Whaley, K. T., Hains, A. H., & Pierce, L. (2001). The evolution of transition policy for young children with special needs and their families. *Topics in Early Childhood Special Education, 21,* 3–16.

Rutter, M. (1978). Diagnosis and definition of childhood autism. *Journal of Autism and Childhood Schizophrenia, 8,* 139–161.

Smith, L., & von Tetzchner, S. (1986). Communicative, sensorimotor, and language skills of young children with Down syndrome. *American Journal of Mental Deficiency, 91,* 57–66.

Stahmer, A. C. (1995). Teaching symbolic play skills to children with autism using pivotal response training. *Journal of Autism and Developmental Disorders, 25,* 123–142.

Starr, E., Foy, J., & Cramer, K. (2001). Parental perceptions of the education of children with pervasive developmental disorders. *Education and Training in Mental Retardation and Developmental Disabilities, 36,* 55–68.

Stone, W. L., Ousley, O. Y., Yoder, P. J., Hogan, K. L., & Hepburn, S. L. (1997). Nonverbal communication in two- and three-year-old children with autism. *Journal of Autism and Developmental Disorders, 27,* 677–696.

Stoner, J. B., Angell, M. E., House, J. J., & Bock, S. J. (2007). Transitions: A parental perspective from parents of young children with autism spectrum disorder (ASD). *Journal of Physical and Developmental Disabilities, 19,* 23–39.

Stoner, J. B., Bock, S. J., Thompson, J. R., Angell, M. E., Heyl, B., & Crowley, E. P. (2005). Welcome to our world: Parent perspectives of interactions between parents of young children with ASD and education professionals. *Focus on Autism and Other Developmental Disabilities, 20,* 39–51.

Sundberg, M. L., & Partington, J. W. (1998). *Teaching language to children with autism and other developmental disabilities.* Pleasant Hill, CA: Behavior Analysts.

Thorp, D. M., Stahmer, A. C., & Schriebman, L. (1995). Effects of sociodramatic play training on children with autism. *Journal of Autism and Developmental Disorders, 25,* 265–282.

Tuchman, R. F., & Rapin, I. (1997). Regression in pervasive developmental disorders: Seizures and epileptiform electroencephalogram correlates. *Pediatrics, 99,* 560–566.

Twatchman-Cullen, D. (2000). More able children with autism spectrum disorders: Socio-communicative challenges and guidelines for enhancing abilities. In A. M. Wetherby & B. M. Prizant, (Eds.), *Autism spectrum disorders: A transactional developmental perspective* (pp. 225–249). Baltimore: Brookes.

Vaughn, B., & Horner, H. (1995). Effects of concrete versus verbal choice systems on problem behavior. *Augmentative and Alternative Communication, 11,* 89–92.

Volkmar, F. R., Klin, A., Siegel, B., Szatmari, P., Lord, C., Campbell, M., et al. (1994). Field trial for autistic disorder in *DSM-IV. American Journal of Psychiatry, 151,* 1361–1367.

Warren, S. F., & Yoder, P. J. (1996). Enhancing communication and language development in young children with developmental delays and disorders. *Peabody Journal of Education, 71,* 118–132.

Wetherby, A., Yonclass, D., & Bryan, A. (1989). Communicative profiles of handicapped preschool children: Implications for early identification. *Journal of Speech and Hearing Disorders, 54,* 148–158.

Wetherby, A. M., & Prizant, B. M. (1992). Profiling young children's communicative competence. In S. F. Warren & J. Reichle (Series & Vol. Eds.), *Communication and language intervention series: Vol. 1. Causes and effects in communication and language intervention* (pp. 217–253). Baltimore: Brookes.

Weatherby, A. M., Prizant, B. M., & Schuler, A. L. (2000). Understanding the nature of communication and language impairments. In A. M. Wetherby & B. M. Prizant (Eds.), *Autism spectrum disorders: A transactional developmental perspective* (pp. 109–141). Baltimore: Brookes.

World Health Organization. (1993). *International classification of mental and behavioral disorders: Diagnostic criteria for research.* Geneva: Author.

Yoder, P. J., & Warren, S. F. (1999). Facilitating self-initiated proto-declaratives and proto-imperatives in prelinguistic children with developmental disabilities. *Journal of Early Intervention, 22,* 79–96.

Yoder, P. J., & Warren, S. F. (2001). Relative treatment effects of two prelinguistic communication interventions on language development in toddlers with developmental delays vary by maternal characteristics. *Journal of Speech, Language, and Hearing Research, 44,* 224–237.

SECTION 7

ASSESSMENT

19

Assessment for Educational Classification

Christine A. Macfarlane

Summary

When a child enters school or transitions from an early-intervention program, the local educational agency must substantiate the presence of a disability and identify the need for special education and related services. The process begins with a referral, may include pre-referral interventions, encompasses a thorough, nondiscriminatory evaluation, leads to determining eligibility and educational classification, and continues on a minimum 3-year cycle. The process is team-driven, collaborative, and must include parents. Despite procedural safeguards and an extensive set of legal regulations, parents or the local educational agency may identify a need for mediation or request a due process hearing. Limited research has been conducted on assessment for educational classification; instead, best practice appears embedded in the legal mandates of federal and state law.

Learning Outcomes

After reading this chapter, you should be able to:

- Identify the difference between diagnosis and educational classification.
- List the steps to determine eligibility for special education services.
- Identify the procedural safeguards associated with educational classification.
- Understand the necessity for collaboration and parental participation.

Introduction

Defining Disability

Disabilities in children and youth can develop in utero, during the birth process, shortly after birth, or at some time during the developmental period (up to age 22). A disability can be genetic or congenital or acquired as a result of an illness, accident, exposure to toxins, or abuse and/or neglect. Disabilities can be apparent or hidden. Determining the presence of a disability may occur before birth, immediately after birth, or at some later point, usually when the child fails to achieve typical developmental milestones or encounters problems with learning in educational environments (La Paro, Olsen, & Pianta, 2002). The Developmental Disabilities Assistance and Bill of Rights Act of 2000 (P.L. 106-402) defines developmental disability (DD) as

> a severe chronic disability of an individual that (i) is attributable to a mental or physical impairment or combination of mental and physical impairments; (ii) is manifested before the individual attains age 22; (iii) is likely to continue indefinitely; (iv) results in substantial limitations in 3 or more of the

following areas of major life activity (self-care, receptive and expressive language, learning, mobility, self-direction, capacity for independent living, economic self-sufficiency; and (v) reflects the individual's needs for a combination and sequence of special, interdisciplinary, or generic services, individualized supports, or other forms of assistance that are of lifelong or extended duration and are individually planned and coordinated. [§102(8)]

The Individuals with Disabilities Education Improvement Act of 2004 (IDEIA-2004) restricts the use of the term *developmental delay* to children ages 3 to 9 or any subset including ages 3 to 5, and who, when measured by appropriate diagnostic instruments and procedures, experience delays in one or more of the following areas: cognitive, physical, communication, social or emotional, or adaptive development [§602(3)(B)(i)]. Individual states then have the option of whether to use developmental delay as a category or not. IDEIA-2004 broadly defines a child with a disability

as having mental retardation, a hearing impairment (including deafness), a speech or language impairment, a visual impairment (including blindness), a serious emotional disturbance (referred to in this part as emotional disturbance), an orthopedic impairment, autism, traumatic brain injury, another health impairment, a specific learning disability, deaf-blindness, or multiple disabilities, and who, by reason thereof, needs special education and related services. [§602(3)(A)(i)]

The terms used in the definition are further delineated into 14 federal categories (see Table 19.1). *Assessment teams* must have sufficient understanding of key factors in each category in order to consider the most probable disability category(s) for a child. The categories most closely associated with the earlier definition of developmental disability are: (a) developmental delay (up to age 9, depending on state regulations), (b) autism spectrum disorder, (c) deaf-blindness, (d) mental retardation (MR), (e) multiple disabilities (depending on state regulations), (f) orthopedic impairment (OI), (g) other health impaired (OHI), and (h) traumatic brain injury (TBI). As a broadly defined category, this subset of disabilities has also been referred to as low-incidence disabilities, with the exception of mild mental retardation (Reschly, 2002).

Determining Need

Diagnosis differs from *educational classification* (Alpert, 2004). Diagnosis may take much time and involve many professionals who have appropriate credentials (e.g., medical doctor, licensed psychologist), or it may be somewhat simple and straightforward. When a licensed psychologist establishes a diagnosis, he or she follows specific guidelines established by a professional organization such as the American Psychiatric Association and set forth in its manual, *Diagnostic and Statistical Manual of Mental Disorders* (DSM-IV, 1994). The language and tenor of the diagnosis are based on a medical model. Educators, with the possible exception of a school psychologist, generally do not have the credentials to make specific diagnoses (e.g., Asperger's syndrome, cerebral palsy, Down syndrome). Further,

TABLE 19.1

Categories of Disability and Possible Assessment Needs

Disability Category	Description of Disability	Exceptions	Possible Assessment Needs to Determine Educational Classification
Autism	Developmental disability significantly affecting verbal and nonverbal communication and social interaction, generally evident before age 3, and adversely affecting child's educational performance	Does not apply if child's educational performance is adversely affected primarily because of emotional disturbance *(see below)*	• Behavioral observation in educational and social settings • Interviews of parents, caregivers, educators, and related service providers • Medical/health assessment • Communication assessment • Educational performance • Developmental progress*
Deaf-blindness	Concomitant hearing and visual impairments that cause such severe communication and other developmental and educational needs that they cannot be accommodated in special education programs solely for children with deafness or children with blindness		• Audiological assessment • Medical/health assessment re: treatment of hearing loss and use of amplification • Medical assessment by an ophthalmologist or optometrist • Educational performance • Developmental progress* • Functional assessment of residual vision acuity or field of vision
Deafness	Severe hearing impairment so that a child cannot process linguistic information through hearing, with or without amplification		• Audiological assessment • Medical/health assessment re: treatment of hearing loss and use of amplification • Educational performance • Developmental progress*
Developmental delay	Child age 3–9 (or any subset, including ages 3–5) experiencing developmental delays in one or more of the following developmental areas: physical, cognitive, communication, social or emotional, adaptive; and who needs special education and/or related services	States have the option to use or not use this category	• Interview/records review to obtain prenatal, birth, and early neonatal history • Interview/records review to obtain developmental history • Medical/health assessment • Vision screening • Hearing screening • Specific assessments as needed in cognitive, communication, motor, and social/emotional areas • Developmental progress*

TABLE 19.1 (*continued*)

Disability Category	Description of Disability	Exceptions	Possible Assessment Needs to Determine Educational Classification
Emotional disturbance	Presence, over a long time period and to a marked degree, that adversely affects a child's educational performance, of one or more of the following characteristics: • Inability to learn that cannot be explained by intellectual, sensory, or health factors • Inability to build or maintain satisfactory interpersonal relationships with peers and teachers • Inappropriate types of behavior or feelings under normal circumstances • General pervasive mood of unhappiness or depression • A tendency to develop physical symptoms or fears associated with personal or school problems • Schizophrenia	Does not apply to children who are socially maladjusted, unless it is determined that the criteria for emotional disturbance are met	• Interview/records review to obtain developmental or social history • Assessment of emotional and behavioral status • Medical/health assessment • Behavior rating scales • Behavioral observation • Educational performance • Developmental progress*
Hearing impairment	Permanent or fluctuating impairment in hearing that adversely affects a child's educational performance but is not included under definition of deafness		• Audiological assessment • Medical/health assessment re: treatment of hearing loss and use of amplification • Educational performance • Developmental progress*
Mental retardation	Significantly subaverage general intellectual functioning, existing concurrently with deficits in adaptive behavior and manifested during developmental period		• Standardized intelligence test • Adaptive behavior scale • Medical/health assessment • Interview/records review to obtain developmental history • Educational performance • Developmental progress*
Multiple disabilities	A combination of concomitant impairments that causes such severe educational needs that the child cannot be accommodated in special education programs solely for one impairment		See specific disability categories
Orthopedic impairment	Severe orthopedic impairment caused by a congenital anomaly, disease, or other factors		• Medical/health assessment • Standardized motor assessment • Educational performance • Developmental progress*

Educational Classification

377

(*continues*)

TABLE 19.1 *(continued)*

Disability Category	Description of Disability	Exceptions	Possible Assessment Needs to Determine Educational Classification
Other health impairment	Limited strength, vitality, or alertness, including a heightened alertness to environmental stimuli, due to chronic or acute health problems & resulting in limited alertness with respect to the educational environment and adversely affecting a child's educational performance		• Medical/health assessment • Educational performance • Developmental progress*
Specific learning disability	A disorder in one or more of the basic psychological processes involved in understanding or in using language, spoken or written, that may manifest itself in the imperfect ability to listen, think, speak, read, write, spell, or to do mathematical calculations	Does not apply to learning problems—primarily the result of visual, hearing, or motor disabilities, mental retardation, emotional disturbance, or environmental, cultural, or economic disadvantage	• Behavioral observation • Interview/records review of developmental history • Standardized intelligence test • Specific assessments as needed in motor, communication, social/emotional, and perception or memory • Records review of cumulative records, previous interventions, and work samples • Medical/health assessment • Educational performance • Developmental progress*
Speech or language impairment	Communication disorder, such as stuttering, impaired articulation, a language impairment, or a voice impairment, that adversely affects a child's educational performance		• Speech/language assessment including a language sample, voice assessment scale, and/or standardized test of expression and comprehension, depending on type of disorder • Behavioral observation • Medical statement from an otolaryngologist for a voice disorder • Medical/health assessment • Hearing acuity • Oral mechanism evaluation • Educational performance • Developmental progress*
Traumatic brain injury	Acquired brain injury caused by external physical force resulting in total or partial functional disability, psychosocial impairment, or both	Congenital or degenerative brain injuries, or brain injuries induced by birth trauma	• Medical/health assessment • Psychological assessment

TABLE 19.1 *(continued)*

Disability Category	Description of Disability	Exceptions	Possible Assessment Needs to Determine Educational Classification
			• Specific assessments as needed in motor, communication, and psychosocial areas • Interview/records review to determine pre-injury performance • Adaptive behavior • Behavioral observation • Educational performance • Developmental progress*
Visual impairment, including blindness	Impairment in vision that, even with correction, adversely affects a child's educational performance; to include both partial sight and blindness		• Medical assessment by an ophthalmologist or optometrist • Educational performance • Developmental progress* • Functional assessment of residual vision acuity or field of vision

*For preschool-age child

Adapted from: Oregon Administrative Rules—581-015-0051: Criteria for Evaluation and Eligibility Determination and Proposed Rules §300.8 Child With a Disability (Federal Register, 2005).

the law does not require diagnosis in order to determine eligibility; instead, educators must determine the educational classification of a child according to one of the federally defined categories (e.g., orthopedic impairment, mental retardation) (Table 19.1) authorized by the state. A child suspected of having a disability must undergo a thoughtful assessment process to determine eligibility, that is, classification. Even if a disability has been diagnosed, once a child enters school, educational assessment for the purpose of classification is necessary. Finally, the documented presence of a disability does not automatically qualify a child to receive special education services. The child must need specially designed instruction (SDI) and/or related services (e.g., physical therapy) in order to benefit from his or her education. However, if a child has a disability and does not qualify for special education services, he or she may be eligible for accommodations and/or modifications (i.e., 504 plan) under Section 504 of the Vocational Rehabilitation Act of 1973.

In addition to defining disability, IDEIA-2004 mandates states to conduct *child find activities* (§612, §635), that is, to seek out infants, toddlers, or children with disabilities in both private and public schools, those who are homeless, and those who are wards of the state to ensure access to special education and/or related services. When children do not have discernible disabilities, medical professionals, social service providers, and/or school district personnel may conduct *screenings* (Woodrich, 1997). Vision, hearing, motor skills, and general readiness for academic skills are typical targets for screening. Assessment conducted for the purpose of screening is generally quick and easy to do but is not always definitive. If screening detects a potential problem, further assessment is warranted. Errors in over-identification and under-identification of possible disabilities in children can create future problems (La Paro et al., 2002). For example, if a child does have a disability and screening does not suggest the need for further assessment, or if screening is not conducted, the child may lose valuable assistance (Scott, Fletcher, & Martell, 2000). If a disability is initially suspected but later unconfirmed, parents may continue to wonder and question whether a disability has been overlooked. Thus screening is an important first step that must be conducted carefully.

Referral

Once screening has been completed and further evaluation appears necessary or when someone identifies or suspects a disability in a child, a *referral* is made. Depending on state regulations, the referral may be written or oral. A parent, a medical provider, someone from a social service agency, a friend, or a concerned person can make a referral for infants and toddlers for early intervention (EI, ages birth–2) or early childhood special education (ECSE, ages 3–5). If an infant or toddler experiences a substantiated case of trauma resulting from exposure to family violence, a referral for evaluation for early-intervention services must be made. For school-age children (ages 5–21) a parent of a child, a state educational agency (e.g., school for the blind), another state agency, or a local educational agency (e.g., school district, teacher) can generate a referral or request for *initial evaluation*. Once a child reaches the age of majority, he or she can make a self-referral.

Early Intervention

The requirement for assessment of infants and toddlers also includes the family. In addition to "a multidisciplinary assessment of the unique strengths and needs of the infant or toddler," IDEIA-2004 requires assessment teams also to identify "services appropriate to meet such needs" [§636(a)(1)]. EI services can begin before assessment is complete.

When a child transitions from ECSE to school-based services or, in some instances, from EI to ECSE, educational classification must occur. When receiving EI and/or ECSE, children are often classified simply as developmentally disabled, even if a more specific diagnosis (e.g., autism) is known. If a specific diagnosis or label has not been identified, the potential exists for parents to revisit the grieving process when a more specific label is applied.

School-Age Services

Pre-Referral

If a child has not received EI or ECSE and a problem is suspected after age 5, the process of determining whether the child would benefit from special education and/or related services begins with pre-referral. When a child experiences academic or social/emotional difficulties in school, a general education teacher will bring the case before a school-based child-study team. Obiakor and Wilder (2003) suggest that pre-referral is the right time to involve parents and begin the collaborative process, particularly if the child in question is a culturally and linguistically diverse (CLD) student. They also suggest that the principal is another key player during the pre-referral process. Interventions are tried in the classroom, and data are gathered to support the effectiveness and number of those interventions. However, "the screening of a student by a teacher or specialist to determine appropriate instructional strategies for curriculum implementation shall not be considered to be an evaluation for eligibility for special education and related services" [§614(a)(1)(E)]. If interventions prove successful, no further action is taken. If interventions fail, a child can then be referred for initial evaluation to determine whether a disability is present. Besides documenting success or failure of interventions, the pre-referral time period provides an opportunity to concisely define the child's problem(s) and generate specific information, which will help during the referral process.

Evaluation

Once a referral has been made, not only must educators engage in the process of trying to determine if the child is a child with a disability, but they must also adhere to extensive laws and regulations related to referral, initial evaluation, timelines, testing instruments, and subsequent decision making (Reschly, 2002). Despite a tremendous effort to ensure that initial evaluation is nondiscriminatory and thorough, once a referral is made, the child most likely will become eligible for special education services (Hosp & Reschly, 2003).

Consent for evaluation must be obtained before any assessment can begin. IDEIA-2004 articulates what can occur in the absence of consent, including children who are wards of the state. As noted in IDEIA-2004:

Section 614 (a)(1)(D)(i) In general—

(I) Consent for initial evaluation.—The agency proposing to conduct an initial evaluation to determine if the child qualifies as a child with a disability as defined in section 602 shall obtain informed consent from the parent of such child before conducting the evaluation. Parental consent for evaluation shall not be construed as consent for placement for receipt of special education and related services.

(ii) Absence of consent.—

(I) For initial evaluation.—If the parent of such child does not provide consent for an initial evaluation under clause (i)(I), or the parent fails to respond to a request to provide the consent, the local educational agency may pursue the initial evaluation of the child by utilizing the procedures described in section 615, except to the extent inconsistent with State law relating to such parental consent.

(iii) Consent for wards of the state.—

(I) In general.—If the child is a ward of the State and is not residing with the child's parent, the agency shall make reasonable efforts to obtain the informed consent from the parent (as defined in section 602) of the child for an initial evaluation to determine whether the child is a child with a disability.

(II) Exception.—The agency shall not be required to obtain informed consent from the parent of a child for an initial evaluation to determine whether the child is a child with a disability if—

(aa) despite reasonable efforts to do so, the agency cannot discover the whereabouts of the parent of the child;

(bb) the rights of the parents of the child have been terminated in accordance with State law;

(cc) the rights of the parent to make educational decisions have been subrogated by a judge in accordance with State law and consent for an initial evaluation has been given by an individual appointed by the judge to represent the child.

The numerous rights guaranteed to parents and children with disabilities by IDEIA-2004 also begin with the request for parental permission to conduct an initial evaluation. At this time parents receive a Notice of Procedural Safeguards from the school district. Districts should provide this notice in the parents' native language or alternative format (e.g., Braille). Parents will also be offered this notice once a year, if they request it, a year before their child's 18th birthday, or if they request a due process hearing or file a complaint with the state. Unfortunately, as Imber and Radclif (2003) noted, "Public education agencies still have a long way to go in providing materials that fully inform parents of their rights in the special education process" (p. 29). Simply reading such documents often requires advanced reading skills. Parental consent for evaluation must be written, and the paperwork and any explanation must be available in the parent's native language. Judicious decisions should be made as to which assessments will be given. Parents should be fully informed as to why and which tests are being given. As noted above, if parents refuse to give permission, school districts may use due process to resolve the issue.

Assessment Team

Following a referral and concurrent with obtaining parental permission to conduct evaluation, an assessment team is put together to pool the expertise necessary to conduct assessments and make decisions. The Individuals with Disabilities Education Act Amendments of 1997 (IDEA 97, P.L. 105-17) strengthened the role of parents as members of the assessment team. In addition to parents, the assessment team generally consists of the child's general education teacher, a special education teacher, and, if needed, a person or persons qualified to give appropriate standardized tests and conduct interviews and behavioral observations. A school administrator and/or school counselor may also be a team member, as well as consultants who have specialized expertise (e.g., autism consultant). Related service personnel (e.g., physical therapist, speech-language pathologist, occupational therapist) should be included as necessary. Most important, the person making the referral and the assessment team should state the child's problem(s) in such a way that meaningful answers can be sought (Woodrich, 1997). For example, saying a child is not "doing well in first grade" is inadequate. Stating behavioral specifics, such as, "The child is unable to write his name and cannot identify any alphabetic characters" provides more meaningful information to the assessor. As noted in IDEIA-2004,

The purpose of the assessment team is to:

(A) review existing evaluation data on the child, including—

    (i) evaluations and information provided by the parents of the child;

    (ii) current classroom-based, local, or State assessments, and classroom-based observations; and

    (iii) observations by teachers and related services providers; and

(B) on the basis of that review, and input from the child's parents, identify what additional data, if any, are needed to determine—

    (i) whether the child is a child with a disability as defined in section 602(3), and the educational needs of the child, or, in case of a reevaluation of a child, whether the child continues to have such a disability and such educational needs;

    (ii) the present levels of academic achievement and related developmental needs of the child;

    (iii) whether the child needs special education and related services, or in the case of a reevaluation of a child, whether the child continues to need special education and related services; and

    (iv) whether any additions or modifications to the special education and related services are needed to enable the child to meet the measurable annual goals set out in the individualized education program of the child and to participate, as appropriate, in the general education curriculum [§614(c)(1)].

Assessment Timeline

Conducting an initial evaluation must be accomplished in a timely manner. Once parental consent for evaluation has been given, the assessment team has 60 days to complete the evaluation and come together to determine eligibility, unless the state establishes an alternate timeline [§614(a)(1)(C)(i)]. Local education agencies are excused from adhering to the timeline if the child moves from a school district where initial assessment began but was not completed to another school district, as long as the current school district makes sufficient progress toward completion and parents agree to a new timeline [§614(a)(1)(C)(ii)(I)]. School districts are also excused from adhering to the timeline if "the parent of a child repeatedly fails or refuses to produce the child for the evaluation" [§614(a)(1)(C)(ii)(II)].

Assessment

Additionally, IDEIA-2004 mandates how local educational agencies will conduct evaluations. The assessment team must:

(A) use a variety of assessment tools and strategies to gather relevant functional, developmental, and academic information, including information provided by the parent, that may assist in determining—

    (i) whether the child is a child with a disability; and

    (ii) the content of the child's individualized education program, including information related to enabling the child to be involved in and progress in the general education curriculum, or, for preschool children, to participate in appropriate activities;

(B) not use any single measure or assessment as the sole criterion for determining whether a child is a child with a disability or determining an appropriate educational program for the child; and

(C) use technically sound instruments that may assess the relative contribution of cognitive and behavioral factors, in addition to physical or developmental factors [§614(b)(2)].

Under additional requirements, the local educational agency must ensure that assessments and other evaluation materials are used in such a way as to produce valid and reliable data [§614(b)(3)(A)(iii)], "administered by trained and knowledgeable personnel" [§614(b)(3)(A)(iv)], and "administered in accordance with any instructions provided by the producer of such assessments" [§614(b)(3)(A)(v)]. Further, "the child is assessed in all areas of suspected disability" [§614(b)(3)(B)]; selected assessment tools and strategies provide relevant information to help determine educational needs [§614(b)(3)(C)]; and should the child transfer during the academic year, coordination occurs between schools to complete a full evaluation as quickly as possible [§614(b)(3)(D)].

Assessment Tools

Depending on areas of suspected disability, the team may need to assess (a) cognitive (i.e., intelligence) ability, (b) achievement levels, (c) adaptive behavior, (d) communication skills, (e) self-help skills, (f) motor skills, (g) vision, and/or (h) hearing (refer to Table 19.1 for some suggested assessment areas). A physician's report may be needed to address medical factors. Assessments may include standardized tests, behavioral observation, and interviews. School records and artifacts related to current school performance should be examined. Psychologists, teachers, and appropriate related service personnel should administer tests and conduct observations and interviews. In specific areas only appropriately licensed personnel may be allowed to administer some assessments. For example, a licensed speech-language pathologist should conduct an articulation assessment. Most important, the assessment team must consider data from multiple sources in making their decision. Pierangelo and Giuliani (2006) developed a guide for special educators to provide a comprehensive overview of frequently used tests for determining eligibility and educational classification across category and age. Another resource may be the test publisher's Web site.

Intelligence Testing

In many cases it is necessary to determine the student's current cognitive ability in order to establish eligibility and decide educational classification. The end result of a standardized intelligence test is an intelligence quotient (IQ). Discussion of a child's IQ score can be fraught with emotion, and historically psychologists, educators, and the general public have debated the wisdom and merit of relying on IQ scores to make educational decisions. What we now know is that "intelligence tests measure a person's genetic potential *and* experiences" (Woodrich, 1997, p. 69), can change over time in children without disabilities (McCall, Appelbaum, & Hogarthy, 1973), and are more stable in children with disabilities and school-age children (Kamphaus, 1993). Cognitive ability and academic performance generally go hand in hand, although not always. When a discrepancy exists between ability and achievement, the assessment team will want to closely examine the data to see if the presence of a disability could explain the difference.

Generally, a licensed psychologist must administer an intelligence test, although it is extremely beneficial for educators to understand the parameters of various tests and their results. The *Wechsler Scale of Intelligence* exists in four forms: (a) *Wechsler Preschool and Primary Scale of Intelligence—Third Edition* (WPPSI-III), ages 2:6 to 7:3, (b) *Wechsler Intelligence Scale for Children—IV* (WISC-IV), ages 6.5 to 16.5, (c) *Wechsler Adult Intelligence Scale—Third Edition* (WAIS-III), ages 16 and over, and (d) *Wechsler Intelligence Scale for Children—IV Spanish* (WISC-IV Spanish), for children who speak Spanish (Wechsler, 1997, 2002, 2003, 2004). These scales are widely used in schools and provide useful information about a child's learning style, potential for learning, organizational skills, processing and reasoning abilities, and adjustment to timed tasks (Pierangelo & Giuliani, 2006). Another well-known test is the *Stanford-Binet Intelligence Scale: Fifth Edition*, for ages 2 to adult (Roid, 2003). Other tests of intelligence were developed for specific purposes. For example, the *Slosson Intelligence Test—Revised* (Slosson, revised by Nicholson & Hibpschman, 1998) screens for verbal intelligence. The *McCarthy Scales of Children's Abilities* (McCarthy, 1972) focuses on preschoolers and young children (ages 2 years 6 months to 8 years 6 months). The *Columbia Mental Maturity Scale* (Burgemeister, Blurn, & Lorge, 1972) is intended for children with disabilities and uses pictures. The *Comprehensive Test of Nonverbal Intelligence* (CTONI; Hammill, Pearson, & Wiederholt, 1996) and the *Test of Nonverbal Intelligence—Third Edition* (TONI-3; Brown, Sherbenou, & Johnsen, 1997) were developed for children who do not speak English, are bilingual, experience other impairments such as motor problems, or are socially/emotionally disadvantaged.

Length of time to give the test and the child's endurance and attention span, the child's age, the child's suspected or known disability, skill of the test administrator, reliability of the instrument, validity, and needed information should factor into an assessment team's decision to select and administer one of these intelligence tests.

Achievement Testing

An intelligence test assesses a child's ability to think, problem-solve, and reason, while an achievement test measures acquisition of academic skills (Woodrich, 1997). Achievement tests can be given to an individual or administered to a group of children. Some are *norm-referenced*, that is, an individual's performance is compared to a group that established norms for the test. Others are *criterion-referenced*; in those tests, a standard or criterion is established and the individual's performance is measured according to progress toward achieving the standard or meeting the criterion. Tests exist to measure specific academic abilities (e.g., reading, math, written language, or spelling) and comprehensive academic abilities. Statewide and district assessments designed to measure academic progress might also be used to determine a child's academic level of achievement. Achievement tests provide a critical piece of information when assessing a child's educational performance. However, while a standardized achievement test will provide information for purposes of educational classification, further assessment may be necessary to determine specific instructional needs and to develop the IEP.

Adaptive Behavior

In order to say that a child should be educationally classified as mentally retarded, the assessment team must consider the child's adaptive behavior. It is also important to look at the adaptive behavior of children who might be classified under another category. The most recent definition of mental retardation put forward by the American Association on Mental Retardation (AAMR) references adaptive behavior "as expressed in conceptual, social, and practical adaptive skills" (Luckasson et al., 2002). Receptive and expressive language and functional academics along with self-determination are examples of conceptual skills. The need for interpersonal skills would be an example of social skills. Practical skills include self-help, work, health and safety, recreation/leisure, domestic, and community. The assessment team can choose to conduct standardized adaptive behavior scales, observe, interview, or review anecdotal records to determine a child's level of adaptive behavior. Two well-known standardized adaptive behavior tests are the *AAMR Adaptive Behavior Scales—School* (Lambert, Nihiri, & Leland, 1993) and the *Vineland Adaptive Behaviors Scales—II* (Sparrow, Cicchetti, & Balla, 2005).

Once a person has been identified as having mental retardation, and particularly as the person enters high school, AAMR advocates that the assessment team determine the level of supports (intermittent, limited, extensive, pervasive) needed for the person to be as independent as possible in the local community. Thompson et al. (2004) developed the *Supports Intensity Scale* to assist teams in deciding the level of support needed in seven areas of competence: community living, employment, health and safety, home living, lifelong learning, protection and advocacy (e.g., protecting self from exploitation, exercising legal responsibilities), and social interaction. The team also gathers information on exceptional medical (e.g., respiratory care, skin care) and behavioral needs (e.g., self-directed destructiveness, sexual). A composite score assists in determining the need for supports and the level of intensity.

Motor Skills

If the assessment team suspects or knows that a child has an orthopedic impairment or the child is young, a motor assessment is needed. Acquisition of gross motor (e.g., crawling, standing, walking) and fine motor (e.g., holding a crayon, putting food into the mouth) skills correlates highly with achievement of developmental milestones. Also, it may be necessary to rule out the possibility of a physical problem in order to consider certain categories for educational classification. Motor assessments are generally conducted by a physical therapist and/or an occupational therapist. However, an adaptive physical education teacher, as well as family members and the classroom teacher, could also provide relevant information. Again, assessment could occur by means of a standardized test, behavioral observations, interviews, or review of records. Frequently, when infants or young children are assessed, the therapists will conduct an *arena assessment* (Overton, 2006), in which several therapists are present and the child is asked to do things or presented with tasks in such a way that each person can gather necessary information. This style of assessment reduces time and is less fatiguing for the child. Further, motor assessment along with communication assessment for young children can often be conducted during play.

Behavioral Observation

Behavioral observation may be necessary because the child exhibits a problem behavior, or a behavioral observation can be conducted to assess a child's ability to interact in a specific setting. For example, if a child is experiencing academic difficulty in the general education classroom, it would be wise to observe the child in the classroom during reading instruction. The observer would thereby have the chance to observe not only the child but also the teacher and the child's peers. The environment may also provide valuable information. Is it noisy? Is the child seated near the back of the room? Does the child appear to be sleepy (and is the room warm)? For purposes of educational classification, the observer should focus on the child; the child's interaction with materials, adults, and peers; and the effects of the environment on the child. It is also a good idea to observe peers, in order to obtain comparative information. Sometimes what a teacher reports as problematic is simply typical behavior for any child and has no bearing on the presence of a disability.

Behavioral observations can be very formal and guided by checklists and/or observational forms or they can be more informal. Observers can count behaviors that occur, use timing devices, or record field notes (i.e., provide a narrative of what he or she observed). Frequently, it is difficult to record notes while observing in the classroom, as it may make the child frustrated to know that someone is watching him or her. In such cases, or even after taking field notes, the observer should enrich the notes or record them as soon as possible. Another decision while observing is whether to interact with the child directly or to simply watch. Since behavioral observation is somewhat subjective, it is wise to conduct several observations over time or to have multiple observers.

Sensory Testing

Sensory testing often falls under the purview of screening when done in educational settings. The school nurse, speech-language pathologist or audiologist, or vision consultant may screen for vision or hearing problems. If a potential problem exists, the child will be referred to the appropriate medical practitioner to conduct more-extensive testing. In the case of sensory impairments, the assessment team will need specific reports to document the level of vision and/or hearing loss. Otherwise, the assessment team will need information about vision and hearing to rule out the possibility of a sensory impairment, thus clearing the way for consideration of other categories. In either case, members of the assessment team will need to acquire the expertise necessary to understand and interpret sometimes sophisticated and complex medical reports.

Possible obstacles to conducting sensory testing can occur if the child also experiences a cognitive delay, has motor problems, or exhibits communication problems. For example, a child with significant cognitive delays might not recognize or be able to follow directions associated with using the standard letter chart as part of a vision screening. In such a case, pictures can be substituted for letters, and the ability to follow directions could become part of the child's IEP. Modifications in the testing may be needed if the child cannot physically perform a requested command (e.g., raise your hand).

Medical Factors

A school nurse or family health-care practitioner may provide routine health information. In many cases the assessment team simply needs to verify that no medical problems exist. However, some disability categories require documentation from a medical practitioner to verify the child's disability. If the family does not have insurance or cannot pay for a medical assessment that is necessary for educational classification, then according to IDEIA-2004, the local education agency must take fiscal responsibility. Again, members of the assessment team may need to acquire the expertise necessary to read and interpret reports prepared by medical personnel.

State-Specific Guidelines

Each state determines the key factors to consider during the evaluation process. These factors will vary from state to state. For example, the Oregon Department of Education (2003) has detailed assessment guidelines for each category (OAR 581-015-0051), while the Iowa Department of Education (2000) uses a systematic problem-solving process to determine eligibility [281—41.47(3)]. The Virginia Department of Education (2005) provides extensive guidelines for conducting evaluations and determining eligibility, but makes specific requirements only for learning disabilities (8 VAC 20-80-56). In addition to variation in guidelines, states also vary in criteria for educational classification. For instance, in classifying children as having mental retardation, some states determine IQ cutoff according to the number of standard deviations below the mean, some set no IQ score cutoff, others specify lower than 70, and still others specify below 75 (Denning, Chamberlain, & Polloway, 2000). Thus, while knowledge and understanding of federal laws and regulations is critical, a thorough understanding of a state's law and regulations is even more essential.

Nondiscriminatory Assessment

One of the most serious and ongoing concerns about assessment is the selection and administration of evaluation materials "so as not to be discriminatory on a racial or cultural basis" [§614(b)(3)(A)(i)]. Further, evaluations must be "provided and administered in the language and form most likely to yield accurate information on what the child knows and can do academically, developmentally, and functionally, unless it is not feasible to so provide or administer" [§614(b)(3)(A)(ii)]. Still, "the disproportionate representation of minority students in special education has been a constant and consistent concern for nearly 4 decades" (Hosp & Reschly, 2004, p. 186). For example, despite a ban on intelligence tests in California since 1986 and tremendous anti-test sentiment, low rates of academic achievement continued among ethnic minority groups (Lopez, 1997). Thus, a focus on testing practices alone does not resolve the issue. Educators must also closely examine instructional practice and cognitive demands.

Evaluation Results

Eligibility Determination Meeting

Upon completion of the administration of assessments and other evaluation measures, the assessment team meets to determine if the child is a child with a disability and what his or her educational needs are [§614(b)(4)(A)]. The parent(s) must receive "a copy of the evaluation report and the documentation of determination of eligibility" [§614(b)(4)(B)]. When the team determines a child's eligibility, the determining factor cannot be (a) lack of appropriate instruction in reading [§614(b)(5)(A)], (b) lack of math instruction [§614(b)(5)(B)], or (c) limited English proficiency [§614(b)(5)(C)]. In addition to determining eligibility, the team also decides educational classification. For example, is this a child who falls under the category of mental retardation?

Examining the various reports and discussing the child's abilities/strengths and lack of ability/weaknesses or deficits is a task that must be completed with sensitivity and awareness of parental and child reactions. Parents should never be "blindsided" by information in a meeting. All participants should keep in mind that child is first and foremost a child; the disability is secondary and not the sum of all the child is. Second, parents may be very relieved to know that their concerns about their child have been acknowledged and confirmed; however, the reality of the disability may cause them to experience grief.

An assessment team and, later, the individualized education program (IEP) team must include someone who is knowledgeable about evaluation and able to explain the results. Explaining standardized test results to persons with little experience in administering or interpreting test results can be somewhat challenging. Parents and even teachers do not always easily understand statistics and standardized scores. It can be very helpful to draw a bell curve or provide a visual representation with standard deviations and scores superimposed on the diagram. Placing scores in a visual context generally increases understanding and helps demystify the results.

In the course of the discussion, disagreements may arise among professionals or between parents and educators about educational classification. The intent of determining eligibility is to identify the child as a child with a disability and to determine the need for special education services and related services, not to engage in "territorial or turf battles" or to "insist on your position." If the process breaks down, or if either party is dissatisfied, *mediation* can be used to resolve differences. If mediation fails, a *due process hearing* can be requested.

Independent Educational Evaluation

One of the procedural safeguards guaranteed by IDEIA-2004 is an *independent educational evaluation* (IEE). If parents want an alternative source of information regarding their child's eligibility for special education services or clarification on specific areas of disability—that is, a second opinion—they can request an IEE at school district expense (Imber & Radclif, 2003). The results of an IEE, whether publicly or privately funded, must be considered by the IEP/assessment team, and independent evaluators must have the same access to student classrooms as school district evaluators.

Despite federal regulation, states have implemented this procedural safeguard unevenly, resulting in numerous due process hearings and court cases (Etscheidt, 2003). School districts must provide technically adequate evaluations, a comprehensive scope of evaluations in the hypothesized area(s) of disability, and useful evaluations for development of an IEP. Otherwise, Etscheidt found, parents prevailed in their requests for an IEE.

Confidentiality

Recently, standards for maintaining the privacy of individually identifiable health information were modified within the Health Insurance Portability and Accountability Act of 1996 (HIPAA, P.L. 104-191). Any mental health, dental, or medical provider must assure patients of their right to privacy and not disclose information to nondesignated parties, including local educational agencies. Permission to share information in either direction (i.e., school to non-school provider, non-school provider to school) has always been required; there is simply a heightened awareness now. Before speaking with someone outside of the local educational agency or sharing written information (e.g., test scores, behavior in classroom), both parties must have explicit written permission to do so.

Reevaluation

The mandate for reevaluation seeks to balance the need for information to determine if a child continues to be a child with a disability with the reality that repeated evaluations over time may not be needed and may not offer new or additional information about a child's eligibility, classification, or educational program. Thus, local educational agencies and parents have the option to determine when a reevaluation should occur, along with appropriate evaluation instruments. A reevaluation should occur at least every 3 years, but not more frequently than once a year. However, a parent, teacher, or the local educational agency can request a reevaluation at any time if both agree that circumstances warrant it. Likewise, if both parent and the local educational agency agree that a reevaluation is not necessary, then it does not have to happen. As a matter of organization, special education teachers or a child's case manager should keep track of impending 3-year reevaluations and begin the process approximately 60 days before the legal due date. This should allow adequate time to collaborate with parents and other team members, obtain informed consent, conduct evaluations, write reports, and process the information.

While planning for a reevaluation, all parties can agree not to repeat certain previous evaluation components. Instead, evaluation can target those areas where current information is needed. Evaluation is not necessary when a child with a disability is graduating or has reached age 22. All procedural safeguards are in effect for a reevaluation. However, if a local educational agency can document reasonable attempts to obtain parental consent for evaluation, informed parent consent is not needed [§614(c)(3)]. At the end of the reevaluation assessment, the IEP/assessment team meets to confirm the educational classification or change it.

Conclusion

In 1995 Jim Ysseldyke received the Council for Exceptional Children Research Award, recognizing more than 25 years of research on assessment and instructional decision-making practices. In 1979 this author sat in her first special education conference session at Utah State University and listened, extremely overwhelmed, to Dr. Ysseldyke's presentation on assessment. Not only did he and his colleagues set the stage for my beginning view of assessment as a special education teacher, they continue to influence my practice in teacher preparation and as a scholar. Ysseldyke (2001) reflected on his years of research and offered the following generalizations in relation to assessment and instructional decision-making:

First, change is difficult. When research demonstrates valid and effective assessment practices, the political nature of schools and educators may resist change and continue ineffective practice.

Second, expectations by educators of students with disabilities drive assessment practices. These expectations are frequently tied to labels and are, far too often, low. We expect children with autism to have difficulty with social interactions and thus, exclude them from opportunities to socialize with peers; or, at best, do not skillfully plan for inclusion.

Third, we still focus more on a search for pathology of a disability; that is, deficit-driven assessment, rather than on information to help the child achieve and succeed.

Fourth, we need to be ever mindful of the purpose of assessment. Tests must be utilized as developed and intended.

Fifth, too many students who are referred are tested and, ultimately, determined to be eligible for special education.

Finally, our current classification practices differ from state to state and even from district to district and frequently change in an effort to "better" identify a child as a child with a disability. Thus, despite increased sophistication of assessment tools and extensive legal requirements to prevent misclassification (Reschly, 2002), we still do not tie assessment for classification to interventions and educational outcomes.

It is critical that we identify students at risk for failure in schools and students with disabilities who need special education and related services in order to receive a free and appropriate education. However, assessment for educational classification is not an end unto itself. Rather, assessment for classification should be the beginning of an ongoing process of gathering information, measuring progress (or lack of progress), and making data-based decisions about educational programs and outcomes for children with disabilities.

Glossary

Assessment team—A group of individuals selected to plan, administer, and review relevant assessment information in order to determine if a child has a disability. Parents must be part of the assessment team, along with a general educator, special educator, and person(s) qualified to give appropriate standardized tests and conduct interviews and behavioral observations.

Child find activities—The federal mandate for school districts to identify, locate, and evaluate all resident preschool and school-age children who may have a disability and need early intervention, early childhood special education, or special education services. Activities may include screening, providing information to medical providers, or conducting awareness activities with parents and the general public.

Child study team—A group of educators selected to support a general education teacher's concerns about a student who has not been identified as having a disability.

Consent—Permission from a parent or other appropriate guardian or the student if over the age of 18 to conduct assessment.

Criterion-referenced—A test designed and administered in order to compare an individual's performance to a preset standard or criterion.

Diagnosis—A determination of a specific disability or condition by a licensed medical or psychological practitioner according to established professional guidelines.

Due process hearing—Legal proceeding initiated by either parents, the student if over the age of 18, or the local education agency to determine if the child is receiving a free and appropriate education or if a procedural violation has occurred. The resulting ruling is binding but can be appealed.

Educational classification—A determination by a school-based assessment team that a child meets the criteria set forth in 1 of the 14 federally defined categories of disability under IDEIA-2004.

Eligibility—A determination that a child is a child with a disability and entitled to receive special education services in the form of specially designed instruction and/or related services.

Independent educational evaluation—An evaluation conducted by a licensed professional who is not employed or contracted by the school district and submitted to the local education agency for use in determining if the child has a disability.

Initial evaluation—The administration of appropriate assessment tools and subsequent data-based analysis to determine if the child's presenting problem(s) is the result of a disability and if the child would benefit from special education.

Intervention—An instructional strategy, educational material, or behavioral strategy utilized with a student who is not responding to current strategies or materials employed in the general education classroom.

Mediation—Proceeding initiated either by parents, by the student he or she is over the age of 18, or by the local education agency and facilitated by a trained person knowledgeable about special education laws in order to reach a mutually agreeable decision on some aspect of a child's IEP or assessment process that has caused tension and disagreement among the parties.

Norm-referenced—A test designed and administered to compare an individual's performance with that of a group.

Pre-referral—Time frame and process during which a school-age child who is experiencing problems in the general education classroom is brought to the attention of a child study team for the purpose of trying various interventions and collecting data to determine if the child's problems are temporary, remediable, or extensive enough to warrant further consideration.

Referral—Process by which a school-age child who is experiencing substantial problems in the general education classroom or an infant or preschool-age child who is experiencing a developmental delay is recommended for assessment to determine if a disability exists.

Screenings—Quick, easy-to-administer assessment to determine whether a child presents as typically developing or warrants further, more sophisticated and complex assessment.

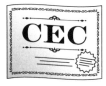

Knowledge and Skills for Entry-Level Special Education Teachers of Students With Developmental Disabilities Standards Addressed in This Chapter

Principle 1: Foundations

DD1K1 Definitions and issues related to the identification of individuals with developmental disabilities.

Principle 2: Development and Characteristics of Learners

DD2K2 Psychological, social/emotional, and motor characteristics of individuals with developmental disabilities.

DD2K3 Identification of significant core deficit areas for individuals with pervasive developmental disabilities, autism, and autism spectrum disorders.

DD2K4 Factors that influence over-representation of culturally/linguistically diverse individuals.

Principle 8: Assessment

DD8K1   Specialized terminology used in the assessment of individuals with developmental disabilities.

DD8K2   Environmental assessment conditions that promote maximum performance of individuals with developmental disabilities.

DD8K3   Adaptive behavior assessment.

DD8K4   Laws and policies regarding referral and placement procedures for individuals with developmental disabilities.

Web Site Resources

Assessment

http://www.education-world.com/special_ed/iep/assessment.shtml

Hosted by Education World, Inc. Provides links to assessment sites, including sections of documents, articles, reviews, and other valuable resources.

President's Commission on Excellence in Special Education Report: A New Era: Revitalizing Special Education for Children and Their Families

http://www.ed.gov/inits/commissionsboards/whspecialeducation/reports/two.html#top

Recommendations regarding assessment practices and needed amendments to IDEA to improve the methods used to locate, identify, and assess children who are suspected of having a disability.

Psychoeducational Assessment for Special Education Placement in School: When Your Child Doesn't Qualify

http://childparenting.about.com/cs/learningproblems/a/specialed.htm

Interesting site oriented toward families and questions they may have regarding the assessment process and their rights.

References

Alpert, D. (2004). Diagnosis versus classification and who can do them. *Special Education Muckraker*. Retrieved April 25, 2005, from http://www.specialeducationmuckraker.com

American Psychiatric Association. (1994). *Diagnostic and statistical manual of mental disorders* (4th ed.). Washington, DC: Author.

Brown, L., Sherbenou, R. J., & Johnsen, S. (1997). *Test of Nonverbal Intelligence—Third Edition*. Austin, TX: PRO-ED.

Burgemeister, B. B., Blurn, L. H., & Lorge, I. (1972). *Columbia Mental Maturity Scale*. San Antonio, TX: Harcourt Assessment.

Denning, C. B., Chamberlain, J. A., & Polloway, E. A. (2000). An evaluation of state guidelines for mental retardation: Focus on definition and classification practices. *Education and Training in Mental Retardation and Developmental Disabilities, 35*, 226–232.

Developmental Disabilities Assistance and Bill of Rights Act of 2000, 42 U.S.C. § 15001 *et seq.*

Etscheidt, S. (2003). Ascertaining the adequacy, scope, and utility of district evaluations. *Exceptional Children, 69*, 227–247.

Hammill, D. D., Pearson, N. A., & Wiederholt, L. (1996). *Comprehensive Test of Nonverbal Intelligence*. Austin, TX: PRO-ED.

Health Insurance Portability and Accountability Act of 1996 (HIPPA), 45 C.F.R. Parts 160 & 164.

Hosp, J. L., & Reschly, D. J. (2003). Referral rates for intervention or assessment: A meta-analysis of racial differences. *Journal of Special Education, 37*(2), 67–80.

Hosp, J. L., & Reschly, D. J. (2004). Disproportionate representation of minority students in special education: Academic, demographic, and economic predictors. *Exceptional Children, 70,* 185–199.

Imber, S. C., & Radclif, D. (2003). Independent educational evaluations under IDEA '97: It's a testy matter. *Exceptional Children, 70,* 27–44.

Individuals with Disabilities Education Act Amendments of 1997, 20 U.S.C. § 1400 *et seq.* (1997).

Individuals with Disabilities Education Improvement Act of 2004, 118 Stat. 2647. (2004).

Iowa Administrative Rules of Special Education, Division VII: Identification, 256B, 34 C.F.R. 300.

Kamphaus, R. W. (1993). *Clinical assessment of children's intelligence.* Boston: Allyn & Bacon.

Lambert, N., Nihiri, K., & Leland, H. (1993). *AAMR Adaptive Behavior Scales—School* (2nd ed.). Austin, TX: PRO-ED.

La Paro, K. M., Olsen, K., & Pianta, R. C. (2002). Special education eligibility: Developmental precursors over the first three years of life. *Exceptional Children, 69,* 55–66.

Lopez, R. (1997). The practical impact of current research and issues in intelligence test interpretation and use for multicultural populations. *School Psychology Review, 26,* 249–254.

Luckasson, R., Borthwick-Duffy, S., Buntinx, W. H. E., Coulter, D. L., Craig, E. M., Reeve, A., et al. (2002). *Mental retardation: Definition, classification, and system of supports* (10th ed.). Washington, DC: American Association on Mental Retardation.

McCall, R. B., Appelbaum, M., & Hogarthy, P. S. (1973). Developmental changes in mental performance. *Monographs of the Society for Research in Child Development, 38*(3), 1–84.

McCarthy, D. (1972). *McCarthy Scales of Children's Abilities.* San Antonio, TX: Harcourt Assessment.

Obiakor, F. E., & Wilder, L. K. (2003). Disproportionate representation in special education. *Principal Leadership* (Middle School Ed.), *4*(2), 16–21.

Oregon Department of Education. (2003). Oregon Administrative Rules, Chapter 581, Rule 581-015-0051.

Overton, T. (2006). *Assessing learners with special needs: An applied approach* (5th ed.). Upper Saddle River, NJ: Pearson/Merrill/Prentice Hall.

Pierangelo, R., & Giuliani, G. (2006). *The special educator's comprehensive guide to 301 diagnostic tests.* San Francisco: Jossey-Bass.

Reschly, D. J. (2002). Change dynamics in special education assessment: Historical and contemporary patterns. *Peabody Journal of Education, 77,* 117–136.

Roid, G. H. (2003). *Stanford-Binet Intelligence Scale: Fifth Edition.* Itasca, IL: Riverside Publishing.

Scott, M. S., Fletcher, K. L., & Martell, B. (2000). Selecting components for a screening test to identify three-year-olds at risk for mild learning problems. *Education and Training in Mental Retardation and Developmental Disabilities, 35,* 208–221.

Section 504 of the Rehabilitation Act of 1973, 29 U.S.C. § 794 *et seq.*

Slosson, R. L., Revised by Nicholson, C. L., & Hibpschman, T. L. (1998). *Slosson Intelligence Test—Revised.* East Aurora, NY: Slosson Educational Publications.

Sparrow, S. S., Cicchetti, D. V., & Balla, D. A. (2005). *Vineland Adaptive Behavior Scales* (2nd ed.). Circle Pines, MN: AGS Publishing.

Thompson, J. R., Bryant, B. R., Campbell, E. M., Craig, E. M., Hughes, C. M., Rotholz, D. A., et al. (2004). *Supports Intensity Scale (SIS).* Washington, DC: American Association on Mental Retardation.

Virginia Department of Education. (2005). Virginia Administrative Code, 8 VAC 20-80-56.

Wechsler, D. (1997). *Wechsler Adult Intelligence Scale* (3rd ed.). San Antonio, TX: Harcourt Assessment.

Wechsler, D. (2002). *Wechsler Preschool and Primary Scale of Intelligence—Third Edition.* San Antonio, TX: Harcourt Assessment.

Wechsler, D. (2003). *Wechsler Intelligence Scale for Children—IV.* San Antonio, TX: Harcourt Assessment.

Wechsler, D. (2004). *Wechsler Intelligence Scale for Children—IV Spanish.* San Antonio, TX: Harcourt Assessment.

Woodrich, D. L. (1997). *Children's psychological testing* (3rd ed.). Baltimore: Brookes.

Ysseldyke, J. (2001). Reflections on a research career: Generalizations from 25 years of research on assessment and instructional decision-making. *Exceptional Children, 67,* 295–309.

20

Measuring Assistive Technology Outcomes in Education:

Theory and Practice

Dave L. Edyburn

Summary

Despite the long-standing interest in technology in special education, interest in measuring the outcomes of assistive technology (AT) is a relatively recent phenomenon. This chapter provides an accessible introduction to theoretical and practical issues associated with measuring AT outcomes in education, placing particular emphasis on the application of principles and practices for professionals' working with students with developmental disabilities. The chapter's four sections discuss the historical context of AT outcomes, the current state of affairs, emerging research and measurement models, and future directions.

Learning Outcomes

After reading this chapter, you should be able to:

- Articulate three events associated with the historical context and emergence of AT outcome measurement.

- Define the term *assistive technology*.

- Give an example of a device that could be considered AT.

- Summarize the concerns associated with the view that "AT is anything."

- Compare and contrast views about how best to measure AT outcomes—by a single variable (e.g., satisfaction) or by a complex construct of variables (e.g., change in performance/function, change in participation, consumer satisfaction, goal achievement, quality of life, and cost).

- Describe design, measurement, analysis, and decision-making factors that need to be addressed in the process of creating an outcomes system for measuring the impact of AT.

- Summarize issues that need to be addressed in future work on AT outcomes relative to theoretical advances and service delivery systems.

Introduction

Technology holds considerable promise for people with disabilities (Blackhurst, 1965). While many people consider the application of technology in special education to be a relatively recent development, in practice the foundations of our field can be traced back well over 100 years (Blackhurst, 1997, 2005). Despite this legacy, we have yet to capture the potential of technology for every individual who could possibly benefit from AT. This chapter provides an accessible introduction to theoretical and practical issues associated with measuring AT outcomes in education, placing particular emphasis on the application of principles and practices for professionals working with students with developmental disabilities.

Historical Context

To establish the historical context of measuring AT outcomes in education it is important to briefly review some critical dates and events within the field of special education. Many readers are aware that the passage of the Education for All Handicapped Children Act of 1975 (P.L. 94-142) was a defining moment in special education. The concept of free appropriate public education (FAPE) provided an important and necessary opportunity for students with disabilities to be educated in public schools. The recent 30th anniversary of this federal law provided an opportunity to reflect on the successes of this landmark legislation (H. Con. Res. 288, 2005), as well as its shortcomings relative to overrepresentation of minorities (Ferri & Connor, 2005) and unfulfilled promises for appropriate funding (Kearns, 2005).

In contrast, establishing a defining event to mark the dawn of AT in special education is not quite as easy. Some observers point to the passage of the Technology Related Assistance for Individuals with Disabilities Act of 1988 (P.L. 100-407), "the Tech Act," as the first large-scale effort to provide AT for every individual with a disability. Other observers believe it was not until the 1997 Amendments to the Individuals with Disabilities Education Act (IDEA, P.L. 105-17), when it was mandated that individualized education program (IEP) teams "consider" AT when planning each student's IEP, that AT came close to reaching every student. Depending on the emphasis that one places on each event, it can be claimed that serious attention to AT in the schools is as young as 10 years or as old as 20 years. Essentially, both figures illustrate the relative youth of the field of special education technology.

What Is Assistive Technology?

The federal definition of AT was first advanced in the Tech Act (P.L. 100-407) and subsequently written into several federal laws and every state's laws associated with technology use by people with disabilities:

§300.5 Assistive technology device.

… Assistive technology device means any item, piece of equipment, or product system, whether acquired commercially off the shelf, modified, or customized, that is used to increase, maintain, or improve the functional capabilities of a child with a disability. [20 U.S.C. 1401(1)]

A second, companion definition outlines a critical component associated with AT. That is, success is dependent on having access not only to a device, but also to several types of supports. These support factors are outlined in the following federal definition of AT services:

§300.6 Assistive technology service.

… Assistive technology service means any service that directly assists a child with a disability in the selection, acquisition, or use of an assistive technology device.

The term includes—

(a) The evaluation of the needs of a child with a disability, including a functional evaluation of the child in the child's customary environment;

(b) Purchasing, leasing, or otherwise providing for the acquisition of assistive technology devices by children with disabilities;

(c) Selecting, designing, fitting, customizing, adapting, applying, maintaining, repairing, or replacing assistive technology devices;

(d) Coordinating and using other therapies, interventions, or services with assistive technology devices, such as those associated with existing education and rehabilitation plans and programs;

(e) Training or technical assistance for a child with a disability or, if appropriate, that child's family; and

(f) Training or technical assistance for professionals (including individuals providing education or rehabilitation services), employers, or other individuals who provide services to, employ, or are otherwise substantially involved in the major life functions of that child. [20 U.S.C. 1401(2)]

The AT service definition is far ahead of its time in that it recognizes that successful AT outcomes are dependent on more than simply acquiring new devices. Indeed, comprehensive "wraparound services" are essential to success in adoption of new technologies.

What Is Meant by "Outcome"?

DeRuyter (1997) clarifies a number of terms associated with AT outcome measurement (bold emphasis added):

An **activity** refers to some specified endeavor, effort or field of action. The purpose toward which such an effort is directed, worked toward or aspired to is referred to as the **goal or objective. The final consequences or end results of that goal is the outcome.** *Goals, objectives, and outcomes are all measurable and change oriented, however, they are not activities.* For example, the creation of a program evaluation system in assistive technology is an activity designed to accomplish the goal/ objective of obtaining increased information regarding assistive technology services that are delivered in order to improve the ultimate outcome of providing the most effective and efficient service or the greatest value at the best cost.

The evaluation process in the service delivery system that is designed to measure and establish a baseline of what works; how well something works; for which clients it works; and, at what level of economic efficiency it works is known as outcomes research. Taking that baseline information to evaluate specific providers to determine how well they perform, either against past performance or amongst one another is referred to as outcomes measurement. Outcomes measurement in the clinical service delivery system has proven to be the most effective and efficient providers for purposes of provider selection, contracting, reimbursement, education, and quality improvement. The process whereby data are managed in an ongoing and systematic manner to improve care is termed outcomes management. By analyzing and evaluating the data as well as disseminating the results it becomes possible to improve the outcomes. (p. 90)

What Type of Variables Might Be Measured to Reflect AT Outcomes?

In focus group research conducted by the Assistive Technology Outcomes Measurement System (ATOMS) Project (Edyburn, 2003c), AT service directors generated the following list of variables that might be measured to understand the outcomes associated with AT use: (a) change in performance/function (body, structure, activity), (b) change in participation, (c) consumer satisfaction (process and devices), (d) goal achievement, (e) quality of life, and (f) cost.

Three other types of variables also need to be tracked and monitored: (a) demographics (age, gender, disability, ethnicity, language, etc.), (b) AT interventions (services and devices), and (c) environmental context.

In the past, single measures (e.g., satisfaction) have served as a proxy for the outcomes associated with AT use. However, the preceding lists raise interesting questions about whether the construct of AT outcomes can be measured in a single dimension or is a complex multidimensional construct. This question brings us to the next issue: Whose outcome is it?

Whose Outcome?

DeRuyter (1995, 1997) raises interesting questions about whose outcome we measure. If an individual reports high satisfaction with a device, is that sufficient outcome data? And, if the individual is satisfied with a device, what if discernible differences in performance or participation cannot be measured? Are these outcomes more or less important than the outcomes a funding source is interested in? Indeed, significant work remains to be done to understand the values held by stakeholders concerning various AT outcomes and how these values might be transformed into weights within a measurement system to give priority to certain factors within the outcome model. It is important to underscore the significance of the underlying theoretical application of self-determination for this critical issue.

Current State of Affairs

Rethinking the Role of AT
in Enhancing Academic Performance

In recent years, concerns have been raised about the broad nature of the definition such that the operative definition is "assistive technology is anything that enhances performance" (Edyburn, 2003f, 2005). Indeed, the broad definition is fraught with significant measurement problems, given estimates that there are more than 26,000 specialized AT products (http://www.abledata.com). As a result, there is an urgent need for definitional clarity with respect to the construct of AT so that researchers can discern what is and isn't AT and can demonstrate differential outcomes for people with developmental disabilities and their non-disabled peers.

For example, if a technology like text-to-speech helps everyone that uses it, is it really AT or universal design? The problem that "AT is anything" takes on new significance in the current context of (a) the mandate to consider AT for each student with a disability, (b) the sheer size of the high-incidence-disability population, and (c) the sanctions associated with failing to demonstrate adequate yearly progress (AYP) within the No Child Left Behind Act of 2001 (NCLB, P.L. 107-110).

Edyburn (2001) has argued that the federal definitions of AT devices and services represent two legs of a three-legged stool. The missing leg is that of outcome. While functional performance is mentioned in the definition of AT, the outcomes achieved through AT use have been overlooked and under-emphasized in federal law. As a result, there are few professional guidelines to inform the decision making associated with using technology to enhance performance. This oversight has resulted in legal exposure for schools such that AT devices and services are federally mandated but there are no recognized guidelines for using outcome data to approve or deny requests for AT.

Practically speaking, if a person is able to complete a task only 20% of the time, does that not provide clear evidence of a performance problem? If so, are systems in place to trigger the assistive technology consideration process? If AT is subsequently provided, what level of performance subsequently should be expected? 30%? 50%? 60%? 80%? 90%?

While the importance of measuring the outcomes of AT is well documented (DeRuyter, 1997; Fuhrer, Jutai, Scherer, & DeRuyter, 2003), limited empirical work has been completed to date, and few measurement instruments are available for assessing outcomes. Why has the field of AT been so slow to measure outcomes? Two perspectives are worth noting. The first involves the youth of the profession. We simply have not been around long enough to build a significant research base. Only within the last 10 years has the profession begun to reexamine the evidence base supporting AT practices. As a result, the evidence base is often found to be inadequate for answering critical questions about the effectiveness of AT (Edyburn, Higgins, & Boone, 2005).

A second perspective suggests an evolving standard of proof. For example, during the explosion of AT devices and services during the 1980s and 1990s, outcomes of AT were of concern to only two stakeholders: the consumer and the provider. Outcomes were not measured in any formal manner; it was obvious that AT helped. A client came to an AT specialist not being able to do a specific task; after an evaluation and location of appropriate AT, he or she was able to complete the task better than before. In hindsight, it seems we were very naive.

A small body of work provides some insight into the role of AT in enhancing academic achievement and ways to measure the outcomes of technology-enhanced performance. Silverman, Stratman, and Smith (2000) examined the role that various assessment instruments play in generating evidence about AT use and outcome. Their findings revealed that practitioners must pay specific attention to the nature of their questions (e.g., does a child need AT?) and the nature of the assessment instrument that they are using to collect data to answer their questions. Denham and Lahm (2001) provide an outstanding example of how IEP objectives guided the use of assistive technology to make accessible curriculum and assessment materials that quantitatively document the educational progress of four students with moderate and severe disabilities. Armstrong (2003) created an example of how to align curriculum standards, instructional technology, AT, and outcome measurement in the context of learning to locate places on a map in a way that allows these interventions to be considered, implemented, and assessed in an inclusive classroom. Edyburn has outlined a series of methodological considerations associated with measuring AT outcomes in the context of academic subjects such as reading (2004b), writing (2003e), and math (2003d). Despite this growing body of literature on measuring AT outcomes in education, much work remains to be done to understand the patterns of performance associated with students' use of AT for learning (Edyburn, 2005).

Essential Components of the Outcome Equation in Education

At the present time, there is little evidence that AT outcomes are routinely measured in K–12 schools. Unfortunately, the data, if collected at all, are associated with issues of compliance (e.g., date of referral, date of assessment, date of follow-up meetings) and acquisition (e.g., date equipment was ordered, date received, price) rather than objective measures of performance outcomes. In the design of an outcome measurement system for a school or a district, attention must be focused on three critical components of the outcome equation: AT consideration, AT intervention, and AT outcome measurement.

Consideration

The IDEA mandate to consider AT provides education with a unique legal requirement among the various service delivery systems (e.g., medical, vocational, independent living) for individuals with developmental disabilities. A number of current practices confound AT outcome measurement:

- *Lack of evidence base*. Little evidence has been provided that all students who could benefit from AT have access to appropriate devices and services, which raises questions about access, bias, and equity for students who are unserved or underserved.

- *Dated service delivery model*. The typical AT service delivery model emulates the special education referral and placement process and therefore is subject to many of the same inherent flaws concerning efficacy, cost, time delay in provision of services, emphasis on front-end activities with little attention to follow-along and follow-up, etc.

- *Paper trail deficiency*. The consideration mandate has been implemented in the form of a yes/no check box that provides virtually no paper trail concerning what has been considered, tried, discarded, and sustained.

- *Lack of training.* IEP teams lack adequate training and tools to support their responsibilities to consider AT that meets the intent of the mandate.

While considerable work remains to achieve the goal of AT consideration, several recent developments show promise. A call for rethinking AT offers the opportunity to advance a unifying theory that links AT, instructional technology, and universal design (Edyburn, 2004). In addition, recognition of the role that assistive technology can play as an cognitive prosthesis to support enhanced cognitive functioning of individuals with disabilities may lead to increased research, development, and policy initiatives (Edyburn, 2004a, 2006a). Finally, new tools are emerging to support the work of IEP teams as they consider AT (Purcell & Grant, 2002, 2004).

Intervention

Few resources are currently available to assist teachers, therapists, and administrators in identifying appropriate AT and instructional technologies that will help students achieve specific academic goals. As a result, it is difficult for the profession to identify a common set of interventions that have been validated as helpful in response to a common set of instructional challenges. This means the profession is characterized by trial and error rather than by a knowledge base that has been established through scientifically based evidence.

Relatively few databases are commonly used for locating appropriate assistive technology interventions. These include (a) CTG Solutions (http://www.closingthegap.com/solutions/), (b) Georgia Tools for Life (http://www.gatfl.org/ldguide/default.htm), and (c) AbleData (http://www.abledata.com).

User perspectives are an important source of information about "what works." For example, Richard Wanderman's LD Resources, at http://www.ldresources.com, is a frequently visited resource for professionals as consumers who are seeking a voice of experience.

Much more work is needed to understand the instructional power of interventions that enhance performance. Particularly problematic are current policy initiatives that seek to negate the use of technology to enhance performance. In many cases, educators, administrators, and policymakers choose to hide behind the cloak of high standards and accountability. If one holds high standards, any requests for using other tools to meet the requirements are viewed as an attempt to lower standards. We must be clear: A one-size-fits-all model that standardizes all variables associated with learning will not produce high performance in all students. While we can hold high standards and expectations, we must recognize the role that technology can play in enhancing the performance of diverse learners such that any number of tools can be used to complete a task successfully. Thus, the variable of intervention must remain flexible and open to multiple means of completing academic tasks. Promising work in this area involves the creation of decision-assist assessment tools for differentiating the need for various assistive and instructional interventions (Dyck & Pemberton, 2002; Edyburn, 2003b).

Outcome Measurement

As mentioned earlier, the measurement of AT outcomes is a recent development. The application of this specialty area in education is still in its infancy. Current available research does, however, support the following:

- *Current service delivery systems do not collect outcome data.* Caseloads are devoted almost exclusively to new evaluations and AT device acquisition, with little attention to ongoing case management.

- *Existing measurement instruments tend to be clinical in nature and not readily applicable to daily classroom use.* The ATOMS Project has created an interactive database to examine an array of outcome measurement instruments. To browse this collection, visit http://www3.uwm.edu/CHS/r2d2/atoms/idata/

Given what we know, some emerging directions include needs for:

1. *Redefining caseload to rebalance effort from new evaluations and device acquisition to increased time allocated to follow-along and follow-up efforts.* The demands of collecting AT outcome data are likely to contribute to the need to redefine caseload such that time is built into one's schedule to allow for routine data collection. It is likely that we will learn that some types of technologies (e.g., augmentative communication devices) will require more-intensive data collection efforts than other forms of AT (e.g., screen readers).

2. *Creation of downloadable tools for measuring AT outcomes.* While commercial protocols are a standard of the assessment industry, the specialized nature of AT outcome measurement may challenge typical commercialization efforts. As a result, the creation and dissemination of standardized data collection protocols that can be downloaded and used might be a viable alternative.

3. *Development of PDA-type tools that facilitate data collection and subsequent uploading of the data for analysis.* Given the time pressures under which professionals work, the availability of handheld data collection tools will increase the likelihood that AT outcome data will be routinely collected. Uploading the data from the device to the computer for analysis will further facilitate the process.

4. *Prototype efforts to create a national database of AT outcome data and decision assist tools.* Creating local databases of AT outcome data is likely to be a developmental progress indicator. However, development of national databases will be important for establishing adequate data sets and sophisticated analyses of AT outcomes (Edyburn & Smith, 2004).

An AT outcome measurement system will need to collect data not only on the specific type of AT but also on various kinds of support services, frequency of service, quality of service, and other important factors. Smith (1996, 2000) argues that the concomitant delivery of services must be isolated in order to understand the unique contribution of AT. Indeed, the task of isolating the unique contributions of AT to improve functional performance has posed formidable research design challenges for AT researchers.

Emerging Research and Measurement Models

In contrast to the abundance of measures and indicators that profile the acquisition of technology, less information is typically available to reflect the impact of AT. Research and development efforts are currently focused on developing frameworks

(Fuhrer et al., 2003; Lenker & Paquet, 2003) for understanding the process of using evidence to inform decision making about the impact of AT.

It is important to distinguish between "claims of effectiveness" and statements that can be supported by evidence and subsequently verified. That is, just because I say a device is effective for a specific child doesn't mean everyone will agree with my statement. As a result, all statements about AT effectiveness should initially be treated simply as claims of effectiveness (Edyburn, 2003a).

The routine scrutiny of each claim of effectiveness of AT is a nondiscriminatory professional practice. That is, vendors are not held to a higher standard simply because they are a for-profit organization versus the standard that an independent engineer would need to meet to show the effectiveness of the product. Similarly, it means that parents are not required to present more "proof" than a professional would present to support a request for AT devices and services.

To judge the validity of a claim that AT is effective, we need to review some evidence. Edyburn (2003c) has viewed the challenges associated with the collection of evidence to support the effectiveness of AT to be a developmental process that moves through three distinct phases: (a) exploratory, (b) descriptive, and (c) empirical. A product that is not commercially available will have less evidence to support claims of effectiveness than one that has been commercially available for many years. Similarly, some devices and services will have been the focus of extensive research efforts, and others will not, which means we may need to rely on general research-based principles of learning to ascertain their potential value for enhancing academic achievement.

As a member of the ATOMS Project, I have helped to identify the following design, measurement, analysis, and decision-making factors that will need to be addressed in the process of creating an outcomes system for measuring the impact of AT: (a) use of repeated measures research designs, (b) standardization of the performance task, (c) standardization of the data collection and coding process, (d) analysis of the results using standardized metrics and benchmarks, and (e) decision making.

Repeated Measures Research Design

Central to the definition of AT is the expectation of enhanced performance. Smith (2000) outlines a theoretical view known as Time Series Concurrent and Differential (TSCD) Approach, which involves a series of performance measures of an individual when she or he is completing a specific task with AT and without AT. Ideally, the results reflect a pattern similar to the one shown in Figure 20.1. As shown, the difference between the two measurements isolates the specific impact of AT and provides evidence of the impact and outcome over time. This approach appears to hold considerable promise for applications of AT in academic content areas (Edyburn, 2003d, 2003e, 2004b).

In general, the repeated measures of performance with and without AT research design utilize the following steps: (a) data collection, (b) data analysis, (c) data interpretation, and (e) decision making.

Data Collection

Data collection with regard to AT outcomes in education is currently very difficult because of the lack of standardization of performance tasks. However, a variety of standard measures are commonly used in education to measure academic performance

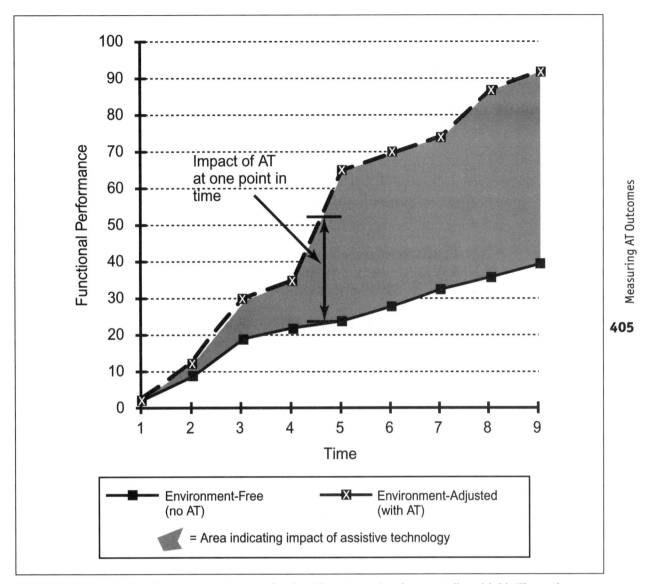

FIGURE 20.1. A graph of performance in environment-free (no AT) context and environment adjusted (with AT) over time.

and therefore may potentially be used here (e.g., mathematics computation, reading comprehension, holistic scoring of writing). Therefore, considerable effort must be devoted to standardizing the performance tasks for which AT outcome measures will be measured. For example, if the outcome of AT in the form of a portable keyboard (e.g., Dana by Alphasmart®) is sought, outcome measures to assess keyboard speed and quality of writing should be used.

At the present time, few standards exist for determining when data should be collected: at the time of initial delivery of the new AT device, daily, weekly, monthly, and so forth. Without agreement about the timeline for data collection, comparisons among outcome data will not be possible. As a result, there is an urgent need for defining and standardizing when AT performance snapshots will be taken (Edyburn, Fennema-Jansen, Hariharan, & Smith, 2005).

Finally, there is little information about the standardization of the data collection procedures and subsequent coding of the data. In work conducted by the ATOMS Project (Edyburn & Smith, 2004), it is very clear that standardizing data collection tools that are scaled to produce scores in multiples of 10 is ideal for computing percentages and other statistical transformations.

Data Analysis

Data collection typically produces what is known as *raw scores*. Raw scores are converted into *standard scores* that allow for the manipulation of the performance data into meaningful units of analysis. Statistical analysis can subsequently be used to make comparisons about data sets.

Science is increasingly relying on visualization tools to reveal meaningful patterns within a data set. Current research efforts are exploring the application of data visualization tools for presenting AT outcome data. At the present time, however, little normative information is available to assist in establishing data analysis standards and protocols. As a result, it is difficult to make comparisons among outcome scores produced by various outcome measurement instruments.

Data Interpretation

Schools routinely evaluate academic performance of students. Every classroom has extensive systems in place to identify failure, adequate performance, and exceptional performance. While traditional grade books serve as convenient containers for collecting academic performance data, they reveal little about trends in academic performance and provide little incentive to intervene. Essentially, grade books serve as a buffer between the teacher and the student and perpetuate the myth that if learning is not occurring, the problem lies with the student.

Figure 20.2 illustrates the daily algebra homework scores of four ninth-grade students.

Which graph illustrates (a) a student who is successfully achieving? (b) a student who is non-engaged? (c) a student with inconsistent performance? (d) a consistently low-performing student? Rather than addressing the issues of poor performance, educators often search for reasons to explain poor performance, become sidetracked, and fail to intervene with appropriate supports. However, without knowing all the reasons, perhaps we can agree that the performance profiles of three of the four students provide clear evidence of a performance problem.

Decision Making

Little is known about individual and group decision making about assistive technology performance data. That is, when viewing a specific set of data, will everyone come to the same conclusion about what the data reflect?

Analysis of the student performance data should reveal several factors that will inform decision making. First, does the graph indicate that performance with AT is higher than performance without assistive technology? If so, the case can be made that the AT is an effective intervention for enhancing performance. If not, the data suggest the need for additional training or a need for a different intervention.

Second, do the data reflect that the student is able to meet the performance standard (i.e., 80% comprehension)? If so, the case can be made that the reading AT effectively compensates for the person's disability. If the performance standard is not met, the IEP team needs to explore whether additional time is needed for developing mastery, whether additional interventions must be applied concomitantly, or whether a different intervention is needed.

Finally, can high levels of performance be maintained over time? That is, will the routine use of the AT result in consistent high-quality performance in reading? Is there any evidence that the assistive technology is closing the achievement gap?

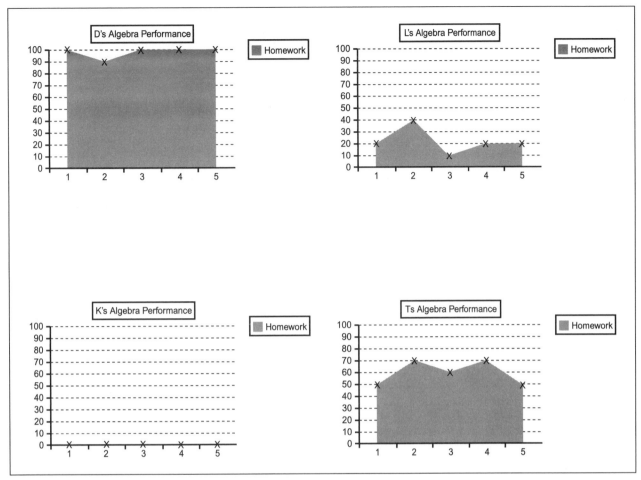

FIGURE 20.2. Four graphs of ninth-grade student performance data from algebra homework. Which graph illustrates (a) a student who is successfully achieving? (b) a student who is non-engaged? (c) a student with inconsistent performance? (d) a consistently low-performing student?

The ATOMS Project has been collecting questions generated by various assistive technology stakeholders (see Table 20.1). The questions are revealing in the sense that they indicate a divergent array of demands concerning what we want an outcome information system to tell us. As a result, question sets such as these are useful in designing AT outcome systems, and they illustrate that a variety of needs must be addressed if the systems are going to yield valuable information for each stakeholder.

Future Directions

In this final section, I outline a series of theoretical and service delivery issues that appear to be important for guiding future directions of the field of developmental disabilities.

TABLE 20.1

Selected Stakeholder Questions Concerning AT Outcomes

Conceptual	• How does cost equate with satisfaction?
	• How long do I keep trying this? (What's the learning curve?)
	• How can change best be measured and then assessed?
	• What is the relationship between AT training (services) and performance? (graph with performance on the Y axis and hours of training on the X axis? S-curve?)
	• Once we have data, what is the interpretation strategy?
Specific	• What organization of vocabulary on a dynamic display communication device promotes communication (e.g., Spontaneous Novel Utterance Generation—SNUG)? What is most effective in promoting function?
Consumer	• How will it help me?
	• Will it ever break down?
	• Will it help me find a job?
Quality of Life	• How can quality of life be assessed for AT?
Parents/Advocates	• Will my child be able to use this to take standardized tests?
	• What will other people think of my child if he or she uses it?
	• Who oversees year-to-year transition of learning needs to make sure the device(s) match the needs? (good outcomes now and in the future)
	• How much training will my child need to be able to use the device?
	• Which device will help my child at the least cost?
Provider	• Has my patient benefited from AT?
	• Did the device meet the goals of the client?
	• Who is responsible for collecting data?
Outcome as It Impacts Selection	• Concerning a specific device: What ones are available?
	• Is this the best device for my client considering cost-effectiveness and performance?
Vendor/Developer	• What difference does our product make?
	• What's the best performance that can be attained?
	• How can we demonstrate the cost-effectiveness of the product?
	• How can I maximize the return on investment?
	• What market segments are we missing?
Payer	• Is it proven to be effective?
	• Is it medically necessary?
	• Who decided it was necessary?

Theoretical Issues

The current definition of AT is problematic when the operational word is *any*. If AT is anything, then how do we determine what isn't AT? While historically this problem was isolated to low-incidence disabilities when AT was considered only for individuals with physical and sensory impairments, it takes on a new magnitude when applied to high-incidence disabilities involving cognition. For example, how does an IEP team respond to requests for the following forms of AT for students with memory impairments (AskJeeves, http://www.askjeeves.com), difficulty generating written text (iDictate, http://www.idictate.com), or the inability to complete math calculations (http://www.webmath.com)? At the present time, little attention has been devoted to applications of technology that serve as a cognitive prosthesis (Edyburn, 2004a, 2006a). As a result, there is a critical need to clarify the theoretical constructs associated with using technology to enhance teaching, learning, and performance. Why is a software product, for example, Inspiration® (Inspiration Software, Inc.), considered to be AT for a student with a disability but instructional technology for everyone else? And how does the design of learning environments and instructional materials that utilize principles of universal design affect the need for AT? Theoretical models that unify these disparate constructs will reduce the artificial boundaries that have developed among these related disciplines and contribute to advances in research, practice, and product development.

If local, state, and federal educational policy is to be informed by data, considerable commitment will be required to establish data collection protocols in order to assemble a body of valid and reliable data concerning the use of technology by students with developmental disabilities. Research is needed to define the essential data set that needs to be collected so as to provide reliable and valid data for decision making but at the same time not overwhelm the professional staff.

Given the paucity of AT outcome data, little attention has been devoted to interpreting performance data. As a result, considerable work must be devoted to understanding the kinds of questions that stakeholders want to be able to answer with an AT outcome system (Edyburn & Smith, 2004). Specific attention needs to be devoted to the ways in which data can be visualized and the impact that these various representations have on the interpretation of performance data.

Little is known about the issues associated with delaying the provision of AT in favor of providing additional instruction and remediation (Edyburn, 2003b, 2005, 2006b). This often means that students are not provided with appropriate AT because of the assumption that they still have time to learn it (or will learn the material if we find the right material, if we provide high-quality instruction, or if they simply try harder). As a result, decision aids that address the balance between remediation and compensation are urgently needed to guide IEP teams in designing interventions that offer the appropriate levels of challenge and support.

Finally, as the AT knowledge base continues to grow in terms of its evidence base, research is needed to demonstrate the power of various interventions for enhancing academic performance. Response-to-intervention protocols (Fuchs & Fuchs, 2005) are a promising development in this regard. These protocols basically use performance on curriculum-based measures to screen for those who are at risk for school failure and then monitor academic progress as interventions are applied. Standardization of the performance measures also allows normative comparisons, an essential task in demonstrating adequate yearly progress (AYP) as required for No Child Left Behind.

Service Delivery Issues

Current professional practices associated with AT consideration will need to be rethought in light of challenges that procedures are biased and discriminatory such that all students who could benefit from assistive technology do not have access to appropriate devices and services. This will necessitate creation of an AT child-find system similar to IDEA-mandated special education child find. In addition, screening protocols will need to be developed to aid in assessing all individuals who could benefit from a specific type of AT. These would replace the current trial-and-error methods currently in use for locating the most appropriate AT.

Given the importance of obtaining evidence to inform AT decision making, data collection will need to be integrated into the daily work of all teachers, administrators, technology specialists, and related service personnel. Acquisition of performance data must become a routine activity. This initiative will involve the clarification of roles and responsibilities within the AT staff, as it is likely to affect caseload, since more time will need to be devoted to follow-up and follow-along than is currently allowed.

When to take data snapshots? The analogy of a snapshot is helpful to consider when discussing assistive technology outcomes (Edyburn et al., 2005; Fenemma-Jansen, 2005). A snapshot provides powerful evidence (i.e., data) about what is going on in the life of the child, where he is, who she is with, and what he is doing. Obviously, if you take 10 snapshots in a day, you have a more complete picture of the child's life than if you take only a single snapshot.

How to collect data? Less information is available about how outcome data collection can be integrated into daily professional practice (Armstrong, 2003; Denham & Lahm, 2001; Laskarewski & Susi, 2003; Reed, Bowser, & Korsten, 2002). Whereas the literature provides little information about the types of AT outcomes data collection systems currently used in K–12 schools, the ATOMS Project staff assembled a list of four strategies that have been implemented by schools in efforts to address questions of assistive technology outcomes. These strategies involve collecting data during AT trials, as part of the IEP development and monitoring process, as part of grant-funded projects, and during year-end loan bank evaluation efforts. Interestingly, the results indicate that each strategy produces a different data profile that is more/less comprehensive. Such efforts suggest the need for more research in the area of AT outcome data collection snapshots (Edyburn et al., 2005).

Data-based decision making is an essential professional practice. The ultimate purpose of this work is to improve data-based decision making about the outcomes of assistive technology (Edyburn & Smith, 2004). In order to achieve a future in which AT outcome data are routinely collected and used to inform decision making, significant theoretical advances will be needed, as well as easy-to-use tools that allow stakeholders to query data sets and provide context-sensitive assistance in interpreting performance data and subsequently modifying interventions and expectations.

Glossary

Assistive technology device—As defined in federal law: "Assistive technology device means any item, piece of equipment, or product system, whether acquired commercially off the shelf, modified, or customized, that is used to increase, maintain, or improve the functional capabilities of a child with a disability."

Cognitive prosthesis—A specialized form of assistive technology that focuses on using technology to enhance cognitive performance (e.g., memory, problem solving, reading, understanding).

Performance measures—Standardized measures of performance that permit quantifiable comparisons (e.g., accuracy, quality, speed) of performance under various conditions.

Technology—Left undefined, technology is often assumed to be computers. In special education, however, several forms of technology are relevant: assistive technology, distance education technology, information technology, instructional technology, medical technology, and productivity technology.

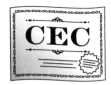

Knowledge and Skills for Entry-Level Special Education Teachers of Students With Developmental Disabilities Standards Addressed in This Chapter

Principle 1: Foundations

DD1K4   Trends and practices in the field of developmental disabilities.

Principle 4: Instructional Strategies

DD4K1   Specialized materials for individuals with developmental disabilities.

DD4K2   Evidence-based practices for teaching individuals with pervasive developmental disabilities, autism, and autism spectrum disorders.

Principle 5: Learning Environments/Social Interaction

DD5S3   Use and maintain assistive technologies.

Principle 8: Assessment

DD8K2   Environmental assessment conditions that promote maximum performance of individuals with developmental disabilities.

Principle 10: Collaboration

DD10K1   Services, networks, and organizations for individuals with developmental disabilities.

Web Site Resources

Assistive Technology Outcomes

http://www.utoronto.ca/atrc/reference/atoutcomes/index.html

An international resource center on assistive technology outcomes. Includes extensive links to people and projects in this area.

Assistive Technology Outcomes Measurement System (ATOMS) Project

http://www.atoms.uwm.edu

A Web site maintained by one of two federally funded research centers focusing on the measurement of assistive technology outcomes. Focuses specifically on measuring assistive technology outcomes in education, vocational, and independent-living environments.

Consortium for Assistive Technology Outcome Research (CATOR)

http://www.atoutcomes.org

A Web site maintained by one of two federally funded research centers focusing on the measurement of assistive technology outcomes. Focuses specifically on measuring assistive technology outcomes in the areas of communication and mobility.

A Primer on Assistive Technology Outcomes

http://www.uwm.edu/CHS/r2d2/atoms/archive/primer.html

An accessible introduction to assistive technology outcomes.

QIATlisterv

http://www.qiat.org

Consortium for Quality Indicators of Assistive Technology (QIAT). Devoted to enhancing the quality of assistive technology services. Offers free subscriptions to the QIAT listserv, as well as access to a historical archive of materials. The Web site also features the latest version of the QIAT indicators.

References

Armstrong, K. (2003). Location of specific places on a map: Assistive technology for learning. *Special Education Technology Practice, 5*(4), 24–27.

Blackhurst, A. E. (1965). Technology in special education: Some implications. *Exceptional Children, 31*, 449–456.

Blackhurst, A. E. (1997). Perspectives on technology in special education. *Teaching Exceptional Children, 29*(5), 41–48.

Blackhurst, A. E. (2005). Historical perspectives about technology applications for people with disabilities. In D. Edyburn, K. Higgins, & R. Boone (Eds.), *Handbook of special education technology research and practice* (pp. 3–29). Whitefish Bay, WI: Knowledge by Design.

Denham, A., & Lahm, E. A. (2001). Using technology to construct alternative portfolios of students with moderate and severe disabilities. *Teaching Exceptional Children, 33*(5), 10–17.

DeRuyter, F. (1995). Evaluating outcomes in assistive technology: Do we understand the commitment? *Assistive Technology, 7*, 3–8.

DeRuyter, F. (1997). The importance of outcome measures for assistive technology service delivery systems. *Technology and Disability, 6*, 89–104.

Dyck, N., & Pemberton, J. B. (2002). A model for making decisions about text adaptations. *Intevention in School and Clinic, 38*(1), 28–35.

Edyburn, D. L. (2001). Public testimony at hearing on the federal reauthorization of the Individuals with Disabilities Education Act (P. L. 105-17) concerning suggested revisions regarding the process of assistive technology consideration, October 23, 2001, Minneapolis, MN.

Edyburn, D. L. (2003a). Assistive technology and evidence-based practice. *ConnSense Bulletin.* Available online at http://www.connsensebulletin.com/edyatevidence.html

Edyburn, D. L. (2003b). Learning from text. *Special Education Technology Practice, 5*(2), 16–27.

Edyburn, D. L. (2003c). Measuring assistive technology outcomes: Key concepts. *Journal of Special Education Technology, 18*(1), 53–55.

Edyburn, D. L. (2003d). Measuring assistive technology outcomes in mathematics. *Journal of Special Education Technology, 18*(4), 76–79.

Edyburn, D. L. (2003e). Measuring assistive technology outcomes in writing. *Journal of Special Education Technology, 18*(2), 60–64.

Edyburn, D. L. (2003f). Rethinking assistive technology. *Special Education Technology Practice, 5*(4), 16–22.

Edyburn, D. L. (2004a). *Cognitive prostheses for students with mild disabilities: Is this what assistive technology looks like?* Paper presented at the Annual Closing the Gap Conference, October 21–23, Minneapolis, MN.

Edyburn, D. L. (2004b). Measuring assistive technology outcomes in reading. *Journal of Special Education Technology, 19*(1), 60–64.

Edyburn, D. L. (2005). Technology-enhanced performance. *Special Education Technology Practice, 7*(2), 16–25.

Edyburn, D. L. (2006a). Cognitive prostheses for students with mild disabilities: Is this what assistive technology looks like? *Journal of Special Education Technology, 21*(4), 62–65.

Edyburn, D. L. (2006b). Failure is not an option: Collecting, reviewing, and acting on evidence for using technology to enhance academic performance. *Learning and Leading With Technology, 34*(1), 20–23.

Edyburn, D., Fennema-Jansen, S., Hariharan, P., & Smith, R. (2005). Assistive technology outcomes: Implementation strategies for collecting data in the schools. *Assistive Technology Outcomes and Benefits, 2*(1), 25–30. Retrieved November 28, 2005, from http://www.atia.org/atob/ATOBWeb/ATOBV2N1/Documents/EdyburnATOBV2N1.pdf

Edyburn, D., Higgins, K., & Boone, R. (Eds.). (2005). *Handbook of special education technology research and practice.* Whitefish Bay, WI: Knowledge by Design.

Edyburn, D. L., & Smith, R. O. (2004). Creating an assistive technology outcomes measurement system: Validating the components. *Assistive Technology Outcomes and Benefits, 1*, 9–15. Retrieved October 26, 2005, from http://www.atia.org/atob/ATOBWeb/ATOBV1N1/Documents/ATOBV1N1A2.pdf

Fenemma-Jansen, S. (2005). *An analysis of assistive technology outcomes in Ohio schools: Special education students' access to and participation in general education and isolating the contribution of assistive technology.* Unpublished doctoral dissertation, University of Wisconsin–Milwaukee, Milwaukee, Wisconsin.

Ferri, B. A., & Connor, D. J. (2005). Tools of exclusion: Race, disability, and (re)segregated education. *Teachers College Record, 107,* 453–474.

Fuchs, D., & Fuchs, L. S. (2005). Responsiveness-to-intervention: A blueprint for practitioners, policymakers, and parents. *Teaching Exceptional Children, 38*(1), 57–61.

Fuhrer, M. J., Jutai, J. W., Scherer, M. J., & DeRuyter, F. (2003). A framework for the conceptual modeling of assistive technology outcomes. *Disability and Rehabilitation, 25,* 1243–1251.

H. Con. Res. 288 (2005). Concurrent resolution, 109th Congress, November 5.

Individuals with Disabilities Education Act Amendments of 1997, 20 U.S.C. § 1400 *et seq.* (1997).

Kearns, T. (2005). *Accountability in IDEA in U.S. education.* Retrieved July 6, 2005, from http://www.icdri.org/Education/ACCOUNTIDEA.htm

Laskarewski, J., & Susi, L. (2003). Tackling a daunting task. *Closing the Gap, 21*(5), 16, 22.

Lenker, J. A., & Paquet, V. L. (2003). A review of conceptual models for assistive technology outcomes research and practice. *Assistive Technology, 15*(1), 1–15.

Purcell, S. L., & Grant, D. (2002). *Using assistive technology to meet literacy standards in grades K–3: An IEP team guide.* Verona, WI: Attainment Company.

Purcell, S. L., & Grant, D. (2004). *Using assistive technology to meet literacy standards in grades 4–6: An IEP team guide.* Verona, WI: Attainment Company.

Reed, P., Bowser, G., & Korsten, J. (2002). *How do you know it? How can you show it?* Oshkosh, WI: Wisconsin Assistive Technology Initiative.

Silverman, M. K., Stratman, K. F., & Smith, R. O. (2000). Measuring assistive technology outcomes in schools using functional assessment. *Diagnostique, 25,* 307–326.

Smith, R. O. (2000). Measuring assistive technology outcomes in education. *Diagnostique, 25,* 273–290.

Smith, R. O. (Ed.). (1996). Measuring assistive technology outcomes: Theoretical and practical considerations. *Assistive Technology, 8,* 71–130.

Technology-Related Assistance for Individuals With Disabilities Act of 1988, 29 U.S.C. § 2201 *et seq.*

21

Alternate Assessment for Students With Developmental Disabilities

Colleen E. Klein-Ezell, Randy LaRusso, and Dan Ezell

Summary

Current legislation requirements for alternate assessment are mandated to guarantee that all students participate and are counted in district- and statewide assessment results. Alternate assessment measures can be used to identify the strengths and needs of students with developmental disabilities. Alternate assessment results can also assist in providing meaningful and appropriate instruction that includes students' future desires and goals. Overall, alternate assessment is used as a means to accurately assess and document educational gains made by students with developmental disabilities.

Learning Outcomes

After reading this chapter, you should be able to:

- Identify the origin of alternate assessments in the United States.

- Understand the limited student population that will require an alternate assessment method.

- Describe the rationale for using alternative assessment methods for students with significant developmental disabilities.

- Describe performance-based assessment.

- Summarize the benefits of using MAPS for future planning and how it relates to the alternate assessment portfolio process.

- Describe the added benefits of using portfolio assessment for students with developmental disabilities.

Alternate Assessment for Students With Developmental Disabilities

Alternate assessments, relatively new in most states, are developed for students who were not included in most large-scale assessments until federal legislation mandated their participation. The requirement for states to develop these assessments first appeared in the Individuals with Disabilities Education Act Amendments of 1997 (IDEA, P.L. 105-17). Regulations for the No Child Left Behind Act of 2001 (NCLB, P.L. 107–110) included the results of these assessments in the areas of reading/language arts, mathematics, and science in its accountability requirements. NCLB regulations clarified that more than one type of alternate assessment may be used by a state and that students with significant developmental disabilities participating in alternate assessments could access alternate achievement standards. As a part of the requirements of the 1997 reauthorization of IDEA and reaffirmed in the Individuals with Disabilities Education Improvement Act of 2004 (IDEIA, P.L. 108-446), states are now reporting data from alternate assessments for those students who cannot participate in large-scale assessment programs because of their disabilities. For the most part, alternate assessments serve two specific purposes: (a) to ensure educational accountability for the purpose of increasing student performance and (b) to fulfill the requirements of federal legislation. IDEIA does not dictate how to construct this assessment or what it should look like, but simply requires it. Since no specific alternate assessment tool and/or reporting measures are mandated by the U.S. Department of Education, states are held responsible for determining the alternate assessment methods that will be used, developing a process to collect student data, and reporting required information on the performance of students with disabilities toward meeting instructional goals.

Alternate assessments are tools used to evaluate the performance of students who are unable to participate in general state assessments even with accommodations. According to federal mandates, this population should represent less than 3% of the total population assessed. Alternate assessments provide a mechanism for students with the most significant developmental disabilities to be included in the accountability system.

According to Ysseldyke and Olsen (1997), "Gathering data on the performance of students with disabilities through alternate assessments requires some re-thinking of traditional assessment methods. An alternate assessment system is neither a traditional large-scale assessment system nor an individualized assessment" (p. 16). Students with significant developmental disabilities require assessments that are both functional and purposeful. These assessments can be a valuable tool to gather critical instructional information on students who differ greatly in their ability to respond to stimuli, solve problems, and provide responses. An alternate assessment should assist in demonstrating what the student is learning, determining whether he or she is able to generalize the learning, and determining the level of assistance required if he or she is to live a productive and fulfilling life with the greatest degree of independence possible given realistic expectations.

Providing all students with an opportunity to truly demonstrate progress toward or mastery of skills and standards and being able to track student performance over time in a variety of situations are essential. Educators have long struggled with the need for using *authentic assessments* to capture the actual skill levels of students with developmental disabilities (Abruscato, 1993; Bullens, 2002; Choate, Enright, Miller, Poteet, & Rakes, 1995; Quenemoen, Thompson, & Thurlow, 2003; Tierney, 1992). Our challenge, therefore, is to use assessment methods that will accurately determine students' instructional needs on demand (situational) as well as over a period of time (sustained).

This chapter addresses the need for and the use of alternate assessment methods to identify and report the performance of students with disabilities when traditional methods of assessment are not appropriate or feasible. Because of various legislative mandates, states have already implemented some form of alternate assessment to track student progress (Burdette & Olsen, 2000; Thompson & Thurlow, 2000; Ysseldyke & Olsen, 1997). A broad continuum exists of alternate assessment systems that are being utilized across the nation, which includes the collection and compilation of evidence. Although alternate assessment can encompass a variety of assessment approaches, the primary focus here will be performance-based assessment and the use of portfolios to gather and document vital information on student achievement.

Performance-Based Assessment Systems

Performance-based assessment systems are best described as formalized approaches to direct observation of student behavior and skill level on tasks commonly required for functioning in the world outside of school (Quenemoen et al., 2003). Performance-based assessment is a measure of actual on-demand student performance of skills and knowledge within clearly identified standards as a way to accurately determine progress. It asks not what the educational system has taught the student but what the student does as a result of his learning.

Performance-based assessment systems allow for an array of meaningful activities to be used to measure what to teach. If curricula are developed that are too narrow—for example, if they focus just on academic skills—valued outcomes like vocational, daily living, and leisure skills are overlooked. These systems are not cookbooks, but processes for teaching curricula and collecting assessment information as part of the learning process.

A performance-based assessment system is typically used one-on-one with a student and measures what that individual knows as a result of his or her learning. Assessment tasks need to be both relevant to the student's curriculum and aligned to the state standards. Learning is evidenced through a student's active response that is relevant to and representative of real-life experiences. The objective in using a performance-based alternate assessment is to be able to clearly measure the student's abilities, strengths, and weaknesses. Performance assessment systems are developed to ensure that progress is being made toward valued educational goals and state standards for this diverse population.

A well-constructed performance-based assessment system provides a mechanism for students who have developmental disabilities so significant that it may be difficult to assess their skills otherwise. This type of systematic assessment allows educators the freedom to design learning environments and experiences that best meet the unique learning needs of each student in a consistent format. This assessment must have a clear relationship to the state standards, curriculum, and classroom instruction, and it also needs to be conceptualized as a unified approach and *not* as separate components. Consistency among education professionals, related service providers, and family members who may be involved in collecting data is vital. Consistency is possible only when all persons working with a student toward the achievement of the state standards share a common understanding of what the expectations mean and how they are exhibited in actual, on-demand performance.

From the beginning, the need for alternate assessment systems to be connected to the state's standards and access the general curriculum has been emphasized (Kleinert & Kearns, 2001; Thompson, Quenemoen, Thurlow, & Ysseldyke, 2001). It is crucial that a system of assessment be instructionally based so that students are measured in areas in which they are being taught, acquiring skills, and moving toward independence at an appropriate level of expectation.

Although performance-based assessment systems can include a variety of methods to obtain data, they are typically scored using a *rubric*. This makes it easier to compare one performance event or performance test to another. The formalization of the performance-based assessment process makes this possible, as the process includes the development of a rubric with which to determine the student's functioning level, identify the goals and state standards being addressed, develop a description of the skill or activity/task, and determine the criteria for mastery at the student's specific level to document the results.

Determination of Student's Functioning Level

Many states clearly define the range of independence at which a student is functioning (Burdette & Olsen, 2000; Quenemoen et al., 2003). Within the population of students who are permitted the use of an alternate assessment, Louisiana, for example, identifies three subgroups (Quenemoen et al., 2003). All three subgroups of student functioning are related to the content standards, regardless of the age or grade level of the student. These subgroups are (a) introductory level, (b) fundamental level, and (c) comprehensive level.

1. Students functioning at the introductory level should be able to demonstrate skills that require basic processing of information to address real-world situations.

2. Students functioning at the fundamental level are expected to demonstrate simple decision making to address real-world situations.

3. Students who are instructed and evaluated at the comprehensive level are working toward skills that require higher-order thinking and complex information-processing skills.

The State of Florida uses a similar identification of levels of functioning for students who are using an alternate assessment. The student's level of functioning is determined by taking into consideration the amount of additional support and assistance needed in order for him or her to be able to accomplish the skill or apply the knowledge. Florida uses the terms *participatory*, *supported*, and *independent* for the levels of functioning, as noted by the Florida Department of Education (2004):

1. Students at the participatory level are so significantly impaired that the IEP team anticipates dependency on others for most or all of their daily needs.

2. Students at the supported level can learn many independent living skills yet require some supervision and support throughout their lives.

3. Students at the independent level of functioning, for the most part, are considered to have the ability to meet their own needs without support from others.

While states may describe the needs of their students with a variety of different terms, the meaning remains the same. It is an acknowledgment that within the population of students with developmental disabilities are subgroups of students who need varying degrees of support.

Identification of Goals and State Standards

As the IEP team considers the state standards for students with developmental disabilities and writes goals and *objectives/benchmarks* to allow for the greatest access to the general curriculum, they must remain student-centered. The team must have clear standards of expected student performance and a long-range focus on the desired outcome for each student. Instructional strategies must be monitored to determine which approaches are the most effective in helping each student reach increased levels of independence and make programmatic decisions with complete and accurate results.

As the team plans for a performance assessment, it is crucial to identify instructional goals specific to an individual student and the context in which the student is being assessed. The teacher must define the context, focus, and environment for which the skills are taught and an assessment is intended. However, it is important that the skills being taught can be generalized across multiple environments (Browder & Snell, 2000; Heward, 2000).

Development of Skills or Activity/Task Description

Since it is difficult to standardize a performance assessment, it is vital that it be written in clearly measurable terms that would allow any individual who is working with a student to duplicate the task. There are many activities in which a student may be able to perform a specified task. One assessment activity may measure a variety of skills in various contexts and across a variety of authentic environments. For example, Patty Sue is a 12-year-old student who has a developmental disability. Some of her IEP objectives are to count to 12, write three simple sentences to form a paragraph, and identify high-frequency sight words. Patty Sue's class is preparing to go on a community-based instructional outing to the local zoo. Patty Sue's assignment for this project includes counting the various animals that have different/same features, totaling the number for each feature, and converting the data into a graph (with peer assistance) for easy interpretation. In preparation for the outing, Patty Sue marked familiar words in a handout on animal features focusing on the concept of "same" and "different" during class reading time. During the trip, Patty Sue collected data on the various animals she saw. On her class project sheet that included pictures of many of the animals at the zoo, she used tally marks to indicate the various feature differences (e.g., long nose, short nose, two legs, four legs, big, little) in the animals she observed. During the outing, Patty Sue, on many occasions, counted the tally marks she had made thus far. The following week, with assistance from one of her peers, she totaled the final tally marks for the various different animal features she had observed and then converted the data to a graph. On her own, Patty Sue was to develop three simple sentences describing one animal of her choice. This performance task involved a variety of skills in various contexts and across a variety of authentic environments and in addition involved a variety of support (independent work versus peer assistance, see Figure 21.1).

Determination of Criteria for Mastery and Documentation

The key to establishing a well-constructed rubric is ensuring that the rater be clearly cognizant of the specifics required for task completion or skill mastery (see Figure 21.2). Having a well-defined, easily understood rubric can be the difference between obtaining good, useful data that can drive instruction and gathering incomplete or useless data. The rubric should measure the ability to perform a task to completion as well as the level of independence at which the task was performed. For instance, a rubric might address questions like these: Is the student able to complete the task independently? Without prompting or support? Did he or she initiate

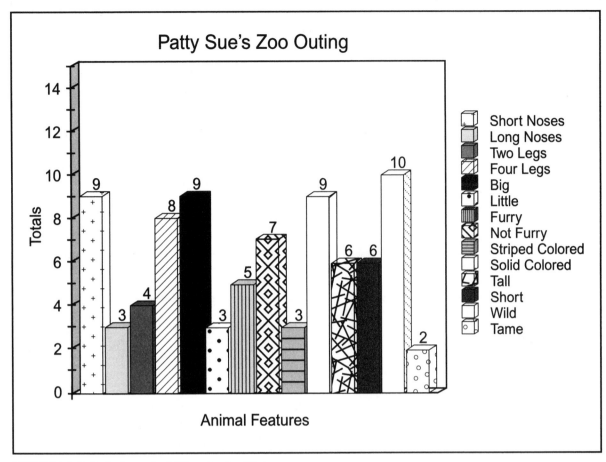

FIGURE 21.1 Patty Sue's graph of different animal features.

independently, require fewer than two prompts, or require more than three? Does the student require repeated direction, redirection, or reminders to stay with the task? If so, to what extent was that support necessary? Did the student remain unengaged, need hand-over-hand assistance to complete the task, or demonstrate complete noncompliance? By incorporating such concepts into the rubric, a distinct level of functioning can be determined and documented.

A rubric can be refined and changed just as the task itself changes. As the student completes a task, the teacher scores the student's level of success. The rubric can then be used to design remediation of a skill or to determine which skill should be taught next and with what level of modifications, supports, and/or assistive technology.

Linking Instruction and Assessment

Performance-based assessment systems allow education professionals an opportunity to measure student success and provide a method with which to gather and report information on the effectiveness of instruction. The most important benefit, and the overall desired outcome in utilizing an alternate assessment for students with significant disabilities, however, is the ability to link instruction and assessment. The ultimate goal should be to focus on a purposeful direction in educating students. The use of

PASS-D Specialized Rubric

Expectation #5:   Participates Effectively in Group Situations

Performance Context: Structured Group Activities

Opportunity Description: During free time, student will initiate playing a group game by choosing a game of his or her choice. Students will have the opportunity to engage in informal conversation with peers and staff. After an appropriate amount of time, or when directed by teacher that game time is up, student will cease activity and return game to designated area.

Performance Requirement

a. Did the student conduct self in safe and appropriate manner?
   0. The student did not attempt activity.
   1. The student required ongoing physical assistance to observe rules of the game, take turns playing, and cease activity.
   2. The student required step-by-step instruction to observe rules of the game, take turns playing, and cease activity.
   3. The student was able to observe good sportsmanship rules of the game, take turns playing, and cease activity at appropriate time with occasional verbal prompts.
   4. The student was able to independently observe good sportsmanship rules of the game, take turns playing, and cease activity at appropriate time.
   N/A – Not applicable.
   NO – No opportunity to observe student.

Performance Requirement

b. Did the student effectively communicate?
   0. The student did not attempt activity.
   1. The student had to be told what to say to others and did not use appropriate tone/volume.
   2. The student used appropriate tone and volume, but required step-by-step instruction to communicate with others and to persist in being understood.
   3. The student was able to use appropriate tone/volume, respond to the communication of others, and persist in being understood when appropriate with occasional verbal prompts.
   4. The student was able to independently use appropriate tone/volume, respond to the communication of others, and persist in being understood when appropriate.
   N/A – Not applicable.
   NO – No opportunity to observe student.

Performance Requirement

c. Did the student advocate for self?
   0. The student did not attempt activity.
   1. The student required physical assistance to make choices of game, others with whom he or she would like to play, indicate his or her turn, request help, and indicate when he or she was finished with the game.
   2. The student required step-by-step instruction to make choices of game, others with whom he or she would like to play, indicate his or her turn, request help, and indicate when he or she was finished with the game.
   3. The student was able to make choices of game, others with whom he or she would like to play, indicate his or her turn, request help, and indicate when he or she was finished with the game with occasional verbal prompts.
   4. The student was able to independently make choices of game, others with whom he or she would like to play, indicate his or her turn, request help, and indicate when he or she was finished with the game.
   N/A – Not applicable.
   NO – No opportunity to observe student.

(Brevard Public Schools, 2000)

FIGURE 21.2 PASS-D specialized rubric.

performance-based assessment systems allows us a means by which to determine the extent of the students' cognitive and physical abilities and how these abilities will factor into the achievement of independence. Students learn best in authentic environments where they can demonstrate what they have learned. Performance-based assessment is an invaluable system when working with students who have a diverse range of needs for instruction and assessment.

Assessment is the process of collecting data for the purpose of making decisions (Salvia & Ysseldyke, 2001). Testing is the process of administering a test to an individual or group to obtain a score. Testing is one way to gather assessment information (Salvia & Ysseldyke, 2001). There is no place in performance assessment for standardized testing. However, when utilizing the portfolio process, test results, functional checklists, teacher observations, IEP reviews, and other pertinent student information can be used to support performance-based assessment activities. Since performance assessment involves a student demonstrating what is understood by performing a skill, task, or activity (Wortham, 1998), portfolios perfectly align with performance assessment and can be used as one way to assemble information to showcase student achievement.

Portfolio Assessment

Portfolio assessment is being used in classrooms today as an alternative means to showcase a student's knowledge in a variety of ways and as an alternate assessment method to meet the requirements of NCLB and IDEIA (Burdette & Olsen, 2000; Thurlow et al., 1996; Ysseldyke & Olsen, 1997). Using portfolio assessment for students with developmental disabilities is becoming a viable alternative means to document individual progress across time for a variety of instructional needs (Burke, Fogarty, & Belgrad, 1994; Ezell & Klein, 2003; Ezell, Klein, & Ezell-Powell, 1999; Swicegood, 1994). With the emphasis on conducting classroom-based assessment that connects assessment to instruction and evaluation that has occured since the passage of the IDEA Amendments of 1997, portfolio assessment has been used to provide valuable data on which to base instructional decisions and to provide much-needed documentation of progress for students with developmental disabilities (Gomez, Grau, & Block, 1991). Student portfolios can include a variety of artifacts that can illustrate a student's instructional progress, such as photographs of the student performing employment or school tasks/activities, teacher-made checklists, copies of student time cards from his or her job site, works in progress, copies of academic tests, and/or bus schedules.

Standardized testing cannot provide the in-depth picture of a student's academic performance and growth. Standardized testing also does not take into account such elements as the student's mental state, health, or motivation at the time of the "one-shot" performance. With portfolio assessment, educators can use a student's portfolio to obtain a "holistic" picture of the student. Portfolios can also substantiate standardized test results and provide more-detailed information concerning a student's strengths and weaknesses.

The use of portfolios proves to be very helpful and beneficial to both teachers and students. Portfolios assist teachers in making decisions about instruction, in documenting IEP goals, in communicating students' strengths and areas of need (Carpenter, Ray, & Bloom, 1995). Portfolio assessment allows teachers to link assessment with their instruction and to allow for individual differences among students' achievement. The current emphasis on inclusion means that general education teachers are expected to focus on the abilities of the student and to provide ways to optimize these abilities. Using portfolio assessment is one possible way to provide for individualization of needs.

One of the major goals of special educators is for their students to manage their own lives with as little assistance as possible—to become self-reliant. Achieving this goal requires numerous skills, such as self-advocacy, self-esteem, self-regulation, and self-determination. Historically, students with developmental disabilities have not had an integral part in making decisions or voicing their preferences for the future. With the mandates of IDEIA, students with disabilities need to be given a more active part in their own educational planning and life choices. Therefore, fostering self-determination skills is an important educational outcome for students with developmental disabilities, and it can be accomplished by using the portfolio assessment process (Ezell et al., 1999).

According to Capper, Frattura, and Keyes, (2000), "Students who challenge schools the most are the ones affected the most by our inability to assess in a way that shows their true abilities" (p. 115). With the emphasis on finding ways of measuring the performance progress of students with disabilities, it is incumbent upon education professionals to consider a greater array of assessment possibilities. As students with disabilities look toward their future, educators need to employ all available information sources to assist in preparing students to transition into the world. To accomplish this, students must leave school with the skills necessary to secure their future desires. One way to accomplish this goal is through self-determination activities (see Chapter 6 for a more detailed discussion of self-determination issues). Educators need to be aware of the student's preferences and plan accordingly to ensure that the student has acquired the necessary skills.

Making Action Plans (MAPS)

To facilitate future planning for students with developmental disabilities, Making Action Plans (MAPS) can be a valuable tool (Falvey, Forest, Pearpoint, & Rosenberg, 2000) and can provide important data to be included in a student's portfolio. The MAPS process involves collecting information about a student to assist in making decisions and planning for his or her future. MAPS focuses on the strengths and positive aspects of the student and uses input from those individuals, family members, and organizations who know the student best. The MAPS process differs from an IEP meeting in that the student is the key person and may choose who participates in the development of the MAPS. The student, when applicable, defines his or her own problems, dreams, and future with assistance from those invited to the MAPS meeting. The purpose of the MAPS team is to guide a student from the present to the future.

According to Forest and Pearpoint (1992), eight questions provide the foundation for a MAPS team meeting:

1. *What is MAPS?* The answer to this question is to help the group focus on the main purpose of the meeting—to help the student get from his or her present situation to where he or she is going (future goals). This question helps group members to focus on the agenda for the meeting and understand that MAPS is to be used to guide the student from one place to another.

2. *What is the person's history or story?* This question is used in order to get the group involved in the MAPS process. As the student's story unfolds, the facilitator/leader of the group can generate a simple graphic to illustrate the story. This step also assists the student in verbalizing his or her history, thereby informing the group of specific details of past and present events, goals, and accomplishments, showing how the student has progressed, and providing a clear perspective and a more complete picture of the student's past and those events and persons who have helped to shape the student's life.

3. *What are your dreams?* This question is pivotal in developing the eventual plan for the future; it is at the core of the process. It is important at this point to remain positive and nonjudgmental. This step is crucial in drawing out the "essence" of the student's eventual outcome of the process. With enough probing by group members, the question should get to the heart of the student's dreams for the future and set the stage for discussing possibilities for the student's short- and long-term goals.

4. *What are your nightmares (fears)?* Even though this question can bring about negative responses, it is an essential component of the process since it can identify barriers to realization of the student's dreams. Overall, it is the "fear" that needs to be avoided, yet voiced and respected.

5. *Who is the person?* This step involves more of a brainstorming session. Everyone in the group is asked to share words that portray who the student "is," and the words are listed for everyone to see. Many categories can be included at this step: dislikes/likes, personal qualities, favorite activities, friends and supports. The student is then asked to identify himself or herself in his or her own words, which are added to the list. The last part of this step is to choose several words and ideas from the entire list to accurately portray who the student "is" at the current time.

6. *What are the person's strengths, gifts, and talents?* This step entails listing the student's strengths either in positive words or graphically—whichever the group prefers. The purpose is to identify strengths that may be fundamental in achieving the student's future goals. This step, which "celebrates" the student's accomplishments and strengths, is unfortunately left out too many times in planning sessions for students.

7. *What does the person need to achieve the dream and avoid the nightmare?* At this step in the process, the group focuses on what resources and formal/informal supports will be needed to make the student's dream become a reality. Items should include not only instructional needs but support people, circle of friends, and assistive devices as well.

8. *What is the plan of action?* This last step entails developing a plan of action that focuses on the dreams of the student while preventing the nightmares (fear), which is the core of the process. Explicit plans pinpoint the person(s) responsible for the action(s) and the timelines involved, taking into consideration everything that has been discussed.

The ultimate goal of conducting a MAPS meeting is to explore the student's personal goals and desires for the future and in turn, to develop an instructional plan that will assist the student in meeting personal goals. It is crucial to stress the need to remain positive and nonjudgmental throughout the entire process. Even though the "dream" specified by the student may seem unrealistic, it can be used to get at the essence of the student's real desire and draw out what may become a feasible "outcome." Once the student's strengths and desires, as well as skill deficits, are identified, a plan for instruction that will assist the student in realizing future plans can be developed and implemented. The entire process involves listening to the student and showing respect for his or her fears, strengths, and dreams, with the ultimate goal of developing a future that is realistic and desired.

Through the use of portfolio assessment, teachers can identify problem areas and adjust the assessment and instructional strategies more appropriately. Portfolio assessment can be the guiding force that encourages a more authentic, valid assessment for students with developmental disabilities.

426 Additional Beneficial Components of Portfolio Assessment

Beyond the appeal of portfolio assessment as an alternative to large-scale assessment, the process involves other beneficial components as well: self-assessment, authentic tasks, and active learning. Students with developmental disabilities who participate in the portfolio assessment process can gain a better understanding of their own strengths and weaknesses and thereby take a more active role in setting their own goals and working toward mastery (Ezell & Klein, 2002).

One of the added benefits of portfolio assessment, particularly with students with developmental disabilities, is an enhanced internal locus of control (Ezell & Klein, 2003). Locus of control pertains to one's perception of control over his or her environment. Educators need to foster internal locus of control in their students with developmental disabilities. Students with developmental disabilities need to have ownership of their learning and be able to attribute their progress to their own personal efforts and hard work. According to Ezell (1995), students involved in the portfolio assessment process were more internally oriented. Ezell and Klein (2003) conducted a study exploring the effects of portfolio assessment on locus of control of students with and without disabilities. The overall results of the study indicated that all individuals in the study who were involved in the portfolio assessment process were more internally oriented than those who were not involved.

Some of the most beneficial elements of portfolio assessment involve students' taking an active part in their learning through self-assessment and self-reflection practices that are embedded in the portfolio assessment process. Students with developmental disabilities should have access to setting goals, self-assessment, and self-reflection.

Conclusion

Legislative mandates require that all students participate and be counted in district- and statewide assessment results. Alternate assessment is a useful tool in fulfilling these mandates and also in accurately assessing the strengths and needs of students with developmental disabilities. When used properly, alternate assessments provide direction concerning instruction, remediation, student desires, and mapping of the student's future. Performance-based assessments can stand alone or be part of the greater picture in the portfolio assessment process. Even though individual states may differ in the methods used in alternate assessments, the overall outcome remains the same—to accurately assess and report the learning gains made by students with developmental disabilities.

Glossary

Alternate assessments—Nontraditional approaches in the assessment of student performance.

Authentic assessments—Methods, used to capture data documented in the alternate assessment process, that naturally occur in the student's environment.

Objectives/benchmarks—Statements of the knowledge and skills that the student must master to achieve the annual goal.

Performance assessment—An alternate assessment method that assesses a whole task, tracks student performance over time in changing contexts, and takes place in authentic/natural environments.

Portfolio assessment—An alternate assessment method of measuring a student's performance by purposefully collecting student's accomplishments over time, thus providing valid information about a student.

Rubrics—The quality criteria and standards used as scoring guides to determine a student's level of success on a particular skill or activity/task.

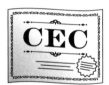

Knowledge and Skills for Entry-Level Special Education Teachers of Students With Developmental Disabilities Standards Addressed in This Chapter

Principal 8: Assessment

DD8S1 Select, adapt, and use instructional assessment tools and methods to accommodate the abilities and needs of individuals with mental retardation and developmental disabilities.

Additional Reading Resources

Almond, P., Quenemoen, R., Olsen, K., & Thurlow, M. (2000). *Gray areas of assessment systems* (Synthesis Report 32). Minneapolis, MN: University of Minnesota, National Center on Educational Outcomes.

Bielinski, J., & Ysseldyke, J. (2000). *Interpreting trends in the performance of special education students* (Technical Report 27). Minneapolis, MN: University of Minnesota, National Center on Educational Outcomes.

Quenemoen, R., Lehr, C. A., Thurlow, M., Thompson, S. J., & Bolt, S. (2000). *Social promotion and students with disabilities: Issues and challenges in developing state policies* (Synthesis Report 34). Minneapolis, MN: University of Minnesota, National Center on Educational Outcomes.

Quenemoen, R., Massanari, C., Thompson, S., & Thurlow, M. (2000). *Alternate assessment forum: Connecting into a whole*. Minneapolis, MN: University of Minnesota, National Center on Educational Outcomes. Retrieved from http://education.umn.edu/NCEO/OnlinePubs/Forum2000/ForumReport2000.htm

Raber, S., & Roach, V. (1998). *The push and pull of standards-based reform: How does it affect local school districts and students with disabilities?* (K. Fraser, Ed.). Alexandria, VA: Center for Policy

Research on the Impact of General and Special Education Reform. Retrieved November 3, 2005, from http://www.nasbe.org/EducationalIssues/Reports/Pushpull.pdf

Thurlow, M., House, A., Boys, C., Scott, D., & Ysseldyke, J. (2000). *State participation and accommodations policies for students with disabilities: 1999 update* (Synthesis Report 33). Minneapolis, MN: University of Minnesota, National Center on Educational Outcomes.

Web Site Resources

Alternate Assessment of Students with Disabilities

http://education.umn.edu/nceo/TopicAreas/AlternateAssessments/StatesAltAssess.htm

Introduction and FAQs section on alternate assessment, plus links to state Web sites for alternate assessment information.

Alternative Performance-Based Assessment

http://www.emtech.net/Alternative_Assessment.html

Links to information concerning performance-based assessment in a variety of subject areas.

Education Topics: Performance and Assessment

http://www.ascd.org/portal/site/ascd/menuitem.7372a5056b2b42fbbfb3ffdb62108a0c/

Links to various sites that address performance-based assessment and its use in the classroom setting.

The Educator's Reference

http://www.eduref.org/cgi-bin/print.cgi/Resources/Evaluation/Alternative_Assessment.html

Links to valuable information concerning alternate assessment, portfolio and performance-based assessment.

Information Center on Disabilities and Gifted Education

http://ericec.org/faq/altassess.html

Selected citations from the ERIC database on alternate assessment and the search terms that were used to find the citations.

Michigan's Parent Training and Information Center

http://www.causeonline.org/iepaltern2.html

Information from the State of Michigan concerning alternate assessment, plus questions and answers for parents about alternate assessment.

National Alternate Assessment Center

http://www.naacpartners.org/Products/products.htm

Downloadable presentations from various conferences on alternate assessment along with additional resource materials.

Prince George's County Public Schools

http://www.pgcps.pg.k12.md.us/~elc/developingtasks.html

Performance-based assessment definition, as well as several useful links, one in particular to the step-by-step process for designing performance assessment tasks and how to score them.

References

Abruscato, J. (1993). Early results and tentative implementation from the Vermont Portfolio Project. *Phi Delta Kappan, 74,* 474–478.

Brevard Public Schools. (2000). *Performance assessment system for students with disabilities (PASS-D) activity guide* (Randy LaRusso—Project Coordinator).

Browder, D., & Snell, M. (2000). Teaching functional academics. In M. Snell & F. Brown (Eds.), *Instruction of students with severe disabilities* (5th ed., pp. 493–542). Columbus, OH: Merrill.

Bullens, D. (2002). *Authentic assessment: Change for the future.* Unpublished master's thesis, Saint Xavier University, Chicago, IL. (ERIC Document Reproduction Service No. ED468067)

Burdette, P. J., & Olsen, K. (2000). *Alternate alternates: A medley of alternate assessments.* (Mid-South Regional Resource Center). (ERIC Document Reproduction Service No. ED452642)

Burke, K., Fogarty, R., & Belgrad, S. (1994). *The mindful school: The portfolio connection. K–college.* Palatine, IL: IRI/Skylight Publishing.

Capper, C. A., Frattura, E., & Keyes, M. W. (2000). *Meeting the needs of students of all abilities: How leaders go beyond inclusion.* Thousand Oaks, CA: Corwin.

Carpenter, C. D., Ray, M. S., & Bloom, L. A. (1995). Portfolio assessment: Opportunities and challenges. *Intervention in School and Clinic, 31,* 34–41.

Choate, J. S., Enright, B. F., Miller, L. J., Poteet, J. A., & Rakes, T. A. (1995). *Curriculum-based assessment and programming* (3rd ed.). Boston: Allyn & Bacon.

Ezell, D. (1995). *A comparative analysis of eighth-grade students' locus of control and their involvement in the portfolio assessment process.* Unpublished doctoral dissertation, University of Alabama, Tuscaloosa, AL.

Ezell, D., & Klein, C. E. (2002). The portfolio assessment criteria checklist for teachers. *Florida Educational Leadership, 2*(2), 38–42.

Ezell, D., & Klein, C. E. (2003). Impact of portfolio assessment on locus of control of students with and without disabilities. *Education and Training in Developmental Disabilities, 38,* 220–228.

Ezell, D., Klein, C. E., & Ezell-Powell, S. (1999). Empowering students with mental retardation through portfolio assessment: A tool for fostering self-determination skills. *Education and Training in Mental Retardation and Developmental Disabilities, 34,* 453–463.

Falvey, M. A., Forest, M., Pearpoint, J., & Rosenberg, R. L. (2000). *All my life's a circle. Using the tools: Circles, MAPS, and PATHS.* Toronto: Inclusion Press.

Florida Department of Education. (2004). *Florida alternative assessment resource manual* (Rev.). Tallahassee, FL: Author. Retrieved November 3, 2005, from http://64.233.167.104/ search?q=cache:EYwpc5kYIuIJ:www.firn.edu/doe/commhome/pdf/faarrm05.pdf+students+ at+the+Participatory+level+are+those,+Florida&hl=en&start=2

Forest, M., & Pearpoint, J. (1992). Everyone belongs: Building the vision with MAPS—the McGill Action Planning System. In D. Wetherow (Ed.), *The whole community catalogue: Welcoming people with disabilities into the heart of community life* (pp. 95–99). Manchester, CT: Communitas.

Gomez, M. L., Grau, M. E., & Block, M. N. (1991). Reassessing portfolio assessment: Rhetoric and reality. *Language Arts, 68,* 620–628.

Heward, W. (2000). *Exceptional children: An introduction to special education* (6th ed.). Columbus, OH: Merrill.

Individuals with Disabilities Education Act (IDEA) Amendments of 1997, 20 U.S.C. § 1400 *et seq.*

Individuals with Disabilities Education Improvement Act of 2004, 20 U.S.C. § 1400 *et seq.*

Kleinert, H. L., & Kearns, J. F. (Eds.). (2001). *Alternate assessment: Measuring outcomes and supports for students with disabilities.* Baltimore: Brookes.

No Child Left Behind Act of 2001, 20 U.S.C. § 6301 *et seq.*

Quenemoen, R., Thompson, S., & Thurlow, M. (2003). *Measuring academic achievement of students with significant cognitive disabilities: Building understanding of alternate assessment scoring criteria* (Synthesis Report 50). Minneapolis, MN: University of Minnesota, National Center on Educational Outcomes. Retrieved from http://education.umn.edu/NCEO/OnlinePubs/ Synthesis50.html

Salvia, J., & Ysseldyke, J. E. (2001). *Assessment* (8th ed.). Boston: Houghton Mifflin.

Swicegood, P. (1994). Portfolio-based assessment practices. *Intervention in School and Clinic, 30,* 6–15.

Thompson, S. J., Quenemoen, R. F., Thurlow, M. L., & Ysseldyke, J. E. (2001). *Alternate assessments for students with disabilities.* Thousand Oaks, CA: Corwin.

Thompson, S. J., & Thurlow, M. L. (2000). *State alternate assessments: Status as IDEA alternate assessment requirements take effect* (National Center on Educational Outcomes Synthesis Report 35). (ERIC Document Reproduction Service No. ED447613)

Thurlow, M., Olsen, K., Elliott, J., Ysseldyke, J., Erickson, R., & Ahearn, E. (1996). *Alternate assessments for students with disabilities* (National Center on Educational Outcomes Policy Directions 5). (ERIC Document Reproduction Service No. ED404800)

Tierney, R. J. (1992). Portfolios: Windows on learning. *Learning, 21*(2), 61–64.

Wortham, S. C. (1998). Introduction. In S. C. Wortham, A. Barbour, & B. Desjean-Perrotta (Eds.), *Portfolio assessment: A handbook for preschool and elementary educators* (pp. 7–13). Olney, MD: Association for Childhood Education International.

Ysseldyke, J. E., & Olsen, K. (1997). *Putting alternate assessments into practice: What to measure and possible sources of data* (National Center on Education Outcomes Synthesis Report 28). (ERIC Document Reproduction Service No. ED416605)

22

Data-Based Decision Making and Students With Developmental Disabilities

Jeffrey P. Bakken

Summary

This chapter focuses on how teachers of students with developmental disabilities can incorporate data-based techniques and decision-making principles into their daily routines to measure how students are performing in terms of content, skills, and behaviors. It discusses the importance of frequent and continuous assessment and explains how assessment and instruction are linked. It also addresses the importance of not only collecting data but also analyzing the data to decide whether to move forward with content or skills since the student has learned the material, to reteach the lesson since the student did not learn the content or skills, or to change or modify the method of instruction. This chapter also discusses the importance of collecting baseline data, setting a goal, and then continuing to collect data during the intervention to assess whether the strategy is effective.

Learning Outcomes

After reading this chapter you should be able to:

- Understand the importance of incorporating frequent and continuous assessment practices into instructional improvement efforts.

- Understand that assessment is a powerful tool to be used through the whole process of teaching and learning, one that demands the same kind of evaluation skills that good teachers use for effective management.

- Understand that frequent and continuous assessment helps schools and teachers to be more effective.

- Understand that successful interventions must be sufficiently powerful to improve the performance of students with disabilities and must also lend themselves to integration with current teaching practices and conceptions of teaching.

- Understand that data help us in our decision making regarding student, teacher, and intervention performance.

- Understand that without data, the proper decisions may not be made and teaching time could be sacrificed.

- Understand that when collecting data, it is important to implement multiple methods of data collection and to view the process as dynamic and continuous.

- Understand the different data collection methods and their associated purposes.

- Understand the importance of collecting baseline data, setting a goal, and then measuring actual progress against expected progress over time to see whether the intervention is effective.

- Understand the importance of choosing the correct method of data collection for the behavior.

- Understand that once data are collected, they must be analyzed and the most appropriate means of intervention determined. It is important that data collection of progress continues while the intervention is being implemented so that the teacher can see if it is effective or not.

- Understand that assistive technology can be an effective intervention, but data must also be collected on it to assess its effectiveness.

- Understand that the goals of data analysis are to find out what the teacher is doing that is effective and should be continued and also to find out what is not effective and should be changed or modified to become more effective.

- Understand that data must be collected and graphed so that student progress, teacher effectiveness, and intervention success can be evaluated.

Introduction

How does a teacher know if his or her students with developmental disabilities are learning what they are being taught? Hopefully, the teacher is administering some type of assessment tool or implementing data collection measures to document student learning. Such data can inform the teacher as to how the students are doing, how he or she is doing as a teacher, and decisions that might need to be made regarding instruction for students with developmental disabilities.

One decision could be to keep moving forward with content or skills since the student has learned the material. Another decision could be to reteach the lesson since the student did not learn the content or skills. Still another decision could be to change or modify the method of instruction in hopes of achieving a better outcome for the students with developmental disabilities. Collecting the data is the easy part; the decision-making process is the part of the task that can be difficult.

Teaching Students With Developmental Disabilities

Characteristics of individuals with developmental disabilities include short attention spans, problems with short-term memory, difficulty in generalizing information to new situations, motor difficulties, and intolerance for frustration, especially with regard to academic learning and abstract instructional activities (Epstein, Cullinan, & Polloway, 1988). To teach these students, we often employ instructional techniques that include a great deal of drill and practice with flash cards and pictures. Repetition of content and skills is essential when teaching students with developmental disabilities. In addition, the transfer of knowledge from the classroom to the community through excursions where the focus is on generalization of skills is also important.

Best Practices Related to Data-Based Decision Making

The National Council for Accreditation of Teacher Education (NCATE, 2000) expects teachers to accurately assess and carefully analyze student learning, make appropriate adjustments to instruction, monitor student learning, and positively affect learning for all students. Teachers who are able to articulate goals and document progress toward achieving these goals through the use of clear data are more likely to earn the confidence of families. Data-based teacher decision making is also more likely to produce positive outcomes for students with developmental disabilities and to lead to greater satisfaction among all stakeholders (Gunter, Callicott, Denny, & Gerber, 2003).

Schools that have incorporated the use of assessment data into their instructional improvement efforts have found that one annual test does not provide enough information to allow teachers to adjust their instruction to students' changing needs throughout the year. Many districts have developed additional short assessments that are directed to the specific needs of their schools and students and that parallel the state-required assessments. The notion of frequent and continuous assessment has come to the forefront of efforts to make schools and teachers more effective. It is also important to remember that in judging how well a lesson went, many teachers rely more on observable student behavior than on quantitative assessment data (Guskey, 1995). For added support, however, more emphasis should be placed on quantitative data.

Characteristics of Effective Interventions

Classroom teachers have direct control of the instructional strategies they employ. *Instructional strategies* refers to the use of highly effective teaching techniques that enhance student learning. The effective teacher not only has a large array of such strategies at his or her disposal but is also adept at determining which strategies to use with specific students and content (Marzano, 2003).

A recurrent finding among researchers is that interventions must not only be sufficiently powerful to improve the performance of students with developmental disabilities but also must lend themselves to integration with current teaching practices and concepts (Gersten, Morvant, & Brengelman, 1995). For sustained use, instructional routines must be perceived by teachers as being effective for typical students as well as for students with disabilities. Research further indicates that merely providing teachers with access to innovative instructional strategies through in-service opportunities is insufficient for effecting change in patterns of teaching (Richardson, 1994).

To build conceptual understanding of an innovation, and to apply this knowledge to their own classrooms, teachers must have opportunities to discuss the new interventions with colleagues, to learn about their underlying concepts and intentions, and to understand changes in student learning resulting from shifts in instruction (Englert & Tarrant, 1995). How do teachers know if an intervention is effective? Research indicates that effective interventions should be supported by outcome data. If an intervention is based on research and has proven to be effective with a certain population, then it can be said that the intervention is effective. Guidelines for the evaluation and implementation of effective instructional practices include (a) student progress that is consistently and regularly monitored (daily and periodically), (b) use of both informal and formal assessment strategies (as appropriate), (c) alignment of all accountability measurements with content and processes involved in the practice, and (d) troubleshooting and/or intervention that is immediately available in response to low performance (Carnine & Granzin, 2001).

The Importance of Using Data

Informal and formal data about student learning not only shape instruction but also determine its effectiveness. It is important to implement multiple methods of data collection and to view the process as dynamic and continuous. The role of a data collector is three-dimensional: to determine students' prior understanding and achievement, to track their responses to moderate challenges, and to measure their outcomes against expected performance goals (Brimijoin, 2002; Bruner, 1963; Tomlinson, 1995).

Assessment is a powerful tool that needs to be integrated throughout the entire process of teaching and learning, and it demands the same kind of evaluation skills that good teachers use for effective management (Brimijoin, Marquissee, & Tomlinson, 2003). Using measures of student learning that are not sensitive to the actual learning occurring in classrooms is the first mistake. This commonly happens when a school or district relies on what is referred to as "indirect" learning data, often provided by off-the-shelf standardized tests and even state-level standards tests. Such measures are indirect because they frequently do not adequately assess the content that is actually taught in a given school. A school might, in fact, be producing impressive student learning gains, but the test data do not pick them up (Marzano, 2003). Notwithstanding the significance of these issues, the most important reason for the collection of educational data on children is to ensure and improve the quality of outcomes.

Reschly, Kicklighter, and McGee (1988a, 1988b, 1988c) identified the following three educative purposes for data collection or assessment: (a) for identification of students as eligible for services, (b) for intervention planning, and (c) for evaluation of program effectiveness. All three purposes share an underlying assumption that the data will be used to modify or make instructional changes of some kind (Gunter et al., 2003). When the generic procedures for measurement are employed with stimulus materials drawn directly from the instructional materials used by teachers in their classrooms, the approach is referred to as curriculum-based (Deno, 2003).

Collecting data is only the beginning, however. The next step is graphing the data. A list of student scores can go unchallenged, but if data are graphed and visually inspected on a continual basis, it is easy to recognize student growth or the lack of it (formative assessment) as well as overall performances (summative assessment). It is important to point out that the *curriculum-based measurement* (CBM) graph, with its multiple references, creates opportunities for clearer communication. It has now become common practice for teachers to use CBM data in parent conferences and at multidisciplinary team meetings to provide a framework for communicating

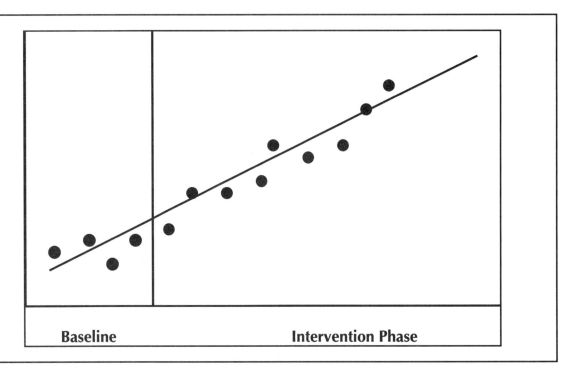

Baseline

Intervention Phase

FIGURE 22.1. Example of a curriculum-based measurement graph.

individual student status. Professional educators and parents can easily use the CBM graph, since little or no interpretation of the scores is necessary (Shinn, Habedank, & Good, 1993). Not only does the collection of student data indicate how a particular student or groups of students are doing, it also tells the teacher how he or she is doing and how effective the intervention is.

Teachers can graph student performance over time to determine whether students are making progress toward achieving instructional goals. When students' performance slopes are relatively flat, teachers can modify instruction to target deficits and then evaluate instructional outcomes. See Figure 22.1 for an example of a CBM graph. This example shows that the intervention is effective at improving the students' performance over time.

The Impact of Making Decisions Without Using Data

When decisions regarding student performance and intervention implementation are not driven by data the effort can turn out to be a hit-and-miss scenario. How does the teacher know how the student is actually performing? How do teachers know if they are doing a good job? How do they know if the chosen interventions are effective? All of these questions arise when data are not collected. If teachers choose an intervention that has no data support, they will be taking a chance on whether it is effective or not. Though not all interventions that have data support will necessarily work with all students, the chances for effectiveness are better.

Data also help teachers to form a rationale or guidelines for decision making regarding student, teacher, and intervention performance. Without the collection of data the proper decisions may not be made and teaching time could be sacrificed.

Outcomes of Using Data in Decision Making

When data are incorporated into the decision-making process, communication among other teachers, school personnel, and parents will be facilitated. If teachers can show that what they are doing in their classroom is effective, or that they are making changes based on data, then other adults involved with the child or children will more easily understand why the teacher is doing what he or she is doing. The collection of data on a continuous, consistent basis will not only provide information about how everyone is doing, but will also communicate to others how everyone is doing.

Madaus, Kellaghan, Rakow, and King (1979) found that when schools used indirect tests to measure student achievement, the schools did not appear to be very effective, but when they used direct tests—tests that actually measured the content being taught in the schools—some schools looked highly effective (Marzano, 2003). The National Research Council concluded that although standardized tests and state tests based on standards certainly have their place in the landscape of K–12 education, schools should not use such instruments as the primary indicator of student learning (Marzano, 2003). A school must use assessments that actually measure the content that teachers teach (Marzano, 2003)—which means schools should go beyond the standardized tests.

Data-Based Decision Making: The Process

The use of data in making decisions means (a) deliberate collection (identifying the critical data to measure), (b) analysis (with a frequency that allows responsive changes in programs or interventions), (c) data-driven decisions (decisions that are made only after questions are answered with data to back up identification of problems and selection of interventions), and (d) data-based evaluation and accountability. Data help us to frame our questions about student performance, to design and implement interventions, and to ask the critical question, "Is there a better way?" Therefore, accountability is a process that includes measurement, data collection, decision making, and evaluation (Isaacs, 2003).

Other questions also need to be asked: What strengths and weaknesses in student performance do the different data sources reveal? Are these the results that were expected? Why or why not? In what areas did the students perform best? What weaknesses are evident? How are different population groups performing on the various assessments? What does this work reveal about student learning and performance? What patterns or changes can be observed over time? Are there any surprises? What results are unexpected? What anomalies exist? Is there evidence of improvement or decline? If so, what might have caused the changes? What questions do these data raise? Are these results consistent with other achievement data? Are there alternative explanations for these results? By what criteria are we evaluating student work? (McTighe & Thomas, 2003). When data are collected it is essential that they be analyzed in detail to see what the results are really telling us about the student(s), the teacher, and instructional practices.

Identifying the Problem

How do teachers know what the problem is? If the student is in your classroom, there are a couple of possibilities regarding how the problem is identified. One option is observation. By observing the student in comparison to peers as well as where he or she should be developmentally, the teacher may be able to identify the problem. Another strategy is collecting student work samples and comparing the student's performance to that of others as well as to where the student should be developmentally. Finally, parents or others involved with the child might raise a concern to the teacher, and then observations, work samples, or both could be used to find out if there is a problem and to document what the actual problem is. Identification of the problem is crucial in order to start the process of remediation.

Setting the Goal

Although writing measurable goals is a critical first step in deciding the nature and scope of services for a student, it is not sufficient to ensure educational benefit to students. Educators must develop a method for measuring progress toward goals. Progress monitoring consists of five steps: (a) establish an annual goal, (b) set the expected rate of progress, (c) measure progress toward that goal at least weekly, (d) compare student's actual progress with the student's expected progress, and (e) make appropriate instructional decisions (Hagan-Burke & Jefferson, 2002). Goal setting and progress monitoring do not need to be time-consuming tasks; they may easily be accomplished using curriculum-based assessment (CBA) and CBM. CBA and CBM measures are sensitive to subtle progress and may be administered at least weekly. CBA includes any measures derived from the student's general education curriculum and typically developed by the teacher, whereas CBM measures are derived from the student's annual curriculum and may be purchased from an existing CBM library or developed according to standard procedures (Shinn, 1997). First, data on individual student performance during an initial baseline phase are collected and plotted on a graph. Second, a goal line is established. A goal line that connects the initial level and the goal shows the rate of improvement necessary for the student to achieve the goal. Third, for every five data points a vertical line is drawn on the graph. The vertical lines indicate the point at which a decision is made regarding a possible change in the student's program. At each point, judgments are made regarding the effectiveness of the instruction being provided. This systematic approach to setting goals, monitoring growth, changing programs, and evaluating the effects of changes is the formative evaluation model. Research on the achievement effects of using this approach has revealed that the students of teachers who use systematic formative evaluation based on CBM have greater achievement rates (Fuchs, Deno, & Mirkin, 1984) than the students of teachers who choose not to implement it. See Figures 22.2–22.4 for examples of the baseline, goal setting, and progress monitoring.

In Figure 22.2 the teacher has collected baseline data and plotted it on the graph. These data are collected before implementation of any intervention and serve to establish the student's current level of performance, providing important information to help the teacher document whether or not an intervention is effective.

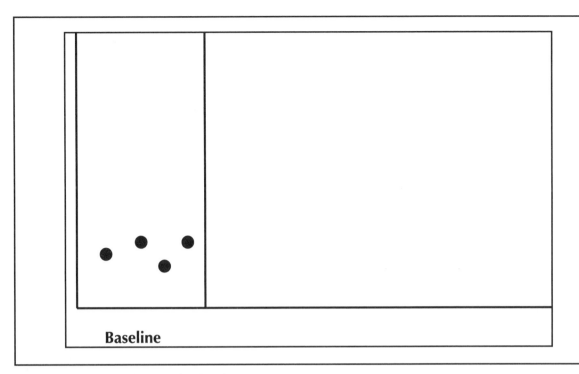

FIGURE 22.2. Example of graphed baseline data.

In Figure 22.3 the teacher has collected baseline data and plotted it on the graph. In addition, the teacher has drawn a goal line, which indicates intended progress over time. This line is important when collecting intervention data, as it will help the teacher determine whether or not the intervention is effective and whether any changes need to be made.

In Figure 22.4 baseline data were collected and plotted on the graph along with a goal line. As noted, after the teacher collected five data points (after baseline), the data indicated the student was *not* making progress toward the goal. Therefore the

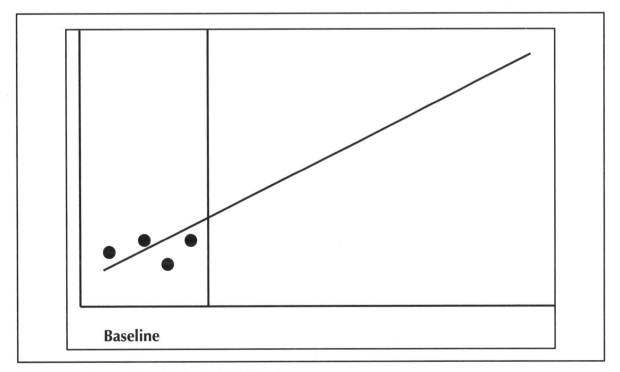

FIGURE 22.3. Example of baseline data and goal line.

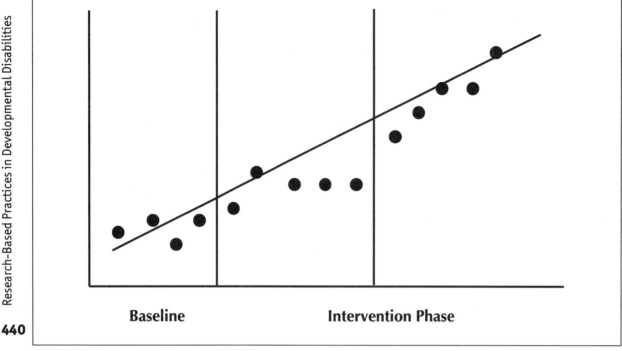

FIGURE 22.4. Example of baseline data, goal line, and progress monitoring.

intervention was modified or another intervention was selected. Data collected after this change indicate that the new intervention is effective and the student is on track toward reaching the desired goal.

Deciding What Data to Collect

Gunter (2001) defined data collection in school settings as the systematic gathering of information designed to verify that student learning occurs. Many types of data are gathered for this purpose, including grades, work samples, and anecdotal notes (Gunter et al., 2003). Data collection is the foundation of informed teacher decision making and is the basis for the individualized education program (IEP) (Gunter et al., 2003). It is important that the correct data are collected so that any problems the student is having are addressed.

Once the behavior is specifically identified and an operational definition of it is formulated, the correct data collection technique can be identified. It is important to choose the correct method of data collection for the behavior; otherwise, the actual behavior, as well as progress and teacher and intervention effectiveness, could be sacrificed. Choosing the wrong data collection method could have serious consequences. If the incorrect method is chosen, the teacher may not accurately record the behavior he or she is trying to observe.

Data Collection Methods and Their Purposes

Tawney and Gast (1984) describe formative evaluation as an ongoing process with frequent (at least weekly) measurement of student performance. They indicate that such evaluation can be used to guide instruction and confirm achievement of objectives. Formative assessment is critical in telling teachers how they are doing as well as how the students are doing. Without formative assessment, teachers' perceptions of student performance compared to actual student performance are often erroneous (Fuchs et al., 1984). In addition, teachers trained in formative assessment procedures may be more open to changing instructional methods and making more frequent instructional changes to promote achievement (Bloom, Hursh, Wienke, & Wold, 1992; Fuchs et al., 1984).

Fuchs and Fuchs (1986) presented three aspects of formative evaluation procedures that directly relate to achievement of students with disabilities. First, effect sizes—the statistical description of the educational impact—increased significantly when behavior modification procedures such as incorporating reinforcement were paired with systematic measurement. Second, when data evaluation rules were used to make decisions about when educational programs should be changed, effect sizes increased significantly. Finally, when data were graphed rather than simply recorded, student outcomes showed significant increases.

Among the many ways of recording observed behaviors are *anecdotal recording*, *event recording*, *latency recording*, *duration recording*, *interval recording*, and *time sampling*. Anecdotal recording is writing down everything that happens regarding a specific student in a particular environment or setting. This method might be used if a teacher is not really sure what behaviors are problems, as it can help the teacher to focus on what is actually happening. Often the collection of data in this way will lead to further data collection using another method to identify precisely what is happening. With respect to all of the data collection methods described here, it is important to note that the person observing the student and the behavior should have a specific behavioral definition of the particular behavior that is being observed.

For example, on-task behavior could be defined as behavior that shows the student doing what the teacher has instructed the student to do (e.g., engaging in independent practice activities, listening to a lecture, taking notes). Event recording is noting the frequency (number of times) of a behavior during a given time period. Typically, the observer would simply tally the number of times the behavior is observed. For example, the student got out of his or her seat four times during the 30-minute science lesson.

Latency recording is noting how long it takes a student to start an activity or to exhibit a particular behavior after being given a teacher prompt. Typically, the observer would record the amount of time that passes before the student exhibits the behavior prompted by the teacher. For example, it took the student 2 minutes and 45 seconds to start the homework assignment after being instructed to do so.

Duration recording is noting how long a behavior lasts. Typically, the observer would record the amount of time the student exhibits the behavior during a given period. For example, the student had a temper tantrum that lasted 3 minutes and 22 seconds.

Teachers who want to find the proportion of a specified time period during which the behavior occurs may select interval recording or time sampling. Both of these data collection methods record an approximation of the actual number of times a behavior occurs. In interval recording a set interval is chosen (say every 30 seconds) and if the behavior occurs at any time during the interval it is marked. For time sampling a set time is also chosen (say 1 minute) and if the behavior occurs at the end of the interval it is marked. See Table 22.1 for a description and comparison of different data collection methods and associated purposes.

Establishing a Baseline

Establishing a baseline simply means measuring a student's skills before intervention (e.g., instruction). Once established, the baseline becomes the yardstick against which a teacher can measure the effectiveness of any intervention (Hagan-Burke & Jefferson, 2002). For example, establishing a baseline for Tony can be accomplished by having him read aloud for 1 minute from each of three second-grade CBM

TABLE 22.1
Data Collection Methods and Associated Purposes

Data Collection Methods	Uses
Anecdotal recording	A brief narrative description of an event or events that the observer felt was important to observe
Permanent product recording	Analysis of student products or work that has been completed that focuses on the process (what and how the student did to get the answer) as well as the product (the correct answer)
Running record (continuous record)	A description of events written as they occur. Everything that the student does is written down
Event recording	The number of times something happens or that a behavior occurs
Duration recording	A measure of the length of time a specific event or behavior lasts
Intensity recording	A measure of the degree of a behavior expressed as high, medium, or low.
Latency recording	Amount of time between a request to begin a behavior or event and beginning the requested behavior or event
Interval recording	An observational method that involves recording specific events or behaviors (that occur frequently) during a prespecified time interval (e.g., 1 minute)
Time sampling	An observational method that involves recording specific events or behaviors at the end of a prespecified time interval (e.g., 1 minute)
Error analysis	Beyond marking answers as correct or incorrect, analyzes the mistakes to see if there is an error pattern for the student; might help teacher to focus instruction differently

reading passages. The teacher notes how many words Tony read correctly in each 1-minute sample and how many errors he made. These three 1-minute samples of reading behavior provide a starting point for setting goals and measuring progress.

The next step is to plot the information on a graph and decide how much progress Tony is expected to make within a 20-week time period. To determine an expected rate of progress for Tony, the teacher considers his baseline rate of 20 words read correctly per minute for each of the three reading passages. Next the teacher decides how much progress Tony should make in 20 weeks, given effective instruction. As a starting point, it might be anticipated that Tony would gain 2 correct words per week—or 40 words in 20 weeks (2 words per week times 20 weeks) (Hagan-Burke & Jefferson, 2002).

Deciding When to Collect Data

So when and how often should teachers collect data? That is really up to the teacher, but the more often and the more consistently a teacher collects data, the better off the student(s) and the teacher will be. The decision of how often the teacher collects data can have serious implications for intervention implementation, as well as for student and teacher progress and effectiveness of teaching time. For example, assume that a teacher collects three to five intervention data samples before making a decision about whether the student(s) are performing up to goals previously set and whether the teacher and the intervention are being effective. If the teacher collects formal data once a week, a decision could be made after 3 to 5 weeks. If the same teacher collected formal data only once a month, it would be 3 to 5 months before the teacher would be able to make a decision. If the student is doing well and the intervention is effective, the timing might not make a difference, but if the student is not doing well and the intervention is not effective, a great deal of time is wasted on something that is not working.

In the first scenario the teacher could make a change in 3 to 5 weeks, whereas in the second scenario the time lapse before the change would be 3 to 5 months. That means a total of 7 to 15 weeks when the teacher is actually implementing something that is not effective—resulting in an extreme waste of student and teacher time.

Choosing the Intervention

Once the baseline and the expected rate of progress have been established, an intervention to remediate Tony's reading skill deficit is developed. As soon as the intervention is enacted, Tony's teacher begins to monitor how well that intervention is working to move him toward his annual reading goal (60 words read correctly in 20 weeks). As a general rule, 1-minute CBM reading probes once weekly are sufficient (Fuchs, 1989). Tony's progress, however, should probably be measured twice weekly, since his skills are significantly below those of his peers (Hagan-Burke & Jefferson, 2002).

Once the problem is clearly defined, a specific intervention plan to help the student achieve the goal needs to be established. The teacher will analyze the problem and develop hypotheses regarding the cause(s) of the problem. This work will inform the structure of the intervention. The intervention plan must be realistic in terms of its ability to be implemented within the context of normal classroom routines and to achieve the goal. Teachers may want to consider the interventions that are supported by research, are easy to implement, and have the best chance of helping the student reach the goal. There is no need to choose the most complicated intervention when a simpler one might work just as well.

Intervention Types

Interventions can be either academic or behavioral. Academic interventions teach skills or processes strategically in small, concrete steps and can focus on areas such as reading, mathematics, written expression, or work-related skills. Some interventions are more general in scope (e.g., self-monitoring, mnemonics, attribution training), while others are specific to a certain content area and process (e.g., teaching the acronym POWER—P = Plan, O = organize, W = write, E = edit, R = Revise—for writing a paper, teaching paragraph restatements for understanding narrative text).

Behavioral interventions also focus on teaching skills or processes strategically in small, concrete steps, but the emphasis is on non-academic areas, such as on-task behavior, use of appropriate language, ability to follow directions, and social skills. The baseline data and knowledge of the student help the teacher to choose an appropriate intervention. It is important that data collection continue while the intervention is being implemented so that the teacher can determine whether it is effective or not. The teacher should be sure that the student understands why it is important to learn the strategy. Students need to be aware of their own deficits (if possible) and how the particular strategy could benefit them. When implementing an intervention, whether academic or behavioral, the teacher must remember to teach the student and to provide enough practice opportunities. When presenting information, the teacher should model what he or she wants the student to learn. The teacher should go through examples and non-examples (talking through the steps out loud), making sure the student has opportunities to discriminate what is being taught. The student should listen and watch the instructor if at all possible. Depending on the teacher's sample population, he or she may need to incorporate more or fewer examples. For students with developmental disabilities, it is highly probable that the teacher will need to spend more time in the instructional phase and the guided practice phase before students will be able to independently implement the intervention. To clarify the steps in the delivery of the information the teacher may find the following acronyms helpful:

The first acronym is PASS (*P*rioritize information to be presented, *A*dapt or modify information for students, *S*CREAM, and *S*ystematically evaluate what was done). All lessons should be planned before they are delivered. First, the lesson should be outlined so that the information to be delivered is prioritized. Information should be organized so that it is meaningful and understandable to the learner. Second, the teacher should review the entire group of students and identify any students who may need adaptations or modifications. For example, if the teacher is delivering a highly verbal lecture, a student who has listening difficulties may need some type of recording device to tape the lecture or even a copy of the instructor's notes. Third, SCREAM (discussed in detail in the next paragraph) refers to the actual lesson being delivered and how teachers can be more effective deliverers of information. Fourth, teachers should systematically evaluate how effective they are as instructors and how students are performing with new concepts and materials.

The second acronym, mentioned in the previous paragraph, is SCREAM. SCREAM stands for *S*tructure (organize the lecture logically so that all pieces mesh together and make sense to the learner), *C*larity (make all points clear and concise with the use of modeling and real-world examples), *R*edundancy (repeat important concepts often to reinforce that what is being said is in fact important; some students may need to be told directly, "This is important"), *E*nthusiasm (be enthusiastic about what is being taught; if the teacher is not excited about what he or she is doing, it is difficult to expect the students to get excited about what they are supposed to be learning), *A*ppropriate pace (move at a comfortable pace through material so students can follow effectively; slow down, speed up, or repeat as necessary), and *M*aximize student engagement (get students involved as much as possible and let them become active rather than passive learners) (Mastropieri & Scruggs, 1994). Teachers who keep this acronym in mind will be able to develop a more meaningful and effective lesson.

Assistive Technology as a Possible Intervention

Assistive technology (AT) can also be considered as a possible intervention for a student with academic or behavioral difficulties. With AT, just as with academic or behavioral interventions, individuals involved in decision making should consider the abilities of the student and the task at hand. Will the AT help the student meet his or her goals and objectives? Is the AT functional for the student? Will the AT be a benefit to the student?

AT should not be implemented just so the teacher is using AT. This decision needs careful consideration and planning for how it will be introduced, maintained, and assessed. As with other interventions, baseline data should be collected before the implementation of the AT and data collection should continue during the implementation so the teacher can decide whether or not the AT is effective (see Chapters 10 and 20 for detailed discussions of AT). These steps are very important, and it is also important to realize that AT alone may not benefit the student.

For example, Joe is a third-grade boy who has difficulty with written expression. When given a writing prompt, he typically writes only 2 or 3 words total. His IEP team decided to implement the use of an AlphaSmart® to help him with written expression. Immediately his responses increased to 7 to 9 words total. At weekly prompts, data were recorded and graphed. Inspection of the visual data showed that

Joe was not making any progress. Over a 2-month period, his responses totaled only 10 to 11 words, yet he had many good ideas when speaking. The team met again and decided to implement the use of a tape recorder to capture his thoughts and ideas. Once given the topic, Joe could record all of his ideas and comments with the tape recorder. Then he could listen to the tape and type the words into the AlphaSmart®. With this intervention his writing output increased from 10 to 11 words total to two to three pages. In this case the original AT was not sufficient and through data collection and reflection the team was able to implement another type of AT to help the student increase his performance.

The team working with the student must consider the purpose of the AT when they are determining what AT implementation will be best. Is the purpose *remediation* (i.e., additional instructional time, different instructional approaches) or *compensation* (i.e., if remediation has failed, compensatory approaches are needed to produce the desired level of performance)? How do teachers decide between remediation and compensation?

Few guidelines are available for decision making about AT for learning. If a child has repeatedly failed a test of essential knowledge (e.g., adding fractions, states and capitals, steps of the water cycle), how much failure data are needed before there is enough evidence that the child can't perform the task? When do teachers intervene? What do teachers do? Theorists of AT suggest that teachers need to make a critical decision: remediate or compensate.

Teachers are very comfortable with remediation strategies: reteach the information, use alternative instructional strategies, break the tasks down into smaller parts to analyze what the child knows and what components are problematic, reduce the number of items that must be completed, provide additional practice, engage in one-on-one tutoring, and so forth. If this approach always worked, teachers would never see high school students who didn't know the times tables or couldn't read independently beyond the third-grade level. Obviously, remediation is not always successful. At some point in the educational process, teachers must recognize the need for compensatory approaches. If a student doesn't know his or her multiplication facts, why doesn't the IEP team allow the student to use a calculator when solving math problems? Some would argue that this solution isn't fair to other students, but it is the process that should be the focus, not the product. In fact, many state assessments allow the use of calculators—why not practice using them in school? The use of calculators would then serve a twofold purpose: preparing students to use them for statewide assessments and preparing students for life outside the classroom, in the "real world."

Determining Intervention Effectiveness

The next step in progress monitoring is to compare the actual rate of progress with the expected rate of progress (Fuchs, 1989; Shinn, 1995, 1997). At this point in the intervention process, data are available to indicate how well the intervention is working. When at least three progress points for the intervention have been plotted on the graph, teachers can draw a trend line, or a line that best fits through these three points. The trend line indicates the actual rate of progress (Fuchs, 1989; Shinn, 1995, 1997).

In the example discussed earlier, progress monitoring can indicate whether Tony's intervention is working sufficiently long before the 20-week mark. Gathering this information early allows his teacher to make modifications in time to ensure that Tony reaches his goal. Once both the expected and the actual rates of progress have been plotted on the progress-monitoring graph, it is time for the final step in progress monitoring—decision making (Hagan-Burke & Jefferson, 2002).

Organizing Data for Analysis

Once the data have been collected, they must be organized and prepared for analysis. Is the information obtained qualitative or quantitative? The teacher must decide what kind of data is available and how the information will be analyzed. Will data be reported by individual student, the entire class, the entire grade level, or some other way?

Once these questions have been answered, the data can be entered into some kind of form or coding sheet to help organize it so that comparisons can be made. If possible, a visual display should also be developed to communicate—to the student, parents, other teachers, and anyone else involved—information about the effectiveness of the intervention(s) and the progress of the student. The clear communication of what the data reveal is very important for those involved with the student, for understanding what interventions are most effective, and for producing the best measurable results for the student. The goals are to find out what the teacher is doing that is effective and keep doing it and also to find out what is not effective and to change or modify that practice so as to have the intervention become more effective.

Using Technology in Data Organization and Analysis

Technology can also be added to the repertoire of behaviors that help teachers to be more effective. Once the data are collected, it is important for the teacher to decide how the information will be reported and used. Technology can help in the analysis of data as well as in the reporting and communication of the results. The Statistical Package for the Social Sciences (SPSS) software is a useful tool for data analysis. SPSS is a suite of products for statistical analysis and data management that enables teachers and researchers to access, prepare, manage, analyze, and report data in order to solve research problems. Once the teacher enters data into this program she or he is able to look at the data in many different ways (individual student, the entire class, the entire grade level, or some other way).

Teachers who are uncomfortable with this type of program, can use other tools, like databases and spreadsheets, to store, organize, and present data effectively and efficiently (Adamy, 2000). Many teachers are already familiar with databases and spreadsheets and are naturally more likely to use what they already know. They do, however, need to seek out the most effective applications, even if they are less familiar. Teachers must reflect on the entire process and make educated decisions as to what is the most effective and beneficial for all involved.

Deciding When an Intervention Needs to Be Stopped

When interventions are being implemented and data collection is under way, teachers need to make appropriate instructional decisions according to the results of the data. Three general patterns between actual and expected rates of progress are possible: (a) actual rate is about the same as expected rate (no progress is being made), (b) actual rate is much higher than expected (student is making progress), or (c) actual rate is much lower than expected (student is doing worse with the intervention than before it was implemented). Monitoring progress toward goals should provide information that helps educators make one of three decisions about an instructional plan: (a) maintain the plan because the student is making good progress toward goals, (b) increase the goal because the student is exceeding goal expectations, or (c) change the plan because the student is not making adequate progress (Fuchs, 1989; Shinn, 1995, 1997). Changing the plan could mean selecting a brand-new intervention or it could mean modifying the existing intervention to make it more effective. Without progress information, students may receive effective instruction, receive ineffective instruction, or be held to a minimum rather than a meaningful goal standard (Hagan-Burke & Jefferson, 2002).

Conclusion

This chapter discussed how teachers of students with developmental disabilities can incorporate data-based techniques and decision-making principles into their daily routines to measure how students are performing on content, skills, and behaviors. Collecting the data is the easiest part, but it is effective only if the most applicable technique is used—the technique that will yield the most reliable and valid data. After successful data collection, it is critical that teachers analyze the data to help them determine the next step. The data can inform the teacher on how the students are doing, as well as supplying information for other important educational decisions. Teachers can continue to move forward with content or skills if the student has learned the material, they can decide to reteach the lesson if the student did not learn the content or skills, or they can decide to change or modify the method of instruction. Data-based decision making can provide teachers a very useful approach for working with students with developmental disabilities.

Glossary

Anecdotal recording—Writing down everything that happens regarding a specific student in a particular environment or setting.

Assistive technology—Any item, piece of equipment, or product system, whether acquired commercially, modified, or customized, that is used to increase, maintain, or improve the functional capabilities of individuals with disabilities.

Curriculum-based measurement—Individualized, direct, and repeated measures of students' proficiency and progress in the curriculum.

Duration recording—Collecting the amount of time a behavior lasts.

Event recording—Collecting the frequency of a behavior for a given time or period.

Formative evaluation—An ongoing process, with frequent and repeated measurement of student performance.

Interval recording—A set time interval is chosen and if the targeted behavior occurs at any time during that interval it is marked.

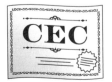

Knowledge and Skills for Entry-Level Special Education Teachers of Students With Developmental Disabilities Standards Addressed in This Chapter

Principle 5: Learning Environments/Social Interaction

    DD5S1   Provide instruction in community-based settings.

    DD5S3   Use and maintain assistive technologies.

DD5S4   Structure the physical environment to provide optimal learning for individuals with developmental disabilities.

DD5S5   Plan instruction for individuals with developmental disabilities in a variety of placement settings.

Principle 7: Instructional Planning

DD7S1   Plan instruction for independent functional life skills relevant to the community, personal living, sexuality, and employment.

DD7S2   Plan and implement instruction for individuals with developmental disabilities that is both age-appropriate and ability-appropriate.

DD7S4   Design, implement, and evaluate specialized instructional programs for persons with developmental disabilities that enhance social participation across environments.

Principle 8: Assessment

DD8S1   Select, adapt, and use instructional assessment tools and methods to accommodate the abilities and needs of individuals with mental retardation and developmental disabilities.

Web Site Resources

Data-Based Decision Making: Resources for Educators
http://www.ael.org/dbdm/

Guides educators through a process to establish a school improvement team, develop a hypothesis, gather data to assess needs, use data, develop a data-based plan, monitor progress, and document success. Also provides an overview, a rationale for the importance of data collection, a glossary, and other related resources.

An Introduction to Data-Based Decision Making
http://www.specialconnections.ku.edu/cgi-bin/cgiwrap/specconn/
main.php?cat=assessment&section=main&subsection=ddm/main

Helps the educator understand what data-based decision making is, how it can be used, what it measures, what the different measurement strategies are, how data collection is initiated, and how strategies and interventions are evaluated. Links to teacher tools, research, case studies, plus an online collaboration component.

3D. Data-Driven Decision Making
http://www.3d2know.org/index.cfm

What data-driven decision making is, why it should be used, what data should be collected, what common report formats are most useful, and why it is important for teachers to implement it; also information or publications, best practices, self-assessment, and other possible resources.

References

Adamy, P. (2000, February). *Using computers to enhance action research*. Paper presented at the Society for Information Technology and Teacher Education International Conference, San Diego, CA.

Bloom, L. A., Hursh, D., Wienke, W. D., & Wold, R. K. (1992). The effects of computer-assisted data collection on students' behaviors. *Behavioral Assessment, 14*, 173–190.

Brimijoin, K. (2002). *A journey toward expertise in differentiation: A preservice and inservice teacher make their way*. Unpublished doctoral dissertation, University of Virginia, Charlottesville.

Brimijoin, K., Marquissee, E., & Tomlinson, C. A. (2003). Using data to differentiate instruction. *Educational Leadership, 60*(5), 70–73.

Bruner, J. (1963). *The process of education*. New York: Vintage Books.

Carnine, D., & Granzin, A. (2001). Setting learning expectations for students with disabilities. *School Psychology Review, 30,* 466–472.

Deno, S. L. (2003). Developments in curriculum-based measurement. *Journal of Special Education, 37,* 184–192.

Englert, C. S., & Tarrant, K. L. (1995). Creating collaborative cultures for educational change. *Remedial and Special Education, 16,* 325–336.

Epstein, M. H., Cullinan, D., & Polloway, E. A. (1988). Patterns of maladjustment among mentally retarded children and youth. *American Journal of Mental Deficiency, 91,* 124–127.

Fuchs, L. S. (1989). Evaluating solutions, monitoring progress, and revising intervention plans. In M. R. Shinn (Ed.), *Curriculum-based measurement: Assessing special children* (pp. 153–181). New York: Guilford Press.

Fuchs, L. S., Deno, S. L., & Mirkin, P. K. (1984). The effects of frequent curriculum-based measurement and evaluation on pedagogy, student achievement, and student awareness of learning. *American Educational Research Journal, 21,* 449–460.

Fuchs, L. S., & Fuchs, D. (1986). Effects of systematic formative evaluation: A meta-analysis. *Exceptional Children, 53,* 199–208.

Gersten, R., Morvant, M., & Brengelman, S. (1995). Closer to the classroom is close to the bone: Coaching as a means to translate research into classroom practice. *Exceptional Children, 62*(1), 52–66.

Gunter, P. L. (2001). Data-based decision-making to ensure positive outcomes for children/youth with challenging behaviors. In L. M. Bullock & R. A. Gable (Eds.), *Addressing social, academic, and behavioral needs within inclusive and alternative settings* (pp. 49–52). Reston, VA: Council for Exceptional Children.

Gunter, P. L., Callicott, K., Denny, R. K., & Gerber, B. L. (2003). Finding a place for data collection in classrooms for students with emotional/behavioral disorders. *Preventing School Failure, 48*(1), 4–8.

Guskey, T. (1995). Professional development in education: In search of the optimal mix. In T. R. Guskey & M. Huberman (Eds.), *Professional development in education* (pp. 114–131). New York: Teachers College Press.

Hagan-Burke, S., & Jefferson, G. L. (2002). Using data to promote academic benefit for included students with mild disabilities. *Preventing School Failure, 46*(3), 112–118.

Isaacs, M. L. (2003). Data-driven decision making: The engine of accountability. *Professional School Counseling, 6,* 288–295.

Madaus, G. F., Kellaghan, T., Rakow, E. A., & King, D. (1979). The sensitivity of measures of school effectiveness. *Harvard Educational Review, 49,* 207–230.

Marzano, R. J. (2003). Using data: Two wrongs and a right. *Educational Leadership, 60*(5), 56–60.

Mastropieri, M. A., & Scruggs, T. E. (1994). *Effective instruction for special education* (2nd ed.). Austin, TX: PRO-ED.

McTighe, J., & Thomas, R. S. (2003). Backward design for forward action. *Educational Leadership, 60*(5), 52–55.

National Council for Accreditation of Teacher Education. (2000). *Professional standards for the accreditation of schools, colleges, and departments of education.* Washington, DC: Author.

Reschly, D. J., Kicklighter, R. H., & McGee, P. (1988a). Recent placement litigation, Part I: Regular education grouping: Comparison of Marshall (1984, 1985) & Hobson (1967, 1969). *School Psychology Review, 17,* 7–19.

Reschly, D. J., Kicklighter, R. H., & McGee, P. (1988b). Recent placement litigation, Part II: Minority EMR overrepresentation: Comparison of Larry P. (1979, 1984) & Marshall (1984, 1985) and S-1 (1986). *School Psychology Review, 17,* 20–36.

Reschly, D. J., Kicklighter, R. H., & McGee, P. (1988c). Recent placement litigation, Part IIII: Analysis of differences in Larry P., Marshall, and S-1 and implications for future practices. *School Psychology Review, 17,* 37–48.

Richardson, V. (1994). Conducting research on practice. *Educational Researcher, 23*(5), 5–10.

Shinn, M. R. (1995). Best practices in curriculum-based measurement and its use in a problem-solving model. In J. Grimes & A. Thomas (Eds.), *Best practices in school psychology* (3rd ed., pp. 547–568). Silver Spring, MD: National Association of School Psychologists.

Shinn, M. R. (1997). Exploring and evaluating solutions. In M. R. Shinn (Ed.), *Curriculum-based measurement: Assessing special children* (pp. 153–181). New York: Guilford Press.

Shinn, M. R., Habedank, L., & Good, R. H. (1993). The effects of classroom reading performance data on general education teachers' and parents' attitudes about reintegration. *Exceptionality, 4*, 205–228.

Tawney, J. W., & Gast, D. L. (1984). *Single subject research in special education.* Columbus, OH: Merrill.

Tomlinson, C. (1995). *Differentiating instruction for mixed-ability classrooms.* Alexandria, VA: ASCD.

SECTION 8

PROFESSIONAL AND ETHICAL PRACTICE

23

The Impact of Attitudes on Individuals With Developmental Disabilities

Ravic P. Ringlaben and Kimberly Griffith

Summary

This chapter reviews the effects of assumptions, biases, stereotypes, and service delivery philosophy on the development of positive and negative attitudes toward persons with developmental disabilities. It also addresses the impact of these attitudes within education, employment, and media environments and presents research-based and emerging strategies that promote positive attitudes toward persons with disabilities.

Learning Outcomes

After reading this chapter you should be able to:

- Identify the major reasons for both positive and negative attitudes toward individuals with developmental disabilities.

- Describe how negative attitudes toward individuals with developmental disabilities can be transformed into positive attitudes.

- Describe how service delivery philosophy can affect attitudes.

- Identify the research-based and emerging trends that can develop positive attitudes among principals, general education teachers, special education teachers, students without disabilities, students with disabilities, interpersonal relationships, post-secondary school environments, employers, employees/coworkers without disabilities, and employees with disabilities.

- Describe how the mass media affect attitudes about individuals with disabilities.

Introduction

Research-based and emerging practices for persons with developmental disabilities are a focus of this text. However, little discussion has been presented relating to *attitudes* about persons with developmental disabilities. Perhaps a typical assumption is that professionals, as well as individuals without disabilities, have the "proper" attitudes concerning people with disabilities. In fact, the most frequently reported barriers for children with disabilities are institutional and attitudinal (Pivik, McComas, & Laflamme, 2002). This chapter will review literature pertaining to the impact of attitudes concerning persons with developmental disabilities and provide research-based strategies for improving those attitudes.

Currently, almost 54 million Americans have disabilities (Jaeger, 2004). This astonishing number makes persons with disabilities the largest minority group in the United

States. Disability knows no boundaries with regard to race, creed, color, national origin, sex, age, religion, economic status, or sexual preference.

Like other minority groups, persons with disabilities, and their advocates, have had to "fight" to receive the same rights as other individuals (Lynch & Thomas, 1994). According of Stubbins (1988), "Changes in the relations between disabled and able-bodied persons are often brought about through a political process" (p. 22). Two main thrusts of this process have been legislation and litigation. Both have expanded access for individuals with disabilities to increase their participation in society, recognizing that individuals with disabilities "have the same needs, desires, and goals for themselves as do all other Americans" (Gerry & Mirsky, 1992, p. 341). Kilbury, Benshoff, and Rubin (1992) noted, "While many legal rights have been acquired by citizens with disabilities in the last 20 years, much needs to be done in advocating for the enforcement of existing legislation" (1992, p. 9).

Once individuals with disabilities gain access to an environment, how are they treated? What are the attitudes of persons without disabilities in the environment? What are some of the assumptions (biases, stereotypes) held by persons without disabilities? What are some of the social and educational policies that evolve from legislation and litigation that perpetuate continued segregation of persons with disabilities in the United States and in the world society (Jahnukainen & Korhonen, 2003; O'Brien, 2003)?

Assumptions, Biases, and Stereotypes

It is well recognized that environmental and social policy variables affect the participation in society of individuals with disabilities (Kilbury et al., 1992; Lynch & Thomas, 1994). Many persons with disabilities believe that the greatest barrier to their full participation in society is not their disability or the inaccessible environments but rather the biased attitudes of, prejudices of, and inappropriate treatment by persons without disabilities (Donaldson, Helmstetter, Donaldson, & West, 1994; Ferri & Connor, 2005; Fine & Asch, 1988; Gordon, Tantillo, Feldman, & Perrone, 2004; Jahoda & Markova, 2004; Quick, Lehmann, & Deniston, 2003).

Attitudes of the public, including educational and other service providers, are a critical component of the environment with which persons with disabilities must continually contend (Hahn, 1988). Stated Westbrook, Legge, and Pennay (1993), "Negative social attitudes toward people with disabilities are most likely expressed in terms of exclusion from, or lack of access to, social roles, activities and facilities" (p. 617). Bogdan and Biklen (1977) used the term *handicapism* and defined it as "a set of assumptions that promote the differential and unequal treatment of people because of apparent or assumed physical, mental or behavioral difference" (p. 14). Numerous investigators (Brantlinger, 2001; Hehir, 2002; McMahon, West, Lewis, Armstrong, & Conway, 2003; Ochs, Kremer-Sadlik, Solomon, & Gainer Sirota, 2001; Pavri, 2001) have reported that negative attitudes and stereotypes regarding persons with disabilities can produce and/or perpetuate prejudice, scorn, rejection, neglect, ableism, discrimination, oppression, exploitation, powerlessness, marginalization, isolation, loneliness, and victimization (including a heightened risk of sexual, physical, and emotional abuse). Even professionals who provide services can unknowingly rely on specious beliefs and stereotypes (Gilmore & Campbell, 2003).

Individuals with disabilities should not only be given access to all facets of society but also be treated with dignity and respect (O'Brien, 2003). More than half a century ago, Barker (1948) wrote that the primary accommodation for persons with disabilities "must involve changes in the values of the physically normal" (p. 37). McCarthy (1988) suggested that accommodation is an attitude that allows for the full expression of human talent. It does so either by removing whatever barriers (attitudinal, physical, procedural) interfere with accomplishing a goal or by providing whatever assistance or support is needed to bring someone to the level at which goals can be approached by standard or alternative means. Accordingly, accommodation should be thought of as a right by which to obtain equal opportunity to participate, not as a special privilege (p. 258).

Historically, persons with disabilities, especially those labeled as having developmental disabilities, have been considered "not quite whole" because they did not meet society's criteria of physical attractiveness or functional independence. Because of this, many pejorative terms evolved and are still used today (Beadles, 2001). People with disabilities produce anxiety in persons without disabilities (Hahn, 1988). People without disabilities often reflect on the following questions when meeting or coming into contact with people with disabilities: How could they lead a satisfactory life? How could they ever really find true happiness? People with disabilities were and continue to be treated differently, devalued, socially stigmatized, and placed in subordinate roles that produce unequal status (Fine & Asch, 1988; Makas, 1988).

Individuals without disabilities seem to go through a sequential process when they come into contact with a person with a disability. This process involves perception, attitude–belief, emotion, and behavior. Hence, one's belief or attitude about individuals with disabilities determines one's behavior: "The perception we have learned and to act the way we have been taught to act; and that is that persons with disabilities tend to be viewed as inferior to those without disabilities" (Lessen, 1991, p. 31). If one believes people with disabilities are "in-valid" or that all people with disabilities are handicapped ("cap-in-hand"), one's behavior will reflect that belief. Members of society, as a whole, and educational or service delivery professionals specifically, need to reflect on their particular attitudes and beliefs, decisions, and policies that may facilitate or harm the integration and participation of people with disabilities in the educational, social, political, and economic mainstream. Correcting negative beliefs and attitudes that are held toward people with disabilities must take place if people with disabilities are to participate effectively in society (Donaldson et al., 1994). Lesson (1991) noted that this "change toward acceptance is a long and difficult process. We need to get over our irrational fears and replace them with thoughts and actions that are based on reason and facts" (p. 36).

Service Delivery Philosophy

The manner in which services are provided to people with disabilities is significantly influenced by "service philosophy." Over time, two main service philosophies have "evolved," based on the beliefs and attitudes about persons with disabilities. *The medical model* and the *social–political model* of service philosophies are described below.

The medical model has focused on the limitations and functional impairments of disability (Hahn, 1988). Disability is viewed as something that needs to be fixed, like any other illness. The individual is considered a victim of the disability: "The concept of victim is entwined with the concept of environment-person interaction and implies helplessness, fate and being at mercy with the environment" (Lynch & Thomas, 1994, p. 9). In fact, much of the literature about people with disabilities indicates that people without disabilities still believe that people with disabilities "are sick or that their disabilities are contagious" (Murray-Seegert, 1989, p. 107). People with disabilities need to be made more "normal." A service delivery philosophy based on the medical model focuses on changing the person with a disability (Olkin, 2002). When the individual with a disability is confronted with a problem, it is assumed that the disability is the cause of the problem (Fine & Asch, 1988; Lynch & Thomas, 1994). The individual with disabilities is devalued and placed in a role that is subordinate or unequal (Makas, 1988). Expectations are developed on the basis of failure. Different is *abnormal*.

A social–political service delivery model focuses on the limitations and functional impairments of the environment. The *environment* is the disability (Hahn, 1988). This service philosophy describes people with disabilities as "an oppressed minority group" that needs to be afforded the same rights as other citizens. The person with a disability is a multidimensional individual, with the disability being only one of the many dimensions of the individual. This philosophy differs from the medical model in that rather than concentrating on the origin of the disability, it focuses on changing the environment to assist the person with the disability to function as effectively and naturally as possible. It also empowers the individual to grow and mature in positive directions (Bolt, 2004; Lynch & Thomas, 1994). Expectations are developed on the basis of success. Different is *normal*. According to Brotherson, Cook, Cunman-Lahr, and Wehmeyer (1995),

> Modifying the physical environment to promote choice and self-determination serves two broad purposes. First, modifications of the physical environment have a direct impact on children with disabilities by permitting greater access to home, school and community settings. . . . A second and more subtle and less well-recognized purpose is that increased accessibility affects the attitudes of persons with and without disabilities. (p. 4)

Models that have evolved from this philosophy include "wraparound services," "neverstreaming" (needs of *all* students and students with disabilities, without special services), and "holistic or amalgamated" services (Bullock, 2002; Stevenson, 2003). This cure-versus-care model dispute is an issue of continued debate in delivering services to individuals with disabilities, and continues to affect attitudes.

Attitudinal Barriers and Bridges

Any philosophy of service delivery is perpetuated one person at a time. There seem to be a number of "environments" in which service delivery philosophy is perhaps more important than in others. In the following section, a number of these environments are described, along with suggestions for attitude improvement.

Education

The educational service delivery system has gone through many changes during the last 30-plus years. At one time, school was for those individuals who could *benefit* from being there. Education for students with disabilities was nonexistent or, at best, limited. With the initiation of litigation and legislation in the 1970s on behalf of students with disabilities, social systems became more accessible. According to Krajewski, Hyde, and O'Keefe (2002), however, "Legal mandates cannot, however, mandate acceptance by peers, neighbors, fellow employees, employers, or any of the other groups of individuals who directly impact the lives of people with disabilities" (p. 27).

The educational service delivery philosophy has evolved from one that believed that students with disabilities should be educated primarily in segregated settings, to one in which students with disabilities were to be "mainstreamed" and "included" to spend part or most of the day with "normal" peers, to one that supports full-time education and inclusion for students with disabilities in general education classes. Gliedman and Roth described this new vision of the education of students with disabilities:

> It is to bring the handicapped child into the mainstream of childhood. It is to end his exclusion from social experiences appropriate to children his age. It is to provide him with an education that no longer reinforces— however inadvertently—society's traditional misconceptions and stereotypes about the abilities of handicapped individuals. It is . . . to improve education by breaking down the barriers of prejudice and misunderstanding that have excluded the handicapped from the mainstream of American life for so long. (1980, p. 218)

In a review of the literature, Wilson (1999) suggested guidelines for inclusion, among then (a) evaluating parent and student preferences, (b) structuring environments in which general education teachers have a sense of empowerment, control, and support, (c) structuring and facilitating friendships among children, and (d) arranging classrooms to maximize learning for all. The manner in which these guidelines are implemented seems to have a direct effect on the attitudes of "all parties involved."

Several investigators (Pivik et al., 2002; Sweeting & West, 2001; Zollers, Ramanathan, & Yu, 1999) described barriers that are intentional (e.g., bullying) and unintentional (e.g., lack of understanding or knowledge). Attitudinal barriers were identified as the most deleterious. Facilitators described were environmental modifications, social/policy changes, and institutional resources.

Interestingly, students both with and without disabilities desire the same teacher attributes and respond similarly when these attributes are implemented (Wallace, Anderson, Bartholomay, & Hupp, 2002). Klingner and Vaughn (1999) report these traits to be appropriate instructional pace, clear explanations, and teaching the same material several different ways. However, Kavale (2002) believes that the requisite attitudes, accommodations, and adaptations for students with disabilities to be successful in school are not yet completely in place, while Kauffman, McGee, and Brigham (2004) indicate that even well-intentioned accommodations can enable students to not persevere to attain more independence. It also appears that students with disabilities are not always given access to the best teachers (Treder, Morse, & Ferron, 2000). Shortages of appropriately trained and certified professionals, including teachers, therapists, and others, exacerbate the problem (Agran, Alper, & Wehmeyer, 2002).

Principals

Investigators are determining that the attitudes and actions of school principals can have a significant impact on whether schools successfully implement inclusion models (Zollers et al., 1999). Praisner (2003) finds that positive experiences with students with disabilities and training in special education concepts are associated with principals' having more-positive attitudes toward inclusion.

General Education Teachers

It has been documented that the attitudes and expectations that teachers hold toward students with disabilities *will* directly affect their behavior and thus affect the manner in which their students are educated and what these students will achieve (Friend & Pope, 2005; Ringlaben & Price, 1981; Smith, Polloway, Patton, & Dowdy, 2004). Positive attitudes and expectations tend to produce positive educational beliefs and experiences regarding students with disabilities, whereas negative attitudes and expectations tend to produce negative beliefs and expectations (Jahnukainen & Korhonen, 2003; Robertson, Chamberlain, & Kasari, 2003). It appears that the development of attitudes, including teacher attitudes, is influenced by several factors, among them knowledge, experiences, and support (Van Reusen, Shoho, & Barker, 2000–2001).

The knowledge about students with disabilities that teachers bring to the classroom is likely acquired in a variety of ways. It may be acquired through information from family, friends, local schools, and the community. Information received during the college years and the teacher training program is especially important. If the information provided in these environments is that individuals with disabilities are sick, hopeless, or less than whole, then the person who becomes a teacher may very well perpetuate these beliefs. However, if the information shared portrays individuals with disabilities as people first and provides facts that emphasize similarities rather than differences, the teacher may treat students with disabilities in a manner that evokes dignity and respect (Garriott, Snyder, Ringlaben, & Tennant, 2004).

Past experience and knowledge also lend much to the development of attitudes and educational programs (Cook, 2001). That is, because of past educational practice, teachers with more than about 25 years of teaching experience may not have had contact with peers with disabilities when they were attending school. However, university students currently in teacher training programs and teachers with fewer than 20 years of teaching experience probably have experienced some contact with peers with disabilities during their education.

Information received during an individual's teacher training program is especially important. There has been a call for teacher preparation programs for general educators to include more information about and experiences with students with disabilities "because teachers in today's public schools must provide instruction and other educational services that meet the needs of a very diverse student population. . . . They must be prepared to deal effectively with all kinds of students" (Smith et al., 2004, p. 5). Traditionally, general educators receive a significant amount of information through one course devoted to principles and practices in educating students with special needs, though frequently candidates pursuing a secondary teaching certificate may not be required to complete this course. Such a course may be the first and only formal professional exposure to information and experiences concerning children with disabilities (Fox & Rotatori, 1986). However, even this one component of a teacher education program can produce positive attitudes in future teachers, according to a review of the literature reported by Hannah (1988) and supported by other investigators (Beattie, Anderson, & Antonak, 1997; Shade & Stewart, 2001; Turner, 2003).

Texts, materials, and activities for such a course tend to follow and perpetuate a disability-labeling format that emphasizes differences in children and the problems of the general educational system. It is suggested that this type of course be structured to emphasize similarities between children, provide information about changing the environment as opposed to changing the student with a disability, provide knowledge about working as a team member, and utilize direct, structured, successful experiences with students with disabilities (Eichinger, Rizzo, & Sirotnik, 1991).

Teacher education candidates, as well as students in other "helping" professional preparation programs, must reflect upon why they have chosen to enter their particular profession. Though wanting to help others is certainly an admirable desire, it can be interpreted as doing for others, holding lowered expectations, and patronizing rather than teaching skills and building confidence in students to help themselves (Asch, 1989; Lynch & Thomas, 1994).

If general educators are to become committed to the concept of integrating and including students with disabilities, they will need to understand the purpose of inclusion, receive additional knowledge and training that meet students' individual needs, and be provided with professional supports (Engelbrecht, Oswald, Swart, & Eloff, 2003; Janney, Snell, Beers, & Raynes, 1995a; McLeskey & Waldron, 2002; Wolery, Werts, Caldwell, Snyder, & Lisowski, 1995). It has been observed that general education teachers go through a process of transformation when they are introduced to and have experiences with the inclusion philosophy (Giangreco, Dennis, & Cloninger, 1993). Teachers get their "rewards" by being *successful* with students, and they are concerned that they might not be able to "reach or teach" students with disabilities. Therefore, teachers often initially are hesitant and resistant to inclusive practices (Van Hoover & Yeager, 2003). However, as their knowledge and skills for having successful experiences with students with disabilities develop, and as they receive specific supports, teachers move to a spirit of cooperation and support that enhances the educational experiences of students with disabilities through a collaborative service delivery system (Janney, Snell, Beers, & Raynes, 1995b). This change is described by Giangreco and colleagues (1993):

> Transformations were gradual and progressive rather than discrete and abrupt. Teachers described an emerging recognition that their initial expectations regarding the student with disabilities were based on unsubstantiated assumptions. Teachers . . . came to the realization they could be successful and that including was not as difficult as they had originally imagined. They developed a willingness to (a) interact with the student, (b) learn skills needed to teach the student, and (c) change their attitude toward the student. (p. 365)

Recent education policies have added another factor: "Not only are teachers being asked to continue to fully *include* students in general education, but they are also being asked to raise their expectations about learning outcomes; that is, align IEP goals with the general curriculum" (Agran et al., 2002, pp. 123–124).

Special Education Teachers

The knowledge and experiences that prepare special education professionals for teaching have a significant impact on their attitudes about including students with disabilities in the general school environment. Traditionally, special education teacher training has been delivered apart from general education, with the exception of several basic courses, such as those on the history of U.S. schools and educational psychology. With the shift to an inclusive philosophy, special educators need to be trained with an emphasis on recognition of the interpersonal and peer-relation needs of students with disabilities. In reflecting on the field of special education, Murray-Seegert (1989) indicated that the

> field's traditional emphasis on the intrapersonal aspects of disability is accompanied by lack of inquiry into the interpersonal aspects of disability. And, in general, the more severe the disability experienced (especially if mental retardation is involved), the less likely it is that interpersonal behavior will be described. . . . Not only do the most severely disabled individuals have the capacity to develop peer relations, but these relations make the difference between surviving in the community and returning to closed institutions. (p. 12)

The special educator's role is also shifting to one of being a support person not only to students but to other professionals as well. This "new" role requires the development of appropriate communication skills, the ability to work as an effective team member, and the ability to work as a co-teacher within the general education classroom. According to Black and Meyer (1992), "Special education teachers are in a unique position to advocate for their students' rights, needs and potential and to have an impact on the attitudes of others" (p. 472). General education teachers have reported that they prefer special education support professionals who engage in at least four practices: (a) a shared framework and goals for inclusion, (b) physical presence (many general education teachers have felt alone in the inclusion of students with disabilities), (c) a validation of effective practices by the general educator, and (d) moral support and a spirit of teamwork (Giangreco et al., 1993).

Students Without Disabilities

Children have attitudes toward individuals with disabilities that are often negative and in need of improvement (Nowicki & Sandieson, 2002). It seems that attitudes about students with disabilities are also related to what students know and have experienced (Krajewski et al., 2002; Krajewski & Hyde, 2000). It is quite natural for "children to go up to persons with disabilities and talk to them. It is when someone drags them away that children begin to believe something is wrong" (Weisman, 1986, p. 66). As Gleason (1991) pointed out, this type of experience can result in negative attitudes and stereotypical thinking, which ultimately can develop into prejudice, discrimination, and lowered expectations. Researchers have emphasized that earlier positive experiences and social contact between children with and without disabilities promote more-positive attitudes (Griffith, Cooper, & Ringlaben, 2003; McDougall, Dewit, King, Mille, & Killip, 2004). Information about the abilities and the positive qualities of children with disabilities, even in the early stages of education, can help to limit later negative attitudes (Cooper & Ringlaben, 1998; Kishi & Meyer, 1994; Morrison & Ursprung, 1987).

Most students without disabilities who have had experience in integration and inclusion programs support the inclusion of students with disabilities, even when those students have severe disabilities (York, Vandercook, MacDonald, Heise-Neff, & Caughney, 1992). It is not merely that students without disabilities "put up with" students with disabilities. A growing body of empirical literature supports the conclusion that integration and inclusion experiences benefit students without disabilities in several ways: Students (a) learn patience, including reduced fears of others who are different; (b) feel good in helping others and successfully meeting a challenge (improved self-concept); (c) gain future benefits in learning how to get along with others who are different; and (d) develop warm and caring friendships based on common interests (Donaldson et al., 1994; Helmstetter, Peck, & Giangreco, 1994; Murray-Seegert, 1989; Staub & Peck, 1995; Staub, Schwartz, Gallucci, & Peck, 1994). Grenot-Scheyer (1994) noted, "As a friend to a child with severe disabilities, a peer without disabilities may be able to elicit socially appropriate behavior, and, further, may be able to reinforce uniquely such positive social behavior" (p. 260).

In a review of the literature, as well as in their own study, Helmstetter and associates (1994) concluded:

> The expanding literature of the outcomes of integration for students without disabilities suggests that a powerful means for addressing these issues exists potentially in every school in which a student with significant disabilities is enrolled. Far from simply helping those with disabilities, the practice of integrating students with highly diverse physical, developmental, and behavioral characteristics may turn out to be "best practice" for all the students involved. (p. 275)

It appears from this review of the literature that (a) the attitudes of students without disabilities can be influenced positively, (b) students without disabilities benefit from educational programs that include peers with disabilities, and (c) students without disabilities can have a positive effect on peers with disabilities (Helmstetter et al., 1994).

Professionals and parents may be concerned about the "perceived" negative effects of inclusion on students without disabilities. Because educators may believe that including students with disabilities in the general education classroom is "harmful" to students without disabilities, it is important that they receive information such as that provided by Staub and Peck (1995), which indicated that students without disabilities involved in "inclusion classrooms" (a) did not decline in academic progress, (b) did not lose significant teacher time and attention, and (c) did not learn undesirable behavior from students with disabilities. Sharpe, York, and Knight (1994) studied the effects of inclusion on students without disabilities in classrooms where students with disabilities were and were not included and found no significant differences between the groups.

Students With Disabilities

A disability in and of itself may not automatically produce negative attitudes. Some literature suggests a relationship between the characteristics or "topography" of the disability and negative reactions and attitudes. Westbrook and colleagues (1993) reported that "less visible disabilities . . . are those which are accepted and that visible disabilities, disabilities involving mental functioning or disabilities for which the person is seen as morally responsible are those most stigmatized" (p. 617). It appears that "those disabilities we cannot see or which are difficult to understand evoke less compassionate responses in us" (Lessen, 1991, p. 32). Students with disabilities may have a limited number of friends "because others view them in terms of their differences, instead of interests and needs they have in common with many nondisabled persons" (Donaldson et al., 1994, p. 233).

Students with and without disabilities may have little contact with each other (Mu, Siegel, & Allinder, 2000). Therefore, "the public school classroom has particular importance as a context for the development of relationships between groups of children who have little contact outside the school setting" (Salisbury, Gallucci, Palombaro, & Peck, 1995, p. 126). This is where all students, if permitted to do so, can discover "common ground" and learn that others who seem different may in actuality be very similar. Zollers et al. (1999) discovered that many youth with disabilities were willing to talk to their peers about their disability. Ochs et al. (2001) discovered that "children whose condition was explained to classmates had positive social interactions with a wider range of classmates" (p. 416). Weinberg (1988) suggested that all students will view disability

> as a difficulty that imposes limits and problems in much the same way that other facets of life impose difficulties. Life has elements of a struggle for everyone, and the struggle of the disabled person is not so different. . . . Disability is a problem and a difficulty, but it is not the only one. (p. 153)

Students with disabilities can learn and apply appropriate skills maximally in a "normalized" environment such as the general education classroom, especially when interactive and interpersonal skill strategies, such as cooperative learning groups, are utilized (Dore, Dion, Wagner, & Brunet, 2002; Hunt, Staub, Alwell, & Goetz, 1994). The classroom must stay as normal as possible so that student differences are minimized and accommodated in the least intrusive manner. It is imperative that teachers reflect on the appropriateness of accommodations, at the very least, because

> the student with a disability deserves to master skills for as much independence as possible, and providing aides or even assigning students as guides, wheelchair pushers, and writers of assignments may needlessly thwart development of self-sufficiency or discourage typical interactions with classmates and adults. (Asch, 1989, p. 187)

According to Donaldson and associates (1994), "Interaction between students with and without disabilities is perhaps the most effective approach to increased understanding of individual differences, creation of new friendships, and greater inclusion of students with moderate or severe disabilities in the life of the school" (p. 236). In a detailed ethnographic study, Murray-Seegert (1989) discovered that "the more severely impaired students . . . were observed to be involved in the same wide range of social relations as the students with more moderate impairments" (p. 140).

Mainstreaming and inclusive programs have a sufficient history that we should begin interviewing graduates with disabilities to determine their perceptions of policies, placements, and programs (Bovee, 2000; Dennis, 2002).

Interpersonal Relationships

According to Ochs et al. (2001), "Although any child may be marginalized within a peer group, children who are institutionally identified as having 'special needs' are particularly vulnerable to social distance" (p. 400). The ability to build and maintain interpersonal relationships is the most salient predictor of the successful transition from school to adult environments for individuals with disabilities, as it is for any individual (Ochs et al., 2001; Strully & Strully, 1992).

"Quality of life" issues are also related to friends and support in the community (Bramston, Bruggerman, & Pretty, 2002; Watson & Keith, 2002; Yazbeck, McVilly, & Parmenter, 2004). Interpersonal relationships, although difficult at times for all of us, present a different set of situations and circumstances for individuals with disabilities (Siperstein, Leffert, & Widaman, 1996). These relationships will happen more often and be more successful if teachers structure opportunities for these students to interact (File & Buzzelli, 1991; Han & Chadsey, 2004; Turnbull, Pereira, & Blue-Banning, 2000; Wang, Reynolds, & Walberg, 1994). This may be extremely important, because merely having students present in the same educational environment may not be effective (McGee & Paradis, 1993; Sale & Carey, 1995; Schnorr, 1990). In fact, "development of friendships is of valid concern for IEP committees" (Boutot & Bryant, 2005, p. 16) and is "considered an important educational outcome" (Han & Chadsey, 2004, p. 205).

An attitude of administrators, teachers, and peers "that expects disabled students to participate and perform on a par with non-disabled students communicates an important message . . . : that regardless of physical characteristics and disabilities, students are more similar than different" (Asch, 1989, p. 191). Murray-Seegert (1989) reported:

> The fact that severely disabled students were not isolated in their self-contained classrooms, but were present in so many school and community areas, had a positive influence on their access to inter-group relations. The special education teachers promoted proximity by scheduling as much instruction as possible outside the special education classrooms, by using common facilities at the same time as regular students, and by making sure that their students participated in special school events. (p. 119)

Students with and without disabilities can enjoy mutual friendships, and each partner can bring something unique to the relationship and receive something unique from it (Baroff, 2000). In fact, positive characteristics in the area of social skills, even for a student with a disability, may have much greater impact in developing friendships. In a study by Grenot-Scheyer (1994), "Characteristics such as developmental level and receptive language ability did not differentiate friends from acquaintances" (p. 259). Green, Schleien, Mactavish, and Benepe (1995) discovered that nondisabled friends of persons with mental retardation were attracted to the friendship not only for altruistic reasons but also because of discovered similarities such as (a) common interests, (b) compatible skill levels in activities, and (c) appropriate social skills.

An emerging strategy is the use of "Peer Buddies" and other "service learning" strategies that promote the inclusion of students with disabilities (Copeland et al., 2004; Copeland, McCall, Williams, Guth, Carter, & Fowler, 2002; Dopp & Block, 2004; Hughes, et al., 2001). Several investigators have determined these strategies to be effective (Burns, Storey, & Certo, 1999; Carter, Hughes, Copeland, & Breen, 2001; Smith, 2003). General education students increase in tolerance and acceptance of diversity, personal growth, and social status among peers. It appears that more contact promotes great positive gains. Copeland et al. (2004) reported that Peer Buddies become more sensitized and perceive the manner in which students with disabilities can be excluded by: "(1) physical and social segregation, (2) differential expectations and treatment, (3) lack of knowledge about disabilities, (4) communication differences, (5) behavioral challenges, (6) negative attitudes, and (7) insufficient or inappropriate support" (p. 345). Copeland et al. also report that Peer Buddies assist students with disabilities by: "(a) taking the lead in interaction opportunities, (b) advocating for students, (c) modeling acceptance for peers without disabilities, (d) improving support skills, and (e) adjusting support roles" (p. 347).

Because "teacher behavior, classroom climate, and instructional practices may differently affect the development and maintenance of friendships in inclusive classrooms" (Staub et al., 1994, p. 324), teachers should attempt to provide experiences for all students with disabilities, even severe disabilities, that promote developing friendships with students without disabilities. Asch (1989) identified the following factors which might be crucial in facilitating these friendships:

1. the amount of integration;

2. the expectation that the disabled student meet class norms of participation, behavior, and cooperation;

3. creation of situations where the disabled student must interact in projects with non-disabled classmates and can make a positive contribution;

4. assertiveness on the part of parents when children are young to create opportunities for children to play with others outside of school;

5. similar assertiveness by the disabled student to create opportunities if others do not initiate them;

6. equipping disabled students with skills to function as independently as possible in the widest range of activities; and,

7. an accessible environment for communication, mobility and transportation. (pp. 196–197)

Salisbury and colleagues (1995) discovered a number of groups of strategies that appeared to be effective for teachers in fostering the development of interpersonal relationships between students with and without disabilities. These included (a) actively facilitating social interactions (cooperative grouping, collaborative problem solving, peer tutoring and classroom roles, and time and opportunities for interaction), (b) valuing insights and contributions of students, (c) building community in the classroom, (d) modeling acceptance, and (e) building and administrative support. Paraeducators can also learn strategies to promote peer interaction utilizing these strategies (Causton-Theoharis & Malmgren, 2005).

Today, individuals with developmental disabilities and mental retardation are living, working, playing, and interacting with their peers without disabilities. As Green et al. (1995) noted, "Friendships between adults with and without mental retardation may be the key to ensuring that transitions from segregated services to community environments are successful" (p. 92).

Post-Secondary Education

Post-secondary education is rapidly becoming an option that more individuals with disabilities are selecting. Thomas (2000) reported an increase from 29% in 1986 to 45% in 1994 of individuals with disabilities who reported some enrollment in post-secondary education. Approximately 45% of post-secondary students with disabilities attend public 2-year institutions, 42% attend public 4-year institutions, and the remaining 13% attend other types of institutions (American Youth Policy Forum and the Center on Education Policy, 2002). It appears that for the education of students with disabilities, a P–16 school organization is replacing the P–12 model, with public schools and post-secondary institutions collaborating to develop effective programs (Grigal, Neubert, & Moon, 2001; Hall, Kleinert, & Kerns, 2000).

In several ways, post-secondary environments have characteristics similar to those of P–12 education 10–20 years ago. Investigators have reported that students with disabilities have not fared well in these environments (Quick et al., 2003). Whitney-Thomas and Moloney (2001) discovered that students leaving the P–12 environment have problems with low self-definition and struggle with post–P–12 choices.

Vasek (2005) discovered that many post-secondary faculty have had little contact with or experience in accommodating for students with disabilities. As with P–12 education, faculty attitudes are one of the main contributors to the success of students with disabilities in post-secondary settings. Rao (2004) and Gordon et al. (2004) report that when post-secondary students without disabilities have positive experiences with peers who are disabled, these experiences will have a direct impact on the choices they make later in adulthood.

Lehman, Davies, and Laurin (2000) indicate that post-secondary students with disabilities report that these environments lack understanding and acceptance and lack adequate academic and non-academic services. As individuals, the students lack financial resources and self-advocacy skills.

Employment

One of the main purposes of education is to prepare an individual for an occupation and employment. For an individual with a disability, the prospect of gainful employment is much different from that for an individual without a disability. It is well documented that individuals with disabilities, when compared with the rest of the population, are significantly more likely to be unemployed and underemployed (e.g., pay rate, length of time employed), with the more severely disabled at most risk (Mank, Cioffi, & Yovanoff, 1998; Yamaki & Fujiura, 2002). In fact, according to Kilbury et al. (1992), "problems of poverty, unemployment and underemployment, and associated social isolation are, in part, attributable to a denial of basic civil rights to citizens with disabilities" (p. 6).

Matkin (1983) and Funk (1987) described some of the "unfounded" perceptions of employers toward workers with disabilities: (a) increased costs are a barrier to hiring disabled workers, especially when the employer behaviors that architectural changes will be necessary; (b) insurance rates for employees will increase when disabled workers are hired; (c) attendance among disabled workers will be substandard, job turnover will be higher, and productivity will be negatively affected; and (d) the disabled employee will be less flexible in the ability to perform a variety of jobs, thereby increasing the associated manpower needs (costs) of the employer.

It seems the business sector follows a process similar to that of the educational sector, and employers and employees without disabilities go through a transformation of attitudes and beliefs similar to that of general education teachers and students without disabilities. Efforts to facilitate the acceptance of people with disabilities into the workplace will apparently be enhanced by improving the attitudes of employers and coworkers and altering the workplace environment (Wehman, West, & Kregel, 1999).

Kiernan (2000) describes the use of *naturally occurring supports* as an emerging and effective practice in the employment of individuals with disabilities. These *universal* supports are typically available to all workers but can also foster the employment of workers with disabilities. Employers and coworkers are often willing and able to assume a primary role in supporting workers with disabilities. When these supports are provided, there is greater job satisfaction and job success (Benz, Yovanoff, & Doren, 1997; Test, Carver, Ewers, Haddad, & Person, 2000).

Employers

Just as general educators who support inclusion efforts in the school often have had previous positive experiences with students with disabilities, employers and coworkers who have had previous positive experiences with employees with disabilities also have a more positive attitude about employing and working with an individual with a disability (Gilbride, Stensrud, Ehlers, Evans, & Peterson, 2000; Unger, 2002). Kilbury et al. (1992) predicts that "the integration into the workplace of citizens with disabilities as a result of the passage of the Americans with Disabilities Act should allow the predominantly non-disabled workforce a chance to modify their attitudes towards this minority group" (pp. 8–9).

Perhaps the business sector has reached a time of readiness to accept persons with disabilities as equal members of the work community, just as the education sector is accepting students with disabilities as equal members of the school community. In a survey of employment executives of the Fortune 500 listing at the time, Levy, Jessop, and Rimmerman (1992) found the attitudes "quite favorable to employment of persons with disabilities, even severe disabilities both in terms of its advantages for the individual and lack of disadvantages for others in the work setting" (p. 71). Similarly, Black and Meyer (1992) concluded that "persons in the business community can adjust their existing conceptions of work and productivity to allow for the . . . intensive supports necessary for employment participation by persons with very severe disabilities" (p. 472). Unger (2002) reports several additional findings regarding employers' attitudes, including a willingness to sacrifice work performance for greater dependability and recognition that hiring persons with disabilities can enhance their community image, strengthen corporate social responsibility, and increase workforce diversity.

Employees/Coworkers Without Disabilities

Just as students without disabilities require appropriate information about and positive experiences with students with disabilities, so do the coworkers of a person with disabilities. Employers can provide "interventions" of knowledge and experience to employees without disabilities to enhance positive attitude change rather than expecting or assuming that the employee with the disability will do all the changing (Butterworth, Hagner, Helm, & Whelley, 2000; Chadsey-Rusch & Heal, 1995; Farris & Stancliffe, 2001). These experiences, as in the general classroom, should be structured and "natural" and presented so that

> experience with persons with disabilities in the work context is associated with positive attitudes . . . and suggest that it is positive contact around work itself that determines attitudes towards employability and that attitudes toward persons with disabilities in general are also similarly affected by such work contact. (Levy et al., 1992, p. 73)

Hagner, Cotton, Goodall, and Nisbet (1992) reported that, after having experiences with coworkers with disabilities, even those who are involved in supportive employment situations, coworkers appeared to treat coworkers with disabilities

> as full-fledged members of the work group and supported them in whatever way was required, as they would do for anyone else, without calculating who received or gave more. Support was perceived as mutual, even when it might appear one-sided to an outsider. (p. 253)

Employees With Disabilities

Certainly any education and training program for students with disabilities will focus on successful skill development. However, successful transition to the work environment should also include, when appropriate, "effective social skills training . . . to enhance the social competence of students" (O'Reilly & Glynn, 1995, p. 187). Individuals with disabilities, even those labeled as "severe," can be successful in the workplace (Hagner & Cooney, 2005). As students with disabilities become employees with disabilities, they must display appropriate interpersonal skills for increased acceptance by coworkers and job fulfillment (Abery & Fahnestock, 1994). Besides these skills, employees with disabilities may often be placed in the role of "educator" about their particular disability.

Mass Media

Because knowledge is a major contributing factor to the attitudes that individuals without disabilities have toward individuals with disabilities, and the majority of citizens receive most of their information through the media, the attitudes that the media perpetuate about individuals with disabilities are extremely important (Safran, 2000; Schleifer & Klein, 1984). Today, people with disabilities appear in all forms of media, from the Sunday advertisement inserts, to comic strips, to being the main characters in children's books, television shows, specials, and films. An important question is whether the disability featured is only one dimension or the *main* dimension of the character.

Several authors believe the media in particular contribute to society's negative attitudes toward individuals with disabilities (Dyches, Prater, & Cramer, 2001; Hardin & Preston, 2001; Prater, 1999; Van Kraayenoord, 2002). Norden (1994) wrote: "The movie industry has perpetuated stereotypes over the years . . . so durable and pervasive that they have become mainstream society's perception of disabled people" (p. 3). Attitudes are affected by the use of language in the media, such as "victim," "suffered," "afflicted," "crippled," and "confined." Several categories of negative stereotypes are perpetuated through the media, including (a) the cap-in-hand/tin-cup image (pleading for help); (b) telethon poster child, when the disability is the focus and the person gets lost; (c) superhero (i.e., "supercrip"), where the focus on "overcoming" the disability has devalued a legitimate claim to fame; and (d) the grisly image of a "fate worse than death" (the terrible accident, illness, condition with which the viewer or reader could never cope). Commenting further on the media, Lynch and Thomas (1994) wrote:

> The concept of a person with a disability as "victim" is embedded in the public press and everyday conversations of the general public. . . . The search for sympathy for "victims" of disease and disability is big business. However, the message promoted does not emphasize a potential for independence or the individuality of each person. . . . People with disabilities are characterized either as victims or as inspirational figures who overcame their disability by some miracle. (p. 8)

The media in general and the broadcast industry specifically can be important sources of accurate information (Hardin & Preston, 2001). In one review of research, Byrd and Elliott (1988) pointed out that accurate depiction of disability by the media may positively influence attitudes of viewers toward persons with disabilities. Marlowe and Maycock (2001) used literary texts, rather than a textbook, in an Introduction to Special Education university course and discovered they were more effective in promoting positive attitude change than traditional text books: "These results imply that the mass media can play a positive role in the formulation of informed, positive attitudes among the public by depicting accurate characterizations of persons with disabilities" (p. 89).

A Review of Suggestions for Improving Attitudes

Although several suggestions have been discussed or implied in this chapter, the following is a brief but important list of the major research-based and emerging practices in improving attitudes toward people with disabilities (File & Buzzelli, 1991; **469** Hehir, 2002; Jorgensen, 1992; McNally, Cole, & Waugh, 2001; Murray-Seegert, 1989; Rimmerman, Hozmi, & Duvdevany, 2000; Zollers et al., 1999):

1. Provide accurate information (education) about individuals with disabilities. Promote disabilities not as deficits, but as a normal part of diversity within humanity.

2. Provide the supports the environment requires for individuals with disabilities to be successful. Select those that are universal.

3. Implement positive and continuing experiences with individuals with disabilities. Do not simply talk about people with disabilities; get involved with repeated interactions, both directly and indirectly, with people with disabilities, in situations that are cooperative and co-equal.

4. Address negative attitudes directly. Implement interventions where they belong. Institute pro-social programs that include disability and sensitivity awareness programs.

5. Expose the inappropriate portrayal of disabilities in the media, social policies, and practices. Do not permit negative portrayals in any form.

Glossary

Ableism—Promoting individuals to depend on others rather than to do for themselves.

Accommodation—Assistance for completing a task.

Attitude—A point of view, belief, or position on a subject.

Handicapism—A set of assumptions that promote the differential and unequal treatment of people because of apparent or assumed physical, mental, or behavioral differences.

Interpersonal relationships—Relationships between individuals or groups that promote positive concepts.

Legislation—A proposed or enacted law or group of laws.

Litigation—A legal case or lawsuit.

Marginalization—The attitude that something is of little value or importance.

Minority—A group of people regarded as different from the larger population.

Patronization—The act of treating someone in a condescending way.

Post-secondary—Educational environments above the high school level. Examples of these are community and junior colleges, colleges and universities, vocational centers.

Service delivery philosophy—The cure vs. care model debate in delivering services to individuals with disabilities

Victimization—The act of taking unfair advantage of some one.

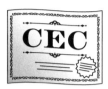

Knowledge and Skills for Entry-Level Special Education Teachers of Students With Developmental Disabilities Standards Addressed in This Chapter

Principle 1: Foundations

DD1K1 Definitions and issues related to the identification of individuals with developmental disabilities.

DD1K4 Trends and practices in the field of developmental disabilities.

Principle 2: Development and Characteristics of Learners

DD2K5 Complications and implications of medical support services.

Principle 5: Learning Environments/Social Interaction

DD5S4 Structure the physical environment to provide optimal learning for individuals with developmental disabilities.

Web Site Resources

American Association on Intellectual and Developmental Disabilities (AAIDD)
http://www.aamr.org

Provides information to AAIDD/AAMR members and those interested in supporting individuals with mental retardation. The Washington Watch newsletter monitors legislation and litigation as it relates to individuals with developmental delays and mental retardation. Resource page for professionals working in this field, addressing attitudes, current programs, training, legislative goals, etc.

Best Buddies International
http://www.bestbuddies.org/site/c.Ij0J8MNIsE/b.933717/k.CBF8/Home.htm

Information concerning individuals with intellectual disabilities, promoting the use of peer buddies beginning in middle school through college and employment, promoting positive attitudes toward individuals with disabilities, and providing insights about the use of peer buddies to enhance interpersonal skills of individuals with disabilities.

Minnesota Governor's Council on Developmental Disabilities
http://www.mncdd.org/

Web site offers features each month on a variety of subjects, such as employer focus, research, ADD, IDEA, etc., and provides links to help employers in creating effective and positive work environments for individuals with developmental disabilities.

References

Abery, B. H., & Fahnestock, M. (1994). Enhancing the social inclusion of persons with developmental disabilities. In M. F. Hayden & B. H. Abery (Eds.), *Challenges for a service system in transition: Ensuring quality community experiences for persons with developmental disabilities* (pp. 83–119). Baltimore: Brookes.

Agran, M., Alper, S., & Wehmeyer, M. (2002). Access to the general curriculum for students with significant disabilities: What it means to teachers. *Education and Training in Mental Retardation and Developmental Disabilities, 37,* 123–133.

American Youth Policy Forum and the Center on Education Policy. (2002). *Educating children with disabilities: The good news and the work ahead.* Washington, DC: Author.

Asch, A. (1989). Has the law made a difference? What some disabled students have to say. In D. Lipsky & A. Gartner (Eds.), *Beyond separate education: Quality education for all* (pp. 181–205). Baltimore: Brookes.

Barker, R. G. (1948). The social psychology of physical disability. *Journal of Social Issues, 4*(4), 28–37.

Baroff, G. (2000). Eugenics, "Baby Doe," and Peter Singer: Toward a More "Perfect" Society. *Mental Retardation, 38*(1), 73–77.

Beadles, Jr., R. J. (2001). How to refer to people with disabilities: A primer for laypeople. *Academic Search Elite, 33*(1), 4–7.

Beattie, J. R., Anderson, R. J., & Antonak, R. F. (1997). Modifying attitudes of prospective educators toward students with disabilities and their integration into regular classrooms. *Journal of Psychology, 131,* 245–254.

Benz, M. R., Yovanoff, P., & Doren, B. (1997). School-to-work components that predict postschool success for students with and without disabilities. *Exceptional Children, 63,* 151–165.

Black, J., & Meyer, L. H. (1992). But . . . is it really work? Social validity of employment training for persons with very severe disabilities. *American Journal on Mental Retardation, 96,* 463–474.

Bogdan, R., & Biklen, D. (1977). Handicapism. *Social Policy, 7*(5), 14–19.

Bolt, D. (2004). Disability and the rhetoric of inclusive higher education. *Journal of Further and Higher Education, 28,* 353–358.

Boutot, E. A., & Bryant, D. P. (2005). Social integration of students with autism in inclusive settings. *Education and Training in Mental Retardation and Developmental Disabilities, 40,* 14–23.

Bovee, J. P. (2000). A right to our own life, our own way. *Focus on Autism and Other Developmental Disabilities, 15,* 250–252.

Bramston, P., Bruggerman, K., & Pretty, G. (2002). Community perspectives and subjective quality of life. *International Journal of Disability, Development, and Education, 49,* 385–397.

Brantlinger, E. (2001). Poverty, class, and disability: A historical, social, and political perspective. *Focus on Exceptional Children, 33*(7), 1–19.

Brotherson, M. J., Cook, C. C., Cunman-Lahr, R., & Wehmeyer, M. L. (1995). Policy supporting self-determination in the environments of children with disabilities. *Education and Training in Mental Retardation and Developmental Disabilities, 30,* 3–13.

Bullock, M. (2002). A systems approach to the provision of services to individuals with disabilities. *Educational Horizons, 81*(1), 21–26.

Burns, M., Storey, K., & Certo, N. (1999). Effect of service learning on attitudes towards students with severe disabilities. *Education and Training in Mental Retardation and Developmental Disabilities, 34,* 58–65.

Butterworth, J., Hagner, D., Helm, D. T., & Whelley, T. A. (2000). Workplace culture, social interactions, and supports for transition-age young adults. *Mental Retardation, 38,* 342–353.

Byrd, E. K., & Elliott, T. R. (1988). Media and disability: A discussion of research. In H. E. Yuker (Ed.), *Attitudes toward persons with disabilities* (pp. 82–95). New York: Springer.

Carter, E., Hughes, C., Copeland, S., & Breen, C. (2001). Differences between high school students who do and do not volunteer to participate in a peer interaction program. *Journal of the Association for Persons With Severe Handicaps, 26,* 229–239.

Causton-Theoharis, J., & Malmgren, K. (2005). Building bridges: Strategies to help paraprofessionals promote peer interaction. *Teaching Exceptional Children, 37*(6), 18–24.

Chadsey-Rusch, J., & Heal, L. W. (1995). Building consensus from transition experts on social integration outcomes and interventions. *Exceptional Children, 62,* 165–187.

Cook, B. (2001). A comparison of teachers' attitudes toward their included students with mild and severe disabilities. *Journal of Special Education, 34,* 203–213.

Cooper, M., & Ringlaben, R. P. (1998). Caring as an essential element for inclusion. *Kappa Delta Pi Record, 34*(2), 56–59.

Copeland, S. R., Hughes, C., Carter, E. W., Guth, C., Presley, J. A., Williams, C. R., & Fowler, S. E. (2004). Increasing access to general education: Perspectives of participants in a high school peer support program. *Remedial and Special Education, 25,* 342–352.

Copeland, S. R., McCall, J., Williams, C. R., Guth, C., Carter, E. W., Fowler, S. E., Presley, J. A., & Hughes, C. (2002). High school buddies: A win-win situation. *Teaching Exceptional Children, 35*(1), 16–21.

Dennis, R. (2002). Nonverbal narratives: Listening to people with severe intellectual disability. *Research and Practice for Persons With Severe Disabilities, 27,* 239–249.

Donaldson, R. M., Helmstetter, E., Donaldson, J., & West, R. (1994). Influencing high school students' attitudes toward and interactions with peers with disabilities. *Social Education, 58,* 233–237.

Dopp, J., & Block, T. (2004). High school peer mentoring that works! *Teaching Exceptional Children, 37*(1), 56–62.

Dore, R., Dion, E., Wagner, S., & Brunet, J. (2002). High school inclusion of adolescents with mental retardation: A multiple case study. *Education and Training in Mental Retardation and Developmental Disabilities, 37,* 253–261.

Dyches, T. T., Prater, M. A., & Cramer, S. F. (2001). Characterization of mental retardation and autism in children's books. *Education and Training in Mental Retardation and Developmental Disabilities, 36,* 230–243.

Eichinger, J., Rizzo, T. L., & Sirotnik, B. (1991). Changing attitudes toward people with disabilities. *Teacher Education and Special Education, 14,* 121–126.

Engelbrecht, P., Oswald, M., Swart, E., & Eloff, I. (2003). Including learners with intellectual disabilities: Stressful for teachers? *International Journal of Disability, Development, and Education, 50,* 293–308.

Farris, B., & Stancliffe, R. (2001). The co-worker training model: Outcomes of an open employment pilot project. *Journal of Intellectual and Developmental Disability, 26*(1), 143–159.

Ferri, B., & Connor, D. J. (2005). Tools of exclusion: Race, disability, and (re)segregated education. *Teachers College Record, 107,* 453–474.

File, N. K., & Buzzelli, C. A. (1991). Gaining respect and understanding: Helping children learn about disabilities. *Day Care and Early Education, 18,* 39–40.

Fine, M., & Asch, A. (1988). Disability beyond stigma: Social interaction, discrimination, and activism. *Journal of Social Issues, 44,* 3–21.

Fox, R., & Rotatori, A. F. (1986). Changing undergraduate attitudes towards the developmentally disabled through volunteering. *College Student Journal, 20,* 162–167.

Friend, M., & Pope, K. (2005). Creating schools in which all students can succeed. *Kappa Delta Pi Record, 41*(2), 56–61.

Funk, R. (1987). Disability rights: From caste to class in the context of civil rights. In A. Gartner & T. Joe (Eds.), *Images of the disabled, disabling images* (pp. 7–30). New York: Praeger.

Garriott, P., Snyder, L., Ringlaben, R. P., & Tennant, L. (2004). It takes a whole village: Reflections on preservice teachers' attitudes toward the inclusion of students with severe disabilities. *Electronic Journal for Inclusive Education, 1*(8). Retrieved November 15, 2005, from http://www.ed.wright.edu/~prenick/Summer_fall04/Village%20Manuscript.htm

Gerry, M. H., & Mirsky, A. J. (1992). Guiding principles for public policy on natural supports. In J. Nesbit (Ed.), *Natural supports in school, at work, and in the community for people with severe disabilities* (pp. 341–346). Baltimore: Brookes.

Giangreco, M. F., Dennis, R. E., & Cloninger, C. J. (1993). "I've counted Jon": Transformational experiences of teachers educating students with disabilities. *Exceptional Children, 59,* 359–372.

Gilbride, D., Stensrud, R., Ehlers, C., Evans, E., & Peterson, C. (2000). Employers' attitudes toward hiring persons with disabilities and vocational rehabilitation services. *Journal of Rehabilitation, 66*(4), 17–24.

Gilmore, L., & Campbell, J. (2003). Developmental expectations, personality stereotypes, and attitudes towards inclusive education: Community and teacher views of Down syndrome. *International Journal of Disability, Development, and Education, 50*(1), 65–76.

Gleason, J. J. (1991). Multicultural and exceptional student education: Separate but equal? *Preventing School Failure, 36,* 47–49.

472

Gliedman, J., & Roth, W. (1980). *The unexpected minority: Handicapped children in America*. New York: Harcourt Brace Jovanovich.

Gordon, P., Tantillo, J. C., Feldman, D., & Perrone, K. (2004). Attitudes regarding interpersonal relationships with persons with mental illness and mental retardation. *Journal of Rehabilitation, 70*(1), 50–57.

Green, E. P., Schleien, S. J., Mactavish, J., & Benepe, S. (1995). Nondisabled adults' perceptions of relationships in the early stages of arranged partnerships with peers with mental retardation. *Education and Training in Mental Retardation and Developmental Disabilities, 30*, 91–108.

Grenot-Scheyer, M. (1994). The nature of interactions between students with severe disabilities and their friends and acquaintances without disabilities. *Journal of the Association for Persons With Severe Handicaps, 19*, 253–262.

Griffith, K., Cooper, M., & Ringlaben, R. P. (2003). A 3-D model for the inclusion of students with disabilities. *Electronic Journal for Inclusive Education, 1*(6). Retrieved November 15, 2005, from http://www.ed.wright.edu/~prenick/kimberly.htm

Grigal, M., Neubert, D. A., & Moon, M. S. (2001). Public school programs for students with significant disabilities in post-secondary settings. *Education and Training in Mental Retardation and Developmental Disabilities, 36*, 244–254.

Hagner, D., & Cooney, B. (2005). "I do that for everybody": Supervising employees with autism. *Focus on Autism and Other Developmental Disabilities, 20*, 91–97.

Hagner, D. C., Cotton, P., Goodall, S., & Nisbet, J. (1992). The perspectives of supportive coworkers: Nothing special. In J. Nesbit (Ed.), *Natural supports in school, at work, and in the community, for people with severe disabilities* (pp. 241–256). Baltimore: Brookes.

Hahn, H. (1988). The politics of physical differences: Disability and discrimination. *Journal of Social Issues, 44*, 39–47.

Hall, M., Kleinert, H. L., & Kerns, J. (2000). Going to college! Postsecondary programs for students with moderate and severe disabilities. *Teaching Exceptional Children, 32*(3), 58–65.

Han, K. G., & Chadsey, J. G. (2004). The influence of gender patterns and grade level on friendship expectations of middle school students toward peers with severe disabilities. *Focus on Autism and Other Developmental Disabilities, 19*, 205–214.

Hannah, M. E. (1988). Teacher attitudes toward children with disabilities: An ecological analysis. In H. E. Yuker (Ed.), *Attitudes toward persons with disabilities* (pp. 154–170). New York: Springer.

Hardin, M., & Preston, A. (2001). Inclusion of disability issues in news reporting textbooks. *Journalism and Mass Communication Educator, 56*(2), 43–54.

Hehir, T. (2002). Eliminating ableism in education. *Harvard Educational Review, 72*(1), 1–32.

Helmstetter, E., Peck, C. A., & Giangreco, M. F. (1994). Outcomes of interactions with peers with moderate or severe disabilities: A statewide survey of high school students. *Journal of the Association for Persons With Severe Handicaps, 19*, 263–276.

Hughes, C., Copeland, S., Guth, C., Rung, L., Hwang, B., Kleeb, G., & Strong, M. (2001). General education students' perspectives on their involvement in a high school peer buddy program. *Education and Training in Mental Retardation and Developmental Disabilities, 36*, 343–356.

Hunt, P., Staub, D., Alwell, M., & Goetz, L. (1994). Achievement by all students within the context of cooperative learning groups. *Journal of the Association for Persons With Severe Handicaps, 19*, 290–301.

Jaeger, P. (2004). The social impact of an accessible e-democracy. *Journal of Disability Policy Studies, 15*(1), 19–27.

Jahnukainen, M., & Korhonen, A. (2003). Integration of students with severe and profound intellectual disabilities into the comprehensive school system: Teachers' perceptions of the education reform in Finland. *International Journal of Disability, Development, and Education, 50*, 169–180.

Jahoda, A., & Markova, I. (2004). Coping with social stigma: People with intellectual disabilities moving from institutions and family home. *Journal of Intellectual Disability Research, 48*, 719–729.

Janney, R. E., Snell, M., Beers, M. K., & Raynes, M. (1995a). Integrating students with moderate and severe disabilities: Classroom teachers' beliefs and attitudes about implementing an educational change. *Educational Administration Quarterly, 31*, 86–114.

Janney, R. E., Snell, M., Beers, M. K., & Raynes, M. (1995b). Integrating students with moderate and severe disabilities into general education classes. *Exceptional Children, 61*, 425–439.

Jorgensen, C. M. (1992). Natural supports in inclusive schools: Curricular and teaching strategies. In J. Nesbit (Ed.), *Natural supports in school, at work, and in the community for people with severe disabilities* (pp. 179–215). Baltimore: Brookes.

Kauffman, J., McGee, K., & Brigham, M. (2004). Enabling or disabling? Observations on changes in special education. *Phi Delta Kappan, 85*, 613–621.

Kavale, K. (2002). Mainstreaming to full inclusion: From orthogenesis to pathogenesis of an idea. *International Journal of Disability, Development, and Education, 49*, 201–214.

Kiernan, W. (2000). Where we are now? *Focus on Autism and Other Developmental Disabilities, 15*, 90–96.

Kilbury, R. E., Benshoff, J. J., & Rubin, S. E. (1992). The interaction of legislation, public attitudes, and access to opportunities for persons with disabilities. *Journal of Rehabilitation, 58*(4), 6–9.

Kishi, G. S., & Meyer, L. H. (1994). What children report and remember: A six-year follow-up of the effects of social contact between peers with and without severe disabilities. *Journal of the Association for Persons With Severe Handicaps, 19*, 277–289.

Klingner, J. K., & Vaughn, S. (1999). Students' perceptions of instruction in inclusion classrooms: Implications for students with learning disabilities. *Exceptional Children, 66*, 23–37.

Krajewski, J. J., & Hyde, M. S. (2000). Comparison of teen attitudes toward individuals with mental retardation between 1987 and 1998: Has inclusion made a difference? *Education and Training in Mental Retardation and Developmental Disabilities, 35*, 284–293.

Krajewski, J. J., Hyde, M. S., & O'Keefe, M. K. (2002). Teen attitudes toward individuals with mental retardation from 1987 to 1998: Impact of respondent gender and school variables. *Education and Training in Mental Retardation and Developmental Disabilities, 37*, 27–39.

Lehmann, J., Davies, T. G., & Laurin, K. (2000). Listening to student voices about postsecondary education. *Teaching Exceptional Children, 32*(5), 60–65.

Lessen, E. (1991). On being different. In S. Schwartz (Ed.), *Exceptional people: A guide for understanding* (pp. 29–49). New York: McGraw-Hill.

Levy, J. M., Jessop, D. J., & Rimmerman, A. (1992). Attitudes of Fortune 500 corporate executives toward the employability of persons with severe disabilities: A national study. *Mental Retardation, 30*, 67–75.

Lynch, R. T., & Thomas, K. R. (1994). People with disabilities as victims: Changing an ill-advised paradigm. *Journal of Rehabilitation, 60*(1), 8–11.

Makas, E. (1988). Positive attitudes toward disabled people: Disabled and nondisabled persons' perspectives. *Journal of Social Issues, 44*, 49–61.

Mank, D., Cioffi, A., & Yovanoff, P. (1998). Employment outcomes for people with severe disabilities: Opportunities for improvement. *Mental Retardation, 36*, 205–216.

Marlowe, M., & Maycock, G. (2001). Using literary texts in teacher education to promote positive attitudes toward children with disabilities. *Teacher Education and Special Education, 24*(2), 75–83.

Matkin, R. E. (1983). Educating employers to hire disabled workers. *Journal of Rehabilitation, 49*(3), 60–63.

McCarthy, H. (1988). Attitudes that affect employment opportunities for persons with disabilities. In H. E. Yuker (Ed.), *Attitudes toward persons with disabilities* (pp. 246–261). New York: Springer.

McDougall, J., Dewit, D., King, G., Mille, L., & Killip, S. (2004). High school-age youths' attitudes toward their peers with disabilities: The role of school and student interpersonal factors. *International Journal of Disability, Development, and Education, 51*, 287–313.

McGee, G. G., & Paradis, T. (1993). Free effects of integration on levels of autistic behavior. *Topics in Early Childhood Special Education, 13*, 57–67.

McLeskey, J., & Waldron, N. L (2002). Professional development and inclusive schools: Reflections on effective practice. *Teacher Educator, 37*, 159–172.

McMahon, B. T., West, S. L., Lewis, A. N., Armstrong, A. J., & Conway, J. P. (2003). Hate crimes and disability in America. *Rehabilitation Counseling Bulletin, 47*(2), 66–75.

McNally, R. D., Cole, P. G., & Waugh, R. F. (2001). Regular teachers' attitudes to the need for additional classroom support for the inclusion of students with intellectual disability. *Journal of Intellectual and Developmental Disability, 26*, 257–273.

Morrison, J. M., & Ursprung, A. W. (1987). Children's attitudes toward people with disabilities: A review of the literature. *Journal of Rehabilitation, 53*, 45–49.

Mu, K., Siegel, E., & Allinder, R. (2000). Peer interactions and sociometric status of high school students with moderate of severe disabilities in general education classrooms. *Journal of the Association for Persons With Severe Handicaps, 25*, 142–152.

Murray-Seegert, C. (1989). *Nasty girls, thugs, and humans like us: Social relations between severely disabled and nondisabled students in high school.* Baltimore: Brookes.

Norden, M. E. (1994). *The cinema of isolation: A history of physical disability in the movies.* New Brunswick, NJ: Rutgers University Press.

Nowicki, E. A., & Sandieson, R. (2002). A meta-analysis of school-age children's attitudes towards persons with physical or intellectual disabilities. *International Journal of Disability, Development, and Education, 49*, 243–265.

O'Brien, P. (2003). Envisioning the future without the social alienation of difference. *International Journal of Disability, Development, and Education, 50*, 17–38.

Ochs, E., Kremer-Sadlik, T., Solomon, O., & Gainer Sirota, K. (2001). Inclusion as social practice: Views of children with autism. *Social Development, 10*, 399–419.

Olkin, R. (2002). Could you hold the door for me? Including disability in diversity. *Cultural Diversity and Ethnic Minority Psychology, 8*, 130–137.

O'Reilly, M. F., & Glynn, D. (1995). Using a process social skills training approach with adolescents with mild intellectual disabilities in a high school setting. *Education and Training in Mental Retardation and Developmental Disabilities, 30*, 187–198.

Pavri, S. (2001). Loneliness in children with disabilities: How teachers can help. *Teaching Exceptional Children, 33*(6), 52–58.

Pivik, J., McComas, J., & Laflamme, M. (2002). Barriers and facilitators to inclusive education. *Exceptional Children, 69*, 97–107.

Praisner, C. (2003). Attitudes of elementary school principals toward the inclusion of students with disabilities. *Exceptional Children, 69*, 135–145.

Prater, M. A. (1999). Characterization of mental retardation in children's and adolescent literature. *Education and Training in Mental Retardation and Developmental Disabilities, 34*, 418–431.

Quick, D., Lehmann, J., & Deniston, T. (2003). Opening doors for students with disabilities on community college campuses: What have we learned? What do we still need to know? *Community College Journal of Research and Practice, 27*, 815–827.

Rao, S. (2004). Faculty attitudes and students with disabilities in higher education: A literature review. *College Student Journal, 38*, 191–198.

Rimmerman, A., Hozmi, B., & Duvdevany, I. (2000). Contact and attitudes toward individuals with disabilities among students tutoring children with developmental disabilities. *Journal of Intellectual and Developmental Disability, 25*, 13–18.

Ringlaben, R. P., & Price, J. R. (1981). Regular classroom teachers' perceptions of mainstreaming effects. *Exceptional Children, 47*, 302–304.

Robertson, K., Chamberlain, B., & Kasari, C. (2003). General education teachers' relationships with included students with autism. *Journal of Autism and Developmental Disorders, 33*, 123–130.

Safran, S. (2000). Using movies to teach students about disabilities. *Teaching Exceptional Children, 32*(3), 44–47.

Sale, P., & Carey, D. M. (1995). The sociometric status of students with disabilities in a full-inclusion school. *Exceptional Children, 62*, 6–19.

Salisbury, C. L., Gallucci, C., Palombaro, M. M., & Peck, C. A. (1995). Strategies that promote social relations among elementary students with and without severe disabilities. *Exceptional Children, 62*, 125–137.

Schleifer, M. J., & Klein, S. D. (1984). Media and attitudes towards people with disabilities. *Exceptional Parent, 14*(2), 15.

Schnorr, R. F. (1990). Peter? He comes and he goes. First graders' perspectives on a part-time mainstream student. *Journal of the Association for Persons With Severe Handicaps, 19*, 231–240.

Shade, R. A., & Stewart, R. (2001). General education and special education preservice teachers' attitudes toward inclusion. *Preventing School Failure, 46*, 37–41.

Sharpe, M. N., York, J. L., & Knight, J. (1994). Effects of inclusion on the academic performance of classmates without disabilities. *Remedial and Special Education, 15*, 281–287.

Siperstein, G. N., Leffert, J. S., & Widaman, K. (1996). Social behavior and the social acceptance and rejection of children with mental retardation. *Education and Training in Mental Retardation and Developmental Disabilities, 31*, 271–281.

Smith, T. E. C., Polloway, E. A., Patton, J. R., & Dowdy, C. A. (2004). *Teaching students with special needs in inclusive settings* (4th ed.). Needham Heights, MA: Allyn & Bacon.

Smith, V. M. (2003). "You have to learn who comes with the disability": Students' reflections on service learning experiences with peers labeled with disabilities. *Research and Practice for Persons With Severe Disabilities, 28*, 79–90.

Staub, D., & Peck, C. A. (1995). What are the outcomes for nondisabled students? *Educational Leadership, 52*(4), 36–40.

Staub, D., Schwartz, I. S., Gallucci, C., & Peck, C. A. (1994). Four portraits of friendship at an inclusive school. *Journal of the Association for Persons With Severe Handicaps, 19*, 314–325.

Stevenson, R. (2003). Wraparound services. *School Administrator, 60*(3), 24–25.

Strully, J. L., & Strully, C. F. (1992). The struggle toward inclusion and the fulfillment of friendship. In J. Nesbit (Ed.), *Natural supports in school, at work, and in the community for people with severe disabilities* (pp. 165–177). Baltimore: Brookes.

Stubbins, J. (1988). The politics of disability. In H. E. Yuker (Ed.), *Attitudes toward persons with disabilities* (pp. 21–32). New York: Springer.

Sweeting, H., & West, P. (2001). Being different: Correlates of the experience of teasing and bullying at age 11. *Research Papers in Education, 16*, 225–246.

Test, D. W., Carver, T., Ewers, L., Haddad, J., & Person, J. (2000). Longitudinal job satisfaction in persons in supported employment. *Education and Training in Mental Retardation and Developmental Disabilities, 35*, 365–373.

Thomas, S. B. (2000). College students and disability law. *Journal of Special Education, 33*, 248–257.

Treder, D. W., Morse, W. C., & Ferron, J. M. (2000). The relationship between teacher effectiveness and teacher attitudes toward issues related to inclusion. *Teacher Education and Special Education, 23*, 202–210.

Turnbull, A. P., Pereira, L., & Blue-Banning, M. (2000). Teachers as friendship facilitators. *Teaching Exceptional Children, 32*, 66–70.

Turner, N. D. (2003). Preparing preservice teachers for inclusion in secondary classrooms. *Education, 12*, 491–495.

Unger, D. (2002). Employers' attitudes toward persons with disabilities in the workforce: Myths or realities? *Focus on Autism and Other Developmental Disabilities, 17*, 2–10.

Van Hoover, S., & Yeager, E. (2003). Secondary history teachers and inclusion of students with disabilities: An exploratory study. *Journal of Social Studies Research, 27*(1), 36–45.

Van Kraayenoord, C. (2002). The media's portrayal of mothers with disabilities. *International Journal of Disability, Development, and Education, 49*, 221–224.

Van Reusen, A. K., Shoho, A., & Barker, K. (2000–2001). High school teacher attitudes toward inclusion. *High School Journal, 84*(2), 7–20.

Vasek, D. (2005). Assessing the knowledge base of faculty at a private, four-year institution. *College Student Journal, 39*, 307–315.

Wallace, T., Anderson, A., Bartholomay, T., & Hupp, S. (2002). An ecobehavioral examination of high school classrooms that include students with disabilities. *Exceptional Children, 68*, 345–359.

Wang, M. C., Reynolds, M. C., & Walberg, H. J. (1994). Serving students at the margins. *Educational Leadership, 52*(4), 12–17.

Watson, S., & Keith, K. (2002). Comparing the quality of life of school-age children with and without disabilities. *Mental Retardation, 40*, 304–312.

Wehman, P., West, M., & Kregel, J. (1999). Supported employment program development and research needs: Looking ahead to the year 2000. *Education and Training in Mental Retardation and Developmental Disabilities, 32*(1), 3–19.

Weinberg, N. (1988). Another perspective: Attitudes of people with disabilities. In H. E. Yuker (Ed.), *Attitudes toward persons with disabilities* (pp. 141–153). New York: Springer.

Weisman, J. (1986). Who wouldn't want me? In F. Weiner (Ed.), *No apologies: A guide to living with a disability* (pp. 66–67). New York: St. Martin's.

Westbrook, M. T., Legge, V., & Pennay, M. (1993). Attitudes towards people with disabilities in a multicultural society. *Social Science and Medicine, 36,* 615–623.

Whitney-Thomas, J., & Moloney, M. (2001). "Who I am and what I want": Adolescents' self-definition and struggles. *Exceptional Children, 67,* 375–389.

Wilson, B. A. (1999). Inclusion: Empirical guidelines and unanswered questions. *Education and Training in Mental Retardation and Developmental Disabilities, 34,* 119–133.

Wolery, M., Werts, M. G., Caldwell, N. K., Snyder, E. D., & Lisowski, L. (1995). Experienced teachers' perceptions of resources and support for inclusion. *Education and Training in Mental Retardation and Developmental Disabilities, 30,* 15–26.

Yamaki, K., & Fujiura, G. (2002). Employment and income status of adults with developmental disabilities living in the community. *Mental Retardation, 40,* 132–141.

Yazbeck, M., McVilly, K., & Parmenter, T. R. (2004). Attitudes toward people with intellectual disabilities. *Journal of Disability Policy Studies, 15,* 97–111.

York, J., Vandercook, T., MacDonald, C., Heise-Neff, C., & Caughney, E. (1992). Feedback about integrating middle-school students with severe disabilities in general education classes. *Exceptional Children, 58,* 244–258.

Zollers, J., Ramanathan, A. K., & Yu, M. (1999). The relationship between school culture and inclusion: How an inclusive culture supports inclusive education. *International Journal of Qualitative Studies in Education, 12,* 157–174.

SECTION 9

SCHOOLS AND COMMUNITY INVOLVEMENT

24

Partnering With Families of Children With Developmental Disabilities to Enhance Family Quality of Life

Ann P. Turnbull, H. R. Turnbull, Jean A. Summers, and Denise Poston

Summary

This chapter focuses on the overarching goal of family-related disability policy in the United States, which is to support the caregiving efforts and enhance the quality of life of all families so that families will remain the core unit of American society. The chapter guides educators on how to enhance the quality of life of families who have children and youth with developmental disabilities. Family quality of life consists of disability-related support, physical/material well-being, parenting, emotional well-being, and family interaction. The chapter suggests how educators can address family quality-of-life outcomes in each of these five domains while simultaneously advancing student outcomes.

Learning Outcomes

After reading this chapter, you should be able to:

- Identify an overarching goal and five supporting goals that are tied to U.S. policy related to families who have members with developmental disabilities.

- Define family quality of life, identify five domains of family quality of life, and identify at least two indicators of each domain.

- Explain the purpose and possible services/supports available from Parent Training and Information Centers, Community Parent Resource Centers, and Parent to Parent.

- Explain the purpose of Supplemental Security Income (SSI) and Medicaid and how educators can help connect families with these economic resources.

- Describe a model system to enable parents to learn how to best help their child with schoolwork and activities.

- Describe three sources of stress for parents of children with disabilities and what educators can to do help reduce or even prevent stress.

- Explain how inviting nuclear and extended-family members to IEP conferences and other school-based conferences/activities might have a positive impact on family interaction.

Introduction

All across America, there are thousands of families who never get information, training, or support in making research-based best practices work in their lives. These families are referred to as the "traditionally underserved." They are families who have become isolated for a number of reasons, including poverty, racism, discrimination, cultural and language differences, geographic location, and socioeconomic factors. These are our families. Many of our families do not even realize the potential that research holds for improving their lives. Others do understand but they are also aware of the huge disconnect between science and solutions for them. They have lost hope for a promising future for their family member with a disability despite the help that research may be able to provide.

—Ursula and DJ Markey, Codirectors, Pyramid Parent Training
Community Parent Resource Center, New Orleans, LA

In January 2003, the Arc of the U.S. (a national organization comprising primarily family members of individuals with intellectual disabilities who advocate for the rights and opportunities for individuals with intellectual disabilities and their families—www.thearc.org), convened a national conference to address the policy promises that the United States has made to its citizens with developmental disabilities and the state of knowledge for keeping those promises. This historic conference had two unique characteristics. First, more than 40 organizations, which included 9 federal agencies, were cosponsors; typically conferences are sponsored by a far more narrow base—often only 1 organization. Second, the participants represented a broad range of constituencies, including self-advocates with developmental disabilities, family members, service providers, researchers, and state/federal agency administrators; typically conferences are focused on a far more narrow constituency—often only 1 group. This broad-based conference included 12 topical groups, each of which addressed a key issue related to developmental disabilities. One of the topics was family life.

The family life group included 18 participants representing the complete range of stakeholder groups previously identified. The quote that you read at the beginning of this chapter was from two of the participants, Ursula and DJ Markey, in the group that addressed family life. As African American community activists and parents of two sons with disabilities (one now deceased), they are passionate and articulate about the particular needs of families from underserved communities.

The members of the family life group reviewed federal law and major court cases to discern the major policy promises that the U.S. government has made to families who have members with developmental disabilities. They then summarized the knowledge base currently available on each of the policy goals and proposed a research agenda for the future to fill in knowledge gaps (Turnbull et al., 2005). Through their comprehensive policy analysis, the family life group identified an overarching goal and five supporting goals. Table 24.1 shows these goals.

TABLE 24.1
Overarching Goal and Five Associated Goals to "Leave No Family Behind"

- **Overarching goal:** To support the caregiving efforts and enhance the quality of life of all families so that families will remain the core unit of American society.

- **Goal A:** To ensure family–professional partnerships in research, policy making, and the planning and delivery of supports and services so that families will control their own destinies with due regard to the autonomy of adult family members with disabilities to control their own lives.

- **Goal B:** To ensure that families fully participate in communities of their choice through comprehensive, inclusive, neighborhood-based, and culturally responsive supports and services.

- **Goal C:** To ensure that services and supports for all families are available, accessible, appropriate, affordable, and accountable.

- **Goal D:** To ensure that sufficient public and private funding will be available to implement these goals and that all families will participate in directing the use of public funds authorized and appropriated for their benefits.

- **Goal E:** To ensure that families and professionals have full access to state-of-the-art knowledge and best practices and that they will collaborate in using knowledge and practices.

This chapter focuses on the educator's role in achieving the overarching goal articulated by the family life group: *To support the caregiving efforts and enhance the quality of life of all families so that families will remain the core unit of American society.* Although policy has been accumulating for decades that has moved the country toward this broad mandate and promise, it was not until this historic conference that the promise to families was so succinctly articulated.

Over the past 30 years, the Individuals with Disabilities Education Act (IDEA) has given legitimacy and substance to the role of parents as educational decision makers, and many special educators now collaborate with families as partners in that task. The primary rationale for family–professional partnerships in terms of student outcomes is to improve the relevance and individualization of special education services and supports and thereby increase the likelihood that students will achieve the goals of IDEA (equality of opportunity, full participation, independent living, and economic self-sufficiency) and the No Child Left Behind Act of 2001 (academic achievement) (Turnbull, Turnbull, Erwin, & Soodak, 2006; Turnbull, Turnbull, Wehmeyer, & Park, 2003).

Establishing family–professional partnerships also benefits the families themselves. The family benefit that is critically important, as delineated by Goal A in Table 24.1, is as follows: *To ensure family–professional partnerships in research, policy making, and the planning and delivery of supports and services so that families will control their own destinies with due regard to the autonomy of adult family members with disabilities to control their own lives.* By subsuming the goal related to partnerships under the overarching goal, however, it is clear that family–professional partnerships, including those focusing on educational decision making, are a *means* to the *end* of the overall goal. That overall goal is to support the caregiving efforts and enhance the quality of life of all families. This chapter addresses the role of educators in enhancing the quality of life of all families who have children and youth with developmental disabilities.

Conceptualization of Family Quality of Life

At the Beach Center on Disability at the University of Kansas (www.beachcenter. org), we and our colleagues have been involved for the last 7 years in research to conceptualize family quality of life and to find ways to work in partnership with families to enhance family quality-of-life outcomes. We started our research by conducting extensive focus groups and interviews with almost 200 individuals, including family members of children and youth with a disability (most of whom had developmental disabilities), individuals with a disability, family members of children without a disability, service providers, and administrators (Poston et al., 2003). We asked families to describe the situations in which things go really well in their family and the situations that are especially tough. From their responses, we then created a preliminary family quality-of-life survey and conducted national field tests in order to identify the specific family quality-of-life domains and indicators that would best enable families to indicate the areas of their family quality of life about which they were satisfied and the areas that they felt needed improvement (Park et al., 2003; Summers et al., 2005).

This qualitative and quantitative research led us to conclude that family quality of life refers to the extent to which family members have their needs met, enjoy their life together, and have a chance to do the things that are important to them (Park et al., 2003). The five domains of family quality of life include (Park et al., 2003; Poston et al., 2003; Summers et al., 2005):

- Disability-related support
- Physical/material well-being
- Parenting
- Emotional well-being
- Family interaction

A mother of a child with a disability shared the challenge that she faces on a daily basis to attain family quality of life:

> You just get to where it gets very difficult to stay joyful, and enjoy your life. I've decided this is a lot of work, but I'm not going to not enjoy my children. And I actually have to make a conscious effort to go put all this behind me. Don't think about how mad I am, I don't think about how stressed I am, don't think about how unjust this all is, don't think about how tired I am and not miss the little things they're doing and enjoy them. Because I could be sitting at the computer writing my hundredth letter of the year to the insurance commissioner and everybody else in the system because of some injustice that's being done, and I'm missing all the wonderful little things they're doing in the next room. Because it's just much more work than when you have, ya know, healthy children.

From this mother's perspective, one of the greatest challenges to family quality of life is not so much the characteristics of the child with a disability but what she perceives to be the injustices of the system that is designed to help the child.

Roles of Educators in Addressing Family Quality-of-Life Outcomes

Many expectations are placed on general and special educators. One wonders how educators can take on responsibility for family quality of life while simultaneously faced with the responsibility of implementing the requirements of both IDEA and NCLB. IDEA alone requires educators to conduct nondiscriminatory evaluations and then to develop and implement IEPs based on the evaluations. NCLB holds schools accountable for adequate yearly progress of students with disabilities. Is it really feasible to suggest that general and special educators also have responsibility to address family quality-of-life outcomes? The answer is yes.

We think that addressing family quality-of-life outcomes is a way to ultimately achieve the IDEA and NCLB goals, and so we are investigating. Our thinking is based on research connecting family strengths and challenges to young children's cognitive and emotional development (Hauser-Cram, Warfield, Shonkoff, & Krauss, 2001; Ran & Hou, 2003) and on other research connecting parent involvement to student academic achievement (Biggam, 2003). Clearly, stronger and more involved families give students the foundation to enable their success in school. Therefore, it makes sense for educators to participate in community-wide efforts to make sure that families are strong and healthy and that they have a high quality of life that assures their ability to support their children in school.

In the meantime, we can only describe each of the five domains of family quality of life and suggest how educators can partner with families to enhance these family quality-of-life outcomes while simultaneously providing an appropriate education to children.

Disability-Related Support

Disability-related support addresses the specific supports and services from family members, professionals, and others to benefit the family member with a disability. The indicators of disability-related support are:

- achieving goals at work or school
- having a good relationship between the family and service providers
- making progress at home
- making friends

Underlying all of these indicators is families' need for information that will enable them to understand their child's special needs and ensure that the supports and services that their child is receiving will enable him or her to progress. For more than a decade, research has clearly indicated the importance of providing relevant and clear information to families (Cooper & Allred, 1992; Shapiro, Monzo, Rueda, Gomez, & Blacher, 2004; Sontag & Schacht, 1994). One parent described the haphazard way that information is often provided as follows:

> It's not simply that people are not getting the information, it's why are they not getting it when they want it or in the form that they can absorb it, or in a way that they can act on it. . . . So it's not enough for services to simply chuck the leaflets across and say there you are, there's the information, because it doesn't work. (Mitchell & Sloper, 2002, p. 78)

Two national networks of parent centers provide information to families: Parent Training and Information Centers (PTIs) and Community Parent Resource Centers (CPRCs), both funded under IDEA.

PTIs typically have a statewide mandate, although some PTIs serve only regions of certain states. There are currently 107 PTIs, and each has a mission of ensuring that parents understand the special needs of their children and have the information that they need to participate as full partners in educational decision making (Summers et al., 2005). PTIs serve families of children and young adults with various disabilities from birth to age 22.

The Technical Assistance Alliance for Parent Centers is a national technical assistance network for PTIs. You can access its Web site (www.taalliance.org) to locate the PTI in your state.

PTIs have a wealth of information for families and professionals about how to best work together on behalf of children and youth with disabilities. PTIs typically offer workshops and have written information on wide-ranging topics, many of which are useful to educators as well as to parents. We encourage you to take advantage of the services and resources available from your PTI both for yourself and for the families of the students you teach so that they will be able to access these valuable resources and services.

To what extent are PTIs successful in achieving their goals? A national report of PTI outcomes from 1997 to 2002 (Technical Assistance Alliance for Parent Centers, 2003) stated that:

- Three-fourths of parents believe that they became more effective as a result of training and that they were helped to resolve conflicts with schools.

- Ninety-four percent indicated that the information learned from the PTI training was useful.

Although PTIs were first funded about 25 years ago, the U.S. Department of Education has more recently funded Community Parent Resource Centers (CPRCs), which are focused at the community rather than the state/regional level. CPRCs have an explicit mandate to reach out to families of children from culturally and linguistically diverse backgrounds. Ursula and DJ Markey, the parent leaders who are quoted at the beginning of the chapter, codirect a CPRC in New Orleans. Table 24.2 provides a brief overview of the work that they do in supporting families who face multiple

TABLE 24.2

Community Parent Resource Centers: Perspectives From Leaders

We are the parents, and that's what makes all the difference for us and for families with whom we work in New Orleans.

Our first son, Duane, was born with epilepsy and autism. We lost him in December 1999, when, at the age of 26, he had a seizure in his bedroom in our house. He died in our arms; for that fact, and for his life, we can only be grateful.

Our other son, Teiko, has some learning disabilities, but he is now launched into adulthood, having graduated from the New Orleans schools and now being enrolled in a postsecondary job-and-life-skills training program in Los Angeles.

We have said that our children have made all the difference in our lives, and that is true. But we also have been heavily involved, since the early 1960s, in the civil rights movement in New Orleans.

As African Americans, we see the disability rights and civil rights movements as one movement, with the disability rights movement being an extension of the civil rights movement.

In New Orleans, discrimination in education takes two forms. First, there's discrimination based on students' races. Second, there's discrimination based on the fact that they have disabilities.

We respond to discrimination by reaching out to the parents of the children, for far too often the parents lack the resources—time, money, and knowledge of the law and the best practices that could benefit their children—to combat discrimination and get an appropriate education for their children.

To reach out to parents and to mediate between them and the schools, we formed Pyramid Parent Training Program. We offer workshops, publish newsletters, refer parents to resources, and provide one-on-one assistance. We attend their children's IEP meetings. We also attend state and local school board meetings. By working on both the individual and the system levels, we mediate—that is, we serve as a go-between. Don't get us wrong: We advocate for the parents and their children, but we can't be successful advocates unless we also understand the school system and what drives it to do what it does.

With these two different cultures and agendas, the question we face as parents and that other families face daily is this. How can we bridge the gaps between the cultures so that the students will get what IDEA promises? For us, the answer was to mediate between the cultures by telling the families, "You are not alone," and then proving it by helping them gain the knowledge and support they need. Whatever help we provide—we call it "leadership development"—we recognize that, within each parent, there is the power to be an effective advocate for his or her child. And we have to acknowledge the parallel: Within every educator there is the power to be an effective teacher of that child.

So cultural mediation consists of recognizing the potential in everyone to become part of a team that works for a child. Thus, team building is an essential part of our work that incorporates the recognition that cultural agendas may differ and that our job is to help both the families and the schools by raising the level of effective parent participation in the education process.

Reprinted from: Turnbull, H. R., Turnbull, A. P., Shank, M., & Smith, S. J. (2004). *Exceptional lives: Special education in today's schools* (4th ed., p. 99). Upper Saddle River, NJ: Merrill/Prentice Hall.

challenges. CPRCs are typically staffed by parents of children with disabilities from diverse backgrounds and have culturally relevant ways to partner with families who have often felt disenfranchised from public schools.

Another valuable national resource is Parent to Parent of the United States (www.p2pusa.org). Parent to Parent programs offer one-to-one matches between a trained "veteran parent" (a parent of a child with a disability who has successfully dealt with a particular issue) and a "referred parent" (a parent of a child with a disability who is facing a particular challenge for the first time). The veteran parent provides informational and emotional support to the referred parent in a casual, informal, family-friendly manner. As of 2000, there were more than 600 local and 33 statewide programs (Santelli, Turnbull, Marquis, & Lerner, 2000). Parents who use Parent to Parent support viewed their circumstances in a more positive light, made progress on goals that were important to them, and perceived that they were able to deal positively with their child and family situations (Singer et al., 1999).

The Internet has increasingly become an invaluable resource in enabling parents of children with developmental disabilities to access critical information. Some of the key Web sites for families are:

- www.beachcenter.org—This Web site of the Beach Center on Disability at the University of Kansas provides research, real stories, and tips for families as well as professionals.

- www.p2pusa.org—The national Parent to Parent Web site provides a clearinghouse of information and links to local and state Parent to Parent programs.

- www.pacer.org—The Minnesota PTI is a national hub of technical assistance, demonstration, and training with relevance to families.

- www.exceptionalparent.com—This Web site by the publishers of *Exceptional Parent* magazine offers breadth and depth of information on numerous topics relevant to families.

- www.familyvillage.wisc.edu—This Web site offers extensive information related to a wide range of topics for families of children with disabilities.

- www.nichcy.org—The Web site of the National Dissemination Center for Children with Disabilities provides information on IDEA, NCLB, and research-based practices.

In addition to Web sites, families of children with disabilities increasingly are participating in chat rooms and on discussion boards to share information with each other. After examining the personal narratives written by parents of children with autism on the Internet, Fleischmann (2004) concluded that the Internet enables "parents to create, if not a full-blown virtual community, then at least a valuable networking system" (p. 41).

Physical/Material Well-Being

The domain of physical/material well-being addresses resources that families need in order to meet their members' needs. Key indicators of physical/material well-being include:

- having a way to take care of expenses
- having transportation to get to the places families need to be
- feeling safe at home, work, school, and in the neighborhood
- getting medical and dental care when needed.

Having a way to take care of expenses is clearly a priority for family quality of life. A mother who was not able to meet her expenses described the impact on family quality of life as follows:

> If you have no money, it's very difficult to be—to do—to be together, to do fun things, to be at peace, to come home to a haven. . . . Because if you have no money, the bills not paid, you not gonna rest when you get home. You might have a good family, you know, a good husband, whatever, whatever. But, you don't have money, all that can go down the drain, so . . . Money provides a way of release. You can go on a vacation, maybe, once a year, whereas if you don't have the money, you won't be able to do that. You can—you can pay your bills. Whereas if you don't have money, you won't be able to do that. And when you can't do those things, you have this feeling of insecurity which floods over into other problems, emotionally. Anger, bitterness, and then it jumps off on the other family members and you got chaos.

Economic challenges become even more problematic for students who have been identified as having mental retardation. There are complex interactions between race, income, and the likelihood of being identified as having mental retardation. As compared to European American students, African American students are more than twice as likely to be identified as having mental retardation (National Research Council, 2002). African American students account for approximately one third of the population of students identified as having mental retardation; however, they account for only 17% of the general student population. In terms of the role of income, poverty among African Americans is three times as high as poverty among European Americans (Blank, 2001). Thus, special educators who teach students with mental retardation can expect a disproportionate number of the students to come from families in which taking care of expenses is a major challenge. This is especially true for special educators who teach in urban schools that are disproportionately attended by African American students.

The impact of poverty on educational outcomes is substantial. This means that meeting NCLB's annual yearly progress requirement is much more challenging when teaching students who experience poverty. Some of the impacts documented through research are as follows:

- As compared to students whose families are in the top 20% with regard to family income, students whose families are in the bottom 20% with regard to family income are five times more likely to drop out of high school (Kaufman, Kwon, Klein, & Chapman, 2000).

- Children from a middle-class background have IQ scores that are 5 to 13 points higher than children who live in poverty (Kaiser & Delaney, 1996; Korenman, Miller, & Sjaasted, 1995).

- Children whose families experience poverty are much more likely to have reduced rates in vocabulary growth and reading, which are highly important predictors of reading success (Hart & Risley, 1995).

What are the other characteristics of families who experience poverty? Families who experience poverty are much more likely to be characterized by having a single parent (usually a single mother) who has less education as compared to families with more adequate family resources (Fujiura & Yamaki, 2000; National Research Council, 2002). It has been found that single parents often are challenged to find time and emotional energy to be actively involved in their child's education (Cigno & Burke, 1997). Additionally, parents who have low educational levels often are intimidated by the expectations to be educational decision makers and to assist their child in being successful in school.

What does all of this mean to you as a special educator in terms of how you can best increase the likelihood that families will be able to meet their expenses and, thereby, have a better family quality of life?

- You can partner with the school social worker and/or school counselor in referring families to community agencies that specialize in assisting families with access to economic resources such as affordable housing, food banks, and job training.

- You can look for organizations in your community that are interested in investing resources in students who have economic needs such as Big Sister/Big Brother programs, religious programs, and community service clubs.

- You can make special efforts to reach out to parents who have low levels of education by providing information to them in ways that are understandable and empowering.

Some economic resources are specifically targeted for children and youth with developmental disabilities and their families. One of these resources is Supplemental Security Income (SSI), which is administered by the Social Security Administration. SSI pays monthly benefits to children and adults who have significant disabilities. To qualify for SSI, a person must meet the federal standard for poverty. This federal standard changes from time to time and is based on a complex formula that takes into account family size, parental income, and whether a child lives at home. To be eligible for SSI on the basis of disability, the child must have a physical or mental condition that results in "marked and severe functional limitations." Second, the disability must be expected to last at least 12 months or to result in the child's death. And third, the disability must be documented by a disability evaluation team, although students with mental retardation qualify for a presumption of disability, which means that payments can start before the evaluation is completed.

Medicaid is another income-support program, but unlike SSI, it provides medical and health-care assistance for people with low incomes, including those with disabilities. Medicaid has two eligibility factors: financial eligibility and group eligibility. In order to meet the financial eligibility criteria, children must be from families whose income and resources fall below the threshold level that is specified in the Medicaid state plan for the state in which they live. Group eligibility is not based on income but rather on qualification of an individual as a member of an intended beneficiary group. These groups include individuals with developmental disabilities.

Medicaid includes a program called Home and Community-Based Services (HCBS) Waivers, which provides funding for a number of services, including "case management, homemaker assistance, home health aids, personal care; residential habilitation; day habilitation, respite care; transportation, supported employment, adapted equipment; home modifications; and occupational, physical, speech and behavioral therapy" (Braddock, Hemp, Parish, & Rizzolo, 2000). The HCBS Waivers program is a source of potential resources for families (Braddock, Hemp, & Rizzolo, 2004).

What can you do to help ensure that families have access to these resources? Perhaps the major barrier that special educators face in assisting families in accessing these resources is the time and effort it takes to find out the details in your own state about the steps that families need to go through to apply. We encourage you to contact the local Social Security Administration office in your community to obtain information about funding availability in your state and community. You can partner with your school counselor and/or school social worker in obtaining this information and making it available to families. Other community partners include advocacy groups such as The Arc (www.thearc.org) and Parent Training and Information Centers.

Parenting

The parenting domain of family quality of life refers to those activities that adult family members do to help children grow and develop. It involves

- knowing how to help their child with schoolwork and activities,
- knowing how to help their child learn to be independent,
- knowing how to help their child get along with others, and
- having time to take care of the individuals needs of every child.

We will focus in this section on what you can do to enable parents to learn how to help their child with schoolwork and activities.

It is clear that one way to help students with disabilities progress more in school, including improving their performance on standards-based assessment, is seeing that they experience more follow-through and success with homework. Research has demonstrated that students in general educational programs who have parental support for homework typically have more-positive attitudes about homework, feel more self-confident, and take greater responsibility for completing their work (Hoover-Dempsey et al., 2001). Additionally, students receiving special education services who complete their homework generally show improvements in their academic achievement (Epstein, Polloway, Foley, & Patton, 1993).

Family involvement with homework for students with disabilities is especially important, since these students often experience more problems than typical students in completing homework successfully (Epstein et al., 1993; Gajria & Salend, 1995). As students with developmental disabilities are increasingly included in the general curriculum, expectations for homework for these students will increase (Salend, Duhaney, Anderson, & Gottschalk, 2004). Ensuring clear home–school communication is one way to enable parents to be more successful in helping their child with schoolwork (Nelson, Jayanthi, Brittain, Epstein, & Bursuck, 2002). Table 24.3 shows tips for increasing the likelihood that families' assistance with homework will be successful in terms of benefits to students and possibly even contribute to family quality of life in a positive way. The last tip in Table 24.3 suggests the use of the Internet to communicate with families. Salend and colleagues provide excellent guidance on ways to design a Web site so that it can facilitate homework communication with families. They describe three phases of developing a full menu for a Homework Assistance Center as follows:

TABLE 24.3

Tips for Supporting Parents to Help With Homework

- Ensure communication among all the students' teachers to avoid homework overload.
  - ✓ Ensure that general education teachers have access to full information on students' preferences, strengths, and needs related to homework modification.
- Increase students' responsibility.
  - ✓ Teach students to use homework planners.
  - ✓ Teach students to graph their homework completion.
- Foster full teacher–student–parent communication about homework.
  - ✓ Use students' graph of homework completion at parent–teacher–student conferences to discuss progress with parents.
  - ✓ Communicate frequently with parents about homework assignments and students' progress.
  - ✓ Use written communication such as notes, progress reports, and forms.
  - ✓ Give parents access to homework assignments by telephone/voice mail with the option for parents to leave messages if they have questions.
  - ✓ Provide parents with teachers' names and their preferred times and methods for being contacted.
  - ✓ Use the Internet to provide guidance to families on homework.

492 Adapted from: Bryan & Sullivan-Burstein, 1998; Epstein et al., 1999; Harniss et al., 2001; Jayanthi et al., 1995; Turnbull et al., 2006.

- Phase 1—Welcome statement, guidelines for using the homework site, index of the site's content, frequently asked questions, homework policies, general recommendations to guide family members in helping with homework, and contact information for the teacher.

- Phase 2—Assignments and directions for completing them, exemplary models and rubrics for evaluation, and a description of the linkage between homework and standards in the general curriculum.

- Phase 3—Online homework resources, a digital drop box to submit assignments and ask questions, cooperative online homework groups, guidelines for evaluating the credibility of Web-based information, online survey for user feedback, and a suggestion box for submitting ideas for improvement.

The authors point out that approximately 90% of students ages 5–17 have access to computers (Nixon, 2002), but there still are families who do not have access. Thus, when using computers to facilitate homework communication with families, teachers can partner with other professionals in the school and community to seek to expand access to personal computers and the availability of computers at libraries, community centers, and other places that are accessible to families who do not have computers.

Emotional Well-Being

Emotional well-being is the domain of family quality of life that involves feelings or affective considerations within the family. It involves families having

- the support that they need to relieve stress
- friends or others who provide support

TABLE 24.4

Tips for Supporting Families to Lower Stress Related to Major Concerns

- Support families to learn state-of-the-art information on positive behavior support and to be able to implement it in home and community settings in order to avoid problem behavior and to increase the likelihood of appropriate behavior.
    - ✓ Have conferences with parents (and encourage them to invite other family members) to explain how you use positive behavior support in the classroom and how they might be able to use similar strategies in home and community settings.
    - ✓ Ask families how they would most like to receive information on positive behavior support and respond accordingly
    - ✓ Build your own resource library on sources of positive behavior support for families including Lucyshyn et al. (2002).
    - ✓ Refer families to state-of-the-art Web sites on positive behavior support (including www.pbis.org and http://challengingbehavior.fmhi.usf.edu/pbs.html).
    - ✓ Seek information on workshops for families through the PTI in your state and through a CPRC, if one is available.
- Seek ways to help students make friends in school settings that will carry over to home, neighborhood, and community settings.
    - ✓ Incorporate opportunities for socialization and peer support in the classroom through peer tutoring and cooperative learning.
    - ✓ Seek opportunities in the school for the involvement of students in extracurricular clubs and activities.
    - ✓ Learn about the Circle of Friends approach and implement it for students with particular challenges related to developing friendships (Falvey et al., 2002).
    - ✓ Support students to develop hobbies consistent with their preferences than can serve as a link for being involved with others.
    - ✓ Invite (with the parent's permission) adult leaders of community activities to come to the IEP conference to learn how to best support the student in a community setting (religious programs, scouting, soccer).

- some time to pursue their own interests

- outside help available to take care of the special needs of all family members

In recent research with large groups of families who have young children with disabilities, family respondents reported lower satisfaction on the domain of emotional well-being than on the other four domains of family quality of life (Jackson & Turnbull, 2004; Mannan, 2005). The indicator in this domain that often receives the lowest score is having the support needed to relieve stress. Although research on the topic of parental stress when children have disabilities has been mixed, the trend indicates that families with children with disabilities have higher stress levels and face more challenges than parents who do not have children with disabilities (Blacher & Lopez, 1997; Hoare, Harris, Jackson, & Kerley, 1998; Olsson & Hwang, 2001; Warfield, Krauss, Hauser-Cram, Upshur, & Shonkoff, 1999).

Two factors that contribute to higher parental stress levels are the child's problem behavior and the lack of friends (Baker et al., 2003; Guralnick, Conner, & Hammond, 1995). Table 24.4 includes tips that you can act on in terms of helping families address challenges in each of these areas that may contribute to their experiencing less stress.

In addition to helping with particular concerns about their children, you can contribute to a family's emotional well-being by providing state-of-the-art services to the student. The lack of quality in many special education programs is a major source of concern and stress for families. Johnson and colleagues (Johnson, Duffett, Farkas, & Wilson, 2002) conducted a national random sample survey of more than 500 parents of children and youth in special education. They reported the following results:

- Forty-five percent of parents believe that their child's special education program is failing or needs improvement to prepare the child for life after high school.

- Thirty-five percent report they were frustrated in seeking special education services that their child needed.

- Thirty-five percent believe that their child's special education program is failing or needs improvements to be a reliable source of information about learning problems and disability.

- Thirty-three percent believe that their child's current school is doing only a fair or poor job when it comes to giving their child the needed help. (Johnson et al., 2002)

Furthermore, approximately 16% of the parents indicated that they have considered legal action because of the lack of quality in their child's special education program. Almost one third of the parents of children with severe disabilities indicated that they had considered suing, as contrasted to 13% of the parents of students with mild disabilities.

What is the most important implication of these findings for you? The message is clear: When you provide the very best education to a student that you can, you do more than make a difference in the life of child. You also have a significant impact on the emotional well-being of the student's whole family. Providing high-quality education eliminates one of the major sources of concern and stress that plague families who have children with disabilities.

Many families experience stress because they have to advocate for quality services. A parent summed up the emotional drain of advocacy as follows:

And so, you have to just use every bit of strength you've got to keep yourself together and just keep advocating and keep chugging and keep going, when you're emotionally drained, physically exhausted spiritually, you know. (Wang, Mannan, Poston, Turnbull, & Summers, 2004, p. 149)

Consider the following quote from a parent who did not need to engage in intense advocacy because the school was doing such a good job:

The last two years have been like in a dream world. It is like I want to call them up and say, "You do not have nothing negative to say?" This educational system—this school itself has worked wonders with my son. It has taken a lot of stress off ME, so that when I go home, I do not have to get into it with him and say, "Oh, you know, the school called me today about this and that." They will call me, but they have already worked it out. Or they will call me to praise him and tell me how wonderful and how positive a role model he is now, and it's because they have worked with us. It is like I said, it has been a dream world to me. (Wang et al., 2004, pp. 149–150)

Parents generally prefer to be partners with educators in implementing quality programs, and they dislike being in the position of an advocate who must engage in adversarial activities in order to obtain services or to ensure that services are high quality (Turnbull et al., 2006). Thus, by offering state-of-the-art, quality services to students and families, you are making a substantial contribution to their emotional well-being.

Family Interaction

The family interaction domain of family quality of life focuses on the relationships among family members. Indicators of family quality of life include:

- enjoying spending time together
- talking openly with each other
- solving problems together
- showing they love and care for each other

When children and youth experience a developmental disability, every family member shares the impact of the disability. That was the message with regard to the families' emotional well-being also. We will focus here on how you can help parents not only to deal with the stress that they experience in raising their child but also to move toward being able to enjoy spending time with the child and involving the child in family activities.

What can you do to increase the likelihood that the family will not only *survive* **495** but will also *prevail* in terms of actually enjoying the time that they spend with their child with a developmental disability? As you learned previously, their child's problem behavior is one of the biggest sources of stress for families in their home setting. Thus, the more you can help families eliminate problem behavior and increase the likelihood of appropriate behavior, the more likely it is that they not only will gain relief from stress but also increasingly enjoy being with their child. You can also work with students to develop hobbies that they can carry out at home in a cooperative way with their family, acquire the necessary communication skills to interact with their family and to say positive things to them, and to develop interests that will enable their families to participate with them in community activities, such as those offered through religious organizations, scouting programs, and community recreation centers.

Family interaction is not limited, however, to the relationship between a child or youth with developmental disabilities and the parents. Research clearly shows that often siblings and grandparents also experience stress (Fisman, Wolf, Ellison, & Freeman, 2000; Hastings, 1997; Sandler, 1998; Stoneman & Waldman-Berman, 1993). In some situations, siblings, grandparents, and other family members need support in learning how to communicate with the child or youth with a developmental disability, and they need to learn about dealing with problem behavior. As you interact with parents, you can encourage them to think about whether it would be helpful to invite nuclear and/or extended family members to the IEP conference or to other conferences or school-based activities that might enable them to learn more about how to achieve the most comfortable interaction with the child or youth with a developmental disability.

A program that has been specifically designed for siblings is Sibshops, developed in Seattle, Washington, by Don Meyer in the 1980s and now offered in many communities throughout the United States (Meyer & Vadasy, 1994). Local and state chapters of The Arc (www.thearc.org) frequently sponsor Sibshops. Sibshops typically focus on a particular age group (elementary, middle, and/or high school) of brothers and sisters of individuals with disabilities. Group meetings are held in which brothers and sisters can talk about topics related to their sibling with a disability that might be especially difficult for them. Among the topics might be embarrassment in public, worry about the future, resentment about the amount of family time and resources devoted to their brother or sister with a disability, and/or feeling guilty because they do not have a disability and their brother or sister does. Research has reported that siblings learn how to improve their relationships with their brother or sister with a disability and have become more aware of his or her special needs through Sibshops (Dyson, 1998). You can learn more details about the program at www.thearc.org/siblingsupport/.

Conclusion

This chapter makes the case that a role of special education teachers is to contribute positively to family quality of life. Teachers can do this by providing supports, resources, and encouragement related to the five domains that make up family quality of life: disability-related support, physical/material well-being, parenting, emotional well-being, and family interaction. Another highly important consideration for teachers is to ensure that they "do no harm" in terms of adding stress and strain to family life by providing poor or mediocre services rather than high-quality services. Related service providers such as school counselors and school social workers, as well as national networks of resources for families, can be helpful to educators in fulfilling this role. A key competency for educators is knowing where to access appropriate information and resources relevant to families.

Glossary

Family quality of life—Refers to the extent to which family members have their needs met, enjoy their life together, and have a chance to do the things that are important to them.

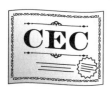

Knowledge and Skills for Entry-Level Special Education Teachers of Students With Developmental Disabilities Standards Addressed in This Chapter

Principle 1: Foundations

DD1K4 Trends and practices in the field of developmental disabilities.

Principle 4: Instructional Strategies

DD4S2 Relate levels of support to the needs of the individual.

Principle 7: Instructional Planning

DD7S2 Plan and implement instruction for individuals with developmental disabilities that is both age-appropriate and ability-appropriate.

Principle 10: Collaboration

DD10K1 Services, networks, and organizations for individuals with developmental disabilities.

Web Site Resources

Beach Center for Disability
www.beachcenter.org

Provides research, real stories, and tips for families as well as professionals.

Exceptional Parent Online Magazine

www.exceptionalparent.com

> Provides parents with information, support, ideas, encouragement, and outreach for parents and families of children with disabilities.

Family Village: A Global Community of Disability-Related Resources

www.familyvillage.wisc.edu

> Extensive information for families of children with disabilities related to a wide range of topics.

Parent Advocacy Center for Educational Rights (PACER)

www.pacer.org

> The Minnesota PTI is a national hub of technical assistance, demonstration, and training with relevance to families.

Parent to Parent of the United States

www.p2pusa.org

> A clearinghouse of information and links to local and state Parent to Parent programs that match experienced parents with parents dealing with challenges for the first time.

National Dissemination Center for Children with Disabilities

www.nichcy.org

> Information on IDEA, NCLB, and research-based practices.

References

Baker, B. L., McIntyre, L. L., Blacher, J., Crnic, K., Edelbrock, C., & Low, C. (2003). Preschool children with and without developmental delay: Behavior problems and parenting stress over time. *Journal of Intellectual and Developmental Disability, 47*, 217–230.

Biggam, S. (2003). Making the most of parent partnerships to strengthen literacy development: Lessons from John and Janet Poeton and recent research. *New England Reading Association Journal, 3*(39), 24–27.

Blacher, J., & Lopez, S. (1997). Contributions to depression in Latina mothers with and without children with mental retardation: Implications for care giving. *Family Relations: Interdisciplinary Journal of Applied Family Studies, 46*, 325–334.

Blank, R. M. (2001). An overview of trends in social economic well-being, by race. In N. J. Smelser, W. J. Wilson, & F. Mitchell (Eds.), *America becoming: Racial trends and their consequences* (Vol. 1, pp. 21–39). Washington, DC: National Academies Press.

Braddock, D., Hemp, R., Parish, S., & Rizzolo, M. C. (2000). *The state of the states in developmental disabilities: 2000 study summary*. Chicago: Department of Disability and Human Development, University of Illinois at Chicago.

Braddock, D., Hemp, R., & Rizzolo, M. C. (2004). State of the states in developmental disabilities: 2004. *Mental Retardation, 42*, 356–370.

Bryan, T., & Sullivan–Burstein, K. (1998). Teacher-selected strategies for improving homework completion. *Remedial and Special Education, 19*, 263–275.

Cigno, K., & Burke, P. (1997). Single mothers of children with learning disabilities: An undervalued group. *Journal of Interprofessional Care, 11*, 177–186.

Cooper, C. S., & Allred, K. W. (1992). A comparison of mothers' versus fathers' needs for support in caring for a young child with special needs. *Infant-Toddler Intervention, 2*, 205–221.

Dyson, L. L. (1998). A support program for siblings of children with disabilities: What siblings learn and what they like. *Psychology in the Schools, 35*(1), 57–63.

Epstein, M. H., Munk, D. D., Bursuck, W. D., Polloway, E. A., & Jayanthi, M. M. (1999). Strategies for improving home–school communication about homework for students with disabilities. *Journal of Special Education, 33*, 166–176.

Epstein, M. H., Polloway, E. A., Foley, R. M., & Patton, J. R. (1993). Homework: A comparision of teachers' and parents' perceptions of the problems experienced by students identified as having behavioral disorders, learning disabilities, or no disabilities. *Remedial and Special Education, 14*(5), 40–50.

Falvey, M. A., Forest, M. S., Pearpoint, J., & Rosenberg, R. L. (2002). Building connections. In J. S. Thousand, R. A. Villa, & A. I. Nevin (Eds.), *Creativity and collaborative learning* (2nd ed., pp. 29–54). Baltimore: Brookes.

Fisman, S., Wolf, L., Ellison, D., & Freeman, T. (2000). A longitudinal study of siblings of children with chronic disabilities. *Canadian Journal of Psychiatry, 45,* 369–375.

Fleischmann, A. (2004). Narratives published on the Internet by parents of children with autism: What do they reveal and why is it important? *Focus on Autism and Other Developmental Disabilities, 19*(1), 35–43.

Fuijiura, G. T., & Yamaki, K. (2000). Trends in demography of childhood poverty and disability. *Exceptional Children, 66,* 187–200.

Gajria, M., & Salend, S. J. (1995). Homework practices of students with and without learning disabilities: A comparison. *Journal of Learning Disabilities, 28,* 291–296.

Guralnick, M. J., Conner, R. T., & Hammond, M. (1995). Parent perspectives of peer relationships and friendships in integrated and specialized settings. *American Journal on Mental Retardation, 99,* 457–476.

Harniss, M. K., Epstein, M. H., Bursuck, W. D., Nelson, J., & Jayanthi, M. M. (2001). Resolving homework–related communication problems: Recommendations of parents of children with and without disabilities. *Reading and Writing Quarterly, 17,* 205–225.

Hart, B., & Risley, T. R. (1995). *Meaningful differences in the everyday experience of young American children.* Baltimore: Brookes.

Hastings, R. P. (1997). Grandparents of children with disabilities: A review. *International Journal of Disability, Development, and Education, 44,* 329–340.

Hauser-Cram, P., Warfield, M. E., Shonkoff, J. P., & Krauss, M. W. (2001). Children with disabilities: A longitudinal study in child development and parent well-being. *Monographs of the Society for Research in Child Development, 66*(3, Serial No. 266).

Hoare, P., Harris, M., Jackson, P., & Kerley, S. (1998). A community survey of children with severe intellectual disability and their families: Psychological adjustment, career distress and the effect of respite care. *Journal of Intellectual Disability Research, 42,* 218–224.

Hoover-Dempsey, K. V., Battiato, A. C., Walker, J. M. T., Reed, R. P., DeJong, J. M., & Jones, K. P. (2001). Parental involvement in homework. *Educational Psychologist, 36,* 195–209.

Individuals with Disabilities Education Act of 1990, 20 U.S.C. § 1400 *et seq.* (1990).

Jackson, C. W., & Turnbull, A. (2004). Impact of deafness on family life: A literature review. *Topics in Early Childhood Special Education, 24*(1), 15–29.

Jayanthi, M., Sawyer, V., Nelson, J. S., Bursuck, W. D., & Epstein, M. H. (1995). Recommendations for homework-communication problems. *Remedial and Special Education, 16,* 212–225.

Johnson, J., Duffett, A., Farkas, S., & Wilson, L. (2002). *When it's your own child: A report on special education from the families who use it.* New York: Public Agenda.

Kaiser, A., & Delaney, E. (1996). The effects of poverty on parenting young children. *Peabody Journal of Education, 71,* 66–85.

Kaufman, P., Kwon, J. Y., Klein, S., & Chapman, C. D. (2000). *Dropout rates in the United States: 1999.* Washington, DC: National Center for Educational Statistics.

Korenman, S., Miller, J. E., & Sjaastad, J. E. (1995). Long–term poverty and child development in the United States: Results from the NLSY. *Children and Young Services Review, 17,* 127–155.

Lucyshyn, J., Dunlap, G., & Albin, R. (2002). *Families and positive behavioral support: Addressing the challenge of problem behaviors in family contexts.* Baltimore: Brookes.

Mannan, H. (2005). *Parents' perceptions of quality family–professional partnerships and family quality of life.* Unpublished doctoral dissertation, University of Kansas, Lawrence.

Meyer, D. J., & Vadasy, P. F. (1994). *Sibshops: Workshops for siblings of children with special needs.* Baltimore: Brookes.

Mitchell, W., & Sloper, P. (2002). Information that informs rather than alienates families with disabled children: Developing a model of good practice. *Health and Social Care in the Community, 10*(2), 74–81.

National Research Council. (2002). *Minority students in special and gifted education.* Washington, DC: National Academies Press.

Nelson, J. S., Jayanthi, M., Brittain, C. S., Epstein, M. H., & Bursuck, W. D. (2002). Using the nominal group technique for homework communication decisions: An exploratory study. *Remedial and Special Education, 23*, 379–386.

Nixon, M. (2002). How the Web keeps parents in the know. *Technological Horizons to Education, 29*(9), 58–60.

No Child Left Behind Act of 2001, 20 U.S.C. 70 § 6301 *et seq.* (2002).

Olsson, M. B., & Hwang, C. P. (2001). Depression in mothers and fathers of children with intellectual disability. *Journal of Intellectual Disability Research, 45*, 535–543.

Park, J., Hoffman, L., Marquis, J., Turnbull, A. P., Poston, D., Mannan, H., Wang, M., & Nelson, L. (2003). Toward assessing family outcomes of service delivery: Validation of a family quality of life survey. *Journal of Intellectual Disability Research, 47*, 367–384.

Poston, D., Turnbull, A., Park, J., Mannan, H., Marquis, J., & Wang, M. (2003). Family quality of life: A qualitative inquiry. *Mental Retardation, 41*, 313–328.

Ran, B., & Hou, F. (2003). Changes in family structure and child outcomes: Roles of economic and familial resources. *Policy Studies Journal, 3*(31), 309–330.

Salend, S. J., Duhaney, D., Anderson, D. J., & Gottschalk, G. (2004). Using the Internet to improve homework communication and completion. *Teaching Exceptional Children, 36*(3), 64–73.

Sandler, A. G. (1998). Grandparents of children with disabilities: A closer look. *Education and Training in Mental Retardation and Developmental Disabilities, 33*, 350–356.

Santelli, B., Turnbull, A., Marquis, J., & Lerner, E. (2000). Statewide parent to parent programs: Partners in early intervention. *Infants and Young Children, 13*(1), 74–88.

Shapiro, J., Monzo, L. D., Rueda, R., Gomez, J. A., & Blacher, J. (2004). Alienated advocacy: Perspectives of Latina mothers of young adults with developmental disabilities on service systems. *Mental Retardation, 42*(1), 37–54.

Singer, G. H. S., Marquis, J., Powers, L., Blanchard, L., DiVenere, N., Santelli, B., & Sharp, M. (1999). A multi-site evaluation of parent to parent programs for parents of children with disabilities. *Journal of Early Intervention, 22*, 217–229.

Sontag, J. C., & Schacht, R. (1994). An ethnic comparison of parent participation and information needs in early intervention. *Exceptional Children, 60*, 422–433.

Stoneman, Z., & Waldman-Berman, P. (1993). *The effects of mental retardation, disability, and illness.* Baltimore, MD: Brookes.

Summers, J. A., Poston, D. J., Turnbull, A. P., Marquis, J., Hoffman, L., Mannan, H., & Wang, M. (2005). Conceptualizing and measuring family quality of life. *Journal of Intellectual Disability, 49*, 777–783.

Technical Assistance Alliance for Parent Centers. (2003). *Parent centers helping families: Data outcomes 1997–2002.* Minneapolis, MN: Alliance National Center.

Turnbull, A. P., Turnbull, H. R., Agosta, J., Erwin, E., Fujiura, G., Singer, G., & Soodak, L. (2005). Support of families and family life across the lifespan. In C. Lakin & A. P. Turnbull (Eds.), *National goals and research for persons with intellectual and developmental disabilities* (pp. 217–256). Washington, DC: American Association on Mental Retardation.

Turnbull, A. P., Turnbull, H. R., Erwin, E., & Soodak, L. (2006). *Families, professionals, and exceptionality: Positive outcomes through partnerships and trust.* Upper Saddle River, NJ: Merrill/Prentice Hall.

Turnbull, H. R., Turnbull, A. P., Wehmeyer, M. L., & Park, J. (2003). A quality of life framework for special education outcomes. *Remedial and Special Education, 24*, 67–74.

Wang, M., Mannan, H., Poston, D., Turnbull, A. P., & Summers, J. A. (2004). Parents' perceptions of advocacy activities and their impact on family quality of life. *Research and Practice for Persons With Severe Disabilities, 29*, 144–155.

Warfield, M. E., Krauss, M., Hauser-Cram, P., Upshur, C., & Shonkoff, J. (1999). Adaptation during early childhood among mothers of children with disabilities. *Journal of Developmental and Behavioral Pediatrics, 43*, 112–118.

25

Roles and Responsibilities of Paraeducators Working With Learners With Developmental Disabilities:

Translating Research Into Practice

Anna Lou Pickett

Summary

As always, educators are respondents to and agents for change. Policy makers and those who implement change are confronted with a multitude of concerns as they seek more effective methods to improve the quality of America's schools for all learners. Over the last 40 years the employment of paraeducators has continued unabated nationwide, the roles and responsibilities of teachers and paraeducators have changed dramatically, and many of the issues that led to the utilization of paraeducators still exist, and in many instances have become more pervasive. Still, "paraeducator issues" receive scant attention, and the policies, standards, and infrastructures required to improve their ability to work with learners who have diverse learning needs, and to be effective members of instructional teams are for the most part not being established (Pickett, Likens, & Wallace, 2003).

The following topics are addressed in the chapter: (a) historical factors that contributed to the employment of teacher aides, (b) changes in teacher roles as supervisors of paraeducators, (c) changes in paraeducator roles that stress participation in different phases of the instructional process and the delivery of other direct services to learners or their families, (d) differences in the roles of principals and teachers in the supervision of paraeducators, and (e) roles of state and local education agency (SEAs and LEAs) policy makers and administrators, personnel developers in institutions of higher education (IHEs) and other stakeholders for developing policies, standards, and systems that prepare teachers and paraeducators for their roles and support their on-the-job performance.

Learning Outcomes

After reading this chapter, you should be able to:

- Describe the impact of court-ordered mandates and provisions in federal laws on paraeducator employment, preparation, and supervision.

- Describe the roles of SEA personnel in creating policies, standards, resources, and systems to ensure that paraeducators are appropriately prepared and supervised.

- Describe the roles of LEA administrators in: (a) establishing personnel practices that include guidelines for paraeducator supervision and monitoring, (b) defining paraeducator roles and responsibilities in the delivery of instructional and related services for learners with developmental disabilities, autism, autism spectrum disorders, and other learning- and language-related needs, (c) developing job descriptions that include educational and experiential criteria for paraeducator employment in different programs, and responsibility for their supervision, and (d) creating structured, standardized systems for career development for paraeducators that recognize differences in the hierarchies of knowledge and skills required for placement in different programs and positions.

- Describe the roles of principals in creating learning environments that support and strengthen the work of teacher and paraeducator teams.

- Identify teacher responsibilities that may not be delegated to paraeducators.

- Describe teacher responsibilities that may be shared with paraeducators who are appropriately prepared to carry them out.

- Describe the distinctions in the roles of principals and teachers* in the day-to-day supervision and monitoring of paraeducators.

Introduction

Paraeducator, paraprofessional, teacher aide, instructional assistant, transition trainer, occupational and physical therapy assistant or aide, speech-language pathology assistant, health-care aide, job coach, and transition trainer: These are just a few of the titles for school district personnel who (a) are supervised by teachers or other licensed practitioners, and (b) assist with the delivery of instructional and related services for learners and/or their families (Pickett, 1989).** "Teacher aides" have been employed in school districts nationwide for more than 40 years. Over time their roles and responsibilities have changed dramatically. They are active members of teams who provide education and other direct services to children and youth who have developmental, sensory, and physical disabilities, as well as other learning- and language-related needs. "In today's schools they are technicians who are more aptly described as paraeducators just as their counterparts in law and medicine are designated as paralegals and paramedics" (Pickett, 1989, p. 1).

This chapter is concerned with one of the many challenges confronting administrators in state education agencies (SEAs) and local education agencies (LEAs), teachers, principals, and personnel developers in institutions of higher education (IHEs) as they seek more effective methods to meet the diverse education needs of all learners. Primary among these challenges are the critical but underrecognized needs for policies, personnel practices, and infrastructures to (a) maintain the integrity of teacher roles in diagnosing learner needs, developing instructional programs and strategies to meet the needs of individual learners, introducing lessons, and assessing learner progress, (b) identify knowledge and skills required by paraeducators to effectively assist teachers or other professional practitioners with their program and classroom management functions, (c) establish career development systems to ensure the availability of a highly skilled paraeducator workforce, and (d) prepare teachers for their expanding roles as team leaders and supervisors of paraeducators.

For the most part, standards for employment, roles, and supervision of paraeducators—whether they work in special, general, or compensatory education programs—have not been established by either SEAs or LEAs, nor have infrastructures been developed that (a) provide a continuum of training experiences for paraeducators and (b) prepare teachers for their changing team roles as front-line directors and monitors of paraeducators (Pickett et al., 2003). Administrators and personnel developers must address several interrelated issues that are central to the development of a

---

* Although other professional practitioners (e.g., occupational and physical therapists, speech-language pathologists, nurses, transitional and early childhood specialists) have supervisory responsibility for paraprofessional personnel, the term *teacher* is used throughout the chapter to designate a person with supervisory responsibility.

** To avoid wordiness, the term *paraeducator* is used throughout this chapter, except when other titles are necessary to maintain historical accuracy or to refer to the terminology of other disciplines.

paraeducator workforce that is well prepared, appropriately supervised, and effectively integrated into education teams. Pickett (1989, 1994, 2003) has identified an ongoing, critical need for policy makers and administrators in SEAs and LEAs to join forces with 2- and 4-year IHEs and professional organizations representing different disciplines, unions, and other stakeholders to (a) define distinctions in teacher and paraeducator responsibilities for diagnosing learner needs, developing instructional plans, adapting curriculum content and instructional strategies to meet the needs of individual learners, engaging students in learning activities, and assessing learner progress, (b) delineate differences in the responsibilities of principals and teachers in the supervision of paraeducators, (c) establish standards for paraeducator employment, roles, preparation, supervision, and performance outcomes, (d) develop curriculum standards and create career development systems to prepare paraeducators for their expanding roles as members of instructional teams, and (e) develop and infuse curriculum standards for teachers into undergraduate and graduate programs to prepare teachers for their roles in directing and monitoring the day-to-day work of paraeducators.

Paraeducators in Education: Historical Perspective— The 1950s to the 1980s

This section provides (a) a foundation that will help answer questions that exist in contemporary education practices in connection with the employment of paraeducators, their roles with respect to the roles of teachers, and their responsibilities in the instructional process and the delivery of other education services and (b) an understanding of why the need for policies and systems concerned with the employment and preparation of paraeducators still require attention in the 21st century. Many of the current policies and personnel practices that contribute to confusion about appropriate roles for paraeducators in the instructional process and the roles of teachers as their supervisors have their roots in policy decisions and events that have and have not taken place over several decades (Pickett, 2003, 1994, 1989). Thus, insight into historical factors that affect the capacity of teacher and paraeducator teams to work well together will enable educators—no matter whether they are administrators, personnel developers, teachers, or teachers in training—to develop strategies for more effectively utilizing the resources provided by paraeducators to support the program and classroom management functions of teachers.

When interest in testing the efficacy of employing "teacher aides" emerged in the latter half of the 20th century, it did not happen by accident. Initially it was fueled by two factors: the need to cope with shortages of licensed teachers created by the baby boom that occurred after World War II, and the beginning of efforts on the part of parents of children and adults with disabilities to gain access to education and community-centered services as alternatives to institutional placement (Gartner, 1971; Pickett, 1994).

During the mid-1950s two research projects examined the value of employing aides to provide teachers with more time for planning, implementing, and evaluating lessons. The first, funded by the Ford Foundation, took place in the Bay City, Michigan, schools. The purpose was to examine the potential of using "teacher aides" to carry out routine administrative functions performed by teachers as a way to reduce the impact of teacher shortages. Women who had attended college but were not licensed teachers were recruited and trained to provide clerical assistance, monitor playgrounds, lunchrooms, and hallways, duplicate instructional materials, help maintain learning centers, and escort students to and from buses (Fund for the Advancement of Education, 1961). The purpose of the second project, carried out at Syracuse University, was to evaluate the effectiveness of teacher aides in special education programs (which were slowly gaining a foothold across the country) in parent-sponsored programs and, to a lesser extent, in public schools (Cruickshank & Herring, 1957). Although the results of both projects showed promise, it was more than 10 years before the employment of teacher aides to support teachers in general, special, and compensatory (remedial) education was more fully explored (Gartner, 1971; Kaplan, 1977).

While the two research projects were under way, parents and civil rights advocates initiated activities that were destined to have a profound impact on schools nationwide. They included challenges to long-standing laws, social customs, and education practices that (a) supported the education of African American students in "separate but equal" schools and (b) denied the right of publicly supported education for children and youth with disabilities. Pickett (2003) identified six primary reasons that led LEAs to employ paraeducators in growing numbers over the last five decades: (a) court-ordered mandates requiring school districts to end the exclusion of children and youth with disabilities from a public school education; (b) provisions in the Education for All Handicapped Children Act of 1975 (P.L. 94-142) and subsequent federal laws requiring individualized education plans, individualized transitional plans for school-age learners with disabilities, and individualized family service plans for infants and toddlers and their parents; (c) amendments to federal laws that created Title I and other compensatory education programs to meet the needs of learners who live in poverty or come from educationally disadvantaged backgrounds and can benefit from personalized attention; (d) increasing enrollment in schools nationwide of learners from diverse racial, cultural, and language minority heritages; (e) continuing shortages of teachers in special and multilingual education, and many academic programs in urban and rural schools across the country; and (f) the addition over the last 20-plus years of new dimensions to traditionally recognized teacher roles.

In the 1950s, the first of a series of events that would have a profound impact on education practices and systems was a suit heard by the Supreme Court of the United States brought by parents of African American children and human and civil rights advocacy organizations. The goal of the landmark case, *Brown v. Board of Education* (1954) was to end segregation in the public schools. In their unanimous decision the justices ruled that social customs and laws that approved of serving African American children and youth in "separate but equal schools" were inherently unequal and that legally sanctioned segregation was unconstitutional.

Although *Brown v. Board of Education* had little direct impact on the employment of teacher aides, in the 1970s it served as a model for two federal lawsuits filed by parents and other advocates who were concerned that the rights of children and youth with disabilities were being overlooked. These cases included *Pennsylvania Association for Retarded Children v. Commonwealth of Pennsylvania* (1972) and *Mills v. Board of Education in the District of Columbia* (1972). These cases challenged the rights of states and local districts to exclude learners with disabilities from public schools. The decisions in both cases recognized the rights of school-age students, regardless of the severity or nature of their "handicap," to a free appropriate public education.

In the 1960s and 1970s, federal laws began to play an important part in ensuring that schools would comply with the mandates established by the court rulings. Provisions in the Elementary and Secondary Education Act of 1965 (ESEA) created Title I to better serve school-age learners from economically and educationally disadvantaged family backgrounds. In 1975, P.L. 94-142 contained federal mandates for programs serving children and youth with developmental, learning, physical, and sensory disabilities who were either underserved or not served by public schools in their community. At the core of each of the laws was a recognition of the value of learner-centered education programs to meet the needs of students with diverse learning- and language-related needs; however, P.L. 94-142 was the only law to require that education services for children and youth with disabilities be based on an individualized education plan (IEP). Thus, to provide teachers with the support that they required to plan and carry out IEPs for learners with disabilities, and to provide personalized attention for students with other learning- and language-related needs, there was a surge in the employment of teacher aides (Gartner, 1971; Kaplan, 1977; Pickett, 1989). In addition, during the 1960s and 1970s, changes in the nature of the roles of teacher aides were recognized by many LEAs, which began to replace the term *teacher aide* with the term *paraprofessional* in describing the newest members of education teams (Gartner, 1971; Pearl & Riessman, 1965).

P.L. 94-142 has been renamed twice, most recently in 2004. It is now known as the Individuals with Disabilities Education Improvement Act (IDEIA). Throughout the 1980s and 1990s IDEA was amended to require schools to provide preschool programs for young children ages 3 to 5 and transition services for teenagers. Other legislative actions encouraged but did not require schools or other provider agencies to develop early-intervention programs for infants and toddlers (ages birth to 2) with disabilities. The services provided by these programs are based on individualized family service plans (IFSPs) for young children and their parents. Individualized transition plans (ITPs) are required to prepare teenagers to move from school to work, or to post-secondary education and to live independently or with support in the community. As a result, the employment of paraprofessionals continued to gain momentum (Pickett, 1989, 1994).

Although the employment of paraprofessionals was increasing steadily and their responsibilities were becoming more complex and demanding, the need to establish or revise policies, personnel practices, and regulatory procedures to improve their ability to support the program and classroom management functions of teachers was rarely systematically scrutinized by SEAs or LEAs (Pickett, 1986, 1994). Moreover, it was even rarer to find examples of SEAs, LEAs, and IHEs working in concert to address an emerging need to prepare teachers to effectively integrate paraprofessionals into instructional teams. Lindemann and Beegle (1988) surveyed teacher education programs preparing students for careers in special education. They discovered that the vast majority did not address the roles of teachers as supervisors of paraeducators at either the undergraduate or the graduate level. Those that did prepare students to plan assignments for paraprofessionals and to direct and monitor their day-to-day performance, usually covered the curriculum content in about 1 hour.

By the late 1980s, only 11 states had certification or other regulatory systems that included standards for paraprofessional roles, preparation, and supervision. The remaining states chose to develop nonbinding administrative guidelines that placed the responsibility with LEAs for identifying roles for paraprofessionals, the skills and knowledge necessary for them to carry out their responsibilities, and standards for their training and supervision (Pickett, 1989). As a result, (a) distinctions in teacher and paraprofessional responsibilities were defined only in general terms or not at all; (b) similarities and differences in the roles and responsibilities of paraprofessionals working in all education programs administered by LEAs were not identified and standards for the core knowledge and skills needed by all paraprofessionals were not established; (c) teacher roles in directing and monitoring the day-to-day performance of paraprofessionals were not defined; and (d) paraeducator training, when it did exist, was sporadic and highly parochial, and did not provide a continuum of opportunities for career development.

Paraeducators in Education: The Present

Translating Research Into Practice

For the most part the issues described previously still remain, and in some cases they have become more pervasive. Over the last two decades, however, an increasing though limited number of researchers have begun to explore these and other issues. One of the most significant findings is that the vast majority of paraeducators spend all or part of their time assisting teachers or other licensed practitioners in the delivery of instructional and other direct services to learners and their parents. Most of the investigations have concentrated on identifying the range of responsibilities assigned to paraeducators in inclusive special education, transition, and early childhood programs for children and youth with developmental and other disabilities (Downing, Ryndak, & Clark, 2000; French, 2003b; Killoran, Templeman, Peters, & Udell, 2001; Passaro, Pickett, Latham, & HongBo, 1994; Riggs & Mueller, 2001; Rueda & Monzo, 2000). Other investigators have assessed the similarities and differences in the roles of paraeducators who (a) work in early childhood, elementary, middle, and secondary schools; and (b) are assigned to inclusive general and special education, Title I, and multilingual programs serving learners of different ages who have different learning needs (Daniels & McBride, 2001; Education and Training Voluntary Partnership, 2003; Pickett, 1999; Pickett & Granik, 2003; Recruiting New Teachers, 2005; Rueda & Monzo, 2000; Snodgrass, 1991). In addition, by the mid-1990s, a few research initiatives were beginning to focus on the emerging roles of teachers as team leaders and supervisors of paraeducators (Drecktrah, 2000; French, 2001, 2003a; French & Pickett, 1997; Pickett, 1999; Vasa & Steckelberg, 1998; Vasa, Steckelberg, & Pickett, 2003; Wallace, Jongho, Bartholomay, & Stahl, 2001). Still other researchers (a) assessed the effectiveness of paraeducator support for learners who have developmental, physical, and sensory disabilities, autism, and behavioral needs; and (b) tested training materials and strategies to prepare paraeducators to effectively facilitate inclusion of learners who have developmental, physical, and sensory disabilities, autism, and autism-like syndromes into general education classrooms, and reduce their social isolation by promoting peer interaction (Broer, Doyle, & Giangreco, 2005; Theoharis-Causton, & Malmgren, 2005; Ghere, York-Barr, & Sommerness, 2002; Giangreco, Backus, Chichoski-Kelly, Sherman, & Mavropoulos, 2003; Giangreco, Edelman, Broer, & Doyle, 2001; Giangreco, Edelman, Luiselli, & MacFarland, 1997; Werts, Zigmond, & Leeper, 2001). The various investigators used different methodologies, including mail surveys and follow-up calls, onsite observations, and structured interviews with administrators and school staff (principals, teachers, and paraeducators), parents, and students. Several themes are shared in many of the studies. A synthesis of the most significant findings includes the following:

1. Nationwide, the roles of paraeducators have continued to expand and are more complex and demanding. Paraeducators, teachers, and principals report that paraeducators participate in all phases of the instructional process and the delivery of other direct services for learners and their parents. In many cases their answers indicate a lack of awareness of the importance of maintaining the distinctions in teacher and paraeducator roles and responsibilities.

2. Studies aiming to identify differences and similarities in paraeducator responsibilities in all programmatic areas found more similarities in the nature of the tasks performed by paraeducators than differences.

3. When asked to describe their responsibilities, paraeducators frequently reported that in addition to engaging individual and small groups of students in learning activities, they also plan lessons and modify lessons and instructional strategies developed by teachers, and perform other tasks that are typically the responsibility of teachers. While this happens in all program areas, it is particularly apparent in classrooms and community-based training sites where paraeducators facilitate the inclusion of learners with disabilities into general education, and in compensatory programs where students receive personalized attention. While some paraeducators report there is time in the schedule for regularly scheduled meetings with teachers, the majority report that there is not.

4. When asked to describe their responsibilities for directing, monitoring, and planning tasks to be carried out by paraeducators, teachers nationwide responded similarly. The most frequent answer was: "We are a team, and we share ideas." In the case of general education teachers in classrooms where learners with disabilities are being educated, it is not unusual for teachers to reply that the paraeducator who has been assigned to support a learner knows what to do. Still other teachers reported that they do not have responsibility for directing and monitoring the day-to-day work of paraeducators; that is the role of the principal. In rare cases, however, teachers indicated that they do plan the instructional and other assignments that paraeducators participate in. Like paraeducators, the majority of teachers report that it is difficult to schedule time to meet with paraeducators.

5. Teachers reported that they have had little or no training at either the undergraduate or the graduate level or through continuing education to prepare them for their roles and responsibilities as team leaders and supervisors of paraeducators. Nor do their district's program descriptions or job descriptions contain information about their supervisory roles.

6. Paraeducators indicated that they receive little or no preparation related to the work they do with learners. Like teachers, their district's program or job descriptions do not contain information about the distinctions in teacher and paraeducator roles in the instructional process. And in some cases, paraeducators reported, districts do not always have job descriptions for instructional paraeducators.

The findings of the researchers who assessed the effectiveness of paraeducators who work with learners with developmental and other disabilities and spend all or part of their day in inclusive general education classrooms have contributed additional information that affects the roles and responsibilities of teachers and paraeducators. Some of these studies have consistently found that unskilled paraeducators, without meaning to, serve as barriers to achieving meaningful peer interaction, expanding self-reliance, and increasing academic performance. The results of the various studies stress the importance of training paraeducators to use positive interventions to facilitate and strengthen interactions among learners who have disabilities and their peers. Some, but not all, studies identify the need for more teacher involvement with the learners in order to reduce situations in which students with the greatest needs spend all or most of their school day with the personnel who have the least training. The problem is that few studies have moved beyond stressing the importance of direct involvement of teachers with learners who have disabilities in inclusive environments to developing policies and practices that assure that teachers: (a) are prepared for their roles as team leaders and supervisors of paraeducators, (b) are aware of teacher responsibilities that may not be delegated to paraeducators and those that may be shared with paraeducators, and (c) are prepared to plan tasks for paraeducators that include working with other students who can benefit from personalized instruction either individually or in small groups (thus enabling teachers to spend time with the learners who have disabilities) and developing learning activities to encourage and support interactions among *all* learners in the classroom.

For the first time, amendments to IDEA in 1997 recognized the need for SEAs to establish standards to ensure that *all* educators (including paraeducators) have the skills and knowledge necessary to meet the identified needs of learners with disabilities; moreover, provisions also recognized the need for more-effective supervision of paraeducators: "Paraeducators who are appropriately trained and supervised in accordance with state law, regulations or written policy may assist teachers with the delivery of special education and related services to children and youth with disabilities" [612(a)(15)]. Provisions in IDEIA 2004 concerned with assuring that paraeducators are highly skilled and well supervised are similar to those in IDEA 1997.

In 2001 the ESEA was given a new title—the No Child Left Behind Act (NCLB). Amendments to NCLB concerned with improving the performance of paraeducators are more specific than those in IDEA. Section 1119 of NCLB requires SEAs or LEAs to establish standards for the employment, roles and responsibilities and career development systems for paraeducators. The standards must include:

1. *Education and experiential requirements.* All paraeducators employed after the enactment of NCLB are required to have completed at least 2 years of study at an IHE; OR earned an associate's degree; OR met a rigorous standard of quality that demonstrates through a formal state or local academic assessment their ability to assist in instructing: (a) reading, language arts, writing, and mathematics, or (b) reading readiness, writing readiness, and mathematics readiness. All paraeducators, no matter when they were employed, must have a high school diploma, or its equivalent;

2. *Timelines for meeting standards.* All paraeducators employed prior to the passage of the new amendments to NCLB were required to meet the same standards by spring of 2006.

3. *Specifications regarding supervision.* NCLB is the first federal law to specify that paraeducators are to be directed by "qualified" teachers.

Although the provisions in NCLB concerned with paraeducator employment, preparation, and supervision do not necessarily apply to those employed in programs serving learners with developmental disabilities, it is important to note that many LEAs are using the standards when they employ new paraeducators and have asked paraeducators who were employed when NCLB was passed and signed into law to meet the same standards.

Changes in Teacher Roles and Responsibilities

It is not possible to discuss the roles and responsibilities of paraeducators without first looking at the evolution of the traditionally recognized responsibilities of teachers. Over the last two decades, intensive efforts have been made to reform education practices and restructure systems to improve the quality of education for all learners. Many of these initiatives have centered on empowering teachers, increasing their accountability for learner progress, and enhancing the status of the profession (Bauch & Goldring, 1998; Carnegie Forum on Education and the Economy, 1987; Daniels & McBride, 2001; Hammond, 1997; Lieberman & Miller, 2000; Pipho, 2000). One of the most significant outcomes of the reform efforts has been a redefinition of teacher roles: Just

TABLE 25.1

Teacher Roles in the Instructional Process

Teachers are responsible for:

- Developing lesson plans to meet curriculuma requirements and education objectives for learners

- Adapting lessons, instructional methods, and curricula to meet the learning needs of individual learners

- Developing behavior management and disciplinary plans

- Creating learner-centered, inclusive environments that respect the cultures, religions, lifestyles, and human rights of children, youth, parents, and staff

- Implementing district policies and procedures for protecting the health, safety, and well-being of learners and staff

- Involving parents in all aspects of their child's education

- Analyzing in collaboration with other licensed professional personnel results of standardized tests

- Developing functional (informal) assessment tools to document and evaluate learner progress and instructional needs

Adapted from: Pickett, A. L. (1999). *Strengthening teacher and paraeducator teams: Guidelines for paraeducator roles, supervision, and preparation.* New York: National Resource Center for Paraprofessionals, Center for Advanced Study in Education, Graduate Center, City University of New York.

510

as "teacher aide" no longer describes the roles of paraeducators, "classroom teacher" no longer adequately describes the roles of teachers. As members of school-based management teams, teachers join principals, parents, and other school staff to: (a) identify the learning needs of students in "their school," (b) establish program priorities to meet the identified needs, and (c) decide how to allocate limited fiscal, personnel, and technological resources to achieve program goals for all learners. In addition, general and special education teachers along with representatives of other professional disciplines and parents serve on program planning teams with responsibilities for developing IEPs, ITPs, or IFSPs for learners with disabilities.

Regardless of the level at which teachers work (preschool, elementary, middle, or secondary) or populations served (learners in inclusive general and special education classrooms, multilingual, Title I, and other compensatory programs), they are responsible for (a) diagnosing learner needs, (b) planning lessons to meet learning requirements, (c) adapting curriculum content and instructional strategies to meet the needs of individual learners, (d) engaging learners in instructional activities, (e) evaluating the effectiveness of the lessons on learner progress, and (f) establishing supportive learning environments that respect the rights of learners, their parents, and school personnel. Table 25.1 provides an overview of teacher roles in the different components of the instructional process and classroom management.

While paraeducators still perform clerical, monitoring, and other routine tasks, in most of their assignments they may spend as much as 90% of their time participating in different components of the instructional process (Education and Training Voluntary Partnership, 2003; Passaro et al., 1994; Pickett, 1999; Pickett & Granik, 2003; Study of Personnel Needs in Special Education, 2001). Currently in many programs administered by LEAs, teachers and paraeducators work in environments where distinctions in their roles are blurred. All too frequently paraeducators are viewed as assistant teachers and are assigned tasks that are teacher responsibilities and that should not be delegated. The primary distinction between teacher and paraeducator roles is that paraeducators serve as assistants to teachers in order to provide teachers with more time to diagnose learning needs and determine how best to meet the needs of individuals and groups of learners (French, 2003b; French & Pickett, 1997; Pickett & Safarik, 2003). For example, paraeducators assist teachers (a) in achieving the learning goals for children and youth by carrying out tasks developed and assigned to them by teachers, (b) with implementing district policies and procedures for protecting the health, safety, and well-being of learners and staff, (c) by providing individual or small-group

TABLE 25.2

Level 1 Paraeducator Roles

Working under the direction of teachers, Level 1 paraeducators:

- Assist teachers with the implementation of district policies and procedures for protecting the safety, health, and well-being of learners and staff.
- Carry out strategies developed by teachers that maintain supportive and inclusive environments, respect individual differences among learners, their parents, and school staff.
- Duplicate learning materials, prepare bulletin boards, and perform other routine tasks.
- Monitor learners in non-academic settings (lunchrooms, playgrounds), halls, and escort learners to and from other classrooms, media centers, buses.
- Reinforce learning activities initiated by teachers.

Adapted from: Pickett, A. L. (1999). *Strengthening teacher and paraeducator teams: Guidelines for paraeducator roles, supervision, and preparation.* New York: National Resource Center for Paraprofessionals, Center for Advanced Study in Education, Graduate Center, City University of New York.

instruction following plans developed by teachers, and (d) with documenting relevant information about learner performance (French, 2003a; French & Pickett, 1997; Pickett, 1999; Pickett & Safarik, 2003; Wallace et al., 2001).

Tables 25.2–25.4 show a model career ladder that recognizes a hierarchy of knowledge and skills paraeducators should demonstrate in order to advance through the different position levels. The roles of paraeducators in Level 1 positions (see Table 25.2) emphasize assisting teachers to maintain, safe, healthy, and supportive learning environments, performing routine clerical tasks, and maintaining learning centers. Paraeducators in Level 1 positions do not act independently. They typically work under the direction of more than one teacher, and the individual teachers are responsible for planning and monitoring the tasks they perform.

The tasks performed by Level 2 paraeducators (see Table 25.3) are primarily instructional in nature. Depending on SEA or LEA policy, Level 2 paraeducators usually work under the supervision of one teacher, or in some cases they may be directed by occupational or physical therapists. The responsibilities of the supervising teachers are to plan and schedule paraeducator tasks, provide on-the-job coaching,

TABLE 25.3

Responsibilities for Level 2 Paraeducators

Working under the direction of teachers, Level 2 paraeducators:

- Carry out team decisions as assigned by teachers or other professional practitioners.
- Participate in staff and team meeting as assigned by teachers.
- Assist teachers with implementing district policies and procedures for protecting the safety, health, and well-being of learners and staff.
- Share relevant information about learner performance to support the planning process.
- Follow plans and instructional strategies developed and introduced by teachers to review and reinforce lessons with individual learners or small groups.
- Assist learners with independent study projects assigned by the teacher.
- Implement behavior management programs developed by teachers for individual learners.
- Carry out functional (informal) assessment activities to assist teachers with documenting information about learner strengths and needs.
- Perform clerical and other routine classroom tasks assigned by the teacher.

Adapted from: Pickett, A. L. (1999). *Strengthening teacher and paraeducator teams: Guidelines for paraeducator roles, supervision, and preparation.* New York: National Resource Center for Paraprofessionals, Center for Advanced Study in Education, Graduate School, City University of New York.

TABLE 25.4

Responsibilities of Level 3 Paraeducators

Working under the direction of teachers, Level 3 paraeducators:

- Consult with teachers or other professional practitioners during regularly scheduled meetings to share information that will facilitate the inclusion of learners with disabilities into general education classrooms and support them in community-based learning environments.

- Document data using functional assessment instruments in assist teachers in evaluating learner needs.

- Implement lesson and behavior management plans developed and introduced by teachers to improve academic, social, and communication skills and increase self-esteem and self-reliance.

- Modify instructional activities for individual learners.

- Assist teachers with supporting and engaging parents in their child's education.

- Support students in community-based learning environments to prepare them to make the transition from to school to work, post-secondary education, and participation in the adult world.

- Familiarize employers and other members of the community with the needs of individual learners as required by the program or learner needs.

- Assist occupational and physical therapists, speech-language pathologists, and nurses to provide related services as required by learner needs.

- Assist teachers to maintain learner records required by the SEA or the LEA.

- Participate in IEP, ITP, and IFSP planning team meetings as required by learner or family needs.

Adapted from: Pickett, A. L., (1999). *Strengthening teacher and paraeducator teams: Guidelines for paraeducator roles, supervision, and preparation.* New York: National Resource Center for Paraprofessionals, Center for Advanced Study in Education, Graduate Center, City University of New York.

and monitor paraeducator performance. Level 2 paraeducators may have limited decision-making authority with regard to non-academic activities.

There are fewer restrictions on the participation of Level 3 paraeducators (see Table 25.4) in all phases of the instructional process or the delivery of related services to learners and their parents. Working under the direction of teachers or other licensed practitioners, Level 3 paraeducators engage learners or their families in activities planned by teachers that (a) strengthen physical, cognitive, and social skill development, (b) increase mastery of academic skills, (c) assist in functional and standardized assessment activities, (d) facilitate inclusion of learners with developmental disabilities into general education classrooms using strategies developed by teachers to encourage peer interactions and support development of increased independence, and (e) expand parental participation in their child's education. Level 3 paraeducators may work with more than one teacher or another professional practitioner (occupational therapist, physical therapist, speech-language pathologist, transition specialist) in classrooms or community-based learning environments. If Level 3 paraeducators work with one or more teachers or other professional personnel, it is more efficient to designate one person as the primary supervisor. The responsibilities of the designated supervisor are to coordinate the development of the paraeducators' work plan with the assistance of other team members, monitor the performance of the paraeducator, and provide on-the-job coaching to the paraeducator.

Other changes in paraeducator roles are attributable to growing numbers of children and youth enrolled in schools nationwide who come from diverse racial, cultural, and linguistic heritages (National Center for Education Statistics, 2000; Office of Special Education Programs and Rehabilitative Services, 2000; Recruiting New Teachers, 2005). Many paraeducators live in the neighborhood served by the schools where they work. They speak the languages and come from the same ethnic and cultural backgrounds as the learners and their families. As a result, bilingual paraeducators serve as mentors for teachers and other school personnel to help them understand how different cultural traditions, religious beliefs, and value systems influence the learning preferences and communication styles of children and youth. Paraeducators may also be asked to provide translation services for students, parents, and school staff.

Professional, Ethical, and Legal Responsibilities of Paraeducators

As key members of education teams, paraeducators have special relationships with learners, teachers and other school staff, families, and members of their communities. The effectiveness of these relationships depends not only on their ability to carry out their assigned tasks in a professional manner but also on their understanding of the ethical and legal responsibilities of their jobs. Demonstrating respect for the human and civil rights of learners, their parents, and colleagues; maintaining confidentiality about all information connected with students and their families; following district policies and procedures; being dependable and cooperative; and participating in opportunities for career development are just a few of the areas in which paraeducators have professional, legal, and ethical responsibilities (Heller & Gerlach, 2003). Table 25.5 contains an outline of paraeducator professional, legal, and ethical responsibilities.

TABLE 25.5
Paraeducator Professional, Ethical, and Legal Responsibilities

Paraeducators:

- Practice standards of professional and ethical conduct approved by the LEA.

- Respect the legal and human rights of learners, their families, and staff.

- Recognize and respect the distinctions in the roles of teachers and paraeducators.

- Perform assigned tasks under the direction of teachers and other professional practitioners in a manner consistent with guidelines established by the SEA, LEA, or professional organizations representing different areas of education and related services.

- Share information with parents about their child's performance as directed by the supervising teacher.

- Follow LEA procedures for maintaining confidentiality of written or oral records concerned with learner's academic performance and progress, results of formal and informal assessments, behaviors, lifestyles, health and medical history, and other personal information about students and their families.

- Share confidential information only with supervising teachers or other designated staff.

- Do not use language or actions that discriminate against learners, their families, or staff members based on differences in ability, race, culture, lifestyles, religion, or gender.

- Follow guidelines established by the LEA to protect the safety, health, and well-being of learners and staff.

- Follow the chain of command established by the LEA to address policy questions, systems issues, and personnel practices when problems cannot be resolved by the LEA's grievance procedure.

- Participate with administrators and other stakeholders in creating and implementing opportunities for paraeducator career development.

- Participate in opportunities for continuing education.

Source: Adapted from: Heller, W., & Gerlach, K. (2003). Professional and ethical responsibilities of team members. In A. L. Pickett & K. Gerlach (Eds.), *Supervising paraeducators in education settings: A team approach* (pp. 289–323). Austin, TX: PRO-ED.

TABLE 25.6

District Administrator Responsibilities for Paraeducator Management

District level administrators:

- Develop standards for the employment, preparation, supervision, assessment, and dismissal of paraeducators.

- Define the roles of teachers in directing and monitoring the day-to-day work of paraeducators.

- Develop performance standards for paraeducators.

- Develop job descriptions for paraeducators that (a) recognize differences in teacher and paraeducator roles, (b) include core skills required by all paraeducators and recognize differences in levels of knowledge and skills to carry out tasks in different positions, and (c) include pre- and in-service training and experiential employment requirements for paraeducators.

- Develop and provide a continuum of career development opportunities for paraeducators.

- Negotiate contractual agreements that include salaries, benefits, job descriptions, employment requirements, and reasons for dismissal.

Adapted from: Vasa, S. F., Steckelberg, A., & Pickett, A. L. (2003). Paraeducators in education settings: Administrative issues. In A. L. Pickett & K. Gerlach (Eds.), *Supervising paraeducators in education settings: A team approach* (pp. 289–324). Austin, TX: PRO-ED.

514

Paraeducator Management and Supervision

Tables 25.6 and 25.7 outline the differences in the responsibilities of LEA administrators and principals in the management of paraeducators. District-level personnel have the overall responsibility for developing policies and personnel practices for the employment, preparation, and supervision of paraeducators. The responsibilities of principals connected with supervising paraeducators center on creating school

TABLE 25.7

Principal Roles in the Management of Paraeducators

Principals:

- Implement district policies and personnel practices connected with the employment, preparation, supervision, and dismissal of paraeducators.

- Create school environments that recognize the contributions all staff make to the delivery of effective education for all learners.

- Interview candidates for paraeducator positions and when possible include teachers in the selection process.

- Evaluate the overall performance of paraeducators and their supervising teachers.

- Ensure that teachers and paraeducators are aware of the differences in their roles and responsibilities.

- Ensure that teachers are aware of their responsibilities for directing and monitoring the day-to-day work of paraeducators.

- Schedule times for teachers and paraeducators to meet and discuss: (a) learner goals and plans for achieving the goals, (b) paraeducator assignments, and (c) opportunities for on-the-job coaching and feedback.

- Ensure that teachers and paraeducators are aware of LEA and school procedures for protecting the safety, health, and well-being of learners and staff.

- Share information with paraeducators about training opportunities, resource materials, state or national conferences concerned with issues of interest to them, changes in LEA or SEA policies that affect their employment, job descriptions, training, salaries, benefits, and extracurricular activities and social events for staff, learners, and parents.

- Share information with teachers about training and materials to enhance their ability to effectively integrate paraeducators into instructional teams.

Adapted from: Vasa, S. F., Steckelberg, A., & Pickett, A. L. (2003). Paraeducators in education setting: Administrative issues. In A. L. Pickett & K. Gerlach (Eds.), Supervising *Paraeducators in education settings: A team approach* (pp. 289–324). Austin, TX: PRO-ED.

TABLE 25.8

Teacher Supervisory Roles

Supervising teachers:

- Plan work assignments for paraeducators based on program objectives, learner need, and the readiness of paraeducators to perform instructional tasks.

- Develop daily and weekly schedules for paraeducators.

- Plan and delegate non-instructional activities to paraeducators (e.g., inventorying supplies, filing information, duplicating instructional materials, escorting learners, reviewing parental permission forms for learners to participate in special events.

- Monitor and document the day-to-day performance of paraeducators.

- Provide on-the-job training and feedback to effectively integrate paraeducators into the instructional process and the team.

- Share relevant information with principals about the strengths and any additional training needs paraeducators may require.

Adapted from: Pickett, A. L. (1999). *Strengthening teacher and paraeducator teams: Guidelines for paraeducator roles, supervision, and preparation.* New York: National Resource Center for Paraprofessionals, Center for Advanced Study in Education, Graduate Center, City University of New York.

environments that support and recognize the value of teacher and paraeducator teams and on carrying out district policies that affect the performance of the teams.

Mandates in NCLB and guidelines in IDEA recognize the need for teachers to participate in directing and monitoring the day-to-day work of paraeducators. To work effectively with paraeducators and involve them in instructional and other classroom activities, teachers have several supervisory responsibilities, described in Table 25.8.

Paraeducators in Education: The Future

Addressing the Issues and Establishing the Systems

Currently, reliance on a greater number of paraeducators, with particular emphasis on their learner support and instructional responsibilities, has not resulted in the development of state or local policies, standards, and infrastructures needed to ensure that paraeducators and the teachers they assist are prepared to carry out their team roles. Indeed, ongoing research conducted by the National Resource Center for Paraprofessionals (Pickett et al., 2003) reveals little evidence of significant progress being made toward achieving the intent of NCLB and IDEA that *all* paraeducators be well trained, highly qualified, and appropriately supervised. Nationwide standardized career development programs for paraeducators are almost nonexistent. When they do exist, they remain highly parochial and do not recognize the similarity in paraeducator roles and responsibilities across different programs and learning environments. They also are not linked to advancement through different levels of paraeducator positions or to the professional ranks based on career preferences (Pickett, 2003).

TABLE 25.9

Key Policy Questions That Require the Attention of Stakeholders

- Are distinctions in teacher and paraeducator roles clearly defined by state or local policies?
- Are there statewide or local standards for the employment, roles, and preparation of paraeducators?
- Is there a continuum of opportunities for career development and advancement for paraeducators?
- Is there a statewide credentialing system or other mechanisms to ensure that paraeducators have mastered the skills they need to work in different paraeducator positions or programs? Is it mandatory or nonbinding?
- Are there standards for teacher roles in the supervision of paraeducators? Are the standards part of the state's licensure requirements for teachers in any disciplines?
- What impact do federal mandates and funding, state reimbursement policies, and collective bargaining agreements have on the employment, roles, supervision, and preparation of paraeducators?
- What barriers exist in our state to the development of policies, standards, or systems to support and strengthen the performance of teacher and paraeducator teams? What resources are available to support the development of standards and infrastructures? How can different stakeholders contribute to the development of policies, standards, and systems?

Adapted from: Pickett, A. L. (2003). Paraeducators in education settings: Framing the issues. In A. L. Pickett & K. Gerlach (Eds.), *Supervising paraeducators in educational settings: A team approach*. Austin, TX: PRO-ED.

516

The Roles of State Education Agencies

Each of the policy, systemic, and personnel development issues described in the previous sections needs to be systematically explored, statewide needs identified, and policies and systems developed. Several policy questions and systemic issues are central to the conceptualization and implementation of standards and infrastructures to enhance and support the performance of teacher and paraeducator teams. They cannot be answered in isolation. A primary task of SEA personnel is to create and nurture partnerships among LEAs, IHEs, and professional organizations representing different disciplines, unions, and other stakeholders to identify state and local needs and develop strategies to meet the needs. Table 25.9 contains important policy questions that require collaborative attention of the partnerships, and Table 25.10 presents the benefits of developing credentialing systems to ensure that paraeducators have mastered the skills required by different positions or programs.

TABLE 25.10

Benefits of Paraeducator Certification

- All learners will be better served and the quality of education and related services will be improved with the availability of a highly skilled paraeducator workforce.
- Certification for paraeducators will ensure that paraeducators have mastered skills and knowledge required to support and supplement teacher program and administrative functions.
- Certification will establish clear distinctions in the complexity of the roles and responsibilities that are associated with different paraeducator positions and program assignments.
- Certification will help establish and maintain infrastructures for career development and advancement for paraeducators.
- Certification will serve as a method for recognizing the contributions paraeducators make to the delivery of education and related services for all learners who can benefit from individualized programs and personalized attention.

Adapted from: Pickett, A. L. (1999). *Strengthening teacher and paraeducator teams: Guidelines for paraeducator roles, supervision, and preparation.* New York: National Resource Center for Paraprofessionals, Center for Advanced Study in Education, Graduate Center, City University of New York.

Glossary

Competencies—Specific required skills and knowledge of paraeducators who are assigned to different programs or positions.

Credentialing—Systems designed to certify that paraeducators have mastered the knowledge and skills they require for entry level or advancement to higher-level positions. Such credentialing systems may be called permits, licenses, or certificates.

Institutions of higher education (IHEs)—Two-year colleges that offer AA or AAS degree or certificate programs for paraeducators, and 4-year colleges or universities that prepare teachers or other professional practitioners at the baccalaureate, master's, and doctoral levels.

Local education agencies (LEA)—Local or intermediate school districts that may have responsibility for providing early-childhood, elementary, middle, and secondary education programs and services to children and youth with developmental disabilities and other learning- and language-related needs.

Paraeducator—Paraprofessional, teacher or instructional assistant, teacher aide, transition trainer, job coach, occupational and physical therapy aide or assistant, speech-language pathology assistant, health-care aide or assistant, and home visitor are just a few of the titles for education and related-services support personnel who work under the direction of teachers or other professional practitioners and assist them with delivery of instructional and other direct services for learners or their parents.

Skill standards—Statements that describe job functions and responsibilities related to competency areas established for an occupation or a profession. Standards include skills, knowledge, and performance indicators to ensure that individuals have mastered the skills required by their position. The skills may be learned on the job or during preservice training.

Stakeholders—Agencies or organizations with responsibility for improving the quality of education and related services for children and youth with developmental or other learning needs. They may include state and local education agencies, 2- and 4-year IHEs, unions, professional organizations representing different disciplines, and advocacy groups concerned with protecting the human and civil right of learners and their families.

State education agency (SEA)—A department of education, department of public instruction, or an agency with another title that is responsible for establishing and administering statewide policies, regulations, or guidelines to ensure that all education personnel (including paraeducators) are highly skilled.

Supervisors—Teachers and other professional practitioners who are responsible for integrating paraeducators into instructional and related-services teams. Their supervisory responsibilities include planning, scheduling, and assigning duties to paraeducators on the basis of their training or demonstrated ability to perform the tasks, directing and monitoring the day-to-day work of paraeducators, providing on-the-job training to paraeducators to enhance the performance of paraeducators, and sharing relevant information with principals about the strength and training needs of paraeducators.

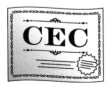

Knowledge and Skills for Entry-Level Special Education Teachers of Students With Developmental Disabilities Standards Addressed in This Chapter

Principle 1: Foundations

DD1K2 Continuum of placement and services available for individuals with developmental disabilities.

DD1K4 Trends and practices in the field of developmental disabilities.

Principle 5: Learning Environments/Social Interaction

DD5S1 Provide instruction in community-based settings.

DD5S5 Plan instruction for individuals with developmental disabilities in a variety of placement settings.

Principle 7: Instructional Planning

DD7K1   Model career/vocational transition programs for individuals with developmental disabilities, including vocational transition.

DD7S2   Plan and implement instruction for individuals with developmental disabilities that is both age-appropriate and ability-appropriate.

DD7S4   Design, implement, and evaluate specialized instructional programs for persons with developmental disabilities that enhance social participation across environments.

Web Site Resources

American Federation of Teachers
http://www.aft.org/pubs-reports/prsp/SkillsStandards.pdf

The Education and Training Volunteer Partnership (ETVP) has established Skill Standards for Frontline Workers in Education and Training. Members of the partnership are the National Education Association and the American Association of Community Colleges.

Council for Exceptional Children (CEC)
www.cec.sped.org

Information on the CEC knowledge and skills standards for beginning paraeducators in special education.

National Resource Center for Paraprofessionals in Special Education (NRCP)
www.nrcpara.org

Located at Utah State University and the University of Minnesota. A database and current information about changes in policies developed by states to meet the requirements of NCLB and IDEA, technical assistance, skill standards, instructional and technical assistance materials, online newsletter, and annual conference for administrators, paraeducators, personnel developers, and other stakeholders.

PARA2 Center
http://www.paracenter.org

Located at the University of Colorado in Denver. Information about training based on materials developed by the center to prepare paraeducators.

References

Bauch, P. A., & Goldring, E. R. (1998). Parent-teacher participation in the context of school governance. *Peabody Journal of Education, 73*, 15–35.

Broer, S. M., Doyle, M. B., & Giangreco, M. F. (2005). Perspectives of students with intellectual disabilities about their experiences with paraprofessional support. *Exceptional Children, 71*, 415–430.

Brown v. Board of Education, 374 U.S. 483 (1954).

Carnegie Forum on Education and the Economy. (1987). *A nation prepared: Teachers for the 21st century.* New York: Carnegie Corporation of New York.

Cruickshank, W., & Herring, N. (1957). *Assistants for teachers of exceptional children.* Syracuse, NY: Syracuse University Press.

Daniels, V. I., & McBride, A. (2001). Paraeducators as critical team members: Redefining roles and responsibilities. *National Association of Secondary School Principals Bulletin, 85*(623), 66–74.

Downing, J. E., Ryndak, D. L., & Clark, D. (2000). Paraeducators in inclusive classrooms: Their own perspectives. *Remedial and Special Education, 21*, 171–181.

Drecktrah, M. E. (2000). Preservice teacher preparation to work with paraeducators. *Teacher Education, 23*, 157–164.

Education for All Handicapped Children Act of 1975, 20 U.S.C. § 1400 *et seq.*

Education and Training Voluntary Partnership. (2003). *Skill standards for frontline workers in education and training.* Retrieved October 28, 2005, from http://www.etvp.org

Elementary and Secondary Education Act of 1965, 20 U.S.C. § 7269 *et seq.*

French, N. K. (2001). Supervising paraprofessionals: A survey of teacher practices. *Journal of Special Education, 35*, 41–53.

French, N. K. (2003a). Management of paraeducators. In A. L. Pickett & K. Gerlach (Eds.), *Supervising paraeducators in educational settings: A team approach* (pp. 97–172). Austin, TX: PRO-ED.

French, N. K. (2003b). Paraeducators in special education programs. *Focus on Exceptional Children, 36*(2), 1–16.

French, N. K., & Pickett, A. L. (1997). The utilization of paraprofessionals in special education: Issues for teacher educators. *Teacher Education and Special Education, 20*(1), 61–73.

Fund for the Advancement of Education. (1961). *Decade of experiment.* New York: Ford Foundation.

Gartner, A. (1971). *Paraprofessionals and their performance: A survey of education, health, and social services programs.* New York: Praeger.

Ghere, G., York-Barr, J., & Sommerness, J. (2002). *Supporting students with disabilities in inclusive schools: A curriculum for job embedded development.* Minneapolis, MN: University of Minnesota.

Giangreco, M. F., Backus, L., Chichoski-Kelly, E., Sherman, P., & Mavropoulos, Y. (2003). Paraeducator training materials to facilitate inclusion: Initial field test data. *Rural Special Education Quarterly, 22*(1), 17–27.

Giangreco, M. F., Edelman, S. W., Broer, S. M., & Doyle, M. B. (2001). Paraprofessional support of students with disabilities: Literature from the past decade. *Exceptional Children, 68*, 485–498.

Giangreco, M. F., Edelman, S. W., Luiselli, T. E., & MacFarland, S. C. Z. (1997). Helping or hovering? Effects of instructional assistant proximity on students with disabilities. *Exceptional Children, 64*, 7–18.

Hammond, L. D. (1997). *The right to learn: A blueprint for creating schools that work.* San Francisco: Jossey-Bass.

Heller, W., & Gerlach, K. (2003). Professional and ethical responsibilities of team members. In A. L. Pickett & K. Gerlach (Eds.), *Supervising paraeducators in education setting: A team approach* (pp. 289–323). Austin: PRO-ED.

Individuals with Disabilities Education Act Amendments of 1997, 20 U.S.C. § 1400 *et seq.* (1997).

Individuals with Disabilities Education Improvement Act of 2004, 20 U.S.C. § 1400 *et seq.* (2004).

Kaplan, G. (1977). *From aide to teacher: The story of the career opportunities program.* Washington, DC: U.S. Government Printing Office.

Killoran, J., Templeman, T. P., Peters, J., & Udell, T. (2001). Identifying paraprofessional competencies for early intervention and early childhood special education. *Teaching Exceptional Children, 34*(1), 68–78.

Lieberman, A., & Miller, L. (2000). A new synthesis for a new century. In R. S. Brandt (Ed.), *Education in a new era* (pp. 47–66). Alexandria, VA: Association for Supervision and Curriculum Development.

Lindemann, D. P., & Beegle, G. P. (1988). Preservice teacher training and the use of classroom paraprofessionals. *Teacher Education and Special Education, 11*, 183–186.

Mills v. Board of Education of the District of Columbia, 348 Supp. 866 (DC, 1972).

National Center for Education Statistics. (2000). *Education statistics: Elementary and secondary schools and staffing survey.* Washington, DC: U.S. Department of Education, Office of Education Research.

No Child Left Behind Act of 2001, 20 U.S.C. § 6301 *et seq.* (2001).

Office of Special Education Programs and Rehabilitative Services. (2000). *22nd annual report to Congress on the implementation of the Individuals with Disabilities Education Act.* Washington, DC: U.S. Department of Education.

Passaro, P., Pickett, A. L., Latham, G., & HongBo, W. (1994). The training and support needs of paraprofessionals in rural special education settings. *Rural Special Education Quarterly, 13*(4), 3–9.

Pearl, A., & Riessman, F. (1965). *New careers for the poor: The non-professional in human services.* New York: Free Press.

Pennsylvania Association for Retarded Children v. Commonwealth of Pennsylvania, 343 F. Supp. 279 (ED, PA 1972).

Pickett, A. L. (1986). *Paraprofessionals in education: The state of the art.* New York: National Resource Center for Paraprofessionals, Center for Advanced Study in Education, Graduate Center, City University of New York.

Pickett, A. L. (1989). *Restructuring the schools: The role of paraprofessionals.* Washington, DC: Center for Policy Study, National Governors' Association.

Pickett, A. L. (1994). *Paraeducators in the education workforce.* Washington, D.C.: National Education Association.

Pickett, A. L. (1999). *Strengthening and supporting teacher and paraeducator teams: Guidelines for paraeducator roles, supervision, and preparation.* New York: National Resource Center for Paraprofessionals, Center for Advanced Study in Education, Graduate Center, City University of New York.

Pickett, A. L. (2003). Paraeducators in education settings: Framing the issues. In A. L. Pickett & K. Gerlach (Eds.), *Supervising paraeducators in educational settings: A team approach* (pp. 1–44). Austin, TX: PRO-ED.

Pickett, A. L., & Granik, L. (2003). *Factors related to paraprofessional roles, career development, and preparation.* Albany, NY: New York State United Teachers.

Pickett, A. L., Likens, M., & Wallace, T. (2003). *A state of the art report on paraeducators in education and related services.* Logan, UT: National Resource Center for Paraprofessionals in Education, Utah State University and University of Minnesota.

Pickett, A. L., & Safarik, L. (2003). Team roles in classrooms and other learning environments. In A. L. Pickett & K. Gerlach (Eds.), *Supervising paraeducators in educational settings: A team approach* (pp. 45–96). Austin, TX: PRO-ED.

Pipho, C. (2000). Governing the American dream of universal public education. In R. S. Brandt (Ed.), *Education in a new era* (pp. 5–19). Alexandria, VA: Association for Supervision and Curriculum Development.

Recruiting New Teachers. (2005). *Preparing highly qualified paraeducators: A guidebook for supporting effective career development.* Belmont, MA: Author.

Riggs, C. G., & Mueller, P. H. (2001). Employment of paraeducators in inclusive settings. *Journal of Special Education, 35*(1), 54–62.

Rueda, R. S., & Monzo, L. D. (2000). *Apprentices for teaching: Professional development issues surrounding the collaborative relationship between teachers and paraeducators.* Washington, DC: Center for Research, Diversity, and Excellence.

Snodgrass, A. S. (1991). *Actual and preferred practices of employment, placement, supervision, and evaluation of teacher aides in Idaho school districts.* Unpublished doctoral dissertation, University of Idaho, Moscow.

Study of Personnel Needs in Special Education. (2001). *The role of paraeducators in special education: Study of personnel needs in special education.* Retrieved October 28, 2005, from http://ferdig.coe.ufl.edu/spense/parasFinal.doc

Theoharis-Causton, J. N., & Malmgren, K. W. (2005). Increasing peer interactions for students with severe disabilities via paraprofessional training. *Exceptional Children, 71,* 431–444.

Vasa, S. F., & Steckelberg, A. L. (1998). How paraeducators learn on the Web. *Teaching Exceptional Children, 30,* 54–59.

Vasa, S. F., Steckelberg, A. L., & Pickett, A. L. (2003). Paraeducators in education settings: Administrative issues. In A. L. Pickett & K. Gerlach (Eds.), *Supervising paraeducators in education setting: A team approach* (pp. 255–288). Austin, TX: PRO-ED.

Wallace, T., Jongho, S., Bartholomay, T., & Stahl, B. J. (2001). Knowledge and skills for teachers supervising the work of paraeducators. *Exceptional Children, 67,* 520–533.

Werts, M. G., Zigmond, N., & Leeper, D. C. (2001). Paraprofessional proximity and academic engagement: Students with disabilities in primary aged classrooms. *Education and Training in Mental Retardation and Developmental Disabilities, 36,* 424–440.

26

Creating Inclusive Schools:

Changing Roles and Strategies

Darlene E. Perner and Gordon L. Porter

Summary

This chapter discusses the importance of establishing a vision and a set of values for inclusive education, defines two specific models that provide support to classroom teachers, and gives examples of how they work. The support teacher model offers one way to assist general education teachers in developing practical strategies and activities for their classrooms, and the multilevel instructional approach provides a framework for planning and implementing classroom instruction.

Learning Outcomes

After reading this chapter, you should be able to:

- Describe what is meant by inclusive education for students with disabilities.

- List and describe at least seven important factors identified as facilitating successful inclusion.

- Develop a set of belief statements that reflect the philosophy of inclusion.

- Describe the role of the support teacher in assisting classroom teachers with inclusion.

- Compare and contrast different co-teaching approaches.

- Describe the concept of multilevel instruction and explain how it can be used to support the inclusion of students with developmental disabilities in general education classes.

Introduction

Throughout the world, departments and ministries of education are setting policies on *inclusive education* (van Kraayenoord, 2003). In a 1999 report on inclusive education in eight nations, the Organization for Economic Co-operation and Development (OECD, 1999) concluded:

> From organizational, curriculum and pedagogical perspectives, given certain safeguards, there is no reason to maintain generally segregated provisions for disabled students in public education systems. In fact, the changes to the ways that schools function in areas such as pedagogy and curriculum development, and in how they are supported by outside agencies as a result of inclusive practices seem only to bring benefits to all students, disabled and non-disabled alike. (p. 14)

The segregated special education model still widely in use is becoming outmoded. This is the assertion particularly of those who suggest that inclusion is the only model that meets both the educational and the human rights needs of children with developmental disabilities (Baglieri & Knopf, 2004; Perner, 2004; UNESCO, 2003). Controversy in this area is not new. The educational program and school placement of students with developmental disabilities have been passionate topics for both those who work in special education and those who work in general education.

Major Factors That Facilitate the Successful Inclusion of Students With Disabilities in General Education Classrooms

Over the past two decades, numerous inclusive education programs have been implemented throughout the United States (Burstein, Sears, Wilcoxen, Cabello, & Spagna, 2004; Lipsky & Gartner, 1999; National Center on Educational Restructuring and Inclusion, 1994; Sailor & Roger, 2005) and Canada (Bunch, 1997; Crawford & Porter, 1992; Hansen, 2001; Roeher Institute, 2003), as well as in Britain (Armstrong, Armstrong, & Barton, 2000; Department for Education and Employment, 1997; Rose, 2001), Australia (Ashman & Elkins, 1998; Forlin, 1997), and other countries, such as South Africa, Mexico, and Panama.

Many factors that facilitate inclusion and improve educational programming of all students in inclusive environments have been identified (e.g., CEC Working Forum on Inclusive Schools, 1994; Crawford & Porter, 1992, 2004; Kugelmass, 2006; National Center on Educational Restructuring and Inclusion, 1994; Perner, 1991, 1993, 1997, 1998, 2004; Sapon-Shevin, 1994; Walther-Thomas, Korinek, McLaughlin & Williams, 2000). For example, the CEC Working Forum on Inclusive Schools (1994) described 12 features that characterize inclusive schools: sense of community, leadership, high standards, collaboration and cooperation, changing roles and responsibilities, array of services, partnership with parents, flexible learning environments, strategies based on research, new forms of accountability, access, and continuing professional development. The National Center on Educational Restructuring and Inclusion (1994) identified seven factors for successful inclusion: visionary leadership, collaboration, refocused use of assessment, supports for staff and students, funding, effective parental involvement, and models and classroom practices that support inclusion. Walther-Thomas et al. (2000) more recently distinguished seven essential features: collaborative culture, shared leadership, coherent vision, comprehensive planning, adequate resources, sustained implementation, and continuous development and improvement. Giangreco (1997) identified common features of successful inclusive schools: collaborative teamwork, shared framework, family involvement, general educator ownership, clear role relationships among professionals, effective use of support staff, meaningful individualized education programs (IEPs), and procedures for evaluating effectiveness. Perner (1998) identified critical factors for successful inclusion that cover both school and classroom practices: school-based problem-solving team, support teacher as a collaborative consultant, instructional strategies for accommodating diverse learners (e.g., multilevel instruction and cooperative learning), ongoing professional development, teacher assistants, parent involvement, and student services team. Clearly many features facilitate the successful inclusion of students with disabilities. Table 26.1 shows the most common features found by a number of researchers, among them collaboration and cooperation, roles and responsibilities (changing and clearly defined), partnerships with parents and families, effective practices and flexible learning environments, continuing professional development, supports and resources for staff and students, and accountability and evaluating effectiveness. Although the terminology of the categories assigned by the researchers varies, the descriptions of the categories were the reference for Table 26.1.

Providing appropriate services and effective supports to students with developmental disabilities is of primary concern to special educators. Many practitioners and researchers have stressed the importance of supporting classroom teachers in integrated and inclusive settings (McLeskey & Waldron, 2002a; Mundschenk, Foley, & Swedburg, 2005; Simpson, de Boer-Ott, & Smith-Myles, 2003; Webber, 2005). O'Neil (1994) asked Sapon-Shevin to define inclusion:

> The vision of inclusion is that all children would be served in their neighborhood schools in *regular classrooms* with children their own age. The idea is that these schools would be restructured so that they are supportive, nurturing communities that really meet the needs of all the children within them: rich in resources and support for both students and teachers. (p. 7)

Finally, as we proceed with inclusion we must focus on two areas identified by McLeskey and Waldron (2002b) in terms of the changes that must occur in our schools. After years of working with inclusive schools and change, they indicated that the focus must be on: (a) the needs of all students rather than the needs of only those students with disabilities, and (b) "school improvement" rather than the referent "inclusion."

In this and the following chapter, a foundation for inclusive education is emphasized and supported by strategies for developing and implementing inclusive education for students with developmental disabilities. The focus is on providing various types of support to classroom teachers who are involved in inclusive education and strategies to

TABLE 26.1

Common Features for Successful Inclusion

	CEC (1994)	NCERI (1994)	Walther-Thomas et al. (2000)	Giangreco (1997)	Perner (1998)
Leadership	X	X	X		
Collaboration and cooperation	X	X	X	X	X
Roles and responsibilities	X		X	X	X
Partnership with parents/ family involvement	X	X	X	X	X
Effective practices/flexible learning environments	X	X	X	X	X
Continuing professional development	X		X		X
Supports/resources for staff and students	X	X	X	X	X
Accountability/evaluating effectiveness	X		X	X	

Note: CEC = Council for Exceptional Children; NCERI = National Center on Educational Restructuring and Inclusion.

assist these teachers. The supports and strategies identified are directed to both school administrators and teachers. Also included is a description of the support teacher (collaborative teacher) and multilevel instruction models that have been developed and used successfully in schools (Perner, 1997; Porter, Collicott, & Larsen, 2000; UNESCO, 2004). In the next chapter, a number of strategies are identified related to planning, implementing, and sustaining inclusive schools.

Inclusion and Students With Developmental Disabilities

The discourse about the utility of inclusion for students with developmental disabilities takes two forms. For students with significant developmental disabilities, functional life skills cannot be taught in general education classes where the emphasis is primarily on academic learning. For students with mild developmental disabilities, the fear is that they will be "lost" in the general education classroom and that the extra supports that had been provided in special education classes will be squeezed out of the system in the interests of cost cutting and fiscal restraint (Hastings & Oakford, 2003). Although these concerns are legitimate, many instances have been documented in which barriers have been overcome by the implementation of a sound inclusive program (Burstein et al., 2004; Organization for Economic Co-operation and Development, 1999; Sailor & Roger, 2005).

525

In the case of students with significant developmental disabilities, direct and indirect supports have continued to be available, and new strategies have been developed to ensure that the students benefit from classroom activities and interactions. Systematic planning has been used to help meet the unique needs of students in the context of the general education classroom. Life skills can be taught and reinforced at times when they are connected to their function. For example, toileting skills can be dealt with when the child needs to go to the toilet, with a paraprofessional providing support and instruction at the same time. A student can be taught money skills during lunch or recess time when he or she buys food or a treat at the school cafeteria or canteen. Community-based instruction, an important component for students, can be part of an inclusive school day.

The situation for students with mild disabilities is somewhat different because it is more difficult for the general education teacher to determine individual needs. Some degree of collaborative assistance is helpful to classroom teachers so that they can adequately address these students' needs. The literature (e.g., Crawley, Hayden, Cade, & Baker-Kroczynski, 2002; Dunn, 1968; Idol, 2006; Kilgore, Griffin, Sindelar, & Webb, 2002; Rea, McLaughlin, & Walther-Thomas, 2002) supports general education class placement for students with mild disabilities, while ensuring that teachers have direct assistance from paraprofessionals in their classrooms and from other experienced, supportive professionals. It is apparent that consultative personnel need to be available to general education teachers so that teachers can provide direct service to students with developmental disabilities in their classrooms (Hanko, 2004; Organization for Economic Co-operation and Development, 1999; Perner, Porter, & Padora, 2003; Simpson, Smith-Myles, Simpson, & Ganz, 2005; Webber, 2005; Weiner, 2003; Wolfe & Hall, 2003).

The effective and emerging school and classroom strategies described here support the creation of successful inclusive schools. They are not the only practices needed to ensure successful inclusion of students, but they are among the most critical.

Vision and Beliefs

Accomplishing significant change in any organization rich in history and practices requires a major focus on the process of change itself. Keilty (1994) and Sarason (1982) described the immutable nature of school organization and practice in public school settings and how difficult it is to bring about change. Fullan and Steigelbauer (1991) added a great deal to the discussion of how change in education can be understood and achieved, and McLeskey and Waldron (2002a) and Walther-Thomas et al. (2000) have made substantive contributions with regard to school change and inclusive schools. Burstein et al. (2004) described a change model that was developed and implemented to successfully promote inclusive schools. As cited in Porter and Richler (1991), Fullan suggested that change in special education is particularly complex because of the issues involved and that highly skilled leadership is required to meet this challenge. He noted:

> The solutions to inclusion are not easily achieved. It is complex both in the nature and degree of change required to identify and implement solutions that work. Given what change requires—persistence, coordination, follow-up, conflict resolution, and the like—leadership at all levels is required. (p. ii)

In this context, it is clear that integrating students in general education classes or creating inclusive schools requires strong leadership based on a well-defined vision of the value of integration or inclusion. It is essential that the shared beliefs and principles of a school team are well articulated and communicated both internally and externally.

In her review of research on inclusion, Zeph (1994) identified six values commonly associated with developing successful inclusion models and establishing a sense of school community: respect for diversity, recognition of gifts and talents for all, ability to listen and understand before trying to be understood, spirit of cooperation, desire and ability to collaborate, and ability to establish a positive climate. It is important that schools and classrooms are welcoming to staff, students, families, and the community. It is critical that teachers create a welcoming classroom, a learning environment where all students have a sense that their classroom and school are a community that they belong to (see Perner, 2004, for strategies to create positive learning environments).

Each individual school needs to develop its unique statement of beliefs that will help to facilitate a "sense of community" within the school. Some schools have been able to frame their beliefs based on provincial or state legislation and/or policies. For example, the Department of Education in the Province of New Brunswick, in conjunction with school districts, has developed a set of beliefs and principles that are considered to be the foundation of an inclusive education policy (New Brunswick Department of Education, 1994). Schools and school districts continue to use these beliefs and principles as a basis for their own statements:

1. All children can learn.

2. All children attend age-appropriate regular classrooms in their local schools.

3. All children receive appropriate educational programs.

4. All children receive a curriculum relevant to their needs.

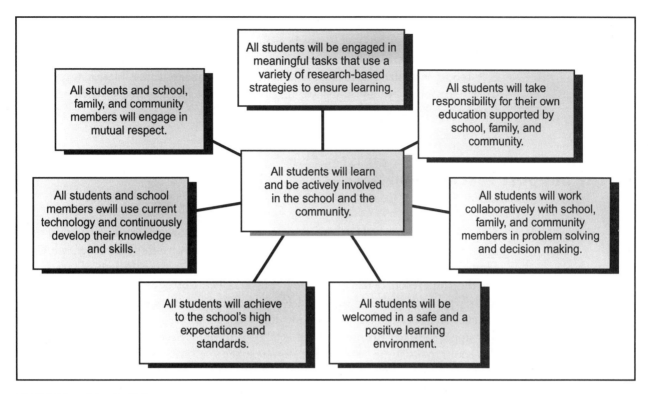

FIGURE 26.1. School belief statements.

5. All children participate in co-curricular and extracurricular activities.

6. All children benefit from cooperation among home, school and community. (New Brunswick Department of Education, 1994, p. 1)

Another example of belief statements that may be used to guide a school in developing a more inclusive setting is provided in Figure 26.1.

The Changing Role of the Special Education Teacher

An inclusive educational program, by definition, mandates a different role for school-based special education staff. Special education teachers and resource teachers no longer provide direct instructional service to students who are now part of the general education class. Several models for a new role have evolved in individual schools and school districts, depending on how the transition to inclusion has been handled. Training and professional development opportunities must be utilized to ensure that teachers master the essentials of the "new" role (Florian, 1998). Collaboration is part of this new role, and it requires teachers to share the interactions and work necessary to achieve their common goal of including all students. Team teaching and co-teaching approaches have been developed on the basis of the concept of collaboration and have been seen as successful (CEC Working Forum on Inclusive Schools, 1994; Dieker & Murawski, 2003; Hourcade & Bauwens, 2003; Hunt, Soto, Maier, & Doering, 2003; Thousand, Villa, & Nevin, 2006; Villa, Thousand, & Nevin, 2004). Whatever model is utilized, it is clear that schools must make it possible for teachers to work collaboratively. By doing so, teachers will not feel isolated in their teaching responsibilities (Corbett, 2001).

The Support Teacher Model

The approach described in this section is less oriented toward direct instruction than other approaches. It is a school-based collaborative consultation model, which is termed the *support teacher model* here, but which has been described elsewhere as the "method and resource teacher model" (Porter, 1991; Porter & Stone, 1998). It is one of the approaches that is preferred for supporting students with disabilities within the general education classroom (Simpson et al., 2005; Webber, 2005). In this model, the support teacher (formerly the special education teacher) gives up his or her own classroom to assist the general education teacher in a variety of ways to help students access the curriculum (Webber, 2005). Among the support teacher's functions are the following: program planning and development, program implementation, assessment and prescriptive services, program monitoring, communication and liaison, and instruction. The collaboration between these support and general education teachers is essential for the success of the effort (Snell & Janney, 2000).

In an inclusive school, the support teacher acts as a collaborative consultant to the general education teacher. The support teacher is responsible for assisting the classroom teacher in developing strategies and activities so that students with disabilities can be effectively included in the general education class. Support teachers do a number of things during the course of a school day to assist teachers and, thus, students. Behind each activity, however, are two key functions. First, the support teacher assists in elaborating pertinent questions about student learning and instructional practices that affect the learning of all students. In practical terms this might be helping to define the instructional issue (or problem) perceived by the teacher. By asking key questions, the support teacher helps the classroom teacher focus on the critical instructional issues and variables at work in the class. Second, the support teacher helps the teacher to solve identified classroom problems or, stated another way, to work out the most promising alternatives for more effective instruction.

In inclusive environments, support teachers provide general education teachers with "(a) information about students and the potential impact of specific disabilities on their learning; and (b) assistance in developing and providing appropriate instruction, accommodations, and modifications" (Lenz, Deshler, & Kissam, 2004, p. 307). According to Lipsky (2003), a support teacher often assists several students with disabilities who are enrolled in different classrooms. As a result, the support teacher's responsibilities to each student and assistance to each teacher may vary.

Time Use

As students with disabilities are being included in general education classrooms, the delivery of services to these students has to be restructured (Bradley & Tessier-Switlick, 1997; Lenz et al., 2004) and requires effective collaboration (Mundschenk et al., 2005). The support teacher serves both the students with disabilities and the general education teacher in a variety of ways. To obtain a better understanding of

TABLE 26.2

Major Activities and Time Commitment of Consulting (Support) Teachers

Activity	Description	% of Time Committed
Collaboration	Collaborating with teachers, teachers' assistants, other consulting teachers, parents, principal, and consulting professionals, such as psychologists and therapists. Done by phone calls or formal and informal meetings.	31
Instructional Support	Providing direct instruction to the whole class so general education teachers can work with the individual student, developing student programs, monitoring and observing individual students or small groups in the general education classroom, evaluating and assisting with classroom management, developing strategies concerning student behavior, providing individual guidance, meeting with students or student groups	29
Teacher Support	Responding to referrals, completing assessments, planning, developing Individualized Education Programs, preparing materials for instruction	20
Direct Instruction	Pulling students out for instruction in the resource or learning support room, assisting students who require extra help, providing individual attention	8
Other	Engaging in all the other teacher activities, such as professional development, staff meetings, and supervision duty	12

Source: Porter, G. L. (1991). The methods and resource teacher: A collaborative consultant model. In G. L. Porter & D. Richler (Eds.), *Changing Canadian schools: Perspectives on disability and inclusion* (pp. 107–154). Toronto: Roeher Institute.

this change in the service delivery role, one district monitored the way support teachers use their time. To do this, the school district had its teachers complete a time-use log over two consecutive work days. The support teachers recorded their major activities for each 15-minute time period while they were at school. These records were used for analysis of their actual work activities (Porter, 1991). The results of this analysis appear in Table 26.2.

The significant change in role for the support teacher in an inclusive system is reflected in the information presented in Table 26.2. Special education teachers spend almost all their time providing direct care and instruction to students with disabilities. Even resource room teachers spend most of their time providing small-group or individual instruction to students with learning difficulties. It is interesting to note that support teachers in this district spent less than 10% of their time on pull-out instruction. They devote their time to collaborating with general education teachers rather than replacing them through the provision of direct instruction.

A common theme emerged from the comments of the support teachers in the Porter (1991) study. Most indicated that it is essential that they visit the classroom frequently to observe student participation in the instructional process and assess student behavior in an authentic manner. This in fact moves their work in the direction of co-teaching models, in which the special education and general education teachers combine their students and work together. However, it is a more informal arrangement and utilized in a much more flexible way.

Providing Support to Teachers and Students

Most support teachers in the Porter (1991) study identified numerous qualities a teacher should have to be successful in this position. They reported that support teachers must be optimistic, confident, and persistent, and have a positive approach. They must be able to accept people for who they are and show genuine concern for the student. Being diplomatic, flexible, observant, creative, and innovative are also considered assets of support teachers. Problem solving, keeping things in perspective, knowing about the education system, and pushing for change are reported to be key qualities as well.

Support teachers must not be seen as "experts" who take over responsibility for student learning from the general education teacher. A challenge for the support teacher is to find workable solutions to problems that occur in the class that are welcomed by the general education teacher and allow them to succeed (Webber, 2005). Choate (2004) also identifies effective collaborators as those who are able to solve the most difficult problems and share in the collective effort. Support teachers who have extensive classroom teaching experience and are regarded by peers as able classroom teachers have the greatest success in this position (Porter, 1991). In the Porter (1991) study most support teachers stated that having general education class teaching experience was essential to their role in support of inclusion. Consulting teachers who provide services to general education teachers usually have experience in both special and general education classrooms (Lewis & Doorlag, 2005). General education teaching experience gives support teachers credibility with other teachers and helps them to be more collaborative in generating solutions (Porter, 1991).

Porter (1991) also found that support teachers work with students, teachers, administrators, and parents, and thus they need to be willing to adjust their plans to the needs of others, even if they have a plan for the day already established. They must work to sustain positive expectations for students with disabilities even when other staff members find their own enthusiasm waning. General education teachers who are teaching students with disabilities for the first time need support from someone with an optimistic and positive perspective. The fact is that general education teachers can and will respond positively to the challenge. The support teacher can help ensure this outcome by maintaining assistance for the teacher throughout the process of finding a solution to a problem.

One aspect of the support teacher role is the requirement for ongoing collaboration with other teachers (Walther-Thomas et al., 2000). This is a new responsibility for most special education teachers. It is also a new experience for the general education teacher (Villa, Thousand, Nevin, & Liston, 2005). As a result, a different set of skills, much more tied to working effectively with other adults, not children, becomes critical to achieving success. In fact, teachers as a whole do not have a lot of experience in sharing responsibility and decision making (Friend & Cook, 2003; Mundschenk et al., 2005). Thus a support teacher must have good communication skills, as well as sound instructional knowledge and experience (Choate, 2004; Friend & Cook, 2003; Walther-Thomas et al., 2000). Support teachers should be committed to ongoing personal development in both knowledge and skills. Teachers who are effective collaborators realize the benefits of collaboration for their own personal growth and seek more knowledge and expertise as a result (Mundschenk et al., 2005).

Schools committed to successful outcomes ensure that all staff members participate in professional development on a regular basis (Keenan, 2005; Mundschenk et al., 2005; Walther-Thomas et al., 2000). School districts implement different types of professional development to help staff understand inclusion and collaboration. The types of professional development implemented are based on the needs of the school system (Keenan, 2005). In one school district the support teacher (special educator) assisted the school system in training of general education teachers by presenting curriculum modifications and strategies that had been successfully used with students (Keenan, 2005). Training sessions were offered as a summer institute, with release days, and after school. The in-service training continued with team support within the school. In the Porter (1991) study, some school districts scheduled a meeting of support teachers for half a day every second week, whereas others met one day per month. The support teachers considered this time to be important for them in fulfilling their role. It allowed for exchanging information with peers, sharing successful strategies, and developing a sense of continuity and collaboration within the school district. Working together, the support teachers were able to keep their goals and vision clear and develop a sense of teamwork and collegiality in their new role. This type of staff development also permitted instruction in new techniques and skills, new materials, and new methods. The support teachers followed through with training sessions for the general education teachers in their respective schools. The school training allowed all teachers to continue developing and sharing skills collaboratively (Porter, 1991). Within-school training also allows teachers to demonstrate effective strategies with individual students (Simpson, Smith-Myles, Simpson, & Ganz, 2005).

Strategies for the Collaborative Role

The support teacher needs to be a good listener and facilitator, and often that means more emphasis on encouragement and confirming the value of the teacher's efforts than on suggesting new practices or approaches. The support teacher can help the general education teacher select an appropriate strategy, but it is the general education teacher who will implement it in the classroom (Porter, 1991).

The constant search for effective ways to work together in support of inclusive education is the major challenge for both the general education teacher and the support teacher. These teachers must find ways to work effectively to collaborate and problem-solve. Open and continuous communication is necessary if the relationship is to work (Choate, 2004; Friend & Cook, 2003; Kugelmass, 2006; Walther-Thomas et al., 2000).

Teaching Together

As teachers become more familiar and comfortable with their new roles, the support teacher and the general education teacher often move toward more co-teaching strategies, sharing responsibilities for instruction within the general education classroom as well as for planning instruction and evaluating students' progress. A number of co-teaching models or approaches have been used successfully by teachers (e.g., Friend & Cook, 2003; Hourcade & Bauwens, 2003; Thousand et al., 2006; Villa et al., 2004; Walther-Thomas et al., 2000). For example, Friend and Cook (2003) identify six co-teaching approaches. In *one teaching, one observing*, the general education teacher or support teacher teaches while the other teacher observes a student, a group of students, or the whole class. *One teaching, one drifting* is similar; however, the one teacher drifts around the room assisting students while the other teacher teaches the whole class. In *station teaching*, the instruction is divided and each teacher teaches his or her part at a station. The students typically move from station to station and often there is a third station that provides an opportunity for students to work independently. *Parallel teaching* allows the teachers to divide the class into two heterogeneous groups of equal size. Each teacher provides the same instruction to his or her designated group. In *alternative teaching*, one teacher teaches the large group of students while the other teacher teaches a small, selective group of students. This selective group may be receiving more intensive or enriched instruction, reviewing missed or unlearned material, or working on a project of interest. *Team teaching* occurs when both teachers are involved together in instructing the whole class, monitoring students during independent work or group activities. Both teachers share in all responsibilities for instruction.

As teachers become more familiar with their students and with their own ability to collaborate, they are more able to incorporate different models including team teaching in their repertoire. It is important for teachers to use a variety of models and to reverse roles within these models so that no one teacher becomes stigmatized (e.g., special education teacher seen as "the assistant"). Similarly, it is imperative that students are grouped flexibly within these approaches and with each teacher so that no one student or group of students becomes labeled as "special" (e.g., the "special needs group").

In the support teacher model special education teachers assist students with and without disabilities in the general education classroom, focusing on instruction and on supporting the general education teacher through collaboration and consultation.

Multilevel Instruction

Once inclusion is well under way, and teachers are beyond the stage of acceptance and attitude change, the emphasis moves from achieving integrated placements to creating inclusive classroom and school environments for students with disabilities. An inclusive classroom should provide age-appropriate and meaningful learning opportunities for all students. A class consisting of 20–30 students is obviously a challenge for the teacher trying to achieve the goal of inclusion for students with varying abilities. Classrooms are more diverse than ever before, and including all students is only one of the many responsibilities that teachers face today.

One of the essential questions in determining how to proceed is to decide how to organize instruction. There are a number of options. One option is to attempt to teach students on an individualized basis; another is to teach by using instructional groups. A third alternative, one that has been viewed as effective in achieving the goals of inclusion, has been for the teacher to establish one key concept and then find ways for each student to participate in the lesson and activities in a meaningful way. Appropriate learning opportunities can thus be provided to all the students.

This third instructional approach has been shown to be a particularly realistic option for teaching students within an inclusive education classroom and is supported by the use of *multilevel instruction* (Campbell, Campbell, Collicott, Perner, & Stone, 1988; Collicott, 1991; Schulz & Turnbull, 1984). A number of other instructional strategies and techniques logically complement multilevel instruction and provide teachers with the means to achieve success. Some of these strategies and techniques include cooperative learning, interactive learning, activity-based learning, and authentic assessment. As well, multilevel instruction is similar to tiered lessons as identified in approaches used to differentiate instruction (e.g., Tomlinson, 1999, 2001).

The Multilevel Instruction Process

Multilevel instruction is a planning strategy that has been adapted by Collicott and Stone (Campbell et al., 1988; Collicott, 1991) from the works of Schulz and Turnbull (1984). The process helps teachers to plan and implement one lesson to accommodate all students and encourages each student to participate at his or her own level in shared class activities. This strategy is particularly useful for including students with developmental disabilities because it focuses on developing concepts by using content as a means for teaching specific skills, rather than teaching the content as an end in itself (Campbell et al., 1988).

TABLE 26.3
The Multilevel Instruction Process

Concept(s)	Methods of Presentation (Process and Activities)
• underlying concept(s) to be taught	• how new information is presented to students
Methods of Practice and Performance (Process and Activities)	**Methods of Assessment (Products)**
• methods used to help students understand the concept on their own terms	• how students show understanding of what they have learned

To develop a unit or lesson, the teacher identifies the objective(s) of the planned instruction. The teacher also includes numerous teaching techniques to accommodate the various levels of ability within any one class. There are a number of considerations that the teacher needs to address when planning for multilevel instruction. According to Collicott (1991), the teacher should (a) consider student learning styles and preferences, (b) involve students in lessons through questioning aimed at different levels, (c) adapt expectations for some students (e.g., include different objectives and outcomes), (d) allow for various levels of participation, (e) give students a choice in methods of practice and in how they will demonstrate understanding of the concept being taught, (f) be aware that each method is of equivalent value, and (g) evaluate students on the basis of their individual differences.

Multilevel instruction also involves a four-step planning process for developing instructional lessons and units. Each of these steps is described in the following section (see Table 26.3).

Underlying Concept

The first step in the multilevel instruction process is for the teacher to identify what concepts are going to be taught. The objectives for students will differ, but the lesson concept should be a shared one. "For example, the study of the novel or short story is not taught for the sake of the content, but is undertaken in order to understand the concepts of plot, character development, setting and atmosphere" (Campbell et al., 1988, pp. 17–18).

Method of Presentation and Method of Practice and Performance

In the next two steps of the multilevel instruction process, the teacher determines the method of presentation and the method of practice and performance. The teacher identifies various ways to present or include the concepts or skills to be taught and for students to practice or use these concepts or skills.

In both of these phases, the teacher considers different presentation and performance modes. For example, as cited in Schulz and Turnbull (1984), Smith and

Written	Oral	Visual
• Advertisement	• Audio tape	• Advertisement
• Book report/review	• Discussion	• Cartoon
• Brochure	• Dramatization	• Collage
• Essay	• Interview	• Computer graphic
• Experiment record	• Oral report	• Data display
• Journal	• Poetry reading	• Design
• Letter	• Rap	• Diagram
• Memo	• Skit	• Display
• Newscast	• Song	• Drawing
• Play	• Speech	• Flyer
• Poem	• Teach a lesson	• Game
• Position paper		• Graph
• Research report		• Map
• Script		• Model
• Story		• Photograph
• Test		• Poster
• Web site		• PowerPoint show
		• Questionnaire
		• Scrapbook
		• Storyboard
		• Videotape/DVD
		• Web site

Figure 26.2 Possible products and performances. Source: Adapted from McTighe, J., & Wiggins, G. (2004). *Understanding by design professional development workbook*. Alexandria, VA: Association for Supervision and Curriculum Development, p. 174.

Bentley identified input and output modes that include a selection of activities categorized under headings such as view, read, make/construct, and solve. Wood (2006) provided a list of activities under modes categorized as expository, inquiry, demonstration, and activity. McTighe and Wiggins (2004) have also developed a number of categories to depict various input and output modes for student performance. An adapted list of their activities is shown in Figure 26.2.

In selecting presentation and practice and performance methods, teachers also should consider variations in questioning techniques and thinking skills (e.g., using the cognitive domain described by Bloom [1956]), student learning styles (e.g., visual, auditory, and/or tactile; seating and lighting; independent or group work), and level of student participation (e.g., partial or total). For example, some students may do parts of an assignment, whereas others may be expected to complete the entire task. Some students may work alone, and others may be paired.

Many instructional methods are planned and used so that students have some choices in how they are going to show their understanding of a concept or their acquisition of a skill. For example, if a novel is being studied and the concept of setting is being taught, then methods of presentation and methods of practice and performance at the middle school level might include those noted in Table 26.4. In this example, the teacher has created a number of activities for students to complete

TABLE 26.4
Methods of Practice for the Concept of Setting

Individual	Pairs	Small Groups
Draws or finds a picture to depict a described setting (e.g., rural setting).	Discuss home setting.	Develop the relationship of setting and atmosphere.
Briefly describes a setting of a television program or rock video.	Find a picture similar to one's home setting.	Construct a diorama of a setting to match a story.
Writes a paragraph describing a setting from an oral reading or a narrated story.	Design a setting for a traditional dance.	Paint a wall mural with a setting that welcomes visitors to the school.
Presents a description of a setting orally.	One describes setting; the other determines plot.	Construct a setting for a class or school play, concert, or other event.

Related Activities for Enrichment

Develop a time line of change of settings in life.

Compare own home setting with setting of story.

In relation to the story, evaluate the effectiveness of the setting as depicted in the movie.

Write a short story that includes a well-developed setting.

to help them "practice" the concept of setting. The teacher assigns one activity for each student to complete. The selected activity for each student is based on his or her prior experiences, interests, and abilities. For example, a student who cannot read can learn about the concept of setting by finding a picture in a magazine or a book that depicts the described setting, or the student can briefly talk about a setting shown in one of his or her favorite television programs. Sometimes the teacher will pair two students or select students to participate in a group so that one student can assist the other(s) in the activity. For example, a student who cannot write can help a group of students construct a diorama of a setting to match the novel being read or a student can help another find a picture that depicts a home setting. As shown in Table 26.4, a number of activities are planned, allowing students to make choices for the other assignments and giving them opportunities for enrichment activities.

Method of Evaluation

The fourth step in the multilevel instruction process is to determine whether students have learned the concept(s) or skill(s) being taught. The teacher identifies a variety of evaluation techniques in order to allow for individual abilities and differences. For example, assessment or evaluation assignments to determine students' understanding of the concept of setting in a story might include completing an oral presentation, constructing a diorama, or creating an illustration. Consistent with the former step, the teacher should allow for a variety of ways to assess or evaluate students' preferences of presentation style. By giving students choices in their preferred mode of performance, the teacher allows each student the best opportunity to demonstrate understanding of the concept.

Teachers who have used multilevel instruction have found that this emerging practice provides for the differentiated needs of students with developmental disabilities and other students in diverse classrooms. It is a practical and realistic way for general education teachers to accommodate the requirements of an inclusive education program (Collicott, 1991; Perner, 1993, 2004). The most compelling factor in using this kind of approach, however, is that it has the potential to improve the quality of instruction for all students.

Conclusion

Schools today need to be creative and responsive places, where collaboration among teachers leads to effective problem solving, shared learning, and a cooperative, welcoming school environment. Innovative school and classroom practices are required if public education is to serve all students, including those with developmental disabilities, in an effective way. Through participation and learning in the general education classroom, students with disabilities will have the opportunity to take their place as contributing citizens of communities.

Glossary

Activity-based learning—Activities that encourage students to be actively involved and engaged in the learning tasks.

Authentic assessments—Informal assessments that help to evaluate student performance within the learning environment and usually relate to instructional objectives. Common authentic assessments are portfolios and checklists.

Collaboration—Two or more people sharing the interactions and work necessary to achieve a common goal.

Cooperative learning—Learning activities that have students work together in small groups (i.e., two to six students per group) to achieve common academic goals. The activities are planned to encourage social interactions and positive goal interdependence. Each member of a group contributes to the learning task.

Co-teaching—Two or more professionals share the planning, teaching, and assessment of a group of diverse students in the general education class.

Inclusion/Inclusive education—A high level of involvement of students with disabilities in age-appropriate general education classes in their home schools, with significant participation in classroom activities and experiences.

Integration—The early steps to move students with disabilities from segregated classes and schools to classrooms and school placements in which they are with their peers who do not have disabilities.

Interactive learning—Activities that encourage students to be actively involved and engaged in the learning tasks and socially interactive with other students.

Multilevel instruction—An approach to classroom instruction and curriculum organization that emphasizes the provision of learning opportunities for students with varying levels of academic skills through the same "core lesson." The approach suggests consideration by teachers of the (a) underlying concept(s) of the lesson, (b) methods of presentation by the teacher, (c) methods of practice and performance by the student, and (d) methods of assessment.

Support teacher—A special education teacher who works collaboratively with general education teachers in providing professional support and assistance for dealing with the issues and challenges of teaching a class that includes students with varying learning strengths and needs. Part of the support teacher's role is in co-teaching with general education teachers. Other terms sometimes used for this role include *method and resource teacher, collaborative teacher, resource teacher,* and *inclusion facilitator.*

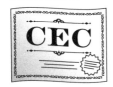

Knowledge and Skills for Entry-Level Special Education Teachers of Students With Developmental Disabilities Standards Addressed in This Chapter

Principle 1: Foundations

DD1K2 Continuum of placement and services available for individuals with developmental disabilities.

DD1K4 Trends and practices in the field of developmental disabilities.

Principle 5: Learning Environments/Social Interaction

DD5S5 Plan instruction for individuals with developmental disabilities in a variety of placement settings.

Web Site Resources

Circle of Inclusion Home Page

http://www.circleofinclusion.org/

Designed for early childhood service providers and families of young children. Useful information (including materials for downloading) about effective practices of inclusive educational programs for children from birth through age 8.

Disabilities Resources Homepage

http://www.disabilityresources.org/INCLUSION.html

Information and resources on and links related to all disabilities. The inclusion page contains links to a variety of Web sites related specifically to inclusive education.

Inclusion.com

http://www.inclusion.com/reslinks.html

Sponsored by the Inclusion Network. Offers workshops, training events, and resources for inclusion, plus links to more than 100 resource Web sites related to inclusion.

Kids Together, Inc.

http://www.kidstogether.org/

Articles, cartoons, video clips, information sheets, and more about inclusion and advocacy. An educational, fun, and inclusive Web site!

Power of 2 Web Site

http://www.powerof2.org/

Designed for online training. Includes resources, articles, and links related to collaboration and co-teaching. Can be used alone or with others to assess and develop collaboration skills.

TASH Homepage

www.tash.org

TASH is an organization that is concerned with the education, dignity, rights, and independence of individuals with disabilities. The Web site contains articles, information, and links to a variety of resources related to inclusion.

United Nations Educational, Scientific and Cultural Organization (UNESCO)

www.unesco.org

International information on inclusive education through the education link to inclusive education. Various inclusive education resources can be downloaded, such as the book *Changing Teaching Practices: Using Curriculum Differentiation to Respond to Students' Diversity* (http://unesdoc.unesco.org/images/0013/001365/136583e.pdf).

University of Canberra in Australia: Educational Support and Inclusion

http://www.canberra.edu.au/special-ed/othersites.html

Inclusive education resource links from the United Kingdom, Canada, the United States, and Europe.

References

Armstrong, F., Armstrong, D., & Barton, L. (2000). *Inclusive education: Policy, contexts, and comparative perspectives*. London: David Fulton Publishers.

Ashman, A., & Elkins, J. (1998). *Educating children with special needs* (3rd ed.). Sydney: Prentice Hall.

Baglieri, S., & Knopf, J. H. (2004). Normalizing difference in inclusive teaching [Electronic version]. *Journal of Learning Disabilities, 37*, 525–529.

Bloom, B. S. (Ed.). (1956). *Taxonomy of educational objectives: The classification of educational goals. Handbook 1: Cognitive domain*. New York: Longman.

Bradley, D. F., & Tessier-Switlick, D. M. (1997). The past and the future of special education. In D. F. Bradley, M. E. King-Sears, & D. M. Tessier-Switlick (Eds.), *Teaching students in inclusive settings* (pp. 1–20). Boston: Allyn & Bacon.

Bunch, G. (1997). From here to there: The passage to inclusive education. In G. Bunch & A. Valeo (Eds.), *Inclusion: Recent research* (pp. 9–23). Toronto: Inclusion Press.

Burstein, N., Sears, S., Wilcoxen, A., Cabello, B., & Spagna, M. (2004). Moving toward inclusive practices [Electronic version]. *Remedial and Special Education, 25*(2), 104–116.

Campbell, C., Campbell, S., Collicott, J., Perner, D., & Stone, J. (1988). Adapting regular class curriculum for integrated special needs students. *Education New Brunswick Journal, 3*, 17–20.

CEC Working Forum on Inclusive Schools. (1994). *Creating schools for all our students: What twelve schools have to say*. Reston, VA: Council for Exceptional Children.

Choate, J. S. (2004). *Successful inclusive teaching: Proven ways to detect and correct special needs*. Boston: Allyn & Bacon.

Collicott, J. (1991). Implementing multi-level instruction: Strategies for classroom teachers. In G. Porter & D. Richler (Eds.), *Changing Canadian schools: Perspectives on disability and inclusion* (pp. 191–218). Toronto: Roeher Institute.

Corbett, J. (2001). *Supporting inclusive education: A connective pedagogy*. London: Routledge/Falmer.

Crawford, C., & Porter, G. L. (1992). *How it happens: A look at inclusive educational practice in Canada for children and youth with disabilities*. Toronto: Roeher Institute.

Crawford, C., & Porter, G. L. (2004). *Supporting teachers: A foundation for advancing inclusive education*. Toronto: Roeher Institute.

Crawley, J. F., Hayden, S., Cade, E., & Baker-Kroczynski, S. (2002). Including students with disabilities into the general education science classroom. *Exceptional Children, 68*, 423–436.

Department for Education and Employment. (1997). *Excellence for all children: Meeting special educational needs* (Green paper). London: Stationery Office.

Dieker, L. A., & Murawski, W. W. (2003). Co-teaching in the secondary level: Unique issues, current trends, and suggestions for success [Electronic version]. *High School Journal, 86*(4), 1–13.

Dunn, L. (1968). Special education for the mildly retarded: Is much of it justifiable? *Exceptional Children, 35*(1), 5–22.

Florian, L. (1998). Inclusive practice: What, why, how? In C. Tilstone, L. Florian, & R. Rose (Eds.), *Promoting inclusive practice* (pp. 13–26). London: Routledge/Falmer.

Forlin, C. (1997). Inclusive education in Australia. *Special Education Perspectives, 6*(1), 21–26.

Friend, M., & Cook, L. (2003). *Interactions: Collaboration skills for school professionals* (4th ed.). Boston: Allyn & Bacon.

Fullan, M. G., & Steigelbauer, S. (1991). *The new meaning of educational change*. New York: Teachers College Press.

Giangreco, M. F. (1997). Key lessons learned about inclusive education: Summary of the 1996 Shonell memorial lecture [Electronic version]. *International Journal of Disability, 44*, 193–206.

Hanko, G. (2004). Towards inclusive education: Interprofessional support strategies within and across schools and school services [Electronic version]. *Education Review, 17*, 60–66.

Hansen, J. (2001). *Each belongs*. Hamilton, Ontario: Hamilton-Wentworth Catholic District School Board.

Hastings, R. P., & Oakford, S. (2003). Student teachers' attitudes towards the inclusion of children with special needs [Electronic version]. *Educational Psychology, 23*, 87–94.

Hourcade, J., & Bauwens, J. (2003). *Cooperative teaching: Sharing the new schoolhouse.* Austin, TX: PRO-ED.

Hunt, P., Soto, G., Maier J., & Doering, K. (2003). Collaborative teaming to support students at risk and students with severe disabilities in general education classrooms. *Exceptional Children, 69*, 315–332.

Idol, L. (2006). Toward inclusion of special education students in general education. *Remedial and Special Education, 27*, 77–94.

Keenan, S. M. (2005). Program elements that support teachers and students with learning and behavior problems. In P. Zionts (Ed.), *Inclusion strategies for students with learning and behavior problems* (2nd ed., pp. 135–155). Austin, TX: PRO-ED.

Keilty, G. C. (1994, August). *Turning the corner: Effective strategies for educational change.* Paper presented at the Excellence and Equity in Education International Conference, Toronto, Ontario.

Kilgore, K., Griffin, C. C., Sindelar, P. T., & Webb, R. B. (2002). Restructuring for inclusion: Changing teaching practices (Part II) [Electronic version]. *Middle School Journal, 33*(3), 7–13.

Kugelmass, J. W. (2006). Sustaining cultures of inclusion: The value and limitation of cultural analyses [Electronic version]. *European Journal of Psychology of Education, 21*, 279–292.

Lenz, B. K., Deshler, D. D., & Kissam, B. R. (2004). *Teaching content to all: Evidence-based inclusive practices in middle and secondary schools.* Boston: Allyn & Bacon.

Lewis, R. B., & Doorlag, D. H. (2005). *Teaching special students in general education classrooms* (3rd ed.). Upper Saddle River, NJ: Merrill/Prentice Hall.

Lipsky, D. K. (2003). The coexistence of high standards and inclusion [Electronic version]. *School Administrator 60*(3), 32–35.

Lipsky, D. K., & Gartner, A. (1999). Inclusive education: A requirement of a democratic society. In H. Daniels & P. Garner (Eds.), *World yearbook of education 1999: Inclusive education* (pp. 12–23). London: Kogan Page.

McLeskey, J., & Waldron, N. L. (2002a). Inclusion and school change: Teacher perceptions regarding curricular and instructional adaptations [Electronic version]. *Teacher Education and Special Education, 25*(1), 41–54.

McLeskey, J., & Waldron, N. L. (2002b). Professional development and inclusive schools: Reflections on effective practice. *Teacher Educator, 37*, 159–173.

McTighe, J., & Wiggins, G. (2004). *Understanding by design professional development workbook.* Alexandria, VA: Association for Supervision and Curriculum Development.

Mundschenk, N. A., Foley, R. M., & Swedburg, K. A. (2005). Collaboration: Building teams to facilitate inclusive practices. In P. Zionts (Ed.), *Inclusion strategies for students with learning and behavior problems* (2nd ed., pp. 57–91). Austin, TX: PRO-ED.

National Center on Educational Restructuring and Inclusion. (1994). *National survey on inclusive education* (Bulletin No. 1). New York Graduate Schools and University Center, City of New York.

New Brunswick Department of Education. (1994). *Best practices for inclusion.* Fredericton, New Brunswick: Author.

O'Neil, J. (1994). Can inclusion work? A conversation with Jim Kauffman and Mara Sapon-Shevin. *Educational Leadership, 52*(4), 7–11.

Organization for Economic Co-operation and Development. (1999). *Inclusive education at work: Students with disabilities in mainstream schools.* Paris: Author.

Perner, D. (1991). Leading the way: The role of school administrators in integration. In G. L. Porter & D. Richler, (Eds.), *Changing Canadian schools: Perspectives on disability and inclusion* (pp. 155–171). Toronto: Roeher Institute.

Perner, D. (1993, December). *All students attend regular classes in neighbourhood schools: A case study of three schools* in *Woodstock, New Brunswick, Canada* (Research report for the Organization for Economic Co-operation and Development/Centre for Educational Research and Innovation International Conference on Active Life for Disabled Youth—Integration in the School Project, Dissemination conference, Vaals, The Netherlands).

Perner, D. (1997). Supporting the classroom teacher in New Brunswick. In Organization for Economic Co-operation and Development (OECD)/Centre for Educational Research and Innovation (CERI), *Implementing inclusive education* (pp. 75–80). Paris: OECD Publications.

Perner, D. (1998, October). *An analysis of the roles of teachers and supports needed in inclusive education settings: A look at inclusive education 12 years later.* Paper presented at the Northeast Educational Research Association Annual Conference, Ellensville, NY.

Perner, D. (2004). *Changing teaching practices, using curriculum differentiation to respond to students' diversity.* Paris: UNESCO.

Perner, D., Porter, G., & Padora, J. (2003, February). *Reviewing inclusive education practices that support general education teachers.* Paper presented at the Council for Exceptional Children–Division on Developmental Disabilities 8th International Conference, Kauai, HI.

Porter, G. L. (1991). The methods and resource teacher: A collaborative consultant model. In G. L. Porter & D. Richler (Eds.), *Changing Canadian schools: Perspectives on disability and inclusion* (pp. 107–154). Toronto: Roeher Institute.

Porter, G. L., Collicott, J., & Larsen, J. (2000). New Brunswick School Districts 10, 12, and 13: The story continued. . . . In R. Villa & J. Thousand (Eds.), *Restructuring for caring and effective education: Piecing the puzzle together* (2nd ed., pp. 484–492). Baltimore: Brookes.

Porter, G. L., & Richler, D. (Eds.). (1991). *Changing Canadian schools: Perspectives on disability and inclusion.* Toronto: Roeher Institute.

Porter, G. L., & Stone, J. (1998). The inclusive school model: A framework and key strategies for success. In J. W. Putnam (Ed.), *Cooperative learning and strategies for inclusion: Celebrating diversity in the classroom* (2nd ed., pp. 229–248). Baltimore: Brookes.

Rea, P. J., McLaughlin, V. L., & Walther-Thomas, C. (2002). Outcomes for students with learning disabilities in inclusive and pullout programs. *Exceptional Children, 68,* 203–222.

Roeher Institute. (2003). *Not enough: Canadian research into inclusive education* (Summary report). Toronto: Roeher Institute.

Rose, R. (2001). Primary school teacher perceptions of the conditions required to include pupils with special educational needs [Electronic version]. *Educational Review, 53,* 147–156.

Sailor, W., & Roger, B. (2005). Rethinking inclusion: Schoolwide applications (Electronic version). *Phi Delta Kappan, 86,* 503–510.

Sapon-Shevin, M. (1994). Why gifted students belong in inclusive schools. *Educational Leadership, 52*(4), 64–67.

Sarason, S. B. (1982). *The culture of school and the problem of change* (Rev. ed.). Needham Heights, MA: Allyn & Bacon.

Schulz, J., & Turnbull, A. (1984). *Mainstreaming handicapped students: A guide for classroom teachers.* Needham Heights, MA: Allyn & Bacon.

Simpson, R. L., de Boer-Ott, S. R., & Smith-Myles, B. (2003). Inclusion of learners with autism spectrum disorders in general education settings [Electronic version]. *Topics in Language Disorders, 23,* 116–133.

Simpson, R. L., Smith-Myles, B., Simpson, J. D., & Ganz, J. B. (2005). Inclusion of students with disabilities in general education settings: Structuring for successful management. In P. Zionts (Ed.), *Inclusion strategies for students with learning and behavior problems* (2nd ed., pp. 193–216). Austin, TX: PRO-ED.

Snell, M., & Janney, R. (2000). *Teachers' guides to inclusive practices: Collaborative teaming.* Baltimore: Brookes.

Thousand, J. S., Villa, R. A., & Nevin, A. I. (2006). The many faces of collaborative planning and teaching. *Theory Into Practice, 45,* 239–248.

Tomlinson, C. A. (1999). *The differentiated classroom: Responding to the needs of all learners.* Alexandria, VA: Association for Supervision and Curriculum Development.

Tomlinson, C. A. (2001). *How to differentiate instruction in mixed-ability classrooms* (2nd ed.). Alexandria, VA: Association for Supervision and Curriculum Development.

van Kraayenoord, C. (2003). The task of professional development [Electronic version]. *International Journal of Disability, Development, and Education, 50,* 363–366.

Villa, R., Thousand, J., & Nevin, A. (2004). *A guide to co-teaching: Practical tips for facilitating student learning.* Thousand Oaks, CA: Corwin.

Villa, R., Thousand, J., Nevin, A., & Liston, A. (2005). Successful inclusive practices in middle and secondary schools [Electronic version]. *American Secondary Education, 33*(3), 33–50.

Walther-Thomas, C., Korinek, L., McLaughlin, V. L., & Williams, B. (2000). *Collaboration for inclusive education: Developing successful programs.* Boston: Allyn & Bacon.

Webber, J. (2005). Responsible inclusion: Key components for success. In P. Zionts (Ed.), *Inclusion strategies for students with learning and behavior problems* (2nd ed., pp. 29–55). Austin, TX: PRO-ED.

Weiner, H. M. (2003). Effective inclusion, professional development in the context of the classroom. *Teaching Exceptional Children, 35*(6), 12–18.

Wolfe, P. S., & Hall, T. E. (2003). Making inclusion a reality for students with severe disabilities. *Teaching Exceptional Children, 35*(4), 56–61.

Wood, J. (2006). *Teaching students in inclusive settings* (5th ed.). Upper Saddle River, NJ: Pearson/Prentice Hall.

Zeph, L. (1994, August). *Assessing the quality of education in inclusive schools: Research and rationale.* Paper presented at the Excellence and Equity in Education International Conference, Toronto, Ontario.

27

Creating Inclusive Schools:

Strategies for Change—
Administrators and Teachers

Darlene E. Perner

Summary

Inclusion of students with disabilities within the general education classroom is a multifaceted undertaking. This chapter discusses the crucial role played by principals and teachers who are implementing inclusive education. Through effective leadership, principals provide critical support for teachers who are working to achieve successful inclusive practices. The collaboration of both general education and special education teachers is also essential for the success of inclusion.

Principals and teachers can choose numerous ways to facilitate the inclusion of students with developmental disabilities within general education classes. This chapter describes some of those that have been found successful in developing and maintaining inclusive school practices. Some of the strategies focus on practices that school administrators are able to implement in support of teachers to facilitate inclusion. Others are practices that teachers perform directly to facilitate the process of including students with development disabilities in general education classes.

Learning Outcomes

After reading this chapter the reader should be able to:

- Define the role of school administrators in inclusive education.

- Describe actions that school administrators can take to support the development and operation of inclusive schools.

- Define the role of teachers (general and special education) in inclusive education.

- Describe actions that teachers can take to facilitate the inclusion of students with developmental disabilities into their classrooms.

- Describe the importance of school-based teams and their function.

- Examine functional ways to include families in the inclusion decision-making and planning process.

Introduction

Policy guidelines and initiatives for integration or inclusive education at the state or provincial level, as well as at the school district level, can be instrumental in bringing about changes in school and classroom practices. However, these guidelines and initiatives do not necessarily mean that the new practices will be implemented in the school (Office of Special Education Programs, 2003). In the end, it is the leadership provided in the individual school and the collaboration of the "whole school" that will determine the extent to which the vision of inclusion will become a reality. "School principals and teachers are in especially critical positions to influence the change process" (Walther-Thomas, Korinek, McLaughlin, &

Williams, 2000, p. 30). Both are seen as change agents and play leadership roles in the development and implementation of inclusive education practices (Kochhar, West, & Taymans, 2000; McLeskey & Waldron, 2002; Walther-Thomas et al., 2000).

Although it may be possible to achieve change in school practice through the efforts of teachers, parents, and the community, principals are in a key leadership position to move integration and inclusive education forward. As school leaders, principals can set an explicit vision for inclusion within their school (Avissar, Reiter, & Leyser, 2003; Friend & Bursuck, 2002; Kochhar et al., 2000). Their commitment and actions can support policies and practices related to inclusion (Avissar et al., 2003; Hammond & Ingalls, 2003; McLeskey & Waldron, 2002). According to Walther-Thomas et al. (2000), school principals not only formulate school missions but are also highly influential in fostering collaboration among teachers and in providing the support necessary to make inclusion happen (e.g., professional development, scheduling time for teacher collaboration). This is consistent with the assertions that a positive and collaborative educational environment is needed and that the school principal is the key to achieving "a sense of community" among students, teachers, parents, and others (CEC Working Forum on Inclusive Schools, 1994; Mundschenk, Foley, & Swedburg, 2005; Simpson, Smith-Myles, Simpson, & Ganz, 2005).

Through effective leadership, principals have been able to implement inclusive educational practices even when a school board or district has not established a philosophy or policy on integration or inclusion (Crawford & Porter, 1992) or has not provided supports to facilitate inclusion (Richardson & Jording, 1999). Crawford and Porter (1992) identified a number of elements that are crucial to visionary leadership:

1. a positive view about the value of education to students with disabilities;

2. an optimistic view of the capacity of teachers and schools to change and to accommodate the needs of all learners;

3. confidence that practices evolve and that everyone benefits from the move toward inclusive education. (pp. 35–36)

Both general education and special education teachers are directly involved in the education of students. When students are integrated or included in the general education classroom, teachers from both specializations play an important role, and their leadership, attitudes, and commitment are crucial to the success of inclusion. Teachers need to become change agents and leaders "who are actively committed to making a difference and capable of doing so" (Walther-Thomas et al., 2000, p. 30).

Inclusion of students with disabilities within the general education classroom is a multifaceted undertaking. Attitudes of school administrators and teachers continue to be investigated. The general consensus has been that having positive experiences with students with disabilities leads to more positive attitudes toward inclusion; both are important components of successful inclusion. Studies related to the attitudes of teachers toward inclusion continue to be conducted (e.g., Ammah & Hodge, 2005; Burke & Sutherland, 2004). Studies related to attitudes and to the process of inclusion have been focusing on ways to help both administrators and teachers develop and improve inclusive practices within their schools (e.g., Keenan, 2005; Lynch & Bruhl, 2005; Simpson et al., 2005).

There are numerous means by which school principals and teachers can facilitate the inclusion of students with developmental disabilities in their schools. In the following sections, a number of strategies are identified and described, drawn from a review of recent research related to inclusion (e.g., Kochhar et al., 2000; McLeskey & Waldron, 2002; Walther-Thomas et al., 2000; Zionts, 2005) and on feedback from school principals and teachers who have had successful experiences with students with disabilities, particularly those students with developmental disabilities, in the general education classroom (Perner, 1991, 1993, 1997; Perner, Porter, & Padora, 2003). Over time, the strategies and recommendations appear to be similar in nature; however, a major change has been to also focus on the use of instructional strategies to include students in the general education curriculum. It appears that over the years, with experience and increased support to move forward with the inclusion process, administrators and teachers have become concerned about instruction and how to best meet the needs of individuals within the general education classroom. It is possible that as teachers gain experience and overcome some of the initial fears of inclusion, they are better able to focus on the need to change their instructional strategies to accommodate all students. Even so, studies have shown that teachers who are integrating and including students with disabilities are not necessarily changing their teaching practices (Scott, Vitale, & Masten, 1998).

It is apparent and integral to the change process that teachers and principals develop ways to implement inclusion and make it successful in their own situations. No single resource or strategy ensures success, but as the principals and teachers enhance their skills, or see a need to do so, they are able to use a variety of sources, such as attending workshops, reading books and articles, visiting inclusive education classrooms, taking courses, sharing and collaborating with colleagues, and gaining practical experience.

Support Strategies for School Administrators

Researchers, teachers, and principals have identified practices that school administrators should implement to facilitate the integration and inclusion of students with disabilities. They include: (a) sharing a vision, strong commitment, and positive attitudes, (b) providing support systems, (c) providing time for collaboration, (d) maintaining natural proportions and reducing class size, (e) providing administrative support, (f) establishing school-based teams, (g) allowing time for visitations and sharing sessions, (h) providing time for transitional planning, (i) supporting the changing roles and responsibilities of staff, and (j) recognizing success and promoting public awareness.

Sharing a Vision, Strong Commitment, and Positive Attitudes

Because the principal is seen as the leader of the school, it is imperative that the commitment to integration and inclusion be reflected in his or her behavior. The school principal is in a key position to set the tone for change and to help school staff have a clear vision and understanding of inclusive education (Friend & Bursuck, 2002; Kugelmass, 2006; McLeskey & Waldron, 2002; Mundschenk et al., 2005; Walther-Thomas et al., 2000). A positive attitude about and a commitment to inclusive education on the part of the school principal will help to enhance the attitudes of others within the school (Simpson, de Boer-Ott, & Smith-Myles, 2003). Schools that have progressed the farthest in the inclusion process are the ones in which the school administrators (principal and vice principal) have a commitment to inclusion. As reported by one group of teachers who had been including students with developmental disabilities for a number of years, "The success of integration in these schools is based on school administrators who planned, promoted, implemented and rewarded" their school staff (Perner, 1991, p. 157). Teachers in another study felt that the principal had to be committed to inclusion in order for it to succeed in their school (Hammond & Ingalls, 2003).

Even though the school principal needs to have a vision of and commitment to inclusion, it is generally agreed that such vision and commitment need to be shared by the whole school. Teachers and other school staff need to be part of creating this vision; in essence, there needs to be a shared vision and a shared commitment—adopted by the entire team (Kochhar et al., 2000; Walther-Thomas et al., 2000; Webber, 2005). It is the school principal's responsibility to facilitate collaboration among the staff so that team members are identified, are valued, and share in the decision-making process related to creating an inclusive education school. It is also crucial that the school principal create opportunities and allow adequate time for staff to discuss their feelings and attitudes about students with developmental disabilities and inclusion. If need be, the principal can use this information to determine what the staff need to enhance their attitudes and move forward with inclusion (Simpson et al., 2005). Burke and Sutherland (2004) recommend that school administrators survey teachers in their school about inclusion and their attitudes and then use the results of the survey to provide professional development opportunities to change teacher attitudes.

In some cases, the attitudes of teachers toward, as well as their expectations of, students with developmental disabilities and inclusion need to be enhanced. To help alleviate confusion and develop realistic expectations, effective practice dictates that the school administrator is responsible for ensuring that all teachers (special education and general education teachers) are involved in the initial planning sessions for including students with disabilities in the general education classroom. Even though secondary school programs involve many teachers and meetings require juggling a number of schedules or hiring substitute teachers, involvement in early meetings allows teachers to be part of the initial planning and to know in advance what is expected of them and their students. The intent is not to diminish the importance of having all teachers meet for subsequent planning, but to stress that the initial meeting helps the teachers and students from being overwhelmed and becoming frustrated because of unclear expectations and goals. Teachers need to be involved from the very beginning.

School administrators do not always agree on how to get all of their staff involved in the inclusion process. For many, it may be a question of the principal's administrative style. Some principals think that, initially, they should allow their staff to volunteer to integrate students with disabilities into their classrooms (Perner, 1991). Provided with many opportunities for sharing, observing, and receiving in-service training, the other teachers will get involved naturally. It is felt that this process gives teachers time to allay their initial fears.

Other principals feel that all teachers on staff should be directly involved early on and responsible for including students with disabilities (Perner, 1991). In these schools, students are automatically placed in their age-appropriate classes. Through direct experience with ongoing in-service and supports, the teachers become less fearful and consequently change their attitudes.

Walther-Thomas et al. (2000) suggest that school administrators create pilot projects. This allows teachers to volunteer without feeling threatened, to make mistakes, and to problem-solve.

Providing Support Systems

Additional support for schools and teachers is needed in order to develop and implement inclusive education programs (McLeskey & Waldron, 2002). Such support varies and may need to be created and funded in different ways; staff should be involved in this process (Webber, 2005). However, it is often the responsibility of the school administrator to identify and expand the use of school resources when including students with disabilities in general education classrooms. For example, a teacher who uses cooperative learning strategies may be the ideal person to help other teachers integrate students along with the support or collaborating teacher. A teacher of physical education or activity-based science may feel comfortable in helping other teachers to adapt a curriculum so that students with disabilities can participate in class instruction. The school administrator should be flexible and creative in using within-school resources and should encourage staff to collaborate in these endeavors.

Also, school principals should advocate at the district level for the support personnel and resources needed to effectively prepare and enhance the skills of school staff. These should include support teachers and paraprofessionals along with professional development resources. The school administrators should facilitate the use of in-school supports, such as volunteer programs, peer support groups, and resource centers.

Providing Time for Collaboration

Planning time for staff to collaborate is one of the most challenging but necessary tasks in establishing and supporting inclusive education (Walther-Thomas et al., 2000). The school administrator, in cooperation with staff, has to be flexible and allow for changes to traditional school operations and schedules in order to accommodate planning time for school collaboration. This may mean providing scheduled time within the school day for meetings. This may include time for (a) discussion and planning related to school improvement (e.g., to develop an inclusive education plan), (b) collaboration meetings between the support/collaborative teacher and general education teachers (e.g., to plan team teaching activities, to adapt instruction for a student with developmental disabilities), or (c) team meetings (e.g., to collaborate as an instructional support team, problem-solving team or school-based team).

Principals who plan for and are able to schedule additional preparation time for their teachers are supported by their staff. Lack of planning time for collaboration can affect teacher attitudes (Hammond & Ingalls, 2003). As stated by Rodriguez and Romaneck (2002), "If staff members don't have time to share about students' special needs, they will quickly become disenchanted with 'inclusion' and see it as 'dumping'" (p. 12). Providing time for planning and collaboration can be done in a variety of ways. How it is accomplished seems to depend on the individual principal and the school district's mode of operation. For example, one principal develops an extensive inclusion plan and presents it as a school improvement project. She requests additional substitute teacher days for the staff so that the classroom and support teachers can meet on a regular basis during the school day. They then use this time for planning and preparing adaptive lessons and materials. Simpson et al.

(2003) reinforce this concept by emphasizing the need for teachers to collaborate on individualizing academic tasks and identifying methods that are appropriate for the student with ASD. Another example of providing planning time is that of a principal who permits his teachers who are involved with inclusion to schedule physical education, art, and music at the times they request. One teacher in the school chooses to have art, music, and physical education "back to back" so that she has at least one long, uninterrupted preparation period per week. Another teacher in the same school requests that her "specials" be scheduled at the end of the day so that she can continue her preparation right after school. In another school, the principal allows his staff to brainstorm ideas for giving extra preparation time for a general education teacher with a newly included student with significant developmental disabilities. The teachers decide that their colleague can be released from lunch and recess duty so she can have additional preparation time. The principal also volunteers to instruct this teacher's class one period every two weeks to provide time for her to collaborate with the support teacher. A popular strategy is for the school administrators and the support teachers to substitute teach for a period while the classroom teachers use that time to meet with their own consulting teacher or to plan for the class. In addition, Mundschenk et al. (2005) offer the following suggestions:

> Scheduling sufficient team planning time may be accomplished through multiple scheduling options, including staggering lunch and extracurricular activity schedules, extending the instructional day, reorganizing the daily sequence of courses and teacher planning periods, or providing team teachers with multiple planning periods. (p. 61)

Maintaining Natural Proportions and Reducing Class Size

Part of an inclusive education philosophy is for all students to attend their neighborhood school or schools in age-appropriate classes that are part of that school area (e.g., magnet schools, vocational schools, charter schools). In this way no one school will have a disproportionate number of students with disabilities in attendance, schools and classes can maintain a natural heterogeneity of students being served, and no teachers should be overburdened with more than the naturally occurring number of students with IEPs in any one class within the school. This approach ensures that "students with special needs do not unduly impact the class" (Halvorsen & Neary, 2001, p. 8). This factor is recognized as being an important component for establishing and maintaining inclusive schools (Halvorsen & Neary, 2001; Rodriguez & Romaneck, 2002), and it is the school principal's responsibility to maintain heterogeneous groupings with an appropriate number of students with disabilities in the general education classrooms (Frederickson, Dunsmuir, Lang, & Monsen, 2004; Mundschenk et al., 2005).

Another recommendation that helps teachers with including students with disabilities is for principals to find ways to reduce class sizes (McLeskey & Waldron, 2002). According to Simpson et al. (2003), a reduced class size helps general education teachers to be more responsive to all students: "Specifically, teachers who have fewer students are often able to better individualize instruction for students and use a wider variety of instructional methods and more effectively manage their classrooms and thereby experience fewer discipline problems" (pp. 120, 123).

Providing Administrative Support

Many teachers feel supported by principals when discussion time is scheduled on a regular basis or at the request of the teacher(s). This discussion time schedule may be either formally or informally arranged. One of the main needs teachers have is for the principal to listen to them in an open-minded way and to interact in a manner that supports teachers' innovative ideas or new approaches to difficult situations. Principals who provide caring and authentic support through personal interest and encouragement using the above approaches do much to support and empower classroom teachers. It is important for the school administrator to offer a variety of ways for teachers and teams to communicate, support, and be part of this collaboration (Downing, Eichinger, & Williams, 1997; Mundschenk et al., 2005; Simpson et al., 2003). Rodriguez and Romaneck (2002) further suggest that administrators provide opportunities for teachers to meet and discuss "the big issues," such as grading, which are involved when establishing inclusion and be allowed to come to consensus on these issues.

Establishing School-Based Teams

School-based teams are consistently recommended as being helpful for teachers involved in the integration or inclusion of students with disabilities (e.g., CEC Working Forum on Inclusive Schools, 1994; Chalfant, Pysh, & Moultrie, 1979; Porter, Collicott, & Larsen, 2000; Walther-Thomas et al., 2000; Webber, 2005). School principals are instrumental in establishing the school-based team(s). Though each team may vary significantly in membership, format, and function, frequent use of collaborative and problem-solving teams has led to successful inclusion programs (Porter et al., 2000; Voltz, Brazil, & Ford, 2001; Walther-Thomas et al., 2000). Although the most frequent and effective use of teams is to help generate specific strategies for particular classroom and instructional situations, practices may vary depending on the needs of the school and the staff members involved. Team members also may help a teacher prepare and plan for the inclusion of a student with developmental disabilities or may assist in establishing a student's IEP. Some school-based teams get started as an inclusion team to facilitate the study of and plan for inclusion (Webber, 2005).

Some administrators feel that it is important for the principal to be involved on the school-based team during the formative years, perhaps even acting as chairperson. Once a team is running smoothly, the principal may remain a member but not necessarily act as chairperson. Some school administrators have included teachers who are not supportive of inclusion as members of the team. When a staff member has become part of an active group responsible for developing strategies and supporting teacher colleagues, attitudes and behaviors have changed in a positive direction.

School administrators who have established school-based teams emphasize the importance of the team meeting schedule. The recommendation is that, if possible, team meetings should be scheduled during the school day rather than before or after school, and reasonable time limits should be established, agreed upon, and adhered to for the meetings. As one administrator stated, "People appreciate knowing that the [teacher assistance team] TAT [problem-solving session] will end on time and usually are not opposed to staying after school if they have participated in making the decision about the meeting time" (Perner, 1991, p. 166).

Allowing Time for Visitations and Sharing Sessions

Effective practice demonstrates that school administrators should facilitate opportunities for teachers and other staff to visit and observe the classes of teachers who have successful experiences with inclusion (Daane, Beirne-Smith, & Latham, 2000; Idol, 2006; McLeskey & Waldron, 2002; Mundschenk et al., 2005). This may be in the teacher's own school or in another school. The school principal should arrange the visitations, ensure that the teachers have a chance to talk to other teachers and school administrators, look for feedback and follow-up, and assist the teachers in drawing constructive strategies from the experience. Krajewski and Krajewski (2000) also suggest that school administrators need to visit schools and meet with other administrators who have been successful in establishing inclusion in their schools. Principals can thereby learn how other administrators initiated and maintained inclusive education practices.

In addition to sharing through visits, principals can use regular staff meetings to share a successful inclusion experience from a specific classroom. Some principals have achieved this by scheduling special "potluck" breakfasts or lunches in which staff can combine a meal and sharing. One principal found more time for teachers to share experiences and to problem-solve by putting all school announcements in a flyer to be read before a staff meeting. Once essential questions about the announcements were answered at the meeting, the staff could then concentrate on talk about teaching (Perner, 1991).

Providing Time for Transitional Planning

Transitional planning is viewed as an important strategy in the inclusion process (Halvorsen & Neary, 2001). It should begin before a student with developmental disabilities enters school or, once the student is in school, at the end of the school year. The school principal should ensure that a process for this planning is in place. Release time needs to be arranged so the teachers receiving a student with disabilities will have adequate time to observe the student in class, meet with the parents, and discuss the student's needs with the current teacher(s). Likewise, the current teacher(s) will need time to prepare the receiving teacher(s). This may include observing the receiving teacher(s) in the classroom environment, meeting with the teacher(s), and following up on observations and meetings once the student has moved to the receiving teacher's class.

This type of planning becomes crucial when a student is entering a new school (e.g., middle or high school). The principals of both schools need to facilitate cooperation among teachers to make transitional planning run smoothly and effectively.

Supporting the Changing Roles and Responsibilities of Staff

The principal is key to supporting teachers in making changes to their roles and responsibilities. School administrators can validate the teachers' new roles and the need to change by focusing on helping students with disabilities to be included in the general education class and accommodated in the general education curriculum. Both the general education and the special education teachers need to examine their roles and responsibilities in light of "changing the school to fit the child" (Mundschenk et al., 2005, p. 60). Traditionally, the most popular model for integrating and including students is the consultation model, in which the "specialists" advise teachers on instructional or behavioral strategies for the students with disabilities (Webber, 2005). However, the collaborative consultation or collaborative model (also referred to as the support teacher model) seems to be preferable, since it denotes "equal status among team members who share information and jointly engage in problem solving" (Simpson et al., 2005, p. 197). In this way, the general education teachers share expertise on curriculum content and standards, while the special education teachers share expertise on teaching and learning strategies (Mundschenk et al., 2005).

The collaborative consultant model, herein referred to as the support teacher model, has been used successfully in several Canadian school districts to support inclusion programs (Crawford & Porter, 1992). This approach has been described in more detail in Chapter 26. It is appropriate to note here, however, that the support teacher needs the assistance of the principal in implementing inclusion in the school. As well, the general education teachers need to work cooperatively with support teachers (i.e., special education teachers) in order for both groups of teachers to mutually define their roles and identify their responsibilities in the teaching of the class (e.g., co-teaching, team teaching) and in supporting individual students. By sharing, general education teachers can learn about specific teaching methods and adaptations, and special education teachers can learn about curriculum content and standards. If teachers collaborate during this process, it will ultimately be the students who benefit from the expanded resources of two teachers working together.

Many principals emphasize the importance of selecting support teachers who can assume a leadership role and effectively collaborate with staff and parents. Because administrators have numerous responsibilities within their school, they tend to rely on the support teacher to facilitate collaboration and inclusion. Once inclusion is under way, principals feel that the support teacher plays a major role in facilitating the inclusion of students. The role of the school administrators then is to provide assistance as needed.

Recognizing Success and Promoting Public Awareness

It is important for school administrators to promote inclusion by ensuring that the positive experiences are shared with staff, parents, and the community at large. In addition to parent meetings, school bulletins, and other internal means, the local media, such as newspapers, radio, and television, should be used. School and school district Web sites should display information about inclusion and promote the school in welcoming and educating students together in positive, supportive environments. Successes also need to be shared with school board members and district administrators because their support can be critical to any school program. It is important to show that communication and collaboration are occurring within the school (Krajewski & Krajewski, 2000; Simpson et al., 2003).

Principals can ensure that the work of effective teachers is recognized (Mundschenk et al., 2005). The school administrators can send staff to other schools to share their successes and can also have teachers from other schools observe and discuss the program with their staff. Administrators have volunteered to have other teachers visit, observe, and discuss the program with their staff. Teachers feel complimented when their principals ask them to share their experiences with others within and outside of the school environment (e.g., presenting at a conference).

Support Strategies for Teachers

Researchers, teachers, and principals who are experienced with inclusive practices have identified specific suggestions for the classroom teacher who is involved in the process of integrating or including students with developmental disabilities into general education classrooms. These suggestions include: (a) making a commitment, (b) collaborating and sharing, (c) working with support personnel, (d) participating in professional development (e.g., having experience and training, visiting inclusive education schools and classes, sharing experiences and problem-solving), and (e) enhancing family support.

Making a Commitment

For most teachers, having students with developmental disabilities included in the classroom is a new experience. Often teachers do not feel prepared for this change, and their greatest concerns (stressors) are that they will not provide appropriate instruction for their students and that the behaviors of students with significant developmental disabilities will be disruptive to the class (Forlin, 2001). Making a commitment to inclusion may require overcoming some fears and prejudices and changing attitudes about students with developmental disabilities. Teachers need to have a better understanding of inclusion, to be prepared, and to have direct, positive experiences with students with disabilities. It also may mean changing attitudes about working with others or sharing a responsibility that is new to them. Therefore, making a commitment to integrating or including students with disabilities also involves making a commitment to collaboration, teaming, and sharing expertise (Frederickson et al., 2004; Kugelmass, 2006; Simpson et al., 2003). For general education and special education teachers alike this can be a difficult task. Generally teachers are not used to working together and sharing students and the traditional teaching responsibilities assigned to their role.

Teacher attitudes affect commitment (Burke & Sutherland, 2004). Teacher attitudes can go beyond feelings and beliefs about students with disabilities. The attitudes and commitment of teachers can also be affected by the many changes that take place when including students with disabilities, such as having to change roles and responsibilities, their "ownership" of students, and their traditional ways of teaching.

To have a better understanding of inclusion, it may be helpful to spend time talking to parents and other teachers who have had experience with students with developmental disabilities. This kind of information sharing can help allay the fears that are a natural part of inexperience. Meeting a student with developmental disabilities and observing the student can also make a difference in teacher attitudes and the commitment to provide instruction. Observing another teacher or working with another teacher can help to diminish fears and give the teacher more confidence through knowing what to expect in different situations and practicing in a nonthreatening way.

Changing attitudes and having a better understanding of inclusion may be helped by other types of input as well, such as visiting classes where students are successfully included, reading articles and books, taking courses, attending conferences, and sharing with others. For example, in the Perner (1991) study, one administrator stated that he finally understood the possibilities for integration after reading an article about curriculum adaptations. He realized that many of the strategies suggested in the article were ones he often used with students in his sixth-grade class and he felt he could apply these techniques with students who have disabilities as well. A teacher in the Perner study stated that he had a better understanding of parents' reasons for wanting their children included after he viewed a television documentary on the subject. He indicated that even though he had been informed in a professional way about integration, he was more deeply affected by the personal nature of the documentary about families and school inclusion. Watching this program made him feel more motivated and committed to the success of the integration effort in his school.

Teachers may have different opportunities to prepare for their first experience with inclusion, but they can still make a commitment. For many teachers, that commitment was to have a positive attitude, to plan and work together as a team, and then to try it and do their best (Perner, 1991).

Collaborating and Sharing

The responsibility for student success in learning is shared by all the members of a school staff. With inclusion, the classroom teacher must accept this "shared" ownership for the learning of students with disabilities who are included in the class. The classroom teacher should be in charge and make decisions regarding the education of the student with disabilities, just as the teacher does for all other students in the class. Accepting this ownership does not mean the teacher should feel alone in the inclusion process; these responsibilities need to be shared with the support teacher. In instances where the support teacher is the "former" special class teacher, clearly transferring some of the responsibility is even more critical. It is easy to simply continue to defer to the "expert" special education teacher. Also, when inclusion is initiated, special education teachers feel a loss of responsibility (Downing et al., 1997) and believe that they should continue to be the main teacher (Daane et al., 2000). This practice tends to erect what may be an unintended barrier to making a student with disabilities a fully included member of the class. This should not detract from the importance of collaboration between the classroom teacher and the support teacher and in the sharing of these responsibilities. As the classroom teacher gains experience and is provided with support, however, acceptance of responsibility for the student's program will increase. Simpson et al. (2003) suggest that the roles of the general teacher and the special education teacher be clarified and responsibilities clearly established. Halvorsen and Neary (2001) recommend that students with disabilities be on the general education teachers' class list and that the special education and general education teachers collaborate

> to ensure (a) students' natural participation as regular members of the class, (b) the systematic instruction of students' IEP objectives, and (c) the adaptation of core curriculum and materials to facilitate student participation and learning. (p. 9)

A collaborative framework should be incorporated to address difficulties so that no one teacher is left on his or her own (Hanko, 2004).

General education teachers who are integrating or including students with developmental disabilities for the first time are often unsure of what is expected of them in terms of teaching and of student outcomes. Teachers also feel that they are not doing enough for their students with disabilities. Therefore, it is important to involve the classroom teacher in all phases of planning. From the beginning it is essential for the general education and special education teachers to collaborate in establishing appropriate goals and outcomes. This should be done after the classroom teacher has had time to observe and work with the student. The general education teacher and the support teacher might want to seek answers to the following questions: What will be expected of the student? What will be expected of each teacher (i.e., classroom teacher and support teacher)? The collaborative discussion of these matters will help to ensure that realistic expectations are part of the process and thus will benefit both the teacher and the student. The teachers also need to collaborate on what parts of the curriculum the student will be involved in and what the specific learning outcomes will be. Part of this step is establishing what portions of the curriculum will be adapted and what specific teaching and learning strategies will be used to accommodate the learning needs of the student. It may be helpful at this point for the teachers to summarize this information using matrices or planning guides (e.g., Giangreco, Cloninger, & Iverson, 1998; Prater, 2003).

Including students with developmental disabilities requires teachers to change their practices. It is essential that the special education and general education teachers collaborate in sharing in this responsibility (Thousand, Villa, & Nevin, 2006; Weiner, 2003) and that they collaborate on "content area integration and for setting achievable goals" (Wolfe & Hall, 2003, p. 57). Instructional accommodations and modifications may need to be designed and a variety of methods shared in order to best meet the instructional needs of the students with developmental disabilities and to ensure that they participate with the other students in the general education class. Many effective strategies have been identified that can assist the general education teacher and the special education teacher in collaborating on making curriculum adaptations and modifications (e.g., Brady, 2005; Fisher & Frey, 2001; Janney & Snell, 2000; Janney & Snell, 2006; Simpson et al., 2005; Perner, 2004; Tomlinson & Edison, 2003a; Tomlinson & Edison, 2003b).

Working With Support Personnel

In support of inclusive education, researchers, administrators, and teachers advocate for having paraprofessional support provided in general education classrooms (e.g., Idol, 2006; Mundschenk et al., 2005; Simpson et al., 2003; Thousand et al., 2006; Walther-Thomas et al., 2000). However, sometimes teachers are fairly reluctant to have another adult in their classroom. They are not familiar with the many roles involved when a paraprofessional is assigned to their class. They now become a supervisor and a team partner. Over time, teachers do realize that the services of the paraprofessional are important and essential to them and to their students. There has also been emphasis on the need to ensure that the paraprofessional's role is to support the teacher and the students within the class, rather than being assigned exclusively to an individual student(s). Students need to have time to be independent and be able to interact with their peers without adult intervention. Teachers and paraprofessionals need to work collaboratively. Opportunities should be provided for this collaboration and for collective professional development so that teachers and paraprofessionals are well prepared for working together.

In some schools, the teachers who initially volunteer to have students with disabilities integrated or included in their classes are so dedicated and committed that they can be described as "super teachers." They try extremely hard to keep things going and hesitate to ask for help or support, even when there is a clear need for it. They are accustomed to working independently and may consider asking for help and assistance as a sign of failure or inadequacy. These teachers may not be sure how to make use of the help available from the support teacher or others who are in a position to assist them, such as their principal, district office staff, and ancillary support personnel (e.g., social workers and therapists).

Over time, teachers realize that they do not need to function in isolation without assistance. There are legitimate reasons to seek support from colleagues who will listen and help them resolve difficult situations. The school principal can take on this role by listening to teachers and offering assistance. In some cases, the principal may be able to teach a class so that the teacher can have an extra period for planning. The support teacher may help in the same way, as well as being there to provide additional resource materials and to assist in adapting the curriculum. In some situations, the support teacher may teach the class while the general education teacher works closely with a student who has developmental disabilities. Once classroom teachers accept assistance from other school staff, they realize how important it is to create a collaborative climate. A positive educational environment facilitates successful integration and inclusion. Halvorsen and Neary (2001) suggest that a transdisciplinary approach be provided to support services for students with disabilities. In this way there is a sharing of support interventions, and the staff works together in the general education classroom.

Participating in Professional Development

For schools to be successful in including students with developmental disabilities, teachers need to develop professionally. Professional development is an extremely important component and appears to be one of the most frequently cited needs of teachers in order to make inclusion work successfully (e.g., Allan, 2003; Daane et al., 2000; Milsom, 2006; Simpson et al., 2005). Professional development can provide teachers with the skills necessary to collaborate with others and to instruct students with disabilities effectively. There is generally agreement that professional development should be ongoing and based on school needs (e.g., Friend & Cook, 2003, McLeskey & Waldron, 2002; Voltz et al., 2001).

Since school staff must have the skills needed for initiating and maintaining the inclusion of students with disabilities, it is the principal's responsibility to ensure that teachers and other staff are provided with effective professional development activities (Idol, 2006; Mundschenk et al., 2005; Walther-Thomas et al., 2000). Teachers, however, should examine their own needs and be accountable for some of their professional development. For example, they may request in-service training on specific topics or instructional strategies. They may propose that such training be made available at the school or district level or they may request support to attend sessions outside the district. Teachers choose and are provided with a variety of activities, including taking university courses, reading articles and books, viewing videotapes and DVDs, or making school visitations. Many teachers, in turn, share this information with other staff members in their school or district. One approach used is forming study groups that meet once a month after school. During these sessions the members help each other through self-selected in-service training, sharing, and problem solving.

School-based in-service training is considered extremely effective because the specific needs of teachers can be assessed and addressed. Barry Bull and Mark Buechler, as cited in McLeskey and Waldron (2002), note:

> These authors suggest that effective professional development should be school-based; should use coaching and other follow-up procedures; should be collaborative; should be embedded in the daily lives of teachers, providing for continuous growth; and should focus on student learning and be evaluated at least in part on that basis. (p. 70)

Van Kraayenoord (2003) provides descriptions and references to a number of unique ways to provide school-based professional development that is continuous and supportive of school improvement initiatives.

Teachers involved in inclusion programs place great value on professional development particularly professional development that includes having direct experience with training, visiting other classrooms and schools, and sharing and problem-solving sessions (Perner et al., 2003).

Having Experience and Training

Direct involvement with the inclusion process has been identified by classroom teachers as a factor in changing their attitudes and feelings about the matter. When a student with disabilities is actually in the class, teachers are provided with a new learning experience from which positive outcomes can flow. Burke and Sutherland (2004) recommend that teachers have more direct experiences with training. To ensure the full benefit of these direct experiences with in-service training, school administrators should provide the teacher with other supports, such as time for planning and collaboration. One suggestion offered by Voltz et al. (2001) is to use "peer coaching teams designed to provide collegial assistance" (p. 29). Time might also be provided for the teacher to work individually with the student with disabilities so the personal level of knowledge of the child's strengths and needs is clear. Teachers who have had experience with inclusive education encourage their peers to "get involved and try" but also to accept that it is all right to make mistakes as you go along. Many teachers have noted that they learned a great deal because they were allowed to try different ways of integrating students. They were able to learn from and be supported by other teachers and support personnel (Perner, 1997).

Over time, as teachers gain more direct experience and school-based in-service training, the focus of the sessions should change from dealing with attitudes and access to learning about effective planning and instructional techniques. Many of these strategies help teachers to meet the individual needs of and set goals for their students with developmental disabilities while also facilitating student participation in regular class instruction and activities. Some examples of team assessment processes used to identify individual strengths, needs, and objectives and to plan for instruction within the class are the McGill Action Planning System (MAPS; Lusthaus & Forest, 1987; Vandercook, York, & Forest, 1989) and the Personal Futures Plan (Hartshorne & Salem-Hartshorne, 2005). The Scheduling Matrix (Giangreco et al., 1998) was developed to help teachers to include individual learning objectives within the context of the general education class curriculum. Many techniques are used to assist teachers in organizing instruction and adapting and enhancing the curriculum for all students. Some of these are multilevel instruction (Campbell, Campbell, Collicott,

Perner, & Stone, 1988; Collicott, 1991; Kochhar et al., 2000; Perner, 1997; Schulz & Turnbull, 1984; Westling & Fox, 2004), differentiated instruction (Perner, 2004; Tomlinson, 1999; 2001; Tomlinson & Edison, 2003a; Tomlinson & Edison, 2003b), direct instruction (Garrison-Kane, Doelling, & Sasso, 2005), cooperative learning (Fore, Riser, & Boon, 2006; Garrison-Kane et al., 2005; Halvorsen & Neary, 2001; Hardin & Hardin, 2002; Putnam, 1998), and peer tutoring (Bond & Castagnera, 2006; Hardin & Hardin, 2002).

Visiting Inclusive Education Schools and Classes

A beneficial professional development activity for teachers who are initiating including students with developmental disabilities in their classes is to visit schools and classes where students are successfully integrated or included. It is important for teachers not only to observe but also to have the opportunity to talk with administrators, teachers, and school staff (Voltz et al., 2001). Initially, these visitations may have to take place outside of one's own school or school district. As more and more schools include students with more significant disabilities in general education classrooms, the need to visit outside of the home school district diminishes greatly. Teachers not only gain knowledge from these visitations but also appreciate being given the opportunity to visit on a school day and learn from their colleagues. With the gradual movement to inclusion, more classes are accessible for visitation and for learning. The availability of various integrated and inclusive settings allows teachers with no integration experience to observe in classrooms close to home, where educational and social conditions are similar to their own.

Sharing Experiences and Problem-Solving

Throughout the process of inclusion, sharing and problem-solving sessions help both general education and special education teachers to make changes and to experience the benefits of inclusion. Teachers and principals who have had both successful and unsuccessful experiences should share these with their colleagues. Successful experiences help to allay the fears of teachers and school administrators who are new to implementing integration or inclusion. Situations that are not going well are discussed and analyzed so that solutions, or at least better alternatives, can be found. This can also help avoid the wasteful practice of repeating mistakes.

One of the most beneficial aspects of inclusion is that it encourages school staff to deal with situation-specific problems by working together in finding solutions (Kugelmass, 2006; McLeskey & Waldron, 2002). Teachers involved with inclusion need the help of their peers to generate the diversity of solutions required for individual or unique situations. These problem-solving sessions or team meetings provide teachers and school administrators an opportunity to choose and implement solutions that best meet their own needs. Teachers must create their own solutions to problematic situations. There are no preset approaches that will exactly fit the situation. There are no "quick fixes," and various team formats (e.g., teacher assistance team, grade-level teams) can be developed within a school to help solve problems (Mundschenk et al., 2005). As one elementary teacher stated, "For us, teaming has avoided many problems—everyone participates in problem solving—from teachers, to the student(s), to the principal" (Perner, 1993, p. 12). School-based teams are one systemic way for teachers and school administrators to share and problem-solve.

Webber (2005) discusses the "transition group team," which helps the school with its inclusive education initiative. The school "team engages in a collaborative effort to share information, solve problems, and plan" (p. 45).

Enhancing Family Support

In any circumstance, the active participation and support of families enhances the prospect for successful outcomes for students. In integration and inclusion programs, families are seen as primary supports in the change process. There is widespread agreement that effective parent–teacher communication is an important component in making inclusion work, and according to the Individuals with Disabilities Education Improvement Act of 2004, parents must be involved in planning and decision making that affects their children. To develop a strong working relationship with parents and families, teachers need to involve parents and families in meaningful ways in the students' educational program. This facilitates families' being more involved in decision making and being participating members of the planning team. Also, many parents and families welcome the opportunity to be members of problem-solving teams and provide a distinct perspective on the situation at issue.

With inclusion it is essential that the general education teacher communicates directly with parents and families of students with developmental disabilities. The general education teacher and the special education teacher should collaborate on this, including sharing in conferences and other interactions with the students' parents and families (Mundschenk et al., 2005). There are many ways to involve families in the education of students. For example, Epstein provides researched strategies and suggestions on how to involve parents and families (Epstein, 2001; Epstein & Salinas, 2004; Epstein et al., 2002). Brady (2005) identifies a number of useful strategies for collaborating with families and other professionals.

Parents and families should be encouraged to visit and observe in the general education class, offer suggestions, and be part of collaborative teams. An extremely useful procedure to help parents and families get involved, resolve conflicts, and make decisions is by using person-centered meetings such as the McGill Action Planning System (MAPS; Lusthaus & Forest, 1987; Vandercook et al., 1989). MAPS was developed initially to help individual students with moderate and severe disabilities be fully included in general education classes. The focus of a MAPS meeting is on the individual student, and the goal is to identify what needs to happen in order for the student to participate successfully with his or her peers in the general education classroom. A MAPS meeting includes the individual with disabilities, friends, family members, general and special education teachers, and others who know the individual well. A facilitator encourages group members to help in the process by interacting and responding to seven questions. The responses are recorded and used to find solutions to help facilitate inclusion and a better quality of life for the individual student. The MAPS questions are as follows:

1. What is the individual's history?

2. What is your dream for the individual?

3. What is your nightmare?

4. Who is the individual?

5. What are the individual's strengths, gifts, and abilities?

6. What are the individual's needs?

7. What would the individual's ideal day at school look like and what must be done to make it happen? (Vandercook et al., 1989, pp. 207–208)

This system has been used extensively by teachers to help plan inclusive programs for students with developmental disabilities and for students with other disabilities.

Conclusion

Many strategies are available to school administrators and teachers for planning, implementing, and sustaining inclusive schools and classrooms. The types of strategies and supports that are used often depend on preferences. In particular, some general education teachers prefer to co-teach; others prefer to work with a teacher assistant or have parent or university students as volunteers in their classroom. Some teachers have requested extra planning time, reduced class size, or access to a support teacher. To ensure the success of an inclusive school, it is imperative that a variety of supports are available and that teachers have some choices based on personal strengths, needs, and preferences. Although a number of strategies were offered, there are many more that can be used to facilitate the inclusion of students with developmental disabilities while helping to support both general education teachers and special education teachers with the inclusion process.

Glossary

Activity-based learning—Activities that encourage students to be actively involved and engaged in the learning tasks.

Authentic assessments—Informal assessments that help to evaluate student performance within the learning environment and usually relate to instructional objectives. Common authentic assessments are portfolios and checklists.

Collaboration—Two or more people sharing the interactions and work necessary to achieve a common goal.

Cooperative learning—Learning activities that have students work together in small groups (i.e., two to six students per group) to achieve common academic goals. The activities are planned to encourage social interactions and positive goal interdependence. Each member of a group contributes to the learning task.

Co-teaching—Two or more professionals share the planning, teaching, and assessment of a group of diverse students in the general education class.

Inclusion/Inclusive education—A high level of involvement of students with disabilities in age-appropriate general education classes in their home schools, with significant participation in classroom activities and experiences.

Integration—The early steps to move students with disabilities from segregated classes and schools to classrooms and school placements in which they are with their peers who do not have disabilities.

Interactive learning—Activities that encourage students to be actively involved and engaged in the learning tasks and socially interactive with other students.

Multilevel instruction—An approach to classroom instruction and curriculum organization that emphasizes the provision of learning opportunities for students with varying levels of academic skills through the same "core lesson." The approach suggests consideration by teachers of the (a) underlying concept(s) of the lesson, (b) methods of presentation by the teacher, (c) methods of practice and performance by the student, and (d) methods of assessment.

Support teacher—A special education teacher who works collaboratively with general education teachers in providing professional support and assistance for dealing with the issues and challenges of teaching a class that includes students with varying learning strengths and needs. Part of the support teacher's role is in co-teaching with general education teachers. Other terms sometimes used for this role include *method and resource teacher, collaborative teacher, resource teacher,* and *inclusion facilitator.*

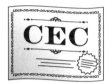

Knowledge and Skills for Entry-Level Special Education Teachers of Students With Developmental Disabilities Standards Addressed in This Chapter

Principle 1: Foundations

DD1K2   Continuum of placement and services available for individuals with developmental disabilities.

DD1K4   Trends and practices in the field of developmental disabilities.

Principle 5: Learning Environments/Social Interaction

DD5S5   Plan instruction for individuals with developmental disabilities in a variety of placement settings.

Web Site Resources

Circle of Inclusion Home Page

http://www.circleofinclusion.org/

Designed for early childhood service providers and families of young children. Useful information (including materials for downloading) about effective practices of inclusive educational programs for children from birth through age 8.

Disabilities Resources Homepage

http://www.disabilityresources.org/INCLUSION.html

Information and resources on and links related to all disabilities. The inclusion page contains links to a variety of Web sites related specifically to inclusive education.

Inclusion.com

http://www.inclusion.com/reslinks.html

Sponsored by the Inclusion Network. Offers workshops, training events, and resources for inclusion, plus links to more than 100 resource Web sites related to inclusion.

Kids Together, Inc.

http://www.kidstogether.org/

Articles, cartoons, video clips, information sheets, and more about inclusion and advocacy. An educational, fun, and inclusive Web site!

Power of 2 Web Site

http://www.powerof2.org/

Designed for online training. Includes resources, articles, and links related to collaboration and co-teaching. Can be used alone or with others to assess and develop collaboration skills.

TASH Homepage

www.tash.org

TASH is an organization that is concerned with the education, dignity, rights, and independence of individuals with disabilities. The Web site contains articles, information, and links to a variety of resources related to inclusion.

United Nations Educational, Scientific and Cultural Organization (UNESCO)
www.unesco.org

> International information on inclusive education through the education link to inclusive education. Various inclusive education resources can be downloaded, such as the book *Changing Teaching Practices: Using Curriculum Differentiation to Respond to Students' Diversity*, at http://unesdoc.unesco.org/images/0013/001365/136583e.pdf.

University of Canberra in Australia: Educational Support and Inclusion
http://www.canberra.edu.au/special-ed/othersites.html

> Inclusive education resource links from the United Kingdom, Canada, the United States, and Europe.

References

Allan, J. (2003). Productive pedagogies and the challenge of inclusion. *British Journal of Special Education, 30,* 175–179.

Ammah, J. O. A., & Hodge, S. R. (2005). Secondary physical education teachers' beliefs and practices in teaching students with severe disabilities: A descriptive analysis [Electronic version]. *High School Journal, 89*(2), 40–54.

Avissar, G., Reiter, S., & Leyser, Y. (2003). Principals' views and practices regarding inclusion: The case of Israeli elementary school principals [Electronic version]. *European Journal of Special Needs Education, 18,* 355–369.

Bond, R., & Castagnera, E. (2006). Peer supports and inclusive education: An underutilized resource. *Theory Into Practice, 45,* 224–229.

Brady, S. J. (2005). Inclusion in the preschool years. In P. Zionts (Ed.), *Inclusion strategies for students with learning and behavior problems* (2nd ed., pp. 363–393). Austin, TX: PRO-ED.

Burke, K., & Sutherland, C. (2004). Attitudes toward inclusion: Knowledge vs. experience [Electronic version]. *Education, 125,* 163–172.

Campbell, C., Campbell, S., Collicott, J., Perner, D., & Stone, J. (1988). Adapting regular class curriculum for integrated special needs students. *Education New Brunswick Journal, 3,* 17–20.

CEC Working Forum on Inclusive Schools. (1994). *Creating schools for all our students: What twelve schools have to say.* Reston, VA: Council for Exceptional Children.

Chalfant, J., Pysh, M., & Moultrie, R. (1979). Teacher assistant teams: A model for within building problem solving. *Learning Disabilities Quarterly, 2,* 85–96.

Collicott, J. (1991). Implementing multi-level instruction: Strategies for classroom teachers. In G. Porter & D. Richler (Eds.), *Changing Canadian schools: Perspectives on disability and inclusion* (pp. 191–218). Toronto: Roeher Institute.

Crawford, C., & Porter, G. L. (1992). *How it happens: A look at inclusive educational practice in Canada for children and youth with disabilities.* Toronto: Roeher Institute.

Daane, C. J., Beirne-Smith, M., & Latham, D. (2000). Administrators' and teachers' perceptions of the collaborative efforts of inclusion in the elementary grades. *Education, 121,* 331–338.

Downing, J., Eichinger, J., & Williams, L. (1997). Inclusive education for students with severe disabilities: Comparative views of principals and educators at different levels of implementation [Electronic version]. *Remedial and Special Education, 18,* 133–42.

Epstein, J. L. (2001). *School, family, and community partnerships: Preparing educators and improving schools.* Boulder, CO: Westview.

Epstein, J. L., & Salinas, K. C. (2004). A well-organized program of family and community partnerships yields many benefits for schools and their students. *Educational Leadership, 61*(8), 12–18.

Epstein, J. L., Sanders, M. G., Simon, B. S., Salinas, K. C., Jansorn, N. R., & Van Voorhis, F. L. (2002). *School, family, and community partnerships: Your handbook for action* (2nd ed.). Thousand Oaks, CA: Corwin.

Fisher, D., & Frey, N. (2001). Access to the core curriculum: Critical ingredients for success. *Remedial and Special Education, 22,* 148–158.

Fore III, C., Riser, S., & Boon, R. (2006). Implications of cooperative learning and educational reform for students with mild disabilities. [Electronic version]. *Reading Improvement, 43*, 3–12.

Forlin, C. (2001). Inclusion: Identifying potential stressors for regular class teachers [Electronic version]. *Educational Research, 43*, 235–245.

Frederickson, N., Dunsmuir, S., Lang, J., & Monsen, J. J. (2004). Mainstream-special school inclusion partnerships: Pupil, parent, and teacher perspectives [Electronic version]. *International Journal of Inclusive Education, 8*, 37–57.

Friend, M., & Bursuck, W. (2002). *Including students with special needs: A practical guide for classroom teachers* (3rd ed.). Needham Heights, MA: Allyn & Bacon.

Friend, M., & Cook, L. (2003). *Interactions: Collaboration skills for school professionals* (4th ed.). Boston: Allyn & Bacon.

Garrison-Kane, L., Doelling, J. E., & Sasso, G. M. (2005). Recent developments in social interaction: Interventions to enhance inclusion. In P. Zionts (Ed.), *Inclusion strategies for students with learning and behavior problems* (2nd ed., pp. 283–308). Austin, TX: PRO-ED.

Giangreco, M., Cloninger, C., & Iverson, V. (1998). *Choosing outcomes and accommodations for children (COACH): A guide to educational planning for students with disabilities* (2nd ed.). Baltimore: Brookes.

Halvorsen, A. T., & Neary, T. (2001). *Building inclusive schools: Tools and strategies for success.* Needham Heights, MA: Allyn & Bacon.

Hammond, H., & Ingalls, L. (2003). Teachers' attitudes toward inclusion: Survey results from elementary school teachers in three southwestern rural school districts [Electronic version]. *Rural Special Education Quarterly, 22*(2), 24–30.

Hanko, G. (2004). Towards inclusive education: Interprofessional support strategies within and across schools and school services [Electronic version]. *Education Review, 17*, 60–66.

Hardin, B., & Hardin, M. (2002). Into the mainstream: Practical strategies for teaching in inclusive environments [Electronic version]. *Clearing House, 75*, 176–180.

Hartshorne, T. S., & Salem-Hartshorne, N. (2005). But he's in 7th grade now! How can he still be included? In P. Zionts (Ed.), *Inclusion strategies for students with learning and behavior problems* (2nd ed., pp. 157–172). Austin, TX: PRO-ED.

Idol, L. (2006). Toward inclusion of special education students in general education. *Remedial and Special Education, 27*, 77–94.

Individuals with Disabilities Education Improvement Act of 2004, 20 U.S.C. § 614 *et seq.* (2004).

Janney, R., & Snell, M. E. (2000). *Modifying schoolwork.* Baltimore: Brookes.

Janney, R. E., & Snell, M. E. (2006). Modifying school work in inclusive classrooms. *Theory Into Practice, 45*, 215–223.

Keenan, S. M. (2005). Program elements that support teachers and students with learning and behavior problems. In P. Zionts (Ed.), *Inclusion strategies for students with learning and behavior problems* (2nd ed., pp. 135–155). Austin, TX: PRO-ED.

Kochhar, C. A., West, L. L., & Taymans, J. M. (2000). *Successful inclusion: Practical strategies for a shared responsibility.* Upper Saddle River, NJ: Prentice Hall.

Kugelmass, J. W. (2006). Sustaining cultures of inclusion: The value and limitation of cultural analyses [Electronic version]. *European Journal of Psychology of Education, 21*, 279–292.

Krajewski, B., & Krajewski, L. (2000). Inclusion planning strategies: Equalizing opportunities for cognitively disabled students [Electronic version]. *NASSP Bulletin, 84*(613), 48–53.

Lusthaus, E., & Forest, M. (1987). The kaleidoscope: A challenge to the cascade. In M. Forest (Ed.), *More education integration* (pp. 1–17). Toronto: Roeher Institute.

Lynch, P., & Bruhl, S. (2005). Inclusive practices in secondary settings. In P. Zionts (Ed.), *Inclusion strategies for students with learning and behavior problems* (2nd ed., pp. 93–109). Austin, TX: PRO-ED.

McLeskey, J., & Waldron, N. (2002). School change and inclusive schools: Lessons learned from practice [Electronic version]. *Phi Delta Kappan, 84*, 65–72.

Milsom, A. (2006). Creating positive school experiences for students with disabilities [Electronic version]. *Professional School Counseling, 10*, 66–72.

Mundschenk, N. A., Foley, R. M., & Swedburg, K. A. (2005). Collaboration: Building teams to facilitate inclusive practices. In P. Zionts (Ed.), *Inclusion strategies for students with learning and behavior problems* (2nd ed., pp. 57–91). Austin, TX: PRO-ED.

Office of Special Education Programs (OSEP). (2003). *Alignment of special and general education reform in comprehensive school reform demonstration programs* (Field initiated study 2003). Washington, DC: Author. Retrieved May 4, 2005, from http://www.dssc.org/CSRD/assets/alignment_01_2003.doc

Perner, D. (1991). Leading the way: The role of school administrators in integration. In G. L. Porter & D. Richler, (Eds.), *Changing Canadian schools: Perspectives on disability and inclusion* (pp. 84–92). Toronto: Roeher Institute.

Perner, D. (1993, December). *All students attend regular classes in neighbourhood schools: A case study of three schools in Woodstock, New Brunswick, Canada* (Research report for Organization for Economic Co-operation and Development/Centre for Educational Research and Innovation International Conference on Active Life for Disabled Youth—Integration in the School Project. Vaals, The Netherlands).

Perner, D. (1997). Supporting the classroom teacher in New Brunswick. In Organization for Economic Co-operation and Development (OECD)/Centre for Educational Research and Innovation (CERI), *Implementing inclusive education* (pp. 75–80). Paris: OECD Publications.

Perner, D. (2004). *Changing teaching practices, using curriculum differentiation to respond to students' diversity*. Paris: UNESCO.

Perner, D., Porter, G., & Padora, J. (2003, February). *Reviewing inclusive education practices that support general education teachers*. Paper presented at the Council for Exceptional Children–Division on Developmental Disabilities 8th International Conference, Kauai, HI.

Porter, G. L., Collicott, J., & Larsen, J. (2000). New Brunswick School Districts 10, 12, and 13: The story continued.... In R. Villa & J. Thousand, (Eds.), *Restructuring for caring and effective education: Piecing the puzzle together* (2nd ed., pp. 484–492). Baltimore: Brookes.

Porter, G. L., Wilson, M., Kelly, B., & den Otter, J. (1991). Problem solving teams: A thirty-minute peer-helping model. In G. Porter & D. Richler (Eds.), *Changing Canadian schools: Perspectives on disability and inclusion* (pp. 219–238). Toronto: Roeher Institute.

Prater, M. A. (2003). She will succeed! Strategies for success in inclusive classrooms. *Teaching Exceptional Children, 35*(5), 58–64.

Putnam, J. W. (Ed.). (1998). *Cooperative learning and strategies for inclusion: Celebrating diversity in the classroom* (2nd ed.). Baltimore: Brookes.

Richardson, M., & Jording, C. (1999). Implementing the inclusion model: Perceptions and observations of elementary principals [Electronic version]. *Journal of At Risk Issues, 6*(1), 14–19.

Rodriguez, J. C., & Romaneck, G. M. (2002). The practice of inclusion. *Principal Leadership, 2*(8), 12–19.

Schulz, J., & Turnbull, A. (1984). *Mainstreaming handicapped students: A guide for classroom teachers*. Needham Heights, MA: Allyn & Bacon.

Scott, B. J., Vitale, R., & Masten, W. G. (1998). Implementing instructional adaptations for students with disabilities in inclusive classrooms: A literature review. *Remedial and Special Education, 19*, 106–119.

Simpson, R. L., de Boer-Ott, S. R., & Smith-Myles, B. (2003). Inclusion of learners with autism spectrum disorders in general education settings. *Topics in Language Disorders, 23*, 116–133.

Simpson, R. L., Smith-Myles, B., Simpson, J. D., & Ganz, J. B. (2005). Inclusion of students with disabilities in general education settings: Structuring for successful management. In P. Zionts (Ed.), *Inclusion strategies for students with learning and behavior problems* (2nd ed., pp. 193–216). Austin, TX: PRO-ED.

Thousand, J. S., Villa, R. A., & Nevin, A. I. (2006). The many faces of collaborative planning and teaching. *Theory Into Practice, 45*, 239–248.

Tomlinson, C. A. (1999). *The differentiated classroom: Responding to the needs of all learners*. Alexandria, VA: Association for Supervision and Curriculum Development.

Tomlinson, C. A. (2001). *How to differentiate instruction in mixed-ability classrooms* (2nd ed.). Alexandria, VA: Association for Supervision and Curriculum Development.

Tomlinson, C. A., & Edison, C. (2003a). *Differentiation in practice: A resource guide for differentiating curriculum, grades K–5*. Alexandria, VA: Association for Supervision and Curriculum Development.

Tomlinson, C. A., & Edison, C. (2003b). *Differentiation in practice: A resource guide for differentiating curriculum, grades 5–9*. Alexandria, VA: Association for Supervision and Curriculum Development.

Vandercook, T., York, J., & Forest, M. (1989). The McGill Action Planning System (MAPS): A strategy for building the vision. *Journal of the Association for Persons With Severe Handicaps, 14*, 205–215.

van Kraayenoord, C. (2003). The task of professional development [Electronic version]. *International Journal of Disability, Development, and Education, 50*, 363–366.

Voltz, D. L., Brazil, N., & Ford, A. (2001). What matters most in inclusive education: A practical guide for moving forward. *Intervention in School and Clinic, 37*(1), 21–23.

Walther-Thomas, C., Korinek, L., McLaughlin, V., & Williams, B. (2000). *Collaboration for inclusive education: Developing successful programs.* Needham Heights, MA: Allyn & Bacon.

Webber, J. (2005). Responsible inclusion: Key components for success. In P. Zionts (Ed.), *Inclusion strategies for students with learning and behavior problems* (2nd ed., pp. 29–55). Austin, TX: PRO-ED.

Weiner, H. M. (2003). Effective inclusion, professional development in the context of the classroom. *Teaching Exceptional Children, 35*(6), 12–18.

Westling, D. L., & Fox, L. (2004). *Teaching students with severe disabilities* (3rd ed.). Upper Saddle River, NJ: Merrill/Prentice Hall.

Wolfe, P. S., & Hall, T. E. (2003). Making inclusion a reality for students with severe disabilities. *Teaching Exceptional Children, 35*(4), 56–61.

Zionts, P. (2005). *Inclusion strategies for students with learning and behavior problems* (2nd ed.). Austin, TX: PRO-ED.

28

Evidence-Based and Emerging Practices for Generating Data-Oriented Results That Matter:

The Continuing Complexity of Transformational Change

Garnett J. Smith, Patricia J. Edelen-Smith, and Robert A. Stodden

Summary

This chapter describes a field-based, operational strategic-planning process that initiates, installs, and supports the creation of transdisciplinary (TD) learning organization teams, a process that the authors have researched and reported on for more than a decade. The TD strategic-planning processes, procedures, and supports described here have been used and evaluated within and across more than 50 SEA, LEA, and IHE settings throughout the United States and the Pacific Basin. The intent of the chapter is to start honest discussions around the "mixed bag" of evidence-based results detailed in the chapter. Six factors identified as being critical to core transformational change in special education and community support systems, programs, and services have by and large stood the test of time and serve to delineate the remaining discussion points in the chapter: (a) provision of actionable knowledge and support study and practice vis-à-vis the dissemination and installation of evidence-based research and performance, (b) importance of obtaining a "critical mass" of stakeholders, (c) importance of involving all relevant educational stakeholders, (d) importance of creating a vision of where the TD team is headed and how to tell when it has arrived, (e) value added through critical-friend associations, and (f) construction of cooperative, collaborative, and congruent networks of stakeholders. The significance of evaluating evidence-based practices *for* creating TD learning organizational teams and the evidence-based effectiveness *of* TD learning organizational teams are also explained.

Learning Outcomes

After reading this chapter, you should be able to:

- Explain why authoritarian-based federal, state, and local strategic-management plans so rarely create the networks and supports necessary to bring about transformational change.

- List four perennial problems that repeatedly confound and impede the installation of transdisciplinary (TD) learning organizations.

- Compare and contrast the premises upon which strategic management and strategic planning are founded.

- Explain the significance of "critical friends" and "critical mass" to TD team development.

- Illustrate how transformational change develops out of the interaction within and between actionable knowledge and stakeholder behavioral change.

- Define what is meant by "big-picture" agents of change

- Provide a rationale for evaluating both "assessment *for*" and "assessment *of*" TD learning organization teams.

Introduction

> Reviews and analyses of any knowledge base must build upon and update previous work in order to provide a current accurate perspective on what works, so there is constantly the need for new synthesis and analysis of research findings. (Cook & Schirmer, 2003, p. 202)

If Special Education Is the Solution, What Is the Problem?

The following appeal was voiced by the mother of Jennifer Felix, lead litigant in a federal class-action lawsuit that became a 15-year court case against the State of Hawai'i:

> And the need for help doesn't end when these kids graduate or are no longer in the public school system. Their problems are lifelong. Just because they graduate from high school doesn't mean they don't have learning problems anymore. If they don't have services for adults [or requisite skills as adults] what do you think happens to these kids? (cited in Shapiro, 2005, p. 2)

This petition reinforces the notion that the long-term (adult and community) educational, social, and vocational well-being of youth with developmental disabilities (DD) and other disabilities is a fundamental obligation of special education and its related adult/community support services and agencies (McTernan & Ward, 2005). The newly authorized Individuals with Disabilities Education Improvement Act of 2004 (IDEIA 2004; P.L. 108-446) clearly renews this obligation in the form of a written mandate for special educators to intensify their efforts to refine and expand the knowledge base of validated and promising practices and procedures shown to improve the attainment of educational, vocational, and social *results that matter* for adolescents and young adults with DD (Cook & Schirmer, 2003; National Council on Disability, 2004).

But is the rhetoric of "results that matter" as articulated in IDEIA 2004 merely what Stodden and Leake (1994) term "old wine in new bottles"? (p. 65). It has been 30 years since P.L. 94-142, the Education for All Handicapped Children Act of 1975, was signed into law. During those 30 years, a multitude of companion initiatives, legislative mandates, court orders, and other external directives has been imposed upon state education agencies (SEAs), local education agencies (LEAs), and institutions of higher education (IHEs) in an attempt to demonstrate improvement in programs and services for children and youth with disabilities (Willis, 2002; Ysseldyke et al., 2004).

In spite of all of the mandates, finger-pointing, name-calling, teacher-proofing of scripts, and the threats and frustration that emanate from external directives, the availability of sufficient and appropriate inclusive community-based services and supports that demonstrably improve adult and community results with youth with DD and other disabilities remains elusive (Brown, 2000; McTernan & Ward, 2005; National Council on Disability, 2004; Nelson, 2004; Scarpati & Peck, 2005;

Sizer, 2004; Sparks, 2004). In general we concur with Edgar, Patton, and Day-Vines (2003) that the current state of special education is a mess. The result of ideological battles, legal issues, and rampant individualism—all coupled with the high-stakes testing movement—has been that children with disabilities are not receiving the multidimensional (i.e., home, community, employment, health, post-secondary education, social, protection, and advocacy) experiences that they require and deserve (cf. Heward, 2003; Kochhar-Bryant & Bassett, 2004; Pearman, Elliott, & Aborn, 2004; Thompson et al., 2002). As noted by deFur (2002):

> If the purpose of schooling is to prepare students to live and work as citizens of this country to the best of their abilities, then educational standards must address competencies beyond academic skills, education must educate beyond the classroom and into the community . . . education for life. (p. 210)

Ironically, the recurring patterns of perceptible confusion, overt inflexibility, and regulated conformity that follow most externally imposed special education/ special services reform efforts may not be the greatest impediment to systemic improvement in general education, vocational education, and special education. The greater impediment seems more closely linked to a widely held (but rarely proven) public and conventional wisdom that SEAs, LEAs, IHEs, and the administrators, teachers, and students within those institutions "don't work hard enough; and that they are lazy, unmotivated, and self serving" (Elmore, 2003, p. 9). The opinion is that members of the educational community are doing whatever they choose to do rather than what they are "supposed" to do. If LEAs and the educators that work in them are offered greater incentives (e.g., merit raises) or threatened with onerous sanctions (e.g., transfer, the educational equivalent of disbarment), the argument goes, then they will be motivated to discover the "new order of things" and to do what needs to be done to improve school and student performance (Smith & Edelen-Smith, 2002). Unfortunately, this classic positive/negative reinforcement predicament is analogous to a cartoon in a recent magazine. The cartoon illustrates galley slaves rowing a ship. Over the heads of these slaves is a plaque inscribed "The beatings will continue until morale improves." As the Roman playwright Lucius Seneca opined nearly 2,000 years ago, "Laws do not persuade just because they threaten" (cited in Stossel, 2004, p. 155). The difficulty with authoritarian models of policy and practice— designed with firm horizontal and vertical boundaries and the dominant principle of "repeat" rather than "create"—is that instead of telling the recipients what to do about crafting a new order of things, they tell the recipients to "just get better" (Beyerlein, Freedman, McGee, & Moran, 2002; Eisler & Montuori, 2001; Elmore, 2003; Joyce, 2004). As Schelling points out, "The problem with incentive [and threat] structures is not getting people to do the right thing. It's getting people to know the right thing to do" (cited in Elmore, 2003, p. 9). For the most part, administrators, teachers, and IHE professionals are devoted and caring advocates for children. They do the best they know how to do. Fatten the pot with incentive carrots or threaten to flay them with sanction sticks, and they still do the best they know how to do, which is what they knew before the new order was mandated (Joyce, 2004; Smith & Edelen-Smith, 2002).

The key to producing results that matter for youth and adults with DD is to invent, implement, refine, and share credible and evidence-based system and structural change models, supports, and practices that demonstrate the power to convert and sustain loosely knit communities of interdependent, transdisciplinary (TD) professionals, family members, individuals with disabilities, agency caregivers, and other education planning partners into *big-picture agents of change* (Barber &

Fullan, 2005; Brady, 2004; Brulle, 2005; Eisler & Montuori, 2001) who are intent on achieving transformational change (Eckel, Hill, & Green, 1998). Big-picture agents of change willingly work within networks and teams; they voluntarily establish sustaining relationships with the other community stakeholders; they regularly examine proven and emerging evidence-based practices; and they make decisions based upon shared promising practices and evidence-based data (Brady, 2004; Brantlinger, Jimenez, Klinger, Pugach, & Richardson, 2005; Dunst, Trivette, & Cutspec, 2002). However, "it's not just a question of explaining the big picture; it's a matter of actively and constantly seeking feedback, refining the [plan] where necessary, and making the big picture come alive on the ground" (Barber & Fullan, 2005, p. 34).

The Details of Transformational Change: Seeking Cooperation, Collaboration, and Congruence

Creating the kind of stakeholder teams that consist of "big-picture" agents requires **571** a fresh understanding about redesigning TD organizations to achieve valued adult community outcomes for children and youth with DD. It requires a fresh understanding of what it takes to achieve "aggressively original, sustained, comprehensive *invention*" (Sizer, 2004, p. 108, italics in original). The big idea at the center of this redesign is a comprehensive consideration of what is required to align a group of interacting, interrelated, and interdependent organizations, facilities, and personnel into a complex but unified whole. In other words, we need to consider ways of understanding the realities that influence and advance transformational cooperative, collaborative, and congruent relationships among the TD organizational constituents (educators, agency personnel, parents, persons with DD, etc.) rather than the constituents themselves (Friend, 2000; Heward, 2006; Senge et al., 2000; Systems Thinker, n.d.).

As Rose (2005) comments, "We are trapped in a language of schooling that stresses economics, accountability, and compliance. These are important issues to be sure, but they are not the stuff of personal dreams and common vision, not a language that inspires [transformational change]" (p. 42).

More than a decade ago, Shanker (1990) warned of perennial problems that repeatedly confound and impede the installation and sustainability of transformational cooperation, collaboration, and congruence if four conditions are not observed. First, there needs to be prior acknowledgment that nothing can change within an organization unless and until the people (human resources) within the organization are willing to change and that people change requires a great deal of internal and external training, persuasion, and support in order for it to be accomplished (Smith & Edelen-Smith, 2002). In short, people need to stop making decisions that affect other people without talking to or including those other people in the decision-making process (Archer, 2005; Sizer, 2004). While seemingly self-evident, this basic tenet is often ignored or overlooked.

Second, there must be the realization that the attainment of transformational congruence is a highly volatile experience. Creating, installing, and sustaining long-term changes in policy, programs, and professional hierarchies and relationships is a high-risk proposition that is sure to result in a considerable amount of chaos, confusion, and resistance (Schmoker, 2004b; Smith & Edelen-Smith, 2002). The problem occurs when this aspect of the process is not recognized and anticipated. In many cases performance or resistance problems can be diminished or avoided simply by communicating information about the capricious nature of organizational change to the involved stakeholders and teams (Center for Effective Performance, 2004; Jentz & Murphy, 2005).

Third, there must be open acknowledgment that the purging of old ways and means requires *reculturing* in addition to restructuring. Decisions that require organizations to "let go" must be thought out carefully as to their "shared community culture" implications (Fullan, 2000). Shared community culture is that intangible "something" that influences the environments and communities in which the stakeholders work and reside every day. According to Systems Thinker (n.d.), "In the area of [stakeholder and team] organizational learning, it refers to the policies, beliefs, activities, and rituals that determine an organization's 'personality'" (p. 2). A shared community culture will not emerge without willingness to change beliefs, activities, and rituals that heretofore determined the way the stakeholders conceptualized and went about their work (Tye, 2000). Suffice it to say that "when you change the way people work it's a big deal" (Center for Effective Performance, 2004, p. 2).

Fourth, it is imperative that the concerned stakeholders involved in building congruent learning-community teams receive long-term technical assistance and supports that help them to function more effectively within and across their newly created TD teams and networks. Time and effort invested in human resources development and technical support have consistently been shown to have a positive effect on the long-term implementation and sustainability of newly evolved big-picture teams (Smith, Stodden, James, Fisher, & Pumpian, 1999; Supovitz & Christman, 2005). Without technical support and assistance, TD teams and networks that are built are not likely to endure.

Confronting Real-Life, on-the-Ground Research: A Decade of Observations

Since the early 1990s we have advocated for, created, and field-tested energetic training and support systems centered on an overriding premise—namely, that enhanced educational, vocational, and social and community outcomes for children and youth with DD will ensue when TD learning communities of educators, rehabilitation counselors, persons with disabilities, parents, and other relevant stakeholders work together as congruent teams to "think big" about the connections to education for "life," not just "school," teaching and learning (Brady, 2004). Enhanced outcomes occur when these teams generate ideas for improving practice that are rooted in such connections, put those ideas into action, observe the long-term results, and refine their team actions according to the results (Kauffman, McGee, & Brigham, 2004; Pearman et al., 2004; Schmoker, 2004a, 2004b; Senge et al., 2000; Smith et al., 1999). Over the past 15 years we have studied and disseminated information on the long-term collaborative efforts and outcomes of more than 50 real-life, on-the-ground TD teams in California, Hawaii, Minnesota, Ohio, and Florida nationally, and in American Samoa and the Republic of the Marshall Islands in the Pacific Basin (cf. Smith, Edelen-Smith, Stodden, 1998). The TD learning communities we have helped to create in hopes that they would "invent" new structures, systems, and supports for youth with DD (and that these new structures, systems, and supports would subsequently flourish within and across their schools and community support systems) have met with limited success. In truth, many, if not most, of the initial TD teams, as well as the transformational modifications they were attempting to generate and sustain, have diminished, disappeared, or regressed to likenesses of their former being. These disappointing results have proven to be "old news" to the majority of researchers attempting to identify, replicate, and disseminate successful evidence-based strategies for producing "learning community" systems change (Joyce, 2004; Sizer, 2004; Supovitz & Christman, 2005). Joyce (2004) confirms that a substantial body of literature now exists that "describes many failed attempts to build learning communities, attempts mounted by sophisticated people, armed with considerable energy and carefully constructed strategies. There are successful cases of course, but generalizable strategies have been elusive" (p. 77). Within this same body of literature, however, there is emerging evidence that at least some versions of TD learning organizations are producing improvements in the adult and community outcomes of persons with DD (cf. Stodden & Zucher, 2004). What follows is an account of strategies and processes that are emerging as quality indicators of TD team development and "education for life" practice(s). These indicators serve as guidelines for (a) individuals who design and construct learning organization research, (b) reviewers who wish to evaluate the "believability" of system restructuring and reform by TD teams, and (c) stakeholders who wish to determine the "useability" of the research on TD learning communities (Odom et al., 2005; Perrin, 2000).

Evidence-Based Use of the TD Protocol

The literal translation of the word *protocol* is "first glue." A protocol acts as an internal adhesive by focusing conversations around community outcomes and stakeholders' work, thus enhancing the possibility that the TD team will undergo new, significant learning together (Thompson-Grove, 2003). The protocol displayed in Figure 28.1 is an updated version of one initially created circa 1993 to serve as a visual bonding agent to the SEAs, LEAs, and IHEs that were involved in developing and improving their state and local school-to-work transition programs. Many of the teams told us that this protocol helped them both to envision the different elements and levels involved in big-picture teaming and to convey those visions to their new and veteran members. We have reworked the protocol to reflect the results-focused transition language of IDEIA 2004 (Smith, Stodden, & Brown, 2005).

The protocol, based on a strategic-planning design, directly and indirectly addresses six fundamental elements consistently identified as being central to the realization of core transformational reform (Cook, 2004).

1. It acknowledges that transformational change is a long-term (three-phase) process that necessitates the provision of *actionable knowledge* and support infrastructures (plans, processes, and practices) that, in turn, will generate the dynamism necessary to alter individual and collective deep-structural behavior within and across the stakeholders on the professional learning organization teams (Tye, 2000).

2. It stresses the importance of achieving a "critical mass" of TD team members, defined as a core of committed disciples willing to speak out, to speak up, to make changes, and—if necessary—to "raise hell" if the restructured system begins to regress to its former structure (Quindlen, 2005).

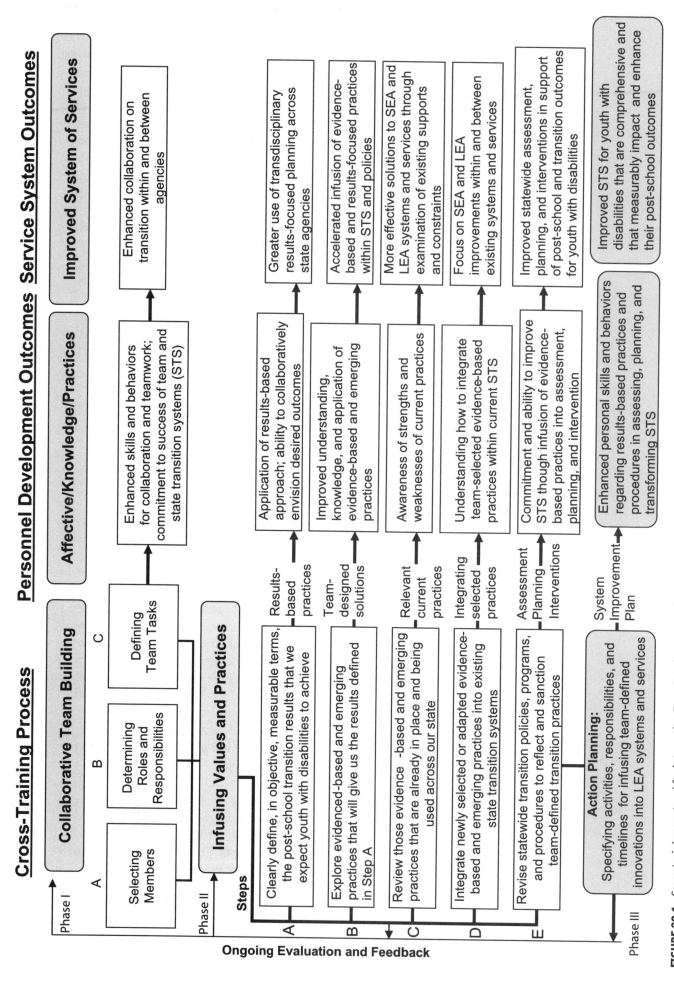

FIGURE 28.1. Cross-training protocol for integrating team development and system improvement (Smith, G. J., Stodden, R. A., & Brown, S. (2005). From Cross-training protocol for integrating team development and system improvement. *National Leadership Summit on Improving Results for Youth*. Washington. DC: Author. Retrieved September 29, 2005, from www.ncset.org.

3. It reinforces the notion that the process of transformational reform needs to begin where it makes the most sense, within the SEA, LEA, and IHE networks and organizations themselves, working in tandem with the external agencies and community support systems that serve those SEAs, LEAs, and IHEs.

4. It supports the opinion that transformational reform (Figure 28.1, column 3) cannot be mandated or externally installed. Rather it must evolve from a clear, collaborative, preferred vision of the future for individuals with DD and the identification of design-down contributions that general and special education systems, programs, services, and the TD planning partners make in order to realize that vision.

5. It sustains the provision of "critical friend" networks of technical experts who assist the TD teams in their work.

6. It authorizes the provision of TD stakeholders and teams with practical and authentic opportunities to work and network with a wide range of professional, family, and community colleagues over time.

Actionable Knowledge, Behavioral Change, and Critical Mass

In the Chinese language, two characters represent the word "learning." The first character means "to study . . . to accumulate knowledge." The second character means "to practice constantly." . . . for the Asian mind, learning is ongoing. "Study" and "practice constantly," together, suggest that learning should mean "mastery of the way of self improvement." (Senge et al., 2000, pp. 10–11)

This Chinese view of learning begins with a simple reality: new ideas are essential if TD team learning is to take place. Sometimes these ideas are created out of necessity, sometimes they are communicated by professional and consumer specialists and consultants who are "in the know," and sometimes they are suggested to the TD teams via IHE critical friend partners. Although these ideas may serve as a catalyst for core transformational improvement and change, they alone are insufficient to create congruent TD learning teams. If ideas are to become realities, the TD stakeholders and teams must be provided concurrently with opportunities to practice implementing their new ideas and to customize them to meet the needs of their particular organizations, agencies, and communities (Allee, 2000; Supovitz & Christman, 2005).

Multidimensional organizational learning is an interactive developmental process that typically requires consideration of three separate factors (Senge et al., 2000) (see Figure 28.2). First, cognitive factors serve as a unifying frame for building TD organization capacity across multiple areas (e.g., how to capture and reuse past experiences, map existing networks of expertise, drive knowledge generation for innovation, etc.) from which stakeholders gain actionable knowledge concerning the adoption and adaptation of proven or promising research-based delivery systems and supports (Allee, 2000). These "how-to and what-to" considerations, generally delivered via professional development seminars, provide the TD stakeholders with menus of field-tested (actionable) knowledge about what we know and what the stakeholder members should know about creating congruent TD learning organizations in the broadest sense (e.g., IHE preparation of TD professionals, effective results-focused planning, promising practices for adapting IDEIA 2004 or NCLB directives, evaluation of multidimensional community outcomes for youth with DD, and effective

Cognition   Behavioral Change   Transformation

Actionable Knowledge   *Collaborative Networks*   *Outcomes and Impacts*

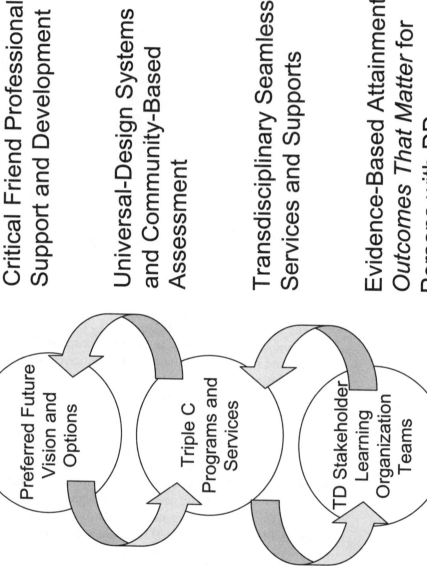

- Preparation   Preferred Future Vision and Options   Critical Friend Professional Support and Development

- Planning   Triple C Programs and Services   Universal-Design Systems and Community-Based Assessment

- Implementation

- Evaluation   TD Stakeholder Learning Organization Teams   Transdisciplinary Seamless Services and Supports

- Sustainability   Evidence-Based Attainment of *Outcomes That Matter* for Persons with DD

FIGURE 28.2. Factors involved in multidimensional organizational learning.

ways to use critical-friend networks to sustain long-term team effort). Study and practice relative to the cognitive factors in TD team development "creates a thriving work and learning environment that fosters the continuous creation, aggregation, use and re-use of both organizational and personal knowledge" (Allee, 2000, p. 2) in pursuit of transformational change. And it prevents precious time being wasted trying to reinvent the wheel (Cook, 2004; Joyce, 2004; Smith, 1998).

The second group of factors for consideration are behavioral. General and special education teachers, parents, IHE critical friends, vocational rehabilitation administrators and counselors, and other stakeholders influential in determining what constitutes "results that matter," are ill equipped by background, training, job description, and inclination to think of the whole of which their narrow areas of expertise or interest are only a part (Brady, 2004). Most stakeholders need to personally experience what it is like to work in self-correcting, cooperative, collaborative, and congruent TD learning communities before they commit to them (Joyce, 2004; Schmoker, 2004a). Just as the TD stakeholders receive initial and ongoing actionable knowledge concerning transformational change, collaborative (behavioral) networking skills also should be taught and nurtured. As Friend (2000) so persuasively argues, collaborative behavior should become a topic that is addressed within and across TD teams as regularly as are approaches for building actionable knowledge. The extraordinary synergy of cooperative, collaborative, and congruent TD teams will be realized only by fostering behavioral skill refinement through promoting a "backward-designed" preferred outcomes dialogue that brings TD stakeholders together to explore how their unique perspectives can contribute to the creation of cultures of continuous improvement (Bassett, 2005). "In addition, the pragmatic and logistical issues that arise in collaborative [TD teams] should be articulated and addressed. The problems that occur in arranging shared planning time, coordinating schedules, and preventing overlapping services are solvable and deserve priority treatment" (Friend, 2000, p. 160).

The third kind of factors for consideration is transformational. Transformational factors involve changes in the core values and assumptions of the TD teams and stakeholders so that they are attuned to the desired revisions generated from the cognitive and behavioral considerations (Anderson & Anderson, 2001; Edgar, Patton, & Day-Vines, 2003). Changes can be considered transformational only if they create a new reality and push existing settings, systems, and supports toward that reality (Cook, 2004). Transformational changes may be "revolutionary"—abrupt (critical mass) tipping points, "the moment when—sometimes quite quickly—people's actions and attitudes change dramatically, and the change spreads like a contagion" (Schmoker, 2004b, p. 431). Or they may be "evolutionary"—slow, deliberate, and methodical. "Both revolutionary and evolutionary change can lead to transformation because it is not the speed of change but its other dimensions—specifically its depth, pervasiveness and impact of culture—that matter most in transformation" (Eckel, Hill, & Green, 1998, p. 6).

We have observed in many TD learning organizations that revolutionary and evolutionary changes frequently interact with each other, growing in intensity until the organization reaches an irreversible critical-mass tipping point—a point at which the TD stakeholders choose new directions that significantly differ from their previous course of action (Tower, 2002). The critical mass of fissile material is the amount needed for a sustained nuclear chain reaction. The critical mass of TD learning organizations is the number of TD team members it takes to reach that irreversible tipping point in team and stakeholder assumptions, actions, and attitudes needed to move the team to results-that-matter changes—changes that, in turn, continuously modify the process, values, incentives, and structures of the TD learning organization (Pryor, n.d.; Quindlen, 2005; Schmoker, 2004b). The idea of critical mass transformation reinforces anthropologist Margaret Mead's exhortation to "never doubt that a small group of thoughtful, committed people can change the world. Indeed, it is the only thing that ever has." Column 3 in both Figure 28.1 and Figure 28.2 illustrate examples of some probable transformational outcomes and impacts.

Involvement of the Planning and Improvement Partners

We stand by our statements of a decade ago that transformational excellence or improvement cannot be created, installed, or mandated through authoritarian directives. It must arise internally out of the collective spirit and experience among teachers, administrators, agency personnel, students, and parents within a local school and community setting (Anderson & Anderson, 2001; Smith, 1998; Smith, Edelen-Smith, & Stodden, 1998). If transformational reforms in education for life systems, services, and supports are to occur, the strategic plans necessary for attaining those reforms must be generated and implemented by TD stakeholders themselves, not delivered from above by outside experts or external authorities.

Ironically, authoritarian-based strategic-management edicts (e.g., NCLB and IDEIA 2004) support the opinion that the locus of control for conceiving, establishing, and evaluating educational excellence and improvement lies outside the TD organization (Edgar, Patton, & Day-Vines, 2002; Sizer, 2004). Cook (2004) emphasizes that strategic-management systems and models are polar opposites of strategic-planning systems and models. While strategic-management plans are generated externally by people in power in an attempt to prevent problems, strategic-planning arrangements are generated internally by people "on the ground" to aid them in dealing with problems. Typically, strategic-management models depict the formulation of strategies leading to program or service restructuring and reform as being independent from implementation, thus separating creation from action. A strategic-planning model, assumes that the locus of control is inside the organization; "it perceives the future not as some received or conjured 'vision,' but as an irrevocable commitment to purpose beyond the ordinary" (Cook, 2004, p. 74). It is understood from the beginning in the TD protocol (Figure 28.1) that the implementers and the planning partners who formulate the restructuring strategies (creation) are the same persons who are charged with carrying out those strategies (action). As Sizer asserts, an external management plan might seem like a good idea in theory, but if the people who are going to live with that plan are not party to its conception and if the plan does not connect stakeholder thinking to stakeholder action, it will fail—if not at first, then in the long run.

Collective Vision

"Create a vision of the thing you want—out of Popsicle sticks, Styrofoam, mud, or your mind's eye. The materials matter little. What matters more is that you start to see the thing more vividly" (Mathis, 2005, p. D-1).

The initial charge to TD community learning teams is as simple as it is complex—create a *collective vision* of a preferred future for the youth and adults that they serve. This vision subsequently drives the strategic-planning process. The shared vision transmits to each stakeholder and to the learning community teams the transformational ideals and values to which they have committed. In brief, a vision is a "picture of the future" that the team and the stakeholders wish to create, described in the present tense, as if it were happening now. A preferred future vision statement confirms where the team wishes to go and what the outcomes for youth and adults with DD will be like once they get there. Because of its tangible and immediate quality, a shared vision gives shape and direction to the TD team's future (Senge et al., 2000).

Overall movement toward a preferred future vision cannot be accomplished by the TD team alone. As mentioned previously, team-invented structures, systems, and supports for youth with DD need to be infused within and across the schools and community support systems as a whole (Smith et al., 1999). External partners who are expected to play an active role through the delivery of additional supports and/or resources (e.g., Social Security administrators, DD councils, protection and advocacy councils, vocational rehabilitation, employers, etc.) are at least tacitly drawn into the visioning process. It is crucial to gain the approval of overall plans of action by stakeholders external to the TD team who are going to be asked to deliver additional (or altered) supports or resources. It is not enough merely to identify these external stakeholders. Each TD team and stakeholder member must be willing to let *team-obligated* external stakeholders become part of the transformational restructuring and improvement process as well. The importance of securing the support and involvement of team-obligated external partners cannot be overstated. Unless these external stakeholders buy in to the vision and mission of the team, halfhearted compliance and covert attacks from dissident stakeholders will likely derail the whole preferred outcome enterprise (Smith & Edelen-Smith, 2002).

Critical Friend Associations

When TD stakeholders regularly get honest, supportive feedback from valued peers and partners, not only does their practice benefit but also the attainment of outcomes that matter for their youth with DD increases too (Cromwell, 2004; Cushman, 1998; Dunne, Nave, & Lewis, 2000). In our work with TD learning organizational teams from across the country we consistently have tried to provide teams access to friendly outsider (i.e., critical friend partner) expertise and support from confident colleagues who assist the team members in putting aside professional rivalries and working cooperatively, collaboratively, and congruently for the benefit of the individuals they serve (Heward, 2006; Pelletier, 2006). As Cushman (1998) explains, critical friend partnerships can aid in the development of new habits of cooperation, collaboration, and congruence in the midst of the action of real life on the ground. However, seeking out and honestly acting upon critical friend advice and feedback takes courage. It is important to remember that new TD team members are not students. They do not need to be supervised. They need honest, clear, collegial information and support from persons who trust them and in turn are trusted by them (Pelletier, 2006). The stakeholder members must feel that it is safe for them to try out new ideas and to experiment with their individual and collective work; they must know that they can rely on critical friend backing that is continual and focused on their own service and support delivery (Dunne et al., 2000). In many ways critical friends serve as mentors to the TD team members in that their role is to guide the team through the protocol processes and phases in a more organized and structured way (Coryell, Edelen-Smith, & Robinson, 2005: Coryell, Edelen-Smith, & Thorpe, 2004).

In summary, the strategic role of a critical friend is to help the TD teams and their stakeholder members to (a) plan, (b) connect, (c) act, (d) reflect, and (e) set goals

(Pelletier, 2006). We have consistently found critical friend associations and supports to be vital to creation, installation, and sustainability of TD learning organization teams. Critical friend associates help the TD team to go beyond the typical multidisciplinary team conversations, in which stakeholders from different disciplines talk to one another, and move to transdisciplinary conversations. In transdisciplinary conversations all members of the TD team, including the critical friend, talk with one another about better ways to provide services and supports in a uniform and integrated fashion, using joint assessments, sharing information and expertise across discipline boundaries, thus selecting outcomes that matter and that are discipline free (Heward, 2006).

Building Networks Through Practice Sessions That Improve the Real Game

In sports and in the performing arts, two settings in which team consistently enhance their capabilities through study and practice, players move regularly between a practice field and the real game, between rehearsal and performance. It is impossible to imagine a basketball team studying evidence-based "moves" without practice, or a chamber music ensemble studying Bach's Brandenburg variations without rehearsal. Yet often that is what is expected from TD learning organizations (teams). As Senge et al. (2000) underscore, TD team members are expected to learn when the costs of failure are high, when personal threat is great, when there is little or no opportunity to "replay" an important decision, and when there is no way to simplify complexity and shorten time delays so as to improve the consequences of team and individual actions. Is it any wonder that generalizable strategies for developing effective TD learning organizations have been elusive (Joyce, 2004)?

Another evidence-based practice that has stood the test of time for our past and present TD teams has been to include opportunities for practice. As we mentioned earlier, knowledge and practice are inseparable elements for TD team learning. As illustrated in Figure 28.2, column 1, knowledge alone cannot produce transformational changes without opportunities to practice that knowledge (Allee, 2000). Likewise, it is futile to expect even teams that exemplify all the elements shown in Figure 28.2, column 2, to achieve visions of preferred adult and community futures for individuals with DD if they are not provided access to, and training in, evidence-based actionable knowledge that can support them in realizing that vision. For this reason, we have attempted consistently to embed the knowledge and practice elements shown in our TD protocol within and across each and every team with whom we have been involved, most recently the statewide TD transition teams attending the 2005 National Leadership Summit (Stodden & Smith, 2005).

What Difference It Makes

"Complexity in special education has several implications for [TD team] research. Researchers cannot just address a simple question about whether a practice in special education is effective; they must specify clearly for whom the practice is effective and in what context" (Odom et al., 2005, p. 139). Early in our research efforts we discovered that assessment of the effectiveness of TD organizational learning teams needed to be addressed from two sometimes contradictory contexts of assessment (Barber & Fullan, 2005). The first or *formative* context of assessment focuses on our analysis of effective practices for creating, installing, and sustaining TD learning organizations: Have our TD team creation efforts assisted stakeholders in analyzing and reflecting upon their teaching and service-delivery methods and upon the strategies that help them to plan, assess, revise, and customize their individual and collective efforts to fit the needs of their particular communities and settings (Supovitz & Christman, 2005)? A second and more vital *summative* context of assessment focuses on our analysis of effective practices of a TD learning organization in practice—that is, have our TD team creation efforts resulted in enhanced educational, vocational, social, and community outcomes for children and youth with DD?

Our answer to the latter question is a hopeful "we think so." Some convincing summative assessment information has emerged that we have gathered and disseminated over an extended period of time and that is concurrently being supported in the literature. This research documents limited but increasing evidence of the value of TD learning organization teams vis-à-vis improved adult and community outcomes for individuals with DD (Black, Smith, Chang, Harding, & Stodden, 2002; Sailor & Roger, 2005; Smith et al., 1999; Stodden & Whelley, 2004; Stodden & Zucker, 2004). Fisher, Sax, and Pumpian (1999) and Morocco and Zigmond (2006) both provide reports of enhanced student outcomes in several inclusive high schools and repeatedly point out that a more personal transdisciplinary learning organization approach as opposed to a more traditional, multidisciplinary bureaucratic one contributes to improved student outcomes across the spectrum of developmental differences. Supovitz and Christman's (2005) report also suggests that when SEA and LEA administrative leaders support and encourage the creation of TD learning teams, the result is quantitative and qualitative improvements in the adult and community outcomes for all youth, including those with DD and other disabilities.

Much of the evidence that we have collected over the years concerning our assistance in practices for creating, installing, and sustaining TD learning organizations has been subjective or qualitative in nature (e.g., anecdotal reports of greater acceptance of diversity, increased confidence, genuine caring, and feelings of individual and collective ownership). We are constantly reminded that TD learning organization teams are unique by their very nature and definition. Because each of the TD teams we have been involved with reflects its own school and community culture and set of assumptions, universal dissemination and adoption of specific models or methods of implementation has proven to be problematic. However, external adaptations of specific models and methods of TD implementation practices and procedures have been documented (cf. www.ncset.org).

We again must concede that the majority of our TD teams failed either to survive (sustain) or to achieve the visions they so valiantly strived to attain. In reality, most of our TD learning organization teams were forced to and continue to exist in what Beyerlein et al. (2002) describe as hostile environments—environments that neither demand nor endorse cooperation, collaboration, or congruence. Still, the most troubling setback we have encountered over the years, and that we still encounter, has to do with the creation of stakeholder sustainability: the creation of TD stakeholders who deliver results and leave behind a legacy of new stakeholders who go even further (Barber & Fullan, 2005; Fullan, 2000). Our original assumption, "If we produce a critical mass of stakeholders who can envision a new reality and do whatever they need to push the existing settings, systems and services toward that new reality, then it will transform them into a self-sustaining TD learning organization" has proven to be largely unwarranted.

Conclusions and Recommendations

Ted Sizer (2004), chairman emeritus of the Coalition of Essential Schools, quips that authoritarian prescriptive directives that "order" change, such as NCLB and IDEIA 2004, are analogous to "ordering" a Model T to drive 60 miles per hour: "You can order all you want, but unless you change the vehicle, right down to how the engine's organized, you're not going to go 60 miles per hour" (as cited in O'Neil, 1995, p. 4). Orders to start picking up speed wrongly assume that the system is basically sound and that it merely needs a tune-up, which can be provided through mandated homogeneity that attempts to force TD stakeholders to do the wrong things better (Brady, 2004; Sizer, 2004). When those in power formulate "transformational" reform policies that do not address core knowledge and social behavior, they fail to understand that transformational reform necessitates a fundamental reculturing of how general and special educators, adult service agencies, parents, and individuals with DD view the way they do business. In other words, when external policy makers perform "tune-ups," the multidisciplinary service vehicle only appears to be changing. At its core it is still a Model T.

The days when a centralized authority could determine and dictate what isolated, compartmentalized "on-the-ground" practitioners need or should do are a thing of the past. Isolated, compartmentalized (multidisciplinary) silos of service must be torn down and replaced with inclusive and adaptable transdisciplinary community-focused webs. If transformational change is to occur, the prescriptive strategic-management forms of planning must give way to more cooperative, collaborative, and congruent strategic-planning TD learning organization forms (Friedman, 2006). We have indicated throughout this chapter that these forms demonstrate evidence of the potential to create new ways and means of learning at all levels and across all groups. Prescriptive, strategic-management advocates say, "'check your brain at the door,'" meaning "'we only want the part of you that can do the simple and repetitive job we have designed'" (Beyerlein et al., 2002, p. 14). Strategic-planning advocates say:

> Here's a chance to start from scratch. Rather than trying to tweak around the edges, let's figure out the best way to attain results that matter for youth with DD in our community, and how we can create the best TD learning organization possible for attaining those results. (Arnold, 2005, p. 1)

Decades of external monitoring have proven that individuals will comply with outside demands either to avoid sanctions and other punishments or to attain some material reward. However, compliance rarely leads to transformation. Individual stakeholders and the teams of which they are members can transform themselves only through their personal and collective commitment (Smith & Edelen-Smith, 2002). Educational researchers have accrued a significant amount of evidence supporting the view that transformational commitment can evolve only out of a genuine sense of vision and purpose—a dream, if you will, of what individuals with DD need in order to ensure their right to a "preferred and enviable life" in their communities and in the world of today and tomorrow. Adherence to democratic principles requires that those persons or stakeholders affected by decisions take a genuine part in debating the issues and making those decisions. Throughout this chapter we have maintained that such debates are necessary to the creation of a multiple intelligence collective mind that, to paraphrase Gardner (2005), is:

- Disciplined—that can think well and appropriately about the game "on the ground"

- Synthesizing—that can sift through a large amount of information, decide what is important, and put it together in ways that make sense to the team stakeholders and to other external stakeholders

- Creative—that can raise new questions, come up with novel solutions, think outside the box

- Respectful—that honors the differences among the individual stakeholders, groups, schools, and agencies and tries to understand them

- Ethical—that thinks beyond selfish interests and uses the power of a team to create the future rather than to predict it

Glossary

Actionable knowledge—A merging of study and practice (knowledge) that assists stakeholders in the know-what and know-how of TD learning organizations across a wide spectrum of situations and settings.

Authoritarian models—Models that epitomize the paradox of compulsory education in a liberal democratic society: "We will force you to learn in order that you may become free."

Big-picture agents of change—Agents willing to include learning (study and practice) beyond the walls of schools—on the street, at jobs, and in the home and community—in their definitions, discussions, and views of "education."

Collective vision—A unifying pledge, stated in measurable terms, that illustrates the kind of outcomes the TD team wants to create together for individuals with DD. A collective vision has no inputs, processes, products, or outputs. It contains only outcomes.

Critical friends—Trusted individuals who ask provocative questions, provide data to be examined from an external viewpoint, and offer an impartial critique of the work of the TD teams as friends.

Protocol—Rules for any procedure; a draft or official illustration of a proceeding or transaction process, as in the University of Hawai'i Cross-Training Protocol.

Real-life, on-the-ground research—Research in which its effectiveness in classroom or naturalistic settings is "established" or "examined" by the natural stakeholders in those settings.

Reculturing—Fundamental changes or alterations in the policies, beliefs, activities, and rituals that influence how people work and interact.

Results that matter—Preferred adult and community outcomes relative to: (a) independence, (b) productivity, (c) community integration, and (e) personal satisfaction.

Strategic management—A management methodology intended to achieve pre-established goals.

Strategic planning—A management methodology intended to create a new "results-that-matter" reality and drive the existing system toward that reality.

Team-obligated stakeholders—Individuals, departments, or agencies that have been obligated by the TD teams, in absentia, to provide additional or altered services or supports to individuals with DD.

Transformational changes—Changes that create a new stakeholder reality of how existing school, agency, and personal infrastructure support will be provided (a) in order to maximize cooperation, collaboration, and congruence, (b) to improve TD service and system efficiency, and (c) to meet consumer (family and individual) expectations.

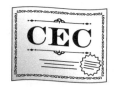

Knowledge and Skills for Entry-Level Special Education Teachers of Students With Developmental Disabilities Standards Addressed in This Chapter

Principle 1: Foundations

DD1K4   Trends and practices in the field of developmental disabilities.

Principle 4: Instructional Strategies

DD4K3   Specialized curriculum specifically designed to meet the need of individuals with pervasive developmental disabilities, autism, and autism spectrum disorders.

Principle 7: Instructional Planning

DD7K1   Model career/vocational transition programs for individuals with developmental disabilities including career/vocational transition.

Principle 10: Collaboration

DD10K1   Services, networks, and organizations for individuals with developmental disabilities.

DD10S1   Collaborate with team members to plan transition to adulthood that encourages full community participation.

Web Site Resources

The Best Evidence Encyclopedia

http://bestevidence.org

Complete descriptions of educational programs and reforms that have been evaluated in valid research.

The Big Picture: One Student at a Time

http://www.bigpicture.org

Complete descriptions of Alternative High School Initiative and big picture–inspired schools. A multitude of avenues to help change the conversation around education.

The Campbell Collaboration

http://www.campbellcollaboration.org

Potentially useful to anyone interested in the effects of social and educational programs and practices in real-life, on-the-ground settings.

National Center on Secondary Education and Transition

http://www.ncset.org

Coordinates national resources, offers technical assistance, and disseminates information related to secondary education and transition for youth with disabilities in order to create opportunities for youth to achieve successful futures.

OD Practitioner: Journal of the Organization Development Network

http://www.odnetwork.org/odponline/

Information and articles on current developments in the "organizational development" field, as well as insights and teachings from practitioners. Members encouraged to submit articles for publication.

Pegasus Communications, Inc.

http://www.pegasuscom.com

Introduction to the basic tools and concepts of systems thinking, building expertise in this essential component of management literacy through a variety of approaches.

The Systems Thinker

www.thesystemsthinker.com

Associated with pegasus.com. Provides a powerful new perspective, a specialized language, and a set of tools that you can use to address the most stubborn problems in your everyday life and work.

What Works Clearinghouse
http://www.whatworks.ed.gov/

The importance of actionable knowledge. Collects, screens, and identifies studies of the effectiveness of educational interventions (programs, products, practices, and policies).

References

Allee, V. (2000). Knowledge networks and communities of practice. *OD Practitioner: Journal of the Organization Development Network, 32*(4), 1–16.

Anderson, D., & Anderson, L. (2001). *Beyond change: Advanced strategies for today's transformational leaders.* San Francisco: Jossey-Bass/Pfeiffer.

Archer, J. (2005, August 31). Leaders go to school on business practices. *Education Week, 25*(1), 1, 20.

Arnold, M. S. (2005, July). *Innovation in education: One student at a time. Blue Sky Rhode Island.* Retrieved October 5, 2005, from http://www.riedc.com/riedc/blue_sky/32/400

Barber, M., & Fullan, M. (2005, March 2). Tri-level development: Putting systems thinking into action. *Educational Week, 24*(25), 32, 34.

Bassett, P. F. (2005). Reengineering schools for the 21st century. *Phi Delta Kappan, 87*(1), 76–78, 83.

Beyerlein, M., Freedman, S., McGee, C., & Moran, L. (2002). *Beyond teams: Building the collaborative organization.* San Francisco: Jossey-Bass/Pfeiffer.

Black, R., Smith, G. J., Chang, C., Harding, T., & Stodden, R. (2002). Provision of educational supports to students with disabilities in two-year postsecondary programs. *Journal for Vocational Special Needs, 24*(2), 3–17.

Brady, M. (2004). Thinking big: A conceptual framework for the study of everything. *Phi Delta Kappan, 86,* 276–281.

Brantlinger, E., Jimenez, R., Klingner, J., Pugach, M., & Richardson, V. (2005). Qualitative studies in special education. *Exceptional Children, 71,* 195–207.

Brown, P. (2000). Linking transition services to student outcomes for students with moderate/severe mental retardation. *Career Development for Exceptional Individuals, 23,* 39–55.

Brulle, A. R. (2005). What can you say when research and policy collide? *Phi Delta Kappan, 86,* 433–437.

Center for Effective Performance. (2004, November). *A holistic approach to introducing new systems.* Retrieved November 17, 2004, from http://www.imakenews.com/cepworldwide

Cook, B. G., & Schirmer, B. R. (2003). What is special about special education? Overview and analysis. *Journal of Special Education, 37,* 200–204.

Cook, W. (2004). When the smoke clears. *Phi Delta Kappan, 86,* 73–75, 83.

Coryell, J., Edelen-Smith, P., & Robinson, C. (2005, February). *University of Hawaii and Hawai'i State Department of Education induction and mentoring partnership model: A five-year implementation model.* Paper presented at the Seventh New Teacher Center Symposium, San Jose, CA.

Coryell, J., Edelen-Smith, P., & Thorpe, M. (2004, November). *Intensive mentoring of uncertified special education teachers.* Paper presented at the Twenty-seventh Annual Teacher Education Division Conference, Albuquerque, NM.

Cromwell, S. (2004). Critical friends groups: Catalysts for school change. *Education World.* Retrieved December 23, 2004, from http://www.educationworld.com

Cushman, K. (1998). How friends can be critical as schools make essential changes. *Horace, 14*(5), 1–11.

deFur, S. H. (2002). Education reform, high-stakes assessment, and students with disabilities. *Remedial and Special Education, 23,* 203–211.

Dunne, F., Nave, B., & Lewis, A. (2000). Critical friends groups: Teachers helping teachers to improve student learning. *Research Bulletins Online.* Retrieved September 28, 2005, from http://www.pdkintl.org

Dunst, C., Trivette, C., & Cutspec, P. (2002). Toward an operational definition of evidence-based practices. *Centerscope, 1(1)*, 1–10.

Eckel, P., Hill, B., & Green, M. (1998). *On change: En route to transformation*. Washington, DC: American Council on Education.

Edgar, E., Patton, J., & Day-Vines, N. (2003). Democratic dispositions and cultural competency: Ingredients for school renewal. *Remedial and Special Education, 23*, 231–241.

Education for All Handicapped Children Act of 1975 (P. L. 94–142). 20 U.S.C. § 1400 *et seq.*

Eisler, R., & Montuori, A. (2001). The partnership organization: A systems approach. *OD Practitioner: Journal of the Organization Development Network, 33*(2), 1–8.

Elmore, R. F. (2003). *Knowing the right thing to do: School improvement and performance-based accountability*. Washington, DC: National Governors Association Center for Best Practices.

Fisher, D., Sax, C., & Pumpian, I. (1999). *Inclusive high schools: Learning from contemporary classrooms*. Baltimore: Brookes.

Friedman, T. L. (2006). *The world is flat: A brief history of the twenty-first century*. New York: Farrar, Stratus and Giroux.

Friend, M. (2000). Perspective: Myths and misunderstandings about professional collaboration. *Remedial and Special Education, 21*, 130–132, 160.

Fullan, M. (2000). The three stories of education reform. *Phi Delta Kappan, 81*, 581–584.

Gardner, H. (2005, September 14). Beyond the herd mentality: The minds that we truly need in the future. *Education Week, 25*(3), 44.

Heward, W. L. (2003). Ten faulty notions about teaching and learning that hinder the effectiveness of special education. *Journal of Special Education, 36*, 186–205.

Heward, W. L. (2006). *Exceptional children: An introduction to special education* (8th ed.). Upper Saddle River, NJ: Pearson/Merrill/Prentice Hall.

Individuals with Disabilities Education Improvement Act of 2004, 20 U.S.C. § 175. (2004).

Jentz, B., & Murphy, J. (2005). Embracing confusion: What leaders do when they don't know what to do. *Phi Delta Kappan, 86*, 358–366.

Joyce, B. (2004). How are professional learning communities created? History has a few messages. *Phi Delta Kappan, 86*, 76–83.

Kauffman, J., McGee, K., & Brigham, M. (2004). Enabling or disabling? Observations on changes in special education. *Phi Delta Kappan, 85*, 613–620.

Kochhar-Bryant, C. A., & Bassett, D. S. (Eds.). (2004). *Aligning transition and standards-based education: Issues and strategies*. Arlington, VA: Council for Exceptional Children.

Mathis, H. (2005, September 15). *Horoscope*. Retrieved September 15, 2005, from http://the.honoluluadvertiser.com

McTernan, M., & Ward, N. (2005). Outcomes that matter: Parents' perspectives. *Mental Retardation, 43*, 214–220.

Morocco, C. C., & Zigmond, N. (2006). Good high schools for students with disabilities [Special issue]. *Learning Disabilities Research and Practice, 21*(3).

National Council on Disability. (2004). *Improving educational outcomes for students with disabilities*. Washington, DC: Author.

Nelson, D. (2004, November 24). Middle mismanagement: It's time to deliver reform to the spot where schools and districts meet. *Education Week, 24*(4), 48 & 38.

No Child Left Behind Act of 2001, 20 U.S.C. 70 § 6301 *et seq.* (2002).

Odom, S., Brantlinger, E., Gersten, R., Horner, R., Thompson, B., & Harris, K. (2005). Research in special education: Scientific methods and evidence-based practices. *Exceptional Children, 71*, 137–148.

O'Neil, J. (1995). On lasting school reform: A conversation with Ted Sizer. *Educational Leadership, 52*(5), 4–9.

Pearman, E., Elliott, T., & Aborn, L. (2004). Transition services model: Partnership for student success. In R. Stodden & S. Zucker (Eds.), *Transition of youth with disabilities to postsecondary education* (pp. 42–56). Arlington, VA: Council for Exceptional Children.

Pelletier, C. (2006). *Mentoring in action*. Boston: Pearson/Allyn & Bacon.

Perrin, B. (2000). Donald T. Campbell and the art of practical "in-the-trenches" program evaluation. In L. Bickman (Ed.), *Donald Campbell's legacy: Validity and social experimentation*. Thousand Oaks, CA: Sage.

Pryor, T. (n.d.). Critical mass. *ICMS.net.* Retrieved September 3, 2005, from http://www.icms.net/news-24.htm

Quindlen, A. (2005, August 22). The barriers, and beyond. *Newsweek, 146*(8), 78.

Rose, M. (2005, September 7). In search of a fresh language of schooling. *Education Week, 25*(2), 42–43.

Sailor, W., & Roger, B. (2005). Rethinking inclusion: Schoolwide applications. *Phi Delta Kappan, 86*, 503–509.

Scarpati, S., & Peck, A. (2005). Middle and secondary curriculum. *Teaching Exceptional Children, 37*(3), 7.

Schmoker, M. (2004a). Learning communities at the crossroads: Toward the best schools we've ever had. *Phi Delta Kappan, 86*, 84–88.

Schmoker, M. (2004b). Tipping point: From feckless reform to substantive instructional improvement. *Phi Delta Kappan, 85*, 424–432.

Senge, P., Cambron-McCabe, N., Lucas, T., Smith, B., Dutton, J., & Kleiner, A. (2000). *Schools that learn: A fifth discipline fieldbook for educators, parents, and everyone who cares about education.* New York: Doubleday-Currency.

Shanker, A. (1990). Staff development and the restructured school. In B. Joyce (Ed.), *Changing school culture through staff development* (pp. 91–103). Alexandria, VA: Association for Supervision and Curriculum Development.

Shapiro, T. (2005, June 1). Decree came too late to help Jennifer. *Honolulu Advertiser, 52*(129), 1 & 2.

Sizer, T. R. (2004). *The red pencil: Convictions from experience in education.* New Haven, CT: Yale University Press.

Smith, G. J. (1998). The consultant from Oz syndrome. *School Administrator, 55*(2), 30–35.

Smith, G. J., & Edelen-Smith, P. J. (2002). The nature of the people: Renewing teacher education as a shared responsibility within colleges and schools of education. *Remedial and Special Education, 23*, 336–349.

Smith, G. J., Edelen-Smith, P. J., & Stodden, R. A. (1998). Effective practice for generating outcomes of significance: The complexities of transformational change. In A. Hilton & R. Ringlaben (Eds.), *Best and promising practices in developmental disabilities* (pp. 331–342). Austin, TX: PRO-ED.

Smith, G. J., Stodden, R. A., & Brown, S. (2005, June). Cross-training protocol for integrating team development and system improvement. *National Leadership Summit on Improving Results for Youth.* Washington, DC: Author. Retrieved September 29, 2005, from www.ncset.org

Smith, G. J., Stodden, R. A., James, R., Fisher, D., & Pumpian, I. (1999). Facilitating and focusing whole-school change. In D. Fisher, C. Sax, & I. Pumpian (Eds.), *Inclusive high schools: Learning from contemporary classrooms* (pp. 132–143). Baltimore: Brookes.

Sparks, D. (2004). The looming danger of a two-tiered professional development system. *Phi Delta Kappan, 86*, 304–306.

Stodden, R. A., & Leake, D. (1994). Getting to the core of transition: A re-assessment of old wine in new bottles. *Career Development for Exceptional Individuals, 17*(1), 65–76.

Stodden, R. A., & Smith, G. J. (2005, June). Four tools for interagency transition teams. *National Leadership Summit on Improving Results for Youth.* Washington, DC. Retrieved September 29, 2005, from www.ncset.org

Stodden, R. A., & Whelley, T. (2004). Postsecondary education and persons with intellectual disabilities: An introduction. *Education and Training in Developmental Disabilities, 39*, 6–15.

Stodden, R. A., & Zucker, S. H. (2004). *Transition of youth with disabilities to postsecondary education.* Arlington, VA: Council for Exceptional Children.

Stossel, J. (2004). *Give me a break.* New York: HarperCollins.

Supovitz, J. A., & Christman, J. B. (2005). Small learning communities that actually learn: Lessons for school leaders. *Phi Delta Kappan, 86*, 649–651.

The Systems Thinker. (n.d.). *What is systems thinking?* Retrieved February 24, 2005, from http://www.thesystemsthinker.com

Thompson, J., Hughes, C., Schalock, R., Silverman, W., Tasse, M., Bryant, B., et al. (2002). Integrating supports in assessment and planning. *Mental Retardation, 40*, 390–405.

Thompson-Grove, G. (2003). Foreword. In D. Allen & T. Blythe (Eds.), *The facilitator's book of questions* (p. i). New York: Teachers College Press.

Tower, D. (2002). Creating the complex adaptive organization: A primer on complex adaptive systems. *OD Practitioner: Journal of the Organization Development Network, 34*(2), 1–12.

Tye, B. B. (2000). *Hard truths: Uncovering the deep structure of schooling.* New York: Teachers College Press.

Willis, S. (2002). Customization and the common good: A conversation with Larry Cuban. *Education Leadership, 59*(7), 6–11.

Ysseldyke, J., Nelson, J., Christenson, S., Johnson, D., Dennison, A., Triezenberg, H., et al. (2004). What we know and need to know about the consequences of high-stakes testing for students with disabilities. *Exceptional Children, 71,* 75–94.

29

Collaboration in the Schools:

Enhancing Success for Students With Developmental Disabilities

Jack J. Hourcade

Summary

America's schools have evolved over the last century from an assembly-line model to one of individualized instruction in inclusive settings.* One particularly promising approach to making this more individualized approach successful is professional collaboration. Though a variety of collaborative approaches have been proposed, most share such similar features as change, sharing, and "voluntariness."

A variety of barriers to collaboration have been identified, including a focus on the present instead of the future, resistance to change, lack of administrative support, lack of knowledge and skills, and lack of perseverance. Collaboration may be categorized as either indirect, in which teachers work together outside of the classroom, or direct, in which they work together inside the classroom, as is the case with cooperative teaching.

Potential issues in collaboration include role changes, interpersonal skills, trust, turf, and flexibility. These and other issues typically can be resolved through collaborative problem solving. The language that collaborative teachers use in discussing their programs and work together often offers insights into the success of that work.

Learning Outcomes

After reading this chapter, you should be able to:

- Describe how U.S. classrooms moved from an assembly-line model to one of individualized, inclusive programs.

- Identify basic features of collaboration in the schools.

- Identify typical barriers to collaboration in the schools.

- Explain the differences between indirect and direct collaboration.

- Define cooperative teaching.

- Identify typical issues in collaboration.

- Explain how issues in collaboration can be resolved through collaborative problem solving.

* The author gratefully acknowledges the contributions of Jeanne Bauwens to this material.

Collaboration in the Schools: Enhancing Success for Students With Developmental Disabilities

"They're not your students. They're not my students. They're OUR students."

In the early 20th century, the conceptual and philosophical foundations of public school programs were tremendously influenced by the emerging assembly-line factories that were changing the face of U.S. industry. These factory assembly lines took in core materials (e.g., steel), modified or changed that material in a standardized way into a new form (e.g., automobile wheels), and then sent the finished products out. In a similar way, schools took in the raw material of new and "uneducated" students, refined those students by making them "educated," and then sent them out as finished products (Friend, 2005).

A problem in this assembly-line model, whether producing automobile wheels or educated students, is the necessity for standardization and uniformity of the raw materials. In factories, if the quality of this material is inconsistent or does not meet certain pre-established standards, the factory is likely to find another supplier. Early in the 20th century, schools quickly learned that student characteristics and needs defied standardization (Friend, 2005). With the advent of compulsory education a century ago, the public schools did not always have the option of rejecting students. The result was tremendous student diversity in language, culture, behavior, and intellectual and academic ability.

Schools then settled on an alternative approach to the problem of inconsistencies in the "raw materials." Students who met some criteria of "typical" were educated in general education classrooms. Students who were perceived as "atypical" (intellectually, developmentally, linguistically, academically, behaviorally, etc.) were "pulled out" of these general education settings and were provided educational services in segregated settings (e.g., ESL classrooms, special education schools or classrooms). Initially this separation was designed with the best interests of the students in mind (Connecticut Special Education Association, 1936). However, by the latter part of the 20th century, substantial concerns about this approach had begun to emerge.

Problems With Separate Educational Programs

Segregated "pull-out" programs are practical only when (a) the numbers of atypical students are relatively small and (b) all concerned individuals are in agreement that segregated programs are effective and desirable. Both of these assumptions are at best highly questionable today.

Growth in Numbers of "Special" Students

In the early 21st century, more than 5.7 million students between the ages of 6 and 21 were receiving special education services (U.S. Department of Education, 2002). These numbers represent approximately 10% of all students in the nation's schools. Growth in other "special" student populations, such as English as a Second Language (ESL), has also been explosive, in some districts now totaling 40% to 60% of all students (Roseberry-McKibbin & Brice, 2005). Pull-out programs clearly become impractical when a majority of students participate.

592 Growth of Inclusive Philosophies

Historically, special education was almost synonymous with "pull-out." Once a student was diagnosed with a disability, he or she typically left the general education classroom for placement in either a special classroom or a special school (Friend, 2005). Over the past two decades, however, this practice has come under increasing attack (Hallahan & Kauffman, 2006). Specific concerns about the pull-out approach often center around two basic themes: (a) the fundamental efficacy of these programs (Walther-Thomas, Korinek, McLaughlin, & Williams, 2000); and (b) the underlying ethics of segregatory practices (Stainback, Stainback, & Ayres, 1996). In response to these concerns, schools have significantly minimized pull-out programs, and moved instead toward more inclusive models (Dore, Dion, Wagner, & Brunet, 2002).

In contemporary conceptualizations of best practice, a student with a developmental disability begins in the general education classroom, specifically the same educational placement in which he or she would have been placed in the absence of disability. The student is to receive in that inclusive setting whatever supplementary aids and services are required for a successful and appropriate educational experience. Only after these resources have been integrated into the general education classroom and found to be ineffective in reaching the goal of an appropriate education for the student should more intensive educational interventions, including those available only in separate programs, be considered (Gargiulo, 2006).

As of 2001, nearly half of all students identified as having disabilities under IDEA received their entire educational programs in general education classrooms. Another 28% received special education programs in resource rooms, while remaining in general education classrooms for the majority of their school day. Thus more than 75% of all students with disabilities spend most or all of their school day in general education classrooms (U.S. Department of Education, 2002). While students with developmental disabilities are more likely to receive segregated specialized services than are students with other kinds of disabilities, again the clear trend is toward greater inclusion of all students in general education classrooms (Gargiulo, 2006).

Making Inclusive Programs Work: Collaboration and the Power of Two

The issue is increasingly not whether students with developmental disabilities should be included in the general education classroom but how inclusive instruction might be provided most effectively for all students, including those with developmental disabilities. Rather than describing *students* as "at risk," it may be more useful to conceptualize some *educators* as "at risk" because of the difficulties teachers face in trying to provide appropriately inclusive educational programs to students with developmental disabilities (Hourcade & Bauwens, 2003).

Historically, teachers and other school professionals have worked in nearly total isolation from each other. The traditional "one teacher–one class of students" organizational structure of the schoolhouse prohibited educators from participating in the sort of collaboration that characterizes most productive and efficient contemporary workplaces (Friend & Cook, 2003; Fullan & Hargreaves, 1991). Thus it is not surprising that much of the present-day effort to renew the nation's schools features greater professional collaboration, in which school professionals share program planning, program implementation, program evaluation, and program accountability (Hourcade, Parette, & Anderson, 2003). In fact, many view collaboration as the most promising way to implement inclusive programs (McCormick, Noonan, Ogata, & Heck, 2001).

Collaboration is a way for people to interact. It is not a process, or an end in and of itself. Rather it is an overall way to think about and structure the shared planning and working relationships through which professionals approach their work. In the schools, collaboration is based on the shared and ongoing commitment of two or more professionals to joint ownership of, and joint obligation to, a larger part of a school's educational responsibilities than either professional individually has assumed in the past (Hourcade & Bauwens, 2003).

Essential Features of Collaboration

There is no single unique approach called "collaboration." Instead, there are a number of different ways in which collaborative efforts might be structured. However, most effective approaches to school collaboration share several basic features.

Collaboration Is Change

First, as school personnel move into collaborative arrangements, they must engage in self-examination and make a commitment to change. Teachers who are unwilling to recognize that substantive changes are necessary are unlikely to be successful collaborators.

After accepting that fundamental changes are in order, educators must then accurately identify those established practices and beliefs that are no longer appropriate. This involves the frequently difficult task of discarding old and dear methods that have become second nature.

Finally, the changes must be translated into actual practice. School professionals may be willing to go through abstract intellectual exercises in identifying the possible changes that collaboration will require. However, in the absence of personal and systemic commitments to actually implementing these changes in practical settings, success is unlikely (Hourcade & Bauwens, 2003).

Successful and adaptive teachers recognize that change is a process, not an event. It is not something to be completed and then never revisited. In dynamic social organizations such as schools, change is inherent in the system (Correa, Jones, Thomas, & Morsink, 2005).

Collaboration Is Sharing

One of the most critical features of collaboration is sharing. Traditionally educators have worked as self-contained instructional units, with great individual autonomy (Lortie, 1975). Each teacher, whether general educator or special educator, had almost complete responsibility for one group of students and minimal-to-no responsibility for any other students. However, the collaborative structures that are evolving in schools throughout the world require school professionals to adopt a very different philosophy and perspective, one in which *all* educators share responsibility for *all* students (e.g., Hourcade & Parette, 2002).

Successful collaborators share responsibility for decisions and for the outcomes of those decisions (Friend & Cook, 2003). Educational activities, and accountability for the outcomes of those activities, are shared. If a problem occurs, it too is shared.

In truly collaborative efforts, resources also are shared. These resources include time, money, materials, and, especially, the skills and ideas of the involved professionals (Friend & Cook, 2003).

Collaboration Is Voluntary

School leaders have an obligation to establish direction. Given the power that collaboration has to dramatically improve teaching and learning in the schools, there is a danger that administrators may arbitrarily impose a collaborative structure upon a school. While such an administrative temptation is understandable, the nature of collaboration requires voluntary commitment of the involved participants. In the absence of this volunteered commitment, any resulting teacher interactions will be collaborative in name only and are unlikely to be successful. The hallmark of a voluntary relationship is that either party has the prerogative of entering or terminating the relationship at any time (Friend & Cook, 2003).

O'Neil (2000) concluded that schools may not fundamentally change when that change is legally imposed by individuals with limited knowledge of how schools work. However, when proposed changes have substantial constituencies supporting them, including teachers in the schools, the changes are more likely to be long-lasting.

Barriers to Collaboration

Changing as massive an enterprise as the nation's education system can be an overwhelming challenge. However, by systematically identifying, considering, and responding to the barriers to this work, the task can begin. Potential barriers to the change of collaboration include the five areas discussed next.

Focus on Present, Not Future

The often overwhelming practical difficulties in simply keeping up with the day-to-day demands of teaching prevent many educators from thinking past "What will I do tomorrow?" It is impossible for them to consider such abstractions as how they might move into collaboration when such a simple task as ensuring that there are enough classroom materials for all students tomorrow seems impossible (Hourcade & Bauwens, 2003).

Resistance to Change

Friend and Cook (2003) concluded that much resistance to change stems from fear. Change is hard. It represents more work (at least initially) and is characterized by inherent uncertainty. Many teachers understandably prefer the "devil one knows" of working alone to the "devil one doesn't know" of collaboration.

Lack of Administrative Support

One powerful factor that is consistently associated with the success or failure of such proposed school changes as moving toward greater collaboration is the support, or the lack thereof, of school administrators (Friend & Cook, 2003). Without substantial administrative leadership and support for systems transformation, few substantial changes toward collaboration can be expected to last or to succeed.

Lack of Knowledge and Skills

A long-standing educational truism holds that most teachers teach essentially as they were taught. A survey of 2000 special and general educators found that veteran teachers' training and experience often are outdated for the new collaborative roles they are expected to assume in the contemporary U.S. school. Unfortunately, even new teachers often reported having received little training in collaborative skills (Sack, 2000). Much like teaching itself, collaboration is a blend of art and science, with any inherent natural inclinations best supported by additional training in specific collaborative knowledge and skills (Dettmer, Thurston, & Dyck, 2005). In order to form productive collaborative relationships with colleagues, teachers must acquire a variety of specific types of collaborative knowledge and skills (Friend & Cook, 2003).

Lack of Perseverance

It takes much more energy to bring about such substantial school change as collaboration than it does to inhibit such development. Developing and implementing substantive change is much harder, and takes substantially more time and energy, than does impeding change. Thus, even when change agents begin with initially large reserves of excitement and energy about their task, over time they become worn down by the barriers to change. Successful change efforts require a substantial reservoir of patience and perseverance (Correa, Jones, Thomas, & Morsink, 2005).

Approaches to Collaboration

One way to conceptualize collaborative efforts in education is to categorize them as indirect collaboration or direct collaboration (Hourcade & Bauwens, 2003). The distinction between the two approaches emerges from where and how the educators interact.

Indirect Collaboration

In indirect collaboration, two (or more) educators work together outside the classroom, meeting and developing educational plans and strategies. However, only one educator, the general education teacher assigned to a class, then returns to the general education classroom to directly provide educational services to the students (Hourcade & Bauwens, 2003).

For example, a general educator might meet with the special educator in the school's conference room to ask for suggestions on developing appropriate accommodations and adaptations for two students with developmental disabilities. Following this meeting, the special educator might also visit the general education classroom for observation. The purpose of this visit is not to directly teach students or assume educational responsibilities in that classroom but simply to gather potentially useful information.

Following a subsequent discussion with the special educator, the general educator then returns alone to the classroom with one or more suggestions and attempts to implement them for the targeted students. In this indirect collaborative approach, ultimate instructional responsibility remains solely with the classroom teacher. This basic model has been the traditional framework for most collaborative efforts, including collaborative consultation, peer collaboration, coaching, and teacher assistance teams.

Direct Collaboration

The key to direct collaboration is the simultaneous presence in the general education classroom of two or more educators who are jointly planning for, instructing, and evaluating heterogeneous groups of students (Hourcade & Bauwens, 2003). In direct collaboration, two (or more) teachers not only meet and plan beforehand but then go on to work together in the classroom, providing instruction to the whole group, small groups, or individual students. This approach contrasts with indirect collaboration, where after meeting with one or more other school professionals the teacher returns to the classroom alone.

Direct collaboration differs from indirect collaboration along a number of other critical dimensions. For instance, indirect collaboration often occurs episodically and "as needed," in response to some difficult situation that has emerged. When that situation has been resolved, the collaborative structure disappears. In direct collaboration, the relationship between the educators is ongoing and sustained over time.

Indirect collaboration is often characterized by professional asymmetry, wherein one partner is the "expert" and the other is in need of assistance. In direct collaboration, the participants function as equals.

Most significantly, in indirect collaboration the teacher returns to the classroom alone, maintaining all instructional responsibility for the students in that classroom. In direct collaboration, two or more educators are in the classroom together, sharing responsibility for all students.

Cooperative Teaching

Over the past decade, one specific approach to direct collaboration, cooperative teaching, has gained great acceptance (Friend & Cook, 2003; Hourcade & Bauwens, 2003). This approach evolved from analyses of weaknesses experienced by educators engaged in indirect approaches to collaboration.

In indirect collaboration teachers do receive assistance in the form of advice or suggestions. Ultimately, however, they still return to their classrooms to "sink or swim" alone. In cooperative teaching, the special educator who is collaborating with the general educator is actually working simultaneously with the general educator in the classroom for at least some part of the instructional day. The most distinctive feature of cooperative teaching, and the one that most differentiates it from indirect collaboration, is this joint and simultaneous direct provision of instruction.

In cooperative teaching, the participants collaboratively determine who teaches what, when, how, and to whom through a shared analysis of the needs of the students in the class at any given time and the specific sets of skills and knowledge that each professional brings to the classroom. For example, traditionally general educators are knowledgeable about curricular sequencing in academic areas and are skilled in large-group instruction. Special educators are especially skilled in such areas as curricular and instructional adaptations and in the development and provision of individualized instruction. The combination of these previously separate sets of skills provides a powerful instructional package for all students in the inclusive general education classroom, including students with developmental disabilities (Hourcade & Bauwens, 2003).

Since both professionals are simultaneously present in the classroom, cooperative teaching avoids the question of who has responsibility for any particular student. Both professionals share the responsibility for the education of all students in that classroom. The relative roles of "expert" and "help-seeker" vary constantly throughout the day, as each professional takes on the function of expert in areas in which he or she has greater competence.

Hourcade and Bauwens (2003) offered the following definition of cooperative teaching:

> Cooperative teaching refers to direct collaboration in which a general educator and one or more support services providers voluntarily agree to work together in a co-active and coordinated fashion in the general education classroom. These educators, who possess distinct and complementary sets of skills, share roles, resources, and responsibilities in a sustained effort while working towards the common goal of school success for all students. (p. 41)

Cooperative teaching offers two distinct advantages over indirect collaboration. First, students in need of support, including those who have developmental disabilities or other disabilities, or simply are academically or behaviorally at risk for school failure, receive early and powerful educational interventions in the general education classroom. Second, each educator can observe and begin to acquire and use the unique strategies and skills that the collaborative partner demonstrates. This set of complementary skills is critical to cooperative teaching.

As Dettmer et al. (2005) noted, an orchestra leader typically would not bring together musicians with many different instruments only to play the same note. That would only make the music louder, not richer or more harmonious. In cooperatively taught classrooms, the integrated combination of two distinctive sets of professional skills provides a powerful instructional package, one that is highly responsive to the diversity of student needs.

Cooperative teaching offers both short-term and long-term benefits. In the short term, all students receive the robust instruction required for educational success in the classroom (Friend & Cook, 2003; Harris et al., 1987; White & White, 1992). In the long term, cooperative teaching builds schoolwide collaborative problem-solving skills and a school culture that supports the ongoing learning of both students and teachers. These outcomes help break the cycle of dependence upon segregated pull-out programs for students with developmental disabilities (Adams & Cessna, 1993; Case, 1992; Friend & Cook, 2003).

(For additional information on specific approaches in cooperative teaching, please see Chapter 26, "Creating Inclusive Schools: Changing Roles and Strategies," by Perner and Porter, in this volume.)

Issues in Collaboration

Historically, teachers largely have been isolated from their colleagues. Many educators see other teachers only briefly before the start of school, again momentarily during lunch, and perhaps again for a short time after school.

In developing and implementing collaborative school programs, this pattern changes dramatically. In direct collaboration, teachers work alongside each other for significant portions of the school day. In this new arrangement, special educators must redefine themselves, especially in the area of interpersonal relationships. A variety of interpersonal issues may emerge that are largely unprecedented in the schools.

Role Changes

As Sarason and his colleagues noted in 1966, teaching is a lonely profession. Rarely do educators have the opportunity to discuss problems or successes with colleagues (Sarason, Levine, Goldenberg, Cherlin, & Bennet, 1966). Similarly, Rudduck (1991) noted that education is among the last vocations where it is still acceptable to work alone. The professional experience of most educators has largely been one of professional and social isolation.

This professional isolation of educators (a) made it difficult for them to share new ideas and better solutions, (b) inhibited the recognition of success, (c) permitted incompetence to exist and persist, to the detriment of both students and educators (Fullan & Hargreaves, 1991), and (d) allowed (if not produced) conservatism and resistance to innovation in teaching (Lortie, 1975).

The combination of isolation, uncertainty, and individualism contributes to and sustains educational conservatism, since educators in such situations have little access to new ideas and the opportunities associated with them. School personnel tend to remain with familiar and safe practices, which may not adequately respond to rapidly changing student needs (Fullan & Hargreaves, 1991).

An especially significant challenge in direct collaboration is that special educators must make significant changes in their well-established professional identities. Establishing new professional roles is stressful and time-consuming (Dettmer et al., 2005). For example, special educators have long administered programs in which students with developmental disabilities were removed from their classrooms into pull-out programs (e.g., resource rooms or self-contained special classes). In these programs the special educator clearly was "in charge."

Now these students increasingly are receiving specialized educational services from special educators in inclusive general education classrooms. This dramatic shift in work role has the potential to cause special educators to experience a loss of professional identity and autonomy (Dettmer et al., 2005; Hourcade, Parette, & Anderson, 2004).

Interpersonal Skills

For most special educators, the single most significant change involved in collaboration is developing new professional relationships with a teaching partner (Friend & Cook, 2003). It takes work and skill to develop and maintain a harmonious and productive working relationship with another professional.

Effective interpersonal skills allow people to initiate, develop, and maintain productive relationships. Johnson (1990) identified four basic interconnected and overlapping components of interpersonal skills: (a) knowing and trusting each other, (b) communicating with each other accurately and unambiguously, (c) accepting and supporting each other, and (d) resolving conflicts and relationship problems constructively.

Trust

Teams of professionals are most productive when the surrounding atmosphere is one of trust (Larson & LaFasto, 1989). When team members trust each other, they can remain focused on problems and goals rather than concentrating on guarding and protecting themselves (Friend & Cook, 2003). In the absence of trust, personal agendas come to the forefront, and considerable energies are expended instigating and protecting against personal attacks. Also, an atmosphere of trust yields a more efficient use of time. Individuals can speak frankly and directly, without others trying to determine "what he's really saying."

When team members trust each other, each feels comfortable in proposing answers or solutions that may be risky. Each is willing to propose possibilities that have some chance of failure. Participants will contribute ideas and suggestions freely, without worrying about potentially hurtful personal criticism. In social interactions characterized by mistrust, people tend either not to propose answers or to propose only those that are conservative and safe (Hourcade & Bauwens, 2003).

Mutual trust builds as two individuals increasingly self-disclose to each other, receiving acceptance and support in return. Trust also builds as a result of successful collaborative experiences with another person (Friend & Cook, 2003). If a colleague meets another's self-disclosures with rejection, violates a shared confidence, or fails to carry through on commitments, any trust that has been built up will be damaged (Friend & Cook, 2003; Hourcade & Bauwens, 2003).

Turf

In moving into collaborative teaching, special educators must shift from professional autonomy to professional sharing. After having had sole responsibility for, control over, and personal and professional privacy within one classroom or with one group of students, special educators in collaborative efforts now are moving into a physically and psychologically different environment, one in which another teacher is present. A potentially unsettling component of this change is sharing one's turf with a colleague (Hourcade & Bauwens, 2003).

There are a number of turfs that partners in cooperative teaching must learn to share. The first of these is the actual physical environment. Many special educators historically have spent most of their school day in resource rooms, where they took great pains to construct and structure an environment in which they felt personally and professionally comfortable. Similarly, most general educators feel ownership over a particular actual classroom and have decorated and personalized that space. Many teachers will confess to a bit of discomfort when another school professional is in that space for any length of time. But in collaborative teaching, both must share and "co-own" the space (Friend & Cook, 2003).

In addition, collaborative educators must share educational materials with each other. Over the years most teachers assemble customized curricular materials, much of it purchased not with school funds but with the educator's personal monies. When teaching collaboratively, the educator must give up personal control of materials that have perhaps been laboriously compiled and assembled over the years.

Typically when a special educator begins working with a general educator, he or she does so in the latter's classroom. While this decision initially appears to be reasonable and logical, the practical reality is that one educator is at "home" and the other is a visitor. Though this fact is covert and often not even recognized (much less stated), it nonetheless can have a negative impact on the desired goal of shared educational ownership and responsibility.

If possible, then, it is a good idea for the two new collaborative teaching partners to move into a new room, one in which neither has previously worked. This new physical environment provides an atmosphere more suitable for the fresh beginning the educators seek in their professional work, while simultaneously avoiding even the suggestion that either is a visitor.

If such a move is not possible, the next best solution is to dramatically rearrange the physical environment of the general education room. Both teachers might substantially rearrange (or even exchange) furniture, work together on room decorations, and so forth. Thus the room becomes less clearly identified as belonging to the previous tenant and instead comes to be viewed as shared space. What is sought is a sense of shared ownership, of the room being not "yours" or "mine" but "ours" (Hourcade & Bauwens, 2003; Hourcade et al., 2004),

Flexibility

As educators move more deeply into direct collaboration, a consistent theme that emerges is the need for mutual professional and personal flexibility. No matter how extensively one plans ahead, it is simply not possible to anticipate and plan for the nearly infinite variety of problems that are possible in human relationships. Realizing beforehand that unexpected developments are virtual certainties makes their inevitable appearance less stressful and disturbing (Hourcade & Bauwens, 2003).

Flexibility includes substantial tolerance for ambiguity. Flexible teachers are able to receive conflicting information without forcing premature closure on the situation. Educators who are flexible are able to look at problems from many different sides and are comfortable moving from one perspective to another. They can drop previous ways of thinking about things and adopt new ones easily. As Dettmer et al. (2005) noted, collaborating educators need not think alike. But they do need to think *together*.

Collaborative teachers who are flexible and adapt to changing situations experience less stress in their professional lives. The ability to respond easily and smoothly to changing situations without worrying endlessly over them helps any educator easily "roll with" the day-to-day surprises that inevitably emerge in collaboration (Hourcade & Bauwens, 2003).

Resolving Conflicts in Collaboration: Collaborative Problem Solving

Conflicts are nearly inevitable in any extended interactions between people, including collaboration between teachers in the schools. Resolving interpersonal conflicts is arguably the most fundamental component of successful collaboration (Friend & Cook, 2003). When conflicts emerge, individuals may engage in any number of flawed conflict resolution strategies, including denial, avoidance, capitulation, domination, and compromise (Hourcade & Bauwens, 2003). None of these approaches consistently generates win–win outcomes. A challenge for many teachers is moving away from the perception of conflicts as win–lose scenarios and toward the belief that all parties can have their needs met effectively and completely at the same time (Hourcade & Bauwens, 2003).

Bolton (1979) outlined an especially effective collaborative problem-solving process, a system based on Dewey's (1916) rules of logic in problem solving. This simple yet effective process involves six steps (Hourcade & Bauwens, 2003; Hourcade, et al., 2004), which are described next.

Step 1. Define the Problem in Terms of Needs, Not Solutions

This is the central step in the process. Much of the tension in conflicts comes about when two individuals propose different solutions to a problem. When these two solutions are incompatible, arguments and animosity develop. Too often the individuals do not realize that their individual needs (frequently unstated) are not necessarily in conflict with each other. Instead, the conflict emerges from the reflexive next step after perceiving a need, wherein people overtly propose solutions to meet those often covert needs.

To avoid or at least minimize conflict, collaborative teachers should describe their issues in terms of primary needs, or the desired outcomes, not in terms of the solutions each came up with to meet those needs. One must be careful to distinguish between the final goal or what one wants out of the situation (the need) and the strategy that one developed to meet that goal (the means to that end). It is easy to get needs and solutions confused. Often conflict is rooted not in the basic needs that each perceives but in the solutions that each has generated to respond to those needs. By returning to the fundamental issues of needs, solutions that effectively respond to the needs of both can be identified (Hourcade & Bauwens, 2003).

For example, assume that a general education teacher has several students with developmental disabilities, each of whom has significant needs in reading. The special educator has proposed that she work with each of these students individually on a pull-out basis in the resource room. However, the general educator is opposed to this proposal, arguing instead that the students should stay in the classroom.

At this point each educator is arguing from a *solutions* perspective. The general educator's thinking is as follows: "The students lose too much instructional time when they leave the room each day. While the resource room time might be useful, it is even more important that they learn the curriculum being presented in my classroom. In addition, they lose the possibility of learning from their more competent peers when they are isolated in the resource room. The solution is for them not to go to the resource room."

The special educator's thinking is as follows: "These students each have reading problems that are significant and severe enough to warrant intensive intervention. The solution is for me to bring them to the resource room so that I can provide the intensive intervention that is required."

Conflict emerges between the solutions that each has generated independently. However, it is only the proposed solutions that are in conflict; it is not the individuals themselves or their basic needs.

Although each teacher is sharing with the other the solutions that she or he individually generated, the basic needs that led to the development of those conflicting solutions in the first place have not been identified or shared. The first (and most critical step) in collaborative problem solving is for each person to share with the other not the solutions that he or she individually generated but the primary needs that the proposed solutions were designed to address.

Thus the general educator might share with the special educator her concern that when students leave the room they miss out on important curricular content and group learning activities. Her need is that students receive these experiences. Similarly, the special educator might explain his belief that the students have reading problems that require intensive intervention. His need is that students receive intensive educational intervention. These two needs may not be in conflict with each other, leading to the possibility of a win–win solution.

One effective way to discover the needs that another person has (which led to the solution that he or she proposed) is to find out *why* he or she wants the particular solution he or she initially proposed. What advantages does it hold for the individual? What need is it meeting?

Each cooperative teaching partner must be able to distinguish between means and ends, between needs and solutions. Once the fundamental "why" underlying a proposed solution is understood by the other, the collaborative problem-solving process can begin in earnest.

Perhaps, needless to say, it is often difficult to identify the underlying needs that led to the particular solutions that are in conflict. The skill of being able to look below the surface of one's proposed solution and discern the underlying need is not one that comes naturally to many people. This first step in collaborative problem solving—defining the problem in terms of the fundamental needs rather than the solutions that have been generated to meet those needs—is the most important and most time-consuming step. However, its value cannot be overstated. Bolton (1979) noted its importance in conflict resolution by quoting the old saying "A problem well-defined is half solved."

Step 2. Brainstorm Possible Solutions

In brainstorming, problem solvers seek to quickly generate as many ideas and solutions as possible without any consideration of the merit or potential of those contributions (Friend & Cook, 2003). The idea is to quickly create a large and diverse pool of possibilities to be more carefully considered and evaluated at a later time.

In the early stages of brainstorming it is important not to slow the rush of ideas by being critical in any way. All proposals and ideas initially are equally valued. They will be recorded for later review and discussion regardless of their apparent feasibility or lack thereof. This approach assures the widest possible beginning pool of ideas. Hourcade and Bauwens (2003) offered several brainstorming guidelines:

- *Don't evaluate.* If each idea is criticized as soon as it is proposed, people soon will stop contributing.

- *Don't explain.* At this early point contributors should not clarify or go into detail about their proposals. This slows down the rapid flow of possibilities.

- *Remove limits.* In brainstorming sessions, participants should understand that there are no constraints whatsoever upon their contributions. Even an apparently foolish proposal may have a germ of an idea within it or may spark someone else to think in a different way to come up with a useful contribution.

- *Prompt.* Someone (perhaps the recorder) should periodically cue the others by saying, "Okay, what else?" or words to that effect.

- *Expand on the ideas of others.* Some of the most effective proposals are made by piggybacking on the ideas of others, using those ideas as springboards for other possible solutions.

- *Record all contributions.* The person serving as recorder should list each person's contribution on a blackboard or large easel, using a few key words to capture the idea so the group can see and use the previously offered ideas for further inspiration.

- *Listen for natural break points.* Often the ideas that ultimately are most useful are proposed early on. A typical pattern of idea production in these sessions is an initial flurry of suggestions for some short period of time, a pause, a second, smaller flurry, another pause, and so on. A useful guideline is to wrap up the brainstorming session after this second lull or pause.

Returning to the aforementioned situation with the special educator and the general educator, after some time they were able to present their positions in terms of needs instead of solutions. They then sat down in the school's conference room to brainstorm possible solutions to their problem. After a few minutes, they had generated the following possible solutions.

- Providing resource room assistance after school.

- Bringing the students into the resource room during nonacademic times in the classroom.

- Providing special education services in the classroom through co-operative teaching.

- Providing resource room assistance on a less frequent basis than initially planned.

- Embedding reading intervention activities within the typical classroom tasks and activities.

They were then ready to move on to the next step in collaborative problem solving.

Step 3. Select the Solution (or Solutions) That Seems to Best Address the Needs of All

When the brainstorming is completed, it is time to begin identifying the most promising solutions. For collaborative problem solving to achieve workable and acceptable solutions, all participants must sense that their needs truly will be met with the selected solution. If not, some sense of compromise will set in and participation will be only halfhearted. The individuals will see themselves as having given in and as not having their needs met (Hourcade & Bauwens, 2003).

After each person has privately identified one or more solutions that appear to meet his or her needs, these individually compiled lists are compared to find the choices selected in common. If the preliminary groundwork on defining the problem in terms of needs was done well, usually one (or more) solutions will be identified by all participants as being good solutions.

In the example of the special educator and the general educator, as they reviewed their list of proposed solutions they found that they had two solutions in common:

- Providing special education services in the classroom through cooperative teaching
- Embedding reading intervention activities within the typical classroom tasks and activities

After some discussion they concluded that both should be chosen and incorporated into the educational program. Each believed that when fully implemented these arrangements could satisfy their previously identified needs.

Step 4. Plan Who Will Do What, Where, and When

At this point the involved parties must develop explicit expectations for each involved party concerning who will do what, and where and when these tasks will be carried out. These expectations must be clear to all concerned. A written record of these determinations and agreements is helpful as a reminder in preventing future questions or problems, since specific details may be overlooked in the excitement of having reached a promising solution.

In the example of the special educator and the general educator, their general agreement was that special education services would be provided in the classroom through cooperative teaching. In addition, ongoing classroom activities would contain special reading intervention activities. They then collaboratively developed the following plan.

Three days a week, from 1:00 p.m. to 2:00 p.m., the special educator would come into the classroom. During this 1-hour period, the students would be divided into small skill groups. These groupings would be based in part on similarity of reading needs of the students.

The general educator, a parent volunteer, and the special educator would each take one group for 20 minutes. Each group's lessons would include specific reading goals and objectives for each student, as well as reading enrichment curricula common to all. During each group's 20 minutes with the special educator, each student with specific reading needs would receive specific attention in the small group and would benefit from similar services being provided to the other students in the group.

The second component of the new plan involved the embedding of reading intervention activities throughout the curriculum. The special educator worked with the general educator to help her identify universal design principles in the typical reading activities and to highlight reading across the curriculum.

This plan met the basic needs identified by both the general educator and the special educator. The general educator saw her needs met, as the students with developmental disabilities would not be leaving the classroom and so would not lose valuable instructional time as well as the opportunity to learn from their peers. The special educator saw his needs met in that during his cooperative teaching times in the classroom, he would be able to provide intensive reading intervention. He also saw the possibility of additional learning occurring as he worked with other students in each group who had similar needs. This win–win outcome is characteristic of successful collaborative problem solving.

Step 5. Implement the Plan

Assuming that the collaborative problem solvers have effectively and completely identified all the necessary steps and have agreed on who will do what and when, the next step is to actually do these things. At this point any lack of clarity in the developed plan will come to light. Even the most carefully developed plans will reveal gaps and oversights at the outset. The involved parties should simply return to the problem-solving system to resolve these issues as they occur.

Step 6. Evaluate the Plan

The final stage in the collaborative problem-solving process is evaluation (Hourcade et al., 2003). Simply put, the most important questions about their collaboration that the special educator and general educator must answer at this point are these: "Is the plan yielding the successful results that were anticipated? Is it meeting our previously identified needs?"

In the ongoing example, the general educator had a need for the students with developmental disabilities to participate in the general education classroom and to experience important curricular content and group learning activities. The special educator expressed a need for these students to receive intensive educational intervention. As the two reviewed their work over the past few weeks, they individually and jointly concluded that their plan was succeeding.

Conclusion

An interesting indicator of the collaborative success of teachers is their use of language. The use of such shared language as "we" and "our," instead of such autonomous language as "I" and "mine," suggests that the cooperative teaching partners have internalized the shared ownership and responsibilities inherent in cooperative teaching (Hourcade & Bauwens, 2003).

At a follow-up training workshop for educators who had been involved in cooperative teaching for a complete academic year, the participants were enthusiastic about the results of their work. One of the cooperative teaching partners had been a general education teacher, while another previously had been a special educator working with students who had mild disabilities. The two educators spoke wonderfully of "our" classroom, "our" curriculum, "our" materials, and "our" program.

The special educator then went on to say, "But on the statewide academic competency testing, my kids did not do as well as I would have liked." This special educator generally demonstrated the shared ownership and responsibility inherent in true collaboration. However, when it came to students with disabilities, she still clearly saw those students as hers and continued to maintain primary educational responsibility for those students. When both teachers similarly identify all students in a classroom as "our" students, sharing responsibility for all, they then move closer to the goal of true collaboration.

Glossary

Brainstorming—A group problem-solving technique that involves the spontaneous contribution of ideas from all members of the group.

Collaboration—Professional working relationships in the schools in which two or more educators (typically a special educator and a general educator) share program planning, program implementation, program evaluation, and program accountability.

Collaborative problem solving—A six-step joint process in which interaction problems are resolved through an initial emphasis on participant needs, not solutions.

Cooperative teaching—The predominant form of direct collaboration, in which two or more educators with complementary sets of skills work together in the general education classroom.

Developmental disability—Cognitive disability/mental retardation, autism, and related disabilities.

Direct collaboration—Two or more educators simultaneously present in the general education classroom, jointly planning for, instructing, and evaluating heterogeneous groups of students.

Flexibility—The capability to adapt to new, different, or changing requirements.

Indirect collaboration—A form of collaboration in which two or more educators meet outside the classroom to solve problems, but only one returns to the classroom to implement proposed strategies.

Needs—The specific personal or professional outcomes one would like to see.

Pull-out—Special education programs in which students with disabilities leave the general education classroom for part or all of the school day to receive special education services in resource rooms or special education classrooms.

Trust—Assured reliance on the character of another.

Turf—A physical environment or set of possessions about which one has developed a sense of ownership.

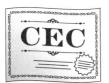

Knowledge and Skills for Entry-Level Special Education Teachers of Students With Developmental Disabilities Standards Addressed in This Chapter

Principle 1: Foundations

DD1K2   Continuum of placement and services available for individuals with developmental disabilities.

DD1K4   Trends and practices in the field of developmental disabilities.

Principle 10: Collaboration

DD10S1   Collaborate with team members to plan transition to adulthood that encourages full community participation.

Web Site Resources

Collaboration

http://www.nwrel.org/nwedu/11-01/ed/

> Different ways that teacher collaboration is happening, including one-to-one mentoring relationships and professional learning teams.

Collaboration: Feedback From Teachers

http://www.yale.edu/ynhti/pubs/A14/polio.html

> Results of a survey on teacher collaboration distributed to fellows of the Yale–New Haven Teachers Institute.

Partners in Pedagogy: Collaboration Between University and Secondary School Foreign Language Teachers. ERIC Digest

http://www.ericdigests.org/2000-3/partners.htm

> A digest that discusses the major issues in collaborative teaching and describes a successful collaborative program.

Teacher Collaboration

http://ericec.org/faq/regsped.html

> Links on collaboration to ERIC digests, mini-bibliographies, frequently asked questions (FAQs), related Internet resources, and Internet discussion groups, as well as selected citations from the ERIC database.

Teacher Collaboration in Secondary Schools

http://ncrve.berkeley.edu/CenterFocus/CF2.html

> Teacher collaboration at the secondary level, notes on barriers and benefits, and recommendations for practical field-tested strategies.

References

Adams, L., & Cessna, K. (1993). Metaphors of the co-taught classroom. *Preventing School Failure*, *37*(4), 28–31.

Bolton, R. (1979). *People skills: How to assert yourself, listen to others, and resolve conflicts*. Englewood Cliffs, NJ: Prentice Hall.

Case, A. D. (1992). The special education rescue: A case for systems thinking. *Educational Leadership*, *50*(2), 32–34.

Connecticut Special Education Association. (1936). *Development and progress of special classes for mentally deficient children in Connecticut*. New Haven, CT: Author.

Correa, V. I., Jones, H. A., Thomas, C. C., & Morsink, C. V. (2005). *Interactive teaming: Enhancing programs for students with special needs*. Upper Saddle River, NJ: Pearson.

Dettmer, P., Thurston, L. P., & Dyck, N. J. (2005). *Consultation, collaboration, and teamwork for students with special needs*. Boston: Allyn & Bacon.

Dewey, J. (1916). *Essays in experimental logic*. New York: Macmillan.

Dore, R., Dion, E., Wagner, S., & Brunet, J. P. (2002). High school inclusion of adolescents with mental retardation: A multiple case study. *Education and Training in Mental Retardation and Developmental Disabilities*, *37*, 253–261.

Friend, M. (2005). *Special education: Contemporary perspectives for school professionals*. Boston: Pearson.

Friend, M., & Cook, L. (2003). *Interactions: Collaboration skills for school professionals*. Boston: Allyn & Bacon.

Fullan, M., & Hargreaves, A. (1991). *What's worth fighting for? Working together for your school*. Andover, MA: Regional Laboratory for Educational Improvement of the Northeast and Islands.

Gargiulo, R. M. (2006). *Special education in contemporary society*. Belmont, CA: Thomson.

Hallahan, D. P., & Kauffman, J. M. (2006). *Exceptional learners* (10th ed.). Boston: Pearson.

Harris, K. C., Harvey, P., Garcia, L., Innes, D., Lynn, P., Munoz, D., Sexton, K., & Stoica, R. (1987). Meeting the needs of special high school students in regular education classrooms. *Teacher Education and Special Education, 10*, 143–152.

Hourcade, J. J., & Bauwens, J. (2003). *Cooperative teaching: Rebuilding and sharing the schoolhouse* (2nd ed.). Austin, TX: PRO-ED.

Hourcade, J. J., & Parette, H. P. (2002, April). *Collaboration in the schools: Relationship problems are solvable*. Paper presented at the 80th Annual International Convention of the Council for Exceptional Children, New York City.

Hourcade, J. J., Parette, H. P., & Anderson, H. (2003). Accountability in collaboration: A framework for evaluation. *Education and Training in Developmental Disabilities, 38*, 398–404.

Hourcade, J. J., Parette, H. P., & Anderson, H. (2004, April). *Collaboration in the schools: Issues and solutions*. Paper presented at the 82nd Annual International Convention of the Council for Exceptional Children, New Orleans, LA.

Johnson, D. W. (1990). *Reaching out: Interpersonal effectiveness and self-actualization* (4th ed.). Englewood Cliffs, NJ: Prentice Hall.

Larson, C. E., & LaFasto, F. M. (1989). *Team work: What must go right/what can go wrong*. Newberry Park, CA: Sage.

Lortie, D. (1975). *School teacher: A sociological study*. Chicago: University of Chicago Press.

McCormick, L., Noonan, M. J., Ogata, V., & Heck, R. (2001). Co-teacher relationship and program quality: Implications for preparing teachers for inclusive preschool settings. *Education and Training in Mental Retardation and Developmental Disabilities, 36*, 119–132.

O'Neil, J. (2000). Fads and fireflies: The difficulties of sustaining change. *Educational Leadership, 57*(7), 6–9.

Roseberry-McKibbin, C., & Brice, A. (2005). *Acquiring English as a second language*. Retrieved October 14, 2005, from http://www.asha.org/public/esl.htm

Rudduck, J. (1991). *Innovation and change*. Bristol, PA: Open University Press.

Sack, J. L. (2000, October 25). CEC report tracks "crisis" conditions in special education. *Education Week*, p. 15.

Sarason, S., Levine, M., Goldenberg, I. I., Cherlin, D., & Bennet, E. (1966). *Psychology in community settings: Clinical, educational, vocational, and social aspects*. New York: Wiley.

Stainback, S., Stainback, W., & Ayres, B. (1996). Schools as inclusive communities. In W. Stainback & S. Stainback (Eds.), *Controversial issues confronting special education: Divergent perspectives* (2nd ed., pp. 29–43). Boston: Allyn & Bacon.

U.S. Department of Education. (2002). *Twenty-fourth annual report to Congress on the implementation of the Individuals with Disabilities Education Act*. Washington, DC: Author.

Walther-Thomas, C., Korinek, L., McLaughlin, V. L., & Williams, B. T. (2000). *Collaboration for inclusive education: Developing successful programs*. Boston: Allyn & Bacon.

White, A. E., & White, L. L. (1992). A collaborative model for students with mild disabilities in middle schools. *Focus on Exceptional Children, 24*(9), 1–10.

Author Index

Subject Index